Comprehensive Management Of

Daily and Long Term Problems in Elderly

K C VERMA

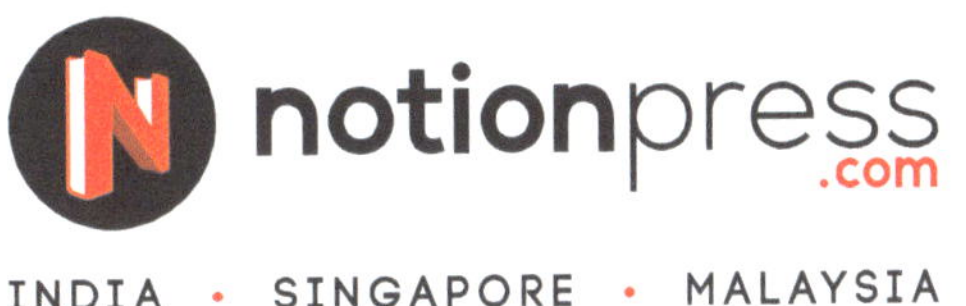

ISBN
Paperback 979-8-89475-398-0
Hardcase 979-8-89498-393-6

Comprehensive Management Of

Daily and Long Term Problems in Elderly

K C VERMA

MBBS, DCH, MD, DM (Cardiology)
FICP(USA), FRSTM&H (Lond), FCSI (India)
Senior Consulting Heart Specialist
Formerly Prof. in Cardiovascular and
Thoracic Unit, Govt. Medical College,
Jammu (J & K)

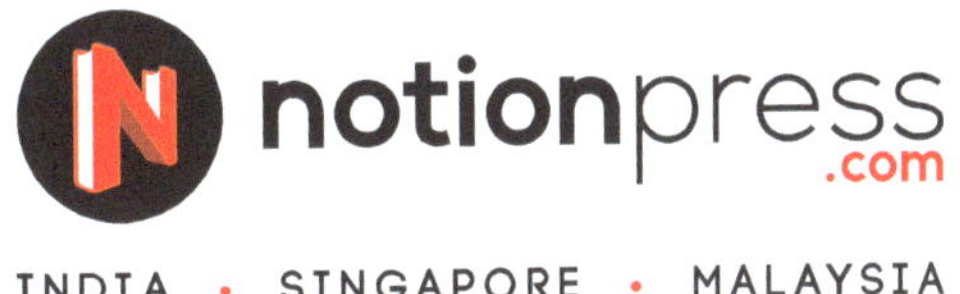

INDIA • SINGAPORE • MALAYSIA

Foreword

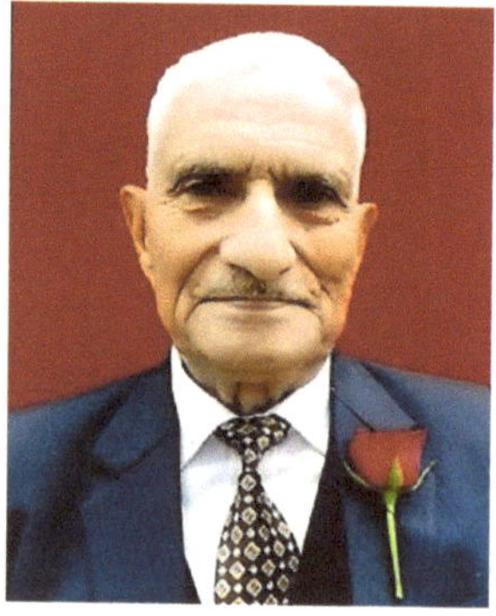

Name ;-**I.D SONI (ISHWAR DASS SONI)**.M.A.B.T & Diploma NCERT

- Formely Dy Director School Education
- Project Director Evaluation of Education in J&K State .
- Formely Commissiner Bharat Scouts and Guides in 1985
- President,of Retired Officers Forum, Jammu and Home for the Aged and Infirm ,Ambphalla, Jammu.
- Best Teacher Award -from Sate Education Department .
- Active Member of Global Gandhi Family J&K ,Branch
- Author of Many Educational and society related books

I, know Prof. (Dr) K.C.Verma for a long time practicing as a cardiologist in the city of Jammu (J&K) and helping all age group people including poor and elderly from all walks of life. As I learn, he has a brilliant record of academic achievements and vast teaching experience in the discipline of Medicine and cardiology. Dr. Verma completed his graduation (MBBS) from medical College, Srinagar, Diploma in Child Health (DCH) from Punjabi University, Patiala and Doctorate in Medicine (MD) from Punjab University Chandigarh. He later showed keen interest towards Cardiovascular Medicine and obtained his Post-Doctoral Degree in cardiology (DM Cardiology). He attained different positions from lecturer to prof. in Medical College, Jammu and worked with full dedication keeping in mind basic objectives of patient care, disease investigation and research. He had been teaching to both under-graduate and post-graduate medical students in the faculty of Medicine

At present Dr. Verma is fully pre-occupied with Private practice in the field of cardiology at Jammu Heart Clinic and is very much interested in Clinical research work and Non-invasive techniques in cardiology. He has to his credit the following honors :-

- He had published more than forty research studies in various reputed medical Indian journals and received due appreciations from different countries of the world..
- Fellow of International College of Physicians from USA (FICP)
- Fellow of Royal Society of Tropical Medicine and Hygiene London. (FRSTM&H)
- Glory of India Award' by India International Friendship Society,
- Best Citizen of India award by International Publishing H selfless ouse New Delhi.
- Fellowship award (FCSI) from cardiological society of India with Gold medal.(FCSI)
- Padama Vibhushan Dr Nirmala Deshpandde Award -2024 for his outstanding contribution to Science and selfless service to the poor and elderly
- He had also published 16 medical books on different aspects of cardiovascular medicine. and public awareness.
- Dr. K.C. Verma is a life-member of Cardiological Society of India.
- He had also taken part in several National and International Cardiology conferences in the capacity of both as a participant and speaker.

Old age will come to every one and brings alongwith many challenges,particularily in socio-economic status,age related health problems ,their shelter, protection from inner and outsider violence and legal rights.

Dr K C Verma has written a book on old age management ,which to my mind is very simple and easy to understand . It is fully colored book spread over thirty chapters highlighting the various difficulties being encountred. by elderly people . Through this manuscript one can also know as to how one can manage socio-ecnomic,,cultural,health and legal problems and take advantage of various Governmental and NGOs:schemes in their benefits

Dated:- 12.6.2024

Place:- Jammu(J&K)

Sd/
I D Soni

Dedication

This illustrative book on"**Comprehensive Management Of Daily and long-term problems In Elderly "** is fully dedicated to Indian elderly and other older people all over the world.

Acknowledgement

The much needed service extended by the Govermental and NGOs for helping Elderly is joyfully acknowledged. The prominent among these are as follows:-

NGOs Supporting and Caring for The Elderly in India

Manavlok is the abbreviation for Marathwada Navnirman Lokayat, where Navnirman means Creation and Lokayat denotes people's opinion. Manavlok symbolizes a new idea or an experiment in rural development. It is actively involved in river rejuvenation, the desilting of dams, and providing seeds and fertilizers to farmers

Abhoy Mission is a non-profit organization started in the year 1988. The organization has an objective of providing multi-dimensional services to disadvantaged groups of people especially destitute senior citizens and persons with disabilities.

Shraddhanand Mahilashram ;-Shraddhanand Mahilashram was started in the year 1927 in memory of Swami Shraddhanand Ji (Munshiram). It was launched as a shelter for women and now has an old age home in Vasai.

Dadidada Foundation DadiDada Foundation is a non-profit organization (NGO) that assists the elderly. Dada-Dadi provides online and community-based assistance to disadvantaged seniors, allowing them to participate in those programs for which they are qualified.

Abhilasha Foundation Abhilasha Foundation was established by a team of social workers who are working in the field of health, education, sustainability, vocational training, empowering women and child development.

VridhCare:- VridhCare is a Delhi-based non-governmental organization (NGO) that works with older citizens. It focuses on their complete well-being and hence attempts to meet all of their needs: financial stability, housing, health care, everyday necessities, and so on.

Agewell Foundation :-Since 1999, the Agewell Foundation has been striving to support the elderly. The NGO engages with old folks and understands their needs and problems, subsequently handled through a network of volunteers. With its team of professionals, volunteers, and social workers, the organization conducts many projects and activities targeted at improving all aspects of the lives of seniors

HelpAge India :-HelpAge India is a not-for-profit organization in India set up in 1978. The organization works for 'the cause and care of disadvantaged older persons to improve their quality of life' HelpAge envisions a society where the elderly have the right to an active, healthy and dignified life.

Asha Kiran :-Asha Kirana Seva Trust (AKST) was established in 1995 to work in the areas of health, education, disability, women & child care, senior citizen care, and other rural developmental activities. The trust works in Bengaluru's urban and rural areas with the support of the government, corporates and donors.

SerudsIndia :-SERUDS is an NGO based in the Kurnool district of Andhra Pradesh, India. It works as a charitable trust for the welfare and development of deprived street children, orphans, destitute women, and senior citizens. SERUDS has been working since 2003 through its need-based programs focused on access to food, livelihood training and healthcare. To date, they have worked in various slums and helped 100s of children and 40 senior citizens.

10 Government Schemes Launched for the Benefit of Senior Citizens

Senior citizens in India are undeniably a vital part of the nation, with their wisdom and experience being invaluable to the younger generations and the economy in general. As such, understanding the senior citizen benefits that are available to the venerable elderly population of the country is an important topic that needs to be discussed.From pension schemes and retirement benefits to healthcare and travel concessions, senior citizens can access a range of services and resources to help them lead a more comfortable and secure life in the arms of their motherland. That said, with ever-changing policies and regulations, it is critical to stay up-to-date on the latest senior citizen benefits available in India.As life expectancy increases, the geriatric population in India is set to experience a dramatic increase. According to statistics given by trusted sources, by 2050, it is estimated that the elderly population will account for around a quarter of the total population. In this situation, savings play a critical role in making their lives merry and content. As one's income diminishes during retirement, it becomes difficult to manage medical expenses. Elderly people are more prone to various ailments, and this increases the need for a steady flow of income to cover the costs of both treatment and prevention. In order to protect the rights of senior citizens and ensure their wellbeing, the Indian government has launched several schemes. The following are some of the best and top government schemes for senior citizens in India 2022 and 2023:

The Senior Citizen Welfare Fund (SCWF) is a fund which provides financial support to the Below Poverty Line (BPL) category senior citizens. It was introduced by the Government of India to help senior citizens who do not have any means of livelihood. The SCWF was instituted by the Finance Act, 2015. It came into effect on 18.03.2016.

Senior Citizens National Helpline "Elderline-14567" Launched In J&K :-Lieutenant Governor Manoj Sinha said the administration is moving towards 100 percent saturation of all 55 public welfare schemes of the central government to reach each and every needy in the UT.

Preface

Old age will come to every one and brings alongwith many challenges .particularily in socio-economic status,age related health problems ,their shelter, protection from inner and outsider violence and legal rights.Elderly, just to exampfly , is like an almost one year old child ,where the former has to be supported through all those processes as one year old or less in age.. Elderly people due to his/her physical and mental imbalance as a result of age related degeneration and younger ones due to their maturational process.
As mentioned above,these two types of physical and mental degeneration and maturation in two groups face equal types of challenges in physical and mental wellbeing ,legal protection,food ,shelter, proper care of their health and education. Undoubetedly ,infants and children are taken care their above mentioned disabilities through a well balanced parenthood.,but on the other hand elderly problems are solved mostly by their,mentally normal grownup children supported by Governmental and non ---Governmental schemes including well established old age homes, Govt legal support and physical and mental training backups
It is well known that as a society we are living much longer thanks to improved living conditions and health care. While being able to reach old age is something to be thankful for, in many ways, there are several challenges facing the elderly, which we all need to pay more attention to. Often it is not until we start to age ourselves or we see a loved one struggling with a problem that we sit up and take notice, but as a society, we can do more to make life easier for our aging population. This article outlines the biggest challenges that elderly people face today and how we can support them and enable them to age with dignity.

Ageism and a lost sense of purpose

There are lots of outdated stereotypes about elderly people, which can lead to isolation and marginalization in a lot of communities. By coming up with innovative ways to involve older people in the community through social events, we can not only help them to maintain a sense of identity and self-esteem but also tap into the wealth of knowledge and experience they have, which is so vital for the development of society.

Financial insecurity

While we are living longer, unfortunately, the world of employment and retirement has not evolved at the same pace. Many elderly people are able and more than willing to work past the standard retirement age, but the opportunities are not there. In addition, managing day to day finances and planning for later life can be challenging for older generations as much is now done online or remotely. This can also leave them more vulnerable to fraud and scams.

Difficulty with everyday tasks and mobility

A person's mobility and dexterity will naturally decline as they age, which makes completing everyday tasks more difficult. This can gradually cause people to care for themselves and prevents them from being social, pursuing interests, or taking part in activities they enjoy. More support is needed to enable elderly people not only to live independently through products and programs which focus on safety, balance, fitness, and mobility but also to ensure they can continue to thrive as an individual.

Finding the right care provision

When complete independence is no longer practical, many elderly people require additional care. Sometimes this care can be provided by family members, but this can place a lot of strain on the caregiver in terms of balancing this with work and other family responsibilities. These caregivers need to be given the training, resources, and emotional support necessary to help them deliver the best care for their loved ones and themselves.
In some cases, it is more appropriate for a professional caregiver to be employed on a regular basis, e.g., when there are complex medical conditions and/or physical disabilities. With a comprehensive elder care service, the elderly person is able to remain in their own home.

Access to healthcare services

Healthcare can be complicated and disjointed for elderly people, especially for those struggling with long-term conditions. The care requires lots of different medical professionals and clinics to coordinate delivery of medication and other types of care.

End of life preparations

We all need to prepare for the inevitable, but death is often a difficult topic for people to discuss or make plans for. Elderly individuals and their families need support when considering the end of life options available, financial implications, and how to ensure that the individual's wishes are respected.

(K C Verma)

Foreword:- Shri D SONI (ISHWAR DASS SONI).M.A.B.T

Dedication:-

- Govermental and NGOs for helping Elderly
- Indian elderly and other older people all overthe world

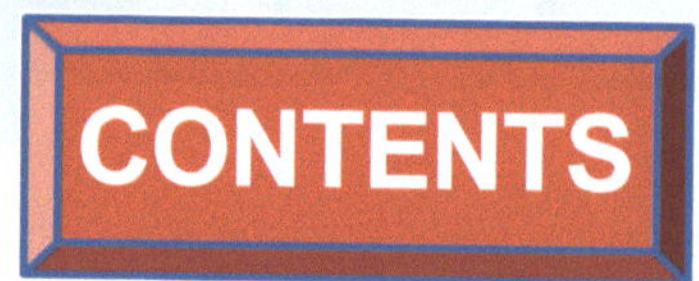

Chapter No.	Name of the Chapter	Page N0.
19	Elderly Suicide vs. Death with Dignity.	129-139
20	Management of Terminal End-stage Medical Conditions in Elderly	140-153
21	Management of Kidney Failure by Grad system and HWI therapy an11 Aternative to Renal dialysis	154-157
22	Health implications of Human body Earthing to the Earth's Surface Electrons	158-174
23	Artificial Intelligence-based Smart Comrade Robot for Elders Healthcare.	175-188
24	Implantable Cardiac and Non- Cardiac Electronic Devices in Elderly	189-201
25	Population Common Diseases in the Elderly	202-208
26	Cardiovascular Diseases in the Elderly	209-242
27	Regulation of long-Term Care Homes for older Adults in India	243-249
28	Long-term Care Insurance for the Elderly	250-252
29	Laws for Protection And National Welfare Programmes For Elderly In India	253-265
30	Summary Of Performing Everyday Routines To Remain Physically & Mentally Fit .	266-310

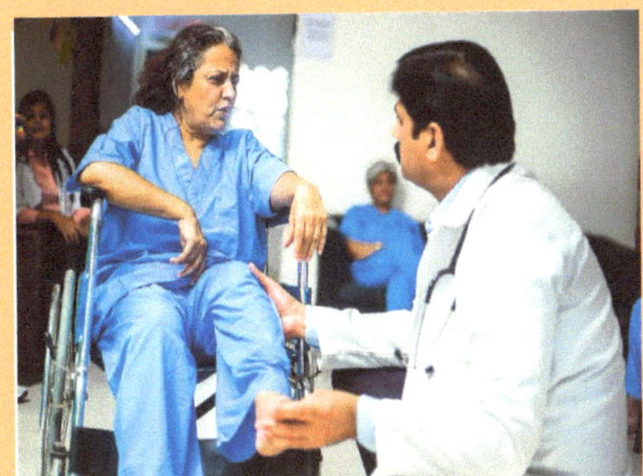

Doctor is examining Elderly women On The Wheel Chair for joint problem.

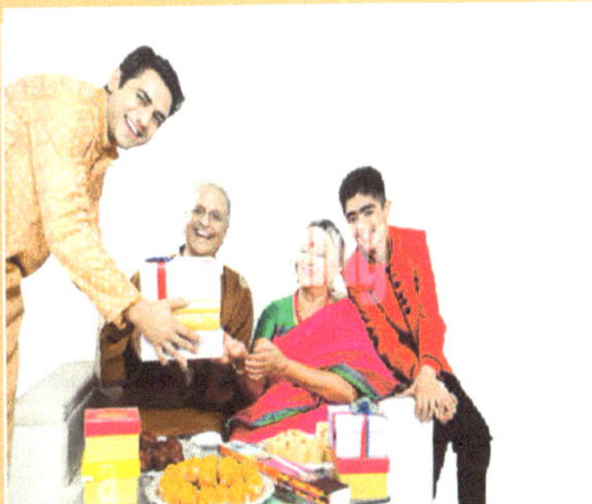

Grand Sons are Offering Dewali GiftsTo their Grand Parents.

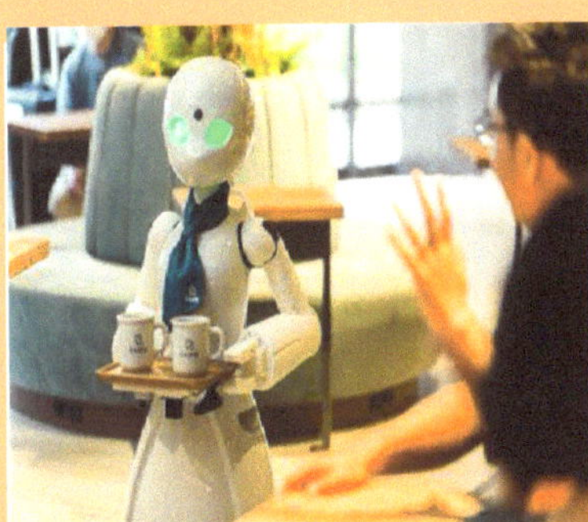

Food serving Robot to elderly who is not able to walk properly

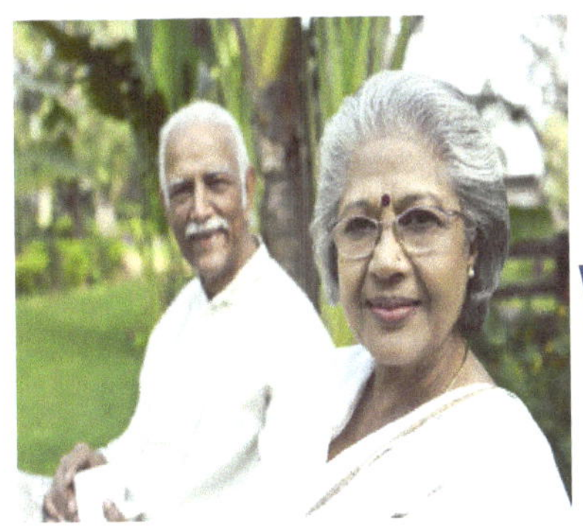

What IsThe Definition of Old Age

The definition of old age varies depending on different factors.The World Health Organisation suggests that most developed world countries characterize old age starting at 60 years and above. The World Economic Forum defines old age based on a measure called “prospective age,” which considers how many more years a person has left to live. In some places, the traditional definition of an elder or elderly person starts between 50 to 65 years of age. Old age is the range of ages for people nearing and surpassing life expectancy. People of old age are also referred to as: old people, elderly, elders, seniors, senior citizens, or older adults Old age is not a definite biological stage: the chronological age denoted as "old age" varies culturally and historically. Some disciplines and domains focus on the aging and the aged, such as the organic processes of aging (senescence) medical studies of the aging process (gerontology) diseases that afflict older adults (geriatrics), technology to support the aging society (gerontechnology), and leisure and sport activities adapted to older people (such as senior sport). Old people often have limited regenerative abilities and are more susceptible to illness and injury than younger adults. They face social problems related to retirement, loneliness, and ageism In 2011, the United Nations proposed a human-rights convention to protect old people. Definitions of old age include official definitions, sub-group definitions, and four dimensions as follows.

Official definitions

Most developed Western countries set the retirement age around the age of 65; this is also generally considered to mark the transition from middle to old age. Reaching this age is commonly a requirement to become eligible for senior social programs Old age cannot be universally defined because it is context-sensitive. The United Nations, for example, considers old age to be 60 years or older. In contrast, a 2001 joint report by the U.S. National Institute on Aging and the World Health Organization [WHO] Regional Office for Africa set the beginning of old age in Sub-Saharan Africa at 50. This lower threshold stems primarily from a different way of thinking about old age in developing nations. Unlike in the developed world, where chronological age determines retirement, societies in developing countries determine old age according to a person's ability to make active contributions to society.

This number is also significantly affected by lower life expectancy throughout the developing world. Dating back to the Middle Ages and prior, what certain scholars thought of as old age varied depending on the context, but the state of being elderly was often thought as being 60 years of age or older in many respects

Sub-group definitions

Gerontologists have recognized that people experience very different conditions as they approach old age. In developed countries, many people in their later 60s and 70s (frequently called "early old age") are still fit, active, and able to care for themselves. However, after 80, they generally become increasingly frail, a condition marked by serious mental and physical debilitation. Therefore, rather than lumping together all people who have been defined as old, some gerontologists have recognized the diversity of old age by defining sub-groups. One study distinguishes the young-old (60 to 69), the middle-old (70 to 79), and the very old (80+) Another study's sub-grouping is young-old (65 to 74), middle-old (75 to 84), and oldest-old (85+) A third sub-grouping is young-old (65 to 74), old (74 to 84), and old-old (85+).

Describing sub-groups in the 65+ population enables a more accurate portrayal of significant life changes. Two British scholars, Paul Higgs and Chris Gilleard, have added a "fourth age" sub-group. In British English, the "third age" is "the period in life of active retirement, following middle age".Higgs and Gilleard describe the fourth age as "an arena of inactive, unhealthy, unproductive, and ultimately unsuccessful ageing".

Dimensions

Chronological age may differ considerably from a person's functional age. The distinguishing marks of old age normally occur in all five senses at different times and at different rates for different people In addition to chronological age, people can be considered old because of the other dimensions of old age. For example, people may be considered old when they become grandparents or when they begin to do less or different work in retirement.

Senior citizen

Senior citizen is a common euphemism for an oldperson used in American English, and sometimes in British English. It implies that the person being referred to is retired. This in turn usually implies that the person is over the retirement age, which varies according to country. Synonyms include old age pensioner or pensioner in British English, and retiree and senior in American English. Some dictionaries describe widespread use of "senior citizen" for people over the age 65

When defined in a legal context, senior citizen is often used for legal or policy-related reasons in determining who is eligible for certain benefits available to the age group. It is used in general usage instead of traditional terms such as "old person", "old-age pensioner", or "elderly" as a courtesy and to signify continuing relevance of and respect for this population group as "citizens" of society, of senior "rank" The term was apparently coined in 1938 during a political campaign. Famed caricaturist Al Hirschfeld claimed on several occasions that his father Isaac Hirschfeld invented the term "senior citizen". It has come into widespread use in recent decades in legislation, commerce, and common speech. Especially in less formal contexts, it is often abbreviated as "senior(s)", which is also used as an adjective.

Age qualifications

The age of 65 has long been considered the benchmark for senior citizenship in numerous countries. This convention originated from Chancellor Otto von Bismarck's introduction of the pension system in Germany during the late 19th century. Bismarck's legislation set the retirement age at 70, with 65 as the age at which individuals could start receiving a pension. This age standard gradually gained acceptance in other nations and has since become deeply entrenched in public consciousness The age which qualifies for senior citizen status varies widely. In governmental contexts, it is usually associated with an age at which pensions or medical benefits for the elderly become available. In commercialcontexts, where it may serve as a marketing device to attract customers, the age is often significantly lowerIn commerce, some businesses offer customers of a certain age a "senior discount". The age at which these discounts are available varies from 55, 60, 62 or 65 upwards, and other criteria may also apply. Sometimes a special "senior discount card" or other proof of age needs to be produced to show entitlement. In the United States, the standard retirement age is currently 66 (gradually increasing to 67) The AARP allows couples in which one spouse has reached the age of 50 to join, regardless of the age of the other spouse

In Canada, the Old Age Security (OAS) pension is available at 65 (the Conservative government of Stephen Harper had planned to gradually increase the age of eligibility to 67, starting in the years 2023–2029, although the Liberal government of Justin Trudeau is considering leaving it at 65), and the Canada Pension Plan (CPP) as early as age 60

Signs of old age

The distinguishing characteristics of old age are both physical and mental.The marks of old age are so unlike the marks of middle age that legal scholar Richard Posner suggests that, as an individual transitions into old age, that person can be thought of as different people "time-sharing" the same identity These marks do not occur at the same chronological age for everyone. Also, they occur at different rates and order for different people. Marks of old age can easily vary between people of the same chronological age. A basic mark of old age that affects both body and mind is "slowness of behavior".The term describes a correlation between advancing age and slowness of reaction and physical and mental task performance However, studies from Buffalo University and Northwestern University have shown that the elderly are a happier age group than their younger counterparts.

Physical characteristics of old age

Physical marks of old age include the following:

- Bone and joint problems: Old bones are marked by "thinning and shrinkage". This might result in a loss of height (about two inches (5 cm) by age 80), a stooping posture in many people, and a greater susceptibility to bone and joint diseases such as osteoarthritis and osteoporosis.
- Chronic diseases: Some older people have at least one chronic condition and many have multiple conditions. In 2007–2009, the most frequently occurring conditions among older people in the United States were uncontrolled hypertension (34%), arthritis

(50%), and heart disease (32%)

Chronic mucus hypersecretion (CMH), defined as "coughing and bringing up sputum", is a common respiratory symptom in elderly people.

Dental problems: Older people may have less saliva and reduced ability to maintain oral hygiene, consequently increasing the chance of tooth decay and infection

Digestive system issues: About 40% of the time, old age is marked by digestive disorders such as difficulty in swallowing, inability to eat enough and to absorb nutrition, constipation and bleeding.

Essential tremor (ET): An uncontrollable shaking in a part of the upper body. It is more common in the elderly and symptoms worsen with age

Eyesight deterioration: Presbyopia can occur by age 50 and it hinders reading, especially of small print in low lighting. The speed with which an individual reads and the ability to locate objects may also be impaired.By age 80, more than half of all Americans either have a cataract or have had cataract surgery.

Falls: Old age increases the risk of injury from fall. .Every year, about a third of those 65 years old and more than half of those 80 years old fall. Falls are the leading cause of injury and death for old people

Gait change: Some aspects of gait normally change with old age. Speed slows after age 70. Time with both feet on the ground ("double stance") increases. Old people sometimes move as if they were walking carefullyonice

Hair usually turns gray and may become thinner About age 50, about 50% of Europeans have 50% grey hair. Many men are affected by balding.

Women enter menopause

Hearing loss: By age 75, 48% of men and 37% of women have lost at least some significant hearing. Of the 26.7 million people [where?] over age 50 with a hearing impairment, one seventh use hearing aids In the 70–79 age range, partial hearing loss affecting communication rises to 65%, mostly in low-income men

Hearts can become less efficient in old age, lessening stamina. Atherosclerosis can constrict blood flow.

Immune-function loss (immunosenescence).

Lungs may expand less efficiently, providing less oxygen.

Mobility impairment or loss: "Impairment in mobility affects 14% of those between 65 and 74, [and] half of those over 85 Loss of mobility is common in old people and has serious "social, psychological, and physical consequences"

Pain: 25% of seniors have chronic pain, increasing with age, up to 80% of those in nursing homes. Most pains are rheumatological or malignant

Decreases in sexual drive in both men and women. Increasing research on sexual behavior and desires in later life is challenging the "asexual" image of older adults. People aged 75–102 do experience sensuality and sexual pleasure Sexual attitudes and identity are established in early adulthood and change little. Sexuality remains important throughout life, and the sexual expression of "typical, healthy older persons is a relatively neglected topic of research".Other known sexual behaviors in older age groups include sexual thoughts, fantasies, and dreams, masturbation; oral sex; and vaginal and anal intercourse.

Skin loses elasticity and gets drier and more lined and wrinkled

Wounds take longer to heal and are likelier to leave permanent scars.

Trouble sleeping and daytime sleepiness affect more than half of seniors. In a study of 9,000 people with a mean age of 74, only 12% reported no sleep complaints. By age 65, deep sleep drops to about 5% of sleep time.

Taste buds diminish by up to half by the age of 80. Food becomes less appealing and nutrition can suffer

Over the age of 85, thirst perception decreases, so that 41% of the elderly don't drink enough.

Urinary incontinence is often found in old age

Vocal cords weaken and vibrate more slowly. This results in a weakened, breathy voice, "old person's voice".

Mental

Mental marks of old age include the following:

Agreeability: Despite the stressfulness of old age, the words "agreeable" and "accepting" are used commonly to describe people of old age. However, in some people, the dependence that comes with old age induces feelings of incompetence and worthlessness from having to rely on others for many different basic living functions.

Caution follows closely with old age. This antipathy toward "risk-taking" often stems from the fact that old people have less to gain and more to lose than younger people.

Depressed mood. According to Cox, Abramson, Devine, and Hollon (2012), old age is a risk factor for depression caused by prejudice. When younger people are prejudiced against the elderly and then become old themselves, their anti-elderly prejudice turns inward, causing depression. "People with more negative age stereotypes will likely have higher rates of depression as they get older." Old age depression results in the over-65 population having the highest suicide rate.

•Fear of crime in old age, especially among the frail, sometimes weighs more heavily than concerns about finances or health and restricts what they do. The fear persists in spite of the fact that old people are victims of crime less often than younger people.

•Increasing fear of health problems.

•Mental disorders affect about 15% of people aged 60+ according to estimates by the World Health Organization.Another survey taken in 15 countries reported that mental disorders of adults interfered with their daily activities more than physical problems

•Reduced mental and cognitive ability: Memory loss is common in old age due to the brain's decreased ability to encode, store, and retrieve information. It takes more time to learn the same amount of new information..The prevalence of dementia increases in old age from about 10% at age 65 to about 50% over age 85.. Alzheimer's disease accounts for 50 to 80 percent of dementia cases. Demented behavior can include wandering, physical aggression, verbal outbursts, depression, and psychosis

•Stubbornness: A study of over 400 seniors found a preference for the routine". Explanations include old age's toll on "fluid intelligence" and the "more deeply entrenched" ways of the old

Successful ageing

The concept of successful ageing can be traced back to the 1950s and was popularized in the 1980s. Traditional definitions of successful ageing have emphasized absence of physical and cognitive disabilities. In their 1987 article, Rowe and Kahn characterized successful ageing as involving three components: a) freedom from disease and disability, b) high cognitive and physical functioning, and c) social and productive engagement. The study cited previous was also done back in 1987 and therefore, these factors associated with successful ageing have probably been changed. With the current knowledge, scientists started to focus on learning about the effect spirituality in successful ageing. There are some differences in cultures which of these components are the most important. Most often across cultures social engagement was the most highly rated but depending on the culture the definition of successful ageing changes

Bibliography and Acknowledgement

- Alam, Moneer, and Armando Barrientos (eds). 2010. Demographics, employment and old age security: Emerging trends and challenges in South Asia. New Delhi: Macmillan Publishers India.
- Aronson L. Elderhood: Redefining Aging, Transforming Medicine, Reimagining Life. 1st ed. New York, USA: Bloomsbury Publishing; 2019.
- Brijnath, Bianca. 2008. The legislative and political contexts surrounding dementia care in India. Ageing & Society 28(07): 913-934.
- Chan, Angelique. 2005. Aging in Southeast and East Asia: issues and policy directions. Journal of Cross- Cultural Gerontology 20(4): 269–284.
- Cohen, L. 1992. "No aging in India: the uses of gerontology," Culture, Medicine and Psychiatry 16(2):
  Compendium. New Delhi: UNESCO and UNICEF.
- Dionigi RA. Stereotypes of aging: their effects on the health of older adults. J Geriatr. 2015; 2015: 1-9
  Fung HH. Aging in culture. Gerontologist. 2013; 53(3): 369-377
- Gopal, Meena. 2006. Gender, ageing and social security. Economic and Political Weekly 41(42): 4477-4486
- Hermalin, Albert I. 2002. Theoretical perspectives, measurement issues, and related research. In The well-being of the elderly in Asia: A four-country comparative study, ed. Albert I Hermalin, 101–142.
- Johnson, Shanthi C., Malathy Duraiswamy, Raani Desai, and Lesley Frank. 2011. Health service
  Journal of Aging & Social Policy 15(2-3): 11-30.
- Kalavar, Jyotsna M., and D. Jamuna. 2011. Aging of Indian women in India: the experience of older
- Lamb, Sarah. 2013. In/dependence, intergenerational uncertainty, and the ambivalent state: Perceptions of old age security in India. South Asia: Journal of South Asian Studies 36(1): 65-78.
- Mathew, E.T. and and Irudaya S. Rajan. 2008. "Employment as old age security."
- Nguyen QD, Moodie EM, Forget M-F, Desmarais P, Keezer MR, Wolfson C. Health heterogeneity in older adults: exploration in the canadian longitudinal study on aging. J Am Geriatr Soc. 2021; 69(3): 678-687
- Ouchi Y, Rakugi H, Arai H, et al. Redefining the elderly as aged 75 years and older: proposal from the Joint Committee of Japan Gerontological Society and the Japan Geriatrics Society. Geriatr Gerontol Int. 2017; 17(7): 1045-1047
- Phelan EA, Anderson LA, LaCroix AZ, Larson EB. Older adults' views of "successful aging" how do they compare with researchers' definitions? J Am Geriatr Soc. 2004; 52(2): 211-216
- Silverstein, Merril, and Roseann Giarrusso. 2010. Aging and family life: A decade review. Journal of social answers from urban India. Ageing & Society 32(4): 697–717.
- Visaria, Pravin. 2001. Demographics of aging in India. Economic and Political Weekly 36(22): 1967-
- Weber R. Basic Content Analysis. Thousand Oaks, USA: SAGE Publications, Inc; 1990. women in formal care homes. Journal of Women & Aging 23(3): 203-215.

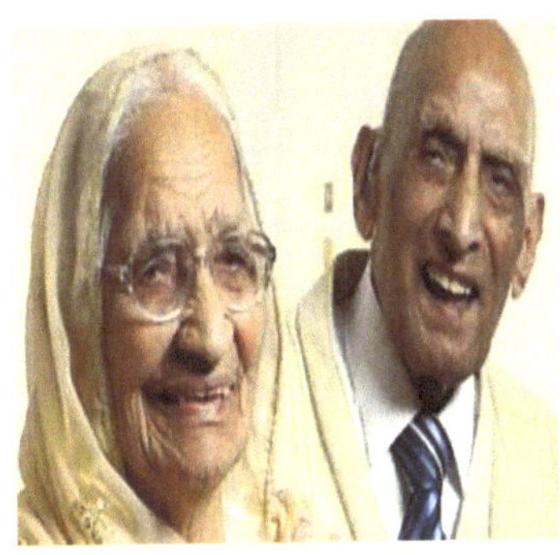

Issues and Challenges Faced by the Elderly and their Management

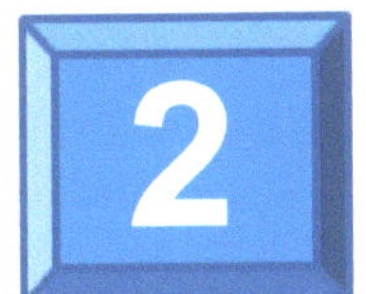

In 2020, Singapore experienced a 26% spike in reported senior suicides, where 154 out of 452 were citizens aged 60 and above. This number has peaked since 1991, and according to the CEO of SOS (Samaritans of Singapore), increased isolation, mental stress, and weak family and social relations are some of the many contributing factors. The present senior population is around 500,000 and is expected to double by 2030, which is why it is extremely integral to provide an environment for the elderly where they are made to be like important members of society rather than a burden. But that can only be done once main problems and challenges are identified. This article covers a list of some of the most common problems faced by the elderly in Singapore.

1. Lack of Engagement and a Sense of Purpose

Ageism and out-of-date social practices have led to the elderly becoming cut off from the Singaporean community. There's not much for them to do rather than sit at home and look forward to an occasional family gathering. On top of that, the pandemic has further halted whatever limited opportunities and activities that were available for the senior citizens, be it finding a new part-time job, indulging in an outdoor hobby, or simply socializing. Stricter and more extended lockdowns have induced depressive symptoms, pushing rates of mental health issues even higher. Fewer opportunities for physical and mental stimulation, infrequent valued interactions with loved ones, and an increased worldwide health fear are bound to bring negative repercussions for the entire population, especially the elderly. Enabling older adults to responsibly indulge in meaningful activities, whether related to employment, community, or home will keep them busy and feeling useful. These can include paid volunteering jobs, movie nights, and other socially enjoyable events.

2. Abuse and Mistreatment

With old age comes physical and mental weakness, resulting in dependency. Increased dependency on responsibility should be assigned to professional care giving, where the family members or inexperienced caregivers could potentially lead to mistreatment if the former isn't aware of proper caregiving measures or just doesn't want to. Similarly, if the caregiver experiences psychological issues, it could result in the possibility of elderly abuse. Neglect by busy family members is also one of the main challenges elderly people face, and it causes a lot of mental distress. For this reason, members of the family who are already juggling with other family and work-related duties should avoid undertaking elderly care. Instead, the responsibility should be assigned to professional caregiving, where the professional caregiver has the right tools and resources and can provide optimal support to care for elderly citizens.

3. Lack of Financial Security

Elderly Singaporeans with limited resources will find it difficult to upgrade their financial status in contrast to their younger counterparts owing to limited job opportunities. Once they enter their retirement age, a lot of elderly Singaporeans live on a fixed stream of income, which is not always enough to support the medical bills and the lifestyle they were used to. Especially in the modern age, as more families are becoming distant and people are choosing to live alone, older parents may have no choice but to live alone and take care of their expenses on their own. For greater financial wellness of the elderly, people should create new job opportunities in the city, catered specifically for retired people, as well as new projects to plan and finance comprehensive senior care systems should be devised.

4. Everyday Struggle with Mobility & Daily Tasks

With older age comes the decline in one's natural dexterity, which can make doing even the simplest tasks much more difficult. This can greatly hinder one's social and work life and prevent one from living life like they once used to. To avoid this, there need to be more policies and programs that involve elderly people in a way that they can enjoy a safe, balanced and happy life. Professional care providers can also make life much more convenient and less stressful.

5. Fear of Becoming a Burden

As people age, they become fearful about becoming a burden on their family, especially if they have failed to receive the necessary support and love in the past. In fact, research suggests that a lot of people who request euthanasia do it out of fear of burdening their loved ones. This usually stems from their loss of independence, health concerns, or a sense of being different than others, which can quickly trigger feelings of guilt, inferiority, and depression.

Choosing the Right Plan for Different Health Conditions

In today's day and age, there is an abundance of different healthcare provision plans for the elderly, and picking the right one can become rather overwhelming. Most of the time, these elderly people are not even consulted and therefore provided with the wrong kind of support. For instance, a family that is not equipped to take care of a senior citizen might deem it best to give in-home care rather than seeking the help of a professional or a care home. For this reason, it is crucial to involve the person in this process so they can actively partake in the decision-making. Encouraging the elderly to seek professional support and help boils down to giving them control. If the decision is imposed on them, they might not react in the most positive way. For this reason, it is best to first give them all the available options and information they need to make an informed decision.

Dementia Care

Dementia is a blanket term used to define different symptoms affecting the memory and impairing the thought process as well as social abilities. In Singapore, dementia impacts around 5.2% of the ageing population above 60, and the numbers continue to rise. Though there is no set cure for this mental disability, there is the possibility of handling dementia with the right tools and increased awareness which can only be done by investing further in the healthcare system. If symptoms of dementia are detected and diagnosed early, and a dementia patient is provided with the right cognitive caregiving, we can expect to tackle this commonly faced challenge quite effectively.

Diversity in Ageing of Seniors

There is no set rule that defines a typical old person. There are certain 90-year olds who are just as physically and mentally capable as 30-year olds, whereas others start experiencing a significant decline in their capabilities during a much younger age. It is also important to note that this diversity in senior age is not random and rather a product of people's social and physical surroundings and the effects of these surroundings on their health. This can include the family, gender, religion, and ethnicity, which can create many health inequalities. To keep this in check, the right public health policy is devised to minimize, rather than encourage, these inequalities.

Lack of Gerontological Data

Gerontology involves the study of physical aging and its effects on the mind as well as society. While the cognitive decline in old age is increasing, the social care resources available for older persons experiencing this decline are inadequate. However, there is still a lot of potential when it comes to home assistive technology that could potentially foster healthy ageing by effectively meeting the needs of senior groups.

What are the Needs of elderlies ?

With the increasing trend in falling birth rates, ageing population and changing living conditions, studies report that growing old in place has become a priority for elderly people once they have retired. Homecare services have become a critical aspect of hassle-free aging and can be provided even if a senior person is living alone or with family. In Singapore, elderly people have various social and personal needs, which include:

Independence

The majority of senior adults are hesitant when it comes to giving up their independence. However, that still doesn't change the fact that their mobility, cognitive and physical abilities deteriorate over time, thereby requiring regular assistance with various tasks. If you as a family member are unable to oversee the daily needs of your loved one, then it is recommended that you hire professional help that will take care of all the important duties, such as medication management, food preparation, transportation, and housekeeping.

Savings

A good percentage of the Singaporean senior population is living on limited finance due to financial incapacity or increased expenses on healthcare services. To put this into perspective, an average senior citizen over the age of 65 who is living alone requires approximately $1,379 a month just for meeting the basic living standards. If they rely on professionals for help on a daily basis, they would be able to save a good amount in the long term. That is because undertaking all household and outside duties with restricted physical and mental capacity opens a window for errors and even health hazards, which could end up costing the person a lot more than expected. Furthermore, hiring a caregiver for several days per week can prove to be quite affordable and can enable aging adults to save up for future use.

Socialization

One of the main reasons behind senior suicides in

Singapore was the result of loneliness and depressionthat can stem from a lack of interaction with peers and family members. The elderly need to be regularly socialized in order to maintain their physical and mental longevity and have something to look forward to each time. During the pandemic, however, going out a lot might not be the best decision. To counter this problem, in-place caretaking is one of the best ways to ensure that your elderly family member is staying stimulated, as well as receiving all the desired help and support. Besides completing daily tasks, caregivers also make great companions who can organize both indoor and outdoor activities, ensuring that your family member maintains a healthy balance in their lives.

Physical & Mental Wellbeing

Older adults experience more stressors as compared to an average adult due to continuous loss in their functional, physical and mental abilities. These might include fragility, immobility, or other health concerns like osteoporosis and heart disease. In addition to that, ageing usually brings along a decline in socioeconomic status and socialization, all of which can ultimately lead to mental distress, which might require professional care. In senior adults, physical health ultimately affects mental health and vice versa. For instance, hypertension might result in depression. For this reason, monitoring and maintaining both the physical and mental wellbeing of a senior loved one becomes extremely crucial. However, this can become a problem if you are unsure of how to manage the symptoms of such health problems are busy with other house or family-related duties, or are simply out of the country. In such a case, home care companies will be your best option. These professionals will make sure that your family member goes through regular check ups, is properly fed, medicated, and stimulated so that they can make the most out of their time at home.

Safe Environment

There are many concerns related to the elderly aging in a space that is not entirely safe, especially in a city. Assisted-living facilities normally provide a very secure environment that is aligned with the physical needs of old people; however, if you do not wish to uproot your elderly loved one from their current lifestyle, then you can create an at-home safe environment with the help of a home care provider. A good place is to start is by installing slip-proof covers on bathroom floors and also shower grab bars for added protection and smoother navigation, moving cabinet contents lower in order to improve access, and decluttering by getting rid of all items that could potentially lead to elderly falls.

Bibliography and Acknowledgement

- Ageing and Health: World Health Organization. 2021Last accessed on 2022 Feb 01 Available from: https://www.who.int/news-room/fact-sheets/detail/ageing-and-health Community Processes: National Health Systems Resource Center; 2021. Last accessed on 2022 Feb 8 Available from: https://nhsrcindia.org/practice-areas/cpc-phc/cpc-about
- Goel A, Raizada A, Agrawal A, Bansal K, Uniyal S, Prasad P, et al Correlates of In-Hospital COVID-19 Deaths: A Competing Risks Survival Time Analysis of Retrospective Mortality Data? Disaster Med Public Health Prep. 2021:1–8 doi: 10.1017/dmp.2021.85
- Gruzieva TS, Diachuk MD, Inshakova HV, Soroka IM, Dufynets VA. Health of the elderly people as the basis for formation of medical and social needs Wiad Lek. 2021;74:658–64
- Hu D, Yan W, Zhu J, Zhu Y, Chen J. Age-related disease burden in China, 1997-2017: Findings from the global burden of disease study Front Public Health. 2021;9:638704
- Kumar P, Singh T. Projection of elderly in India during the census years 2021 to 2051 Int J Curr Adv Res. 2020;6:7463–6
- Mishra AK, Maurya RK, Haque Z, Verma D, Singh N, Kushwaha JP, et al Elderly in India: Government of India, Ministry of Statistics and Programme 2021Last accessed on 2021 Jan 30 Available from: https://www.mospi.gov.in/documents/213904/301563Elderly.in.India.20211627985144626.pdf/a4647f03-bca1-1ae2-6c0f-9fc459dad64c
- Kumar P, Singh T. Projection of elderly in India during the census years 2021 to 2051 Int J Curr Adv Res. 2020;6:7463–6 Mishra AK, Maurya RK, Haque Z, Verma D, Singh N,
- Kushwaha JP, et al Elderly in India: Government of India, Ministry of Statistics and Programme 2021Last accessed on 2021 Jan 30 Available from: https://www.mospi.gov.in/documents/213904/301563Elderly.in.India.20211627985144626.pdf/a4647f03-bca1-1ae2-6c0f-9fc459dad64c
- Nasir Z. M., Ali S. M. (2000). Labour market participation of the elderly. The Pakistan Development Review, 39, 1075-1086.
- National Sample Survey Organization. (1989). Socio-economic profile of the aged persons, report of forty-second round: July 1986-June 1987 (NSS Report No. 367). New Delhi: Government of India.
- Palloni A. (2001). Living arrangements of older persons: Critical issues and policy responses (United Nations Population Bulletin, Special Issue Nos. 42/43). New York, NY: Department of Economic and Social Affairs, Population Division.
- Rajan S. I. (2007). Population ageing, health and social security in India (Discussion Paper No. 3, CREI Discussion Paper Series). Osaka, Japan: Osaka City University, Centre for Research on Economic Inequality.
- Yadava K. N. S., Yadava S. S., Sharma C. L. N. (1996). A study of socioeconomic factors and behavioural problems of the aged persons in rural Northern India. Demography India, 25, 21-34.
- Zimmerman M., Israel B., Schulz A., Checkoway B. (1992). Further explorations in empowerment theory: An empirical analysis of psychological empowerment. American Journal of Community Psychology, 20, 707-727.

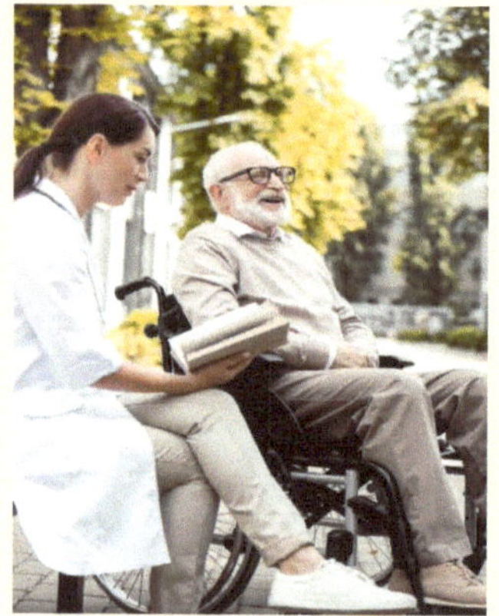

The Common Chronic Health Conditions In Elderly

1.Parkinsons disease

Parkinson's disease starts in the brain. Certain nerve cells break down or die. As a result, the levels of dopamine, a chemical in your brain, begin to fall. When your dopamine levels decrease, it causes your brain to act in unusual ways and leads to impaired movement, among other things. Parkinson's disease affects around 1% of people older than 60 and 5% of people over 85. It is a disease that typically appears after the age of 60. There is still much we have yet to learn about Parkinson's disease. Unfortunately, there is no cure yet. Many of the forms of treatment for the disease only manage the symptoms. The exact cause of Parkinson's is still unclear. Scientists believe that factors like genes and exposure to certain toxins may increase your likelihood for getting Parkinson's. They have also linked the presence of a certain type of protein found in the brain to Parkinson's disease. We also know that younger people rarely experience Parkinson's, having a relative that has Parkinson's increases your chance of getting it, and that men are more likely to get it than women. How to Identify Symptoms of Parkinson's in Older People At first, the symptoms of Parkinson's may be subtle. They usually begin on one side of your body and are more present on that side even when they progress to your whole body. These symptoms could be:• Tremors. You might start to notice that one of your limbs, usually a hand, will start to shake. Sometimes you will rub your thumb and pointer finger together or start to shake even when you are relaxed.

• Slowed movement. As your Parkinson's symptoms progress, you might find that your movements are slowed or delayed. Normal tasks might become challenging or take more time to do than they used to. It can also become difficult to walk.
• Stiff muscles. Parts of your body's muscles might become stiff. This will limit how much you can move and may be painful.
• Balance and posture issues. You might begin to have a stooped back and lose your balance.
• Speech problems. Your voice might become more monotone, quieter, or quicker. You also might slur or hesitate before you speak.

Writing problems. Parkinson's can affect your writing. It can make your handwriting look different and make it harder to write quickly.
• Emotional issues. Some people with Parkinson's experience issues with depression or other emotional changes.
• Difficulty swallowing. It may become more difficult to swallow, and saliva buildup can lead to drooling.
• Urinary and bowel movement issues. Some people experience issues in their urinary tract or constipation.
• Sleep issues. People with Parkinson's often have issues with sleep and waking up at night.
• Chewing and eating difficulties. More advanced cases of Parkinson's affect the mouth and eating becomes hard.

The onset of symptoms differs with different people. It can look like normal signs of aging because the symptoms appear so gradually. You might feel some mild shaking in your hand or have mobility issues at first, or you might start speaking slower or more softly. However, you will eventually start to walk and stand leaning forward and do specific things with your arms. You will also start to experience symptoms on one side of the body. Many people first feel stiff, have a tremor, experience sleep difficulties, have constipation, experience loss of smell, or have restless legs before any other symptom.

How to Treat Parkinson's

Since there is no known treatment for Parkinson's, treatment is all about symptom management. There are different medications, surgeries, and other methods to help with the symptoms.

Medicines used to treat Parkinson's often:

- Increase dopamine levels
- Affect other brain chemicals in your body
- Help control other symptoms not related to movement problems

The most common medication for Parkinson's is called levodopa, or L-dopa. Levodopa helps the brain make more dopamine. Unfortunately, levodopa can cause nausea, vomiting, low blood pressure, and sleep difficulties. That is why people usually take a medication called carbidopa alongside levodopa. Carbidopa helps to reduce those side effects.

People who take these medications should always consult their doctor before they stop taking them. Suddenly stopping these medications can have serious and unwanted effects.

Other medications that people take for Parkinson's include:

- Medications that mimic dopamine in the brain
- MAO-B inhibitors, which slow down a dopamine-killing enzyme
- COMT inhibitors, which break down dopamine
- Amantadine, which helps reduce involuntary movements
- Anticholinergic drugs that reduce tremors and muscle stiffness

Some people may not respond well to these medications. In that case, a surgery called deep brain stimulation, or DBS, could be a good option. This is a procedure where the surgeon places electrodes in the brain that connect to another device in the chest. Together, the device and electrodes help to stop many Parkinson's symptoms like tremors, slow movement, and muscle stiffening.

Other ways to treat Parkinson's symptoms include physical, occupational, and speech therapies. These can help with the physical, vocal, and mental effects of Parkinson's. You can also use exercise and diet to help with muscle and balance issues

2.Depression

Sixteen percent of older adults sought treatment for depression—a treatable medical condition that is not a normal part of aging. Depression causes persistent feelings of sadness, pessimism, hopelessness, fatigue, difficulty making decisions, changes in appetite, a loss of interest in activities, and more.

Steps you can take to help with depression include:

- Manage stress levels. Reach out to family and friends during rough spells and consider regular meditation.
- Eat a healthy diet. What you put into your body can affect your mood, so focus on foods that are high in nutrients and promote the release of endorphins and those "feel good" chemicals, and limit consumption of things like alcohol, caffeine, artificial sweeteners, and highly processed foods.
- Routine exercise. Exercise has a number of physical and psychological benefits, including improving your mood through the release of endorphins and other "feel good" brain chemicals, boosting self-confidence and self-worth through meeting goals and improving your physical appearance, and increased socialization through interactions at gyms and group classes.
- Talk to your doctor. If you've experienced any of the warning signs of depression, talk to your doctor, and ask about your treatment options. Antidepressant medications or psychotherapy could be right for you.

If you're in severe emotional distress, one of the first things you should do is tell someone else about it—such as a trusted friend or family member. You can also dial or text 988 from your phone to speak with a counselor who is specially trained in suicide prevention.

3.Alzheimer's disease and dementia

Nearly 12% of older adults on Medicare were treated for Alzheimer's disease or another form of dementia. Alzheimer's disease is one specific type of dementia—a condition that causes memory loss and difficulty thinking or problem-solving to the point that it interferes with every day activities. Dementia is not a normal part of aging and is caused by changes in the brain over time. The biggest risk factors for these chronic conditions are things you often can't control, including age, family history, and genetics. But studies have suggested incorporating the following habits into your lifestyle could slow or prevent onset:

- Exercise. Staying active isn't just good for your heart; it's also great for your brain.
- Sleep. Your brain does important stuff while you are sleeping, so getting at least 7 hours of deep sleep a night is crucial.
- Be smart about your diet. Research suggests that some foods can negatively affect your brain.

Dementia is the loss of cognitive functioning — thinking, remembering, and reasoning — to such an extent that it interferes with a person's daily life and activities. Some people with dementia cannot control their emotions, and their personalities may change. Dementia ranges in severity from the mildest stage, when it is just beginning to affect a person's functioning, to the most severe stage, when the person must depend completely on others for basic activities of daily living, such as feeding oneself. Dementia affects millions of people and is more common as people grow older (about one-third of all people age 85 or older may have some form of dementia) but it is not a normal part of aging. Many people live into their 90s and beyond without any signs of dementia.

There are several different forms of dementia, including Alzheimer's disease, which is the most common.

What are the signs and symptoms of dementia?

Signs and symptoms of dementia result when once-healthy neurons (nerve cells) in the brain stop working, lose connections with other brain cells, and die. While everyone loses some neurons as they age, people with dementia experience far greater loss.

The signs and symptoms can vary depending on the type and may include:

- Experiencing memory loss, poor judgment, and confusion
- Difficulty speaking, understanding and expressing thoughts, or reading and writing
- Wandering and getting lost in a familiar neighborhood
- Trouble handling money responsibly and paying bills
- Repeating questions
- Using unusual words to refer to familiar objects
- Taking longer to complete normal daily tasks
- Losing interest in normal daily activities or events
- Hallucinating or experiencing delusions or paranoia
- Acting impulsively
- Not caring about other people's feelings
- Losing balance and problems with movement

People with intellectual and developmental disabilities can also develop dementia as they age, and in these cases, recognizing their symptoms can be particularly difficult. It's important to consider a person's current abilities and to monitor for changes over time that could signal dementia.

What causes dementia?

Dementia is the result of changes in certain brain regions that cause neurons (nerve cells) and their connections to stop working properly. Researchers have connected changes in the brain to certain forms of dementia and are investigating why these changes happen in some people but not others. For a small number of people, rare genetic variants that cause dementia have been identified.

Although we don't yet know for certain what, if anything, can prevent dementia, in general, leading a healthy lifestyle may help reduce risk factors.

What are the different types of dementia?

Various neurodegenerative disorders and factors contribute to the development of dementia through a progressive and irreversible loss of neurons and brain functioning. Currently, there is no cure for any type of dementia. Types of dementia include:

- Alzheimer's disease, the most common dementia diagnosis among older adults. It is caused by changes in the brain, including abnormal buildups of proteins known as amyloid plaques and tau tangles.
- Frontotemporal dementia, a rare form of dementia that tends to occur in people younger than 60. It is associated with abnormal amounts or forms of the proteins tau and TDP-43.
- Lewy body dementia, a form of dementia caused by abnormal deposits of the protein alpha-synuclein, called Lewy bodies.
- Vascular dementia, a form of dementia caused by conditions that damage blood vessels in the brain or interrupt the flow of blood and oxygen to the brain.
- Mixed dementia, a combination of two or more types of dementia. For example, through autopsy studies involving older adults who had dementia, researchers have identified that many people had a combination of brain changes associated with different forms of dementia.

Scientists are investigating how the underlying disease processes in different forms of dementia start and influence each other. They also continue to explore the variety of disorders and disease processes that contribute to dementia. For example, based on autopsy studies, researchers recently characterized another form of dementia known as LATE. Further knowledge gains in the underlying causes of dementia will help researchers better understand these conditions and develop more personalized prevention, treatment, and care strategies.

Researchers who investigate what's happening inside the brain after death recently helped characterize a new form of dementia: ***limbic-predominant age-related TDP-43 encephalopathy (LATE).*** LATE causes symptoms similar to Alzheimer's, including problems with thinking, remembering, and reasoning, but has different underlying causes involving abnormal clusters of a protein called TDP-43. This protein is also involved in frontotemporal dementia, but LATE exhibits a different pattern of brain changes and tends to affect people over the age of 80. For example, a team of researchers analyzed the brains of 6,196 people with an average age at death of 88 years and found that almost 40% of them may have had LATE.

Currently, there is no way to diagnose LATE in living people. Researchers are working to further explore the causes of and risk factors for LATE and to identify pathways that could help develop methods for doctors to diagnose LATE.

How is dementia diagnosed?

To diagnose dementia, doctors first assess whether a person has an underlying, potentially treatable, condition that may relate to cognitive difficulties. A physical exam to measure blood pressure and other vital signs, as well as laboratory tests of blood and other fluids to check levels of various chemicals, hormones, and vitamins, can help uncover or rule out possible causes of symptoms.

A review of a person's medical and family history can provide important clues about risk for dementia. Typical questions might include asking about whether dementia runs in the family, how and when symptoms began, changes in behavior and personality, and if the person is taking certain medications that might cause or worsen symptoms.

The following procedures also may be used to diagnose dementia:

- Cognitive and neurological tests. Used to evaluate thinking and physical functioning, these tests include assessments of memory, problem solving, language skills, and math skills, as well as balance, sensory response, and reflexes.
- Brain scans. These tests can identify strokes, tumors, and other problems that can cause dementia. Scans also identify changes in the brain's structure and function. The most common scans are:

1. Computed tomography (CT), which uses X-rays to produce images of the brain and other organs

2.Magnetic resonance imaging (MRI), which uses magnetic fields and radio waves to produce detailed images of body structures, including tissues, organs, bones, and nerves

3.Positron emission tomography (PET), which uses radiation to provide pictures of brain activity — such as energy use — or specific molecules in different brain regions.

- Psychiatric evaluation. If someone is experiencing behavioral or mood changes, a psychiatric evaluation may be recommended to help determine if depression or another mental health condition is causing or contributing to a person's symptoms.
- Genetic tests. Some forms of dementia are caused by a person's genes. In these rare cases, a genetic test ordered by a doctor can help people know if they have the altered genes. It is important to talk with a genetic counselor before and after getting tested, along with family members and the doctor. There are also genetic tests that look for genetic variations that affect someone's risk of developing dementia, but these tests cannot be used to diagnose dementia.
- Cerebrospinal fluid (CSF) tests. CSF is a clear fluid that surrounds the brain and the spinal cord, providing protection, insulation, and nutrients. Doctors collect CSF by performing a lumbar puncture, also called a spinal tap. Measuring the levels of proteins or other substances in CSF may be used to help diagnose Alzheimer's or other types of dementia.
- Blood tests. It is now possible for many doctors, dependent on state-specific availability reflecting U.S.

your health care team to determine what options may work best for you.

Food and Drug Administration guidelines, to order a blood test to measure levels of beta-amyloid, a protein that accumulates abnormally in people with Alzheimer's. Several other blood tests are in development. At present, blood test results alone should not be used to diagnose dementia, but may be taken into consideration along with other tests. However, the availability of these diagnostic tests is still limited.

Some of the tests and procedures used to diagnose dementia may not be covered by health insurance. Check with your insurance provider and talk with your health care team to determine what options may work best for you.

Early detection of symptoms is important as some causes can be successfully treated. However, in many cases, the cause of dementia is unknown and cannot be effectively treated. Still, obtaining an early diagnosis can help with managing the condition and planning ahead. In the early stages of dementia, it may be possible for people to continue with their everyday activities. As the disease progresses, people will need to adopt new strategies to help adjust.Planning ahead may also include deciding what happens if and when the disease becomes more severe. Sometimes, a person with dementia will volunteer to donate their brain after they have died. Brain donation helps researchers study brain disorders such as Alzheimer's disease and related dementias. By studying the brains of people who have died, researchers have already learned a great deal about how types of dementia affect the brain and how we might better treat and prevent them. But much more remains to be understood. When donating as part of a research study or to the NIH NeuroBioBank, there is no cost to the family for the donation and an autopsy report. Learn more about brain donation.

4. Heart failure

About 5% of older adults were treated for heart failure—a condition that occurs when the heart cannot adequately supply blood and oxygen to all of the organs in the body. The heart might become enlarged, develop more muscle mass, or pump faster in order to meet the body's needs, causing you to feel tired, light headed, nauseous, confused, or lack an appetite.Steps you can take to prevent or diminish symptoms of heart failure:

The best prevention is to follow a doctor's recommendations to decrease your risk for coronary heart disease and high blood pressure

5.Chronic kidney disease (CKD)

Nearly 25% of older adults were treated for chronic kidney disease (CKD) or a slow loss in kidney function over time. People dealing with CKD have an increased risk for developing heart disease or kidney failure. Steps you can take to prevent or diminish symptoms of CKD:

- Understand what damages your kidney. Diabetes and high blood pressure are the greatest risk factors for kidney damage, so taking steps to prevent these diseases is your best strategy.
- Early detection and treatment. Talk to your doctor regularly, stay current on screenings, and keep up on prescriptions you need to diminish symptoms.

6.Diabetes

Twenty-seven percent of older adults were treated for diabetes—a disease that occurs when your body is resistant to, or doesn't produce enough, insulin. Insulin is what your body uses to get energy from food, and distributes it to your cells. When this doesn't happen, you get high blood sugar, which can lead to complications such as kidney disease, heart disease, or blindness. Chances of having diabetes increases after age 45.

Steps you can take to keep you from developing diabetes or to manage this condition:

- Eating a healthy diet, including monitoring your carbohydrate and calorie intake, and talking to your doctor about alcohol consumption.
- Exercising for 30 minutes five times a week to keep your blood glucose levels in check, and to control weight gain.
- Safely losing 5-7% of body weight if you are diagnosed with pre-diabetes.

7.Ischemic heart disease

Nearly 29% of older adults were treated for ischemic heart disease—a condition that is caused by a build-up of plaque that narrows the arteries leading to the heart. Narrow or blocked arteries decreases the amount of oxygen-rich blood delivered to the heart. This can cause other complications like blood clots, angina, or a heart attack. Steps you can incorporate to help if you have ischemic heart disease:

1. Avoid saturated and trans fats, and limit sugar and salt intake
2. Get seven to eight hours of sleep each night
3. Keep your stress levels in check
4. Do regular cardio exercises
5. Abstain from smoking
6. Talk to your doctor about the major risk factors, including high cholesterol and high blood pressure

8. Arthritis

About 35% of older adults were treated for arthritis —an inflammation of your joints, which causes pain and stiffness and is more common in women.

Steps you can take to delay the onset of arthritis or manage the symptoms:

- Exercise at least five times per week, for 30 minutes each time, to improve function and decrease pain. Try to include a mixture of aerobic, strength-building, and stretching movements.
- Stay within the recommended weight for your height—losing one pound can remove four pounds of pressure on your knees.
- Make sure your back, legs, and arms are always supported.
- Take precautions to avoid joint injuries.
- Do not smoke.

9.Obesity

About 40% of adults 65 and older are obese. NCOA is pressing to define quality obesity care as a universal right. That includes the right to coverage for treatment with access to the full range of treatment options.

Tips for addressing obesity include:

- Understanding what obesity treatments are covered by Medicare
- Empowering yourself with knowledge about nutrition
- Educating others and being your own advocate

10. High cholesterol

More than 50% of older adults were treated for high cholesterol—a condition that occurs when your body has an excess of bad fats (or lipids), resulting in your arteries getting clogged, which can lead to heart disease.

Steps you can take to prevent or manage high cholesterol:

- Abstain from smoking and excessive alcohol consumption
- Be active each day
- Manage your weight
- Minimize saturated fats and trans fats in your diet

11.Hypertension (high blood pressure)

Nearly 60% of older adults were treated for hypertension—a common condition that involves both how much blood your heart pumps, as well as how resistant your arteries are to the blood flow. When your heart pumps a lot of blood, and you have narrow arteries which resist the flow, that's when you get high blood pressure, also known as hypertension. The danger of hypertension is not

only that you can have it for years and not know it, but it can cause other
serious health conditions, like stroke and heart attacks. Steps you can take to prevent or reduce high blood pressure:

- Maintain a healthy weight. Losing just 10 pounds can reduce blood pressure
- Regulate your stress levels
- Limit salt and alcohol consumption
- Exercise daily, including a combination of moderate to vigorous-intensity aerobic activities, flexibility and stretching, and muscle strengthening
- Check your blood pressure regularly—the quicker you catch pre-hypertension, the more likely you are to prevent high blood pressure

12. Eye Problems;- Your retina is a layer of specialized cells in the back of your eye that converts light into electrical signals that your brain can interpret. Diseases that involve this layer of cells are known as retinal diseases. Many different types of retinal diseases have been identified. Some are caused by inherited genes, and others are caused by retinal damage that develops over time.

These are senile cataracts,Glucoma,retinal hemorrhage ,senile retinal degeration , Macular Degeneration. Talk to your eye specialist regarding the treatment of these diseases

Age-related macular degeneration

Age-related macular degeneration (AMD) accounts for 8.7%Trusted Source of blindness diagnoses worldwide. It's a progressive disease characterized by the breakdown of your macula. The macula is the part of your retina that controls your central vision.

The risk of developing age-related macular degeneration is are over age 55 years have a family history of the eye disease smoke

The first noticeable symptoms often include changes in your central vision and difficulty reading. You may notice that you cannot see fine details in your central vision, whether you're looking at an object close up or at a distance. As it progresses, you may notice that straight lines look wavy. You may also notice dark spots in your vision.

Diabetic retinopathy

Diabetic retinopathy is the most commonTrusted Source cause of blindness in people of typical working ages in the United States. It's characterized by damage to the retina from chronically high blood sugar levels in people with diabetes.

Symptoms often do not appear in the early stages. When they do appear, they may include blurred vision, floaters, and vision loss

Retinal tear

Your eye is filled with a gel-like substance called the vitreous body. As you get older, this gel peels away from your retina. This process is called posterior vitreous detachment. Posterior vitreous detachment is the most common cause of a retinal tear. A retinal tear occurs when the gel pulls part of the retina with it. More rarely, a retinal tear can occur due to injury.

Two of the most common symptoms of a retinal tear are a sudden onset of floaters or seeing sudden flashes of light.

Retinal detachment

Retinal detachment is when your retina is pulled away from its normal position at the back of your eye. You may be at a higher riskTrusted Source for this condition if you have diabetic retinopathy or are extremely myopic (nearsighted). Early symptoms may include an increase in floaters, flashes of light, or a shadow over your field of vision. Retinal detachment is a medical emergency that requires immediate medical attention.

Macular hole

A macular hole is a gap in the central part of your retina called the macula. Most cases have no apparent cause. It develops most often in people ages 60 to 80 years, and more often in women than men. Early symptoms can include blurry or wavy vision. Loss of central vision may occur in the later stages of this disease.

Retinoblastoma

Blastomas are cancers that start in immature cells. Retinoblastoma is an extremely rare cancer that starts in immature cells in your retina. About 90% of cases develop before age 5 years.

About 40% of diagnosed cases develop because of inherited genes, and the rest are caused by gene mutations that arise spontaneously.The most common initial symptoms of a retinoblastoma were eye bulging (proptosis) followed by an abnormal white spot in the pupil (leukocoria).

How are retinal diseases treated?

Treatment depends on which disease you have. For example, doctors sometimes treat age-related macular degeneration with:

1. Anti-VEGF injections into the affected eye

2.Photodynamic therapy, a therapy that uses medications that take effect when exposed to lasers

3.Retinal tears and detachment often require surgical repair. Retinoblastoma is treated with six standard treatments including:

1 .cryotherapy

2. radiation therapy
3. thermotherapy
4. chemotherapy
5. high-dose chemotherapy with stem cell rescue
6. surgery

Diabetic retinopathy is primarily treated with
1.laser treatment
2.injections
3.surgery to remove blood and scar tissue

13. Ear Problems

Understanding Age-Related Hearing Loss;- When a person gets older, their ability to hear may gradually decrease over time. This process is referred to as age-related hearing loss. Age-related hearing loss, otherwise known as presbycusis, is common. Research shows that roughly one-third of people over the age of 65 will deal with some loss of hearing.

What Causes Age-Related Hearing Loss?

There are various factors that can cause age-related hearing loss.

The main cause is the changes that occur in the inner ear and auditory nerve as a person ages.3 The inner ear is deep within the ear and is designed to help transfer the sounds that you hear to the brain with the help of the auditory nerve.

Other factors that can contribute to age-related hearing loss include:
1.Hearing loss that runs in your family
2.Exposure to extremely loud noise on a regular basis
3.Loss of hair cells in the ear that assist in the hearing process
4.Health conditions such as diabetes, heart disease, and high blood pressure
5.Head trauma
6.Ototoxic medications (such as NSAIDs or certain antibiotics) that cause permanent damage to the inner ear

Treatment Options for Age-Related Hearing Loss

The main treatment for age-related hearing loss is hearing aids. A hearing aid is an electronic medical device that is placed either in or around the ear to help improve someone's ability to hear sounds.

People will get one hearing aid per ear and the devices can improve hearing. People that wear hearing aids have to follow up with their otolaryngologist regularly to make sure that there are no issues with the hearing aid and their rehabilitation. Hearing aids are also available over-the-counter for adults with self-perceived mild to moderate hearing loss. Other possible treatment options include:

- Devices that can amplify sounds
- Devices that can translate speech into text so a person can read what a person is saying
- Learning speech-reading techniques, such as sign language

Is surgery an option for age-related hearing loss?

In some rare cases, surgery may be performed if there are any injuries, inflammation, or disease within the ear. However, there are risks associated with surgery, so it is not considered a first-line treatment

How Is Age-Related Hearing Prevented?

There is no true way to prevent-age related hearing loss, but there are ways you can protect your ears from other factors that may contribute to it. This involves keeping your ears healthy and avoiding excessive noise exposure. If you have to be in areas with loud noises, wearing earplugs or earmuffs can help to limit the noise that makes its way into your ears.

14.Chronic obstructive pulmonary disease (COPD)

Another common chronic conditions for adults 65+ is chronic obstructive pulmonary disease (COPD), which includes two main conditions: emphysema and chronic bronchitis. COPD makes it hard to breathe and causes shortness of breath, coughing, and chest tightness.

Steps you can take to manage COPD include:

- The best way to prevent COPD—or slow its progression—is to quit or avoid smoking. Also try to avoid secondhand smoke, chemical fumes, and dust, which can irritate your lungs.
- If you already have COPD, complete the treatments that your doctor has prescribed, get the flu and pneumonia vaccines as recommended by your doctor, and continue to remain active.

pneumonia vaccines as recommended by your doctor, and continue to remain active.

15.Chronic kidney disease (CKD)

Nearly 25% of older adults were treated for chronic kidney disease (CKD) or a slow loss in kidney function over time. People dealing with CKD have an increased risk for developing heart disease or kidney failure. Steps you can take to prevent or diminish symptoms of CKD:

1. Understand what damages your kidney. Diabetes and high blood pressure are the greatest risk factors for kidney damage, so taking steps to prevent these diseases is your best strategy.
2.Early detection and treatment. Talk to your doctor regularly, stay current on screenings, and keep up on prescriptions you need to diminish symptoms.

16.Malignancy in elderly

Elderly people are also prone to various types of cancers due to lowered immunity.The organs involved are colon,stomach,liver, prostate,breast,cervical and brain. If such situation arises talk to your personel physician for proper investigation and treatment.

Bibliography and Acknowledgement

- Ahirwar R, Mondal PR. Prevalence of obesity in India: A systematic review. Diabetes & Metabolic Syndrome: Clinical Research & Reviews. 2019;13: 318–321. doi: 10.1016/j.dsx.2018.08.032 [PubMed] [CrossRef] [Google Scholar]
- Alam M, Karan A. Elderly Health In India: Dimension, Differentiatials and Determinats. UNFPA. 2011. doi: 10.13140/2.1.4232.5128 [CrossRef] [Google Scholar]
- Bhagat RB. Emerging pattern of urbanisation in India. Economic and political weekly. 2011. Aug 20:10–2. [Google Scholar]
- Blinder AS. Wage Discrimination: Reduced Form and Structural Estimates. The Journal of Human Resources. 1973;8: 436–455. doi: 10.2307/144855 [CrossRef] [Google Scholar]
- Chattopadhyay A, Khan J, Bloom DE, Sinha D, Nayak I, Gupta S, et al. Insights into Labor Force Participation among Older Adults: Evidence from the Longitudinal Ageing Study in India. Population Ageing. 2022. [cited 26 Feb 2022]. doi: 10.1007/s12062-022-09357-7 [CrossRef] [Google Scholar]
- Chaurasia H, Srivastava S. Abuse, Neglect, and Disrespect against Older Adults in India. Population Ageing. 2020;13: 497–511. doi: 10.1007/s12062-020-09270-x [CrossRef] [Google Scholar]
- Dandona L, Dandona R, Kumar GA, Shukla DK, Paul VK, Balakrishnan K, et al. Nations within a nation: variations in epidemiological transition across the states of India, 1990–2016 in the Global Burden of Disease Study. The Lancet. 2017;390: 2437–2460. doi: 10.1016/S0140-6736(17)32804-0 [PMC free article] [PubMed] [CrossRef] [Google Scholar]
- Ewing R, Schmid T, Killingsworth R, Zlot A, Raudenbush S. Relationship between Urban Sprawl and Physical Activity, Obesity, and Morbidity. Am J Health Promot. 2003;18: 47–57. doi: 10.4278/0890-1171-18.1.47 [PubMed] [CrossRef] [Google Scholar]
- Geldsetzer P, Manne-Goehler J, Theilmann M, Davies JI, Awasthi A, Vollmer S, et al. Diabetes and Hypertension in India. JAMA Intern Med. 2018;178: 363–372. doi: 10.1001/jamainternmed.2017.8094 [PMC free article] [PubMed] [CrossRef] [Google Scholar
- Hellström Y, Hallberg IR. Perspectives of elderly people receiving home help on health, care and quality of life. Health & Social Care in the Community. 2001;9: 61–71. doi: 10.1046/j.1365-2524.2001.00282.x [PubMed] [CrossRef] [Google Scholar]
- International Institute for Population Sciences (IIPS), NPHCE, MoHFW, Harvard T. H. Chan School of Public Health (HSPH), The University of Southern California (USC). Longitudinal Ageing Study in India (LASI) Wave 1. India Report. Mumbai, India; 2020.
- Jones DA, Peters TJ. Caring for elderly dependants: effects on the carers' quality of life. Age and ageing. 1992. Nov 1;21(6):421–8. doi: 10.1093/ageing/21.6.421 [PubMed] [CrossRef] [Google Scholar]
- Karki P. Living with chronic diseases in India. 2019; 17–21. [Google Scholar]
- Katta VA, Kokiwar PR. A Study of Prevalence of Childhood Obesity among School Children in Karimnagar Town. MRIMS Journal of Health Sciences. 2013;1: 8. doi: 10.4103/2321-7006.301935 [CrossRef] [Google Scholar]
- Kim S, Symons M, Popkin BM. Contrasting socioeconomic profiles related to healthier lifestyles in China and the United States. Am J Epidemiol. 2004;159: 184–191. doi: 10.1093/aje/kwh006 [PubMed] [CrossRef] [Google Scholar]
- Lahariya C. 'Ayushman Bharat' Program and Universal Health Coverage in India. Indian Pediatr. 2018;55: 495–506. doi: 10.1007/s13312-018-1341-1 [PubMed] [CrossRef] [Google Scholar]
- Liu S, Yan Z, Liu Y, Yin Q, Kuang L. Association between air pollution and chronic diseases among the elderly in China. Nat Hazards. 2017;89: 79–91. doi: 10.1007/s11069-017-2955-7 [CrossRef] [Google Scholar]
- Marttila A, Johansson E, Whitehead M, Burström B. Living on social assistance with chronic illness: Buffering and undermining features to well-being. BMC Public Health. 2010;10: 754. doi: 10.1186/1471-2458-10-754 [PMC free article] [PubMed] [CrossRef] [Google Scholar]
- Ng R, Sutradhar R, Yao Z, Wodchis WP, Rosella LC. Smoking, drinking, diet and physical activity—modifiable lifestyle risk factors and their associations with age to first chronic disease. Int J Epidemiol. 2020;49: 113–130. doi: 10.1093/ije/dyz078 [PMC free article] [PubMed] [CrossRef]
- Omran AR. The Epidemiologic Transition: A Theory of the Epidemiology of Population Change. Milbank Q. 2005;83: 731–757. doi: 10.1111/j.1468-0009.2005.00398.x [PMC free article] [PubMed] [CrossRef] [Google Scholar]
- Parmar MC, Saikia N. Chronic morbidity and reported disability among older persons from the India Human Development Survey. BMC Geriatr. 2018;18. doi: 10.1186/s12877-018-0979-9 [PMC free article] [PubMed] [CrossRef] [Google Scholar]
- Rajan I, Risseeuw C, Perera M, editors. Institutional Provisions and Care for the Aged. Anthem Press; 2009. doi: 10.7135/UPO9781843317777 [CrossRef] [Google Scholar]
- Samanta T, Chen F, Vanneman R. Living Arrangements and Health of Older Adults in India. The Journals of Gerontology: Series B. 2015;70: 937–947. doi: 10.1093/geronb/gbu164 [PubMed] [CrossRef] [Google Scholar]
- Tripathy JP, Thakur JS, Jeet G, Chawla S, Jain S, Prasad R. Urban rural differences in diet, physical activity and obesity in India: are we witnessing the great Indian equalisation? Results from a cross-sectional STEPS survey. BMC Public Health. 2016;16: 816. doi: 10.1186/s12889-016-3489-8
- Verma R, Khanna P. National Program of Health-Care for the Elderly in India: A Hope for Healthy Ageing. Int J Prev Med. 2013;4: 1103–1107. [PMC free article] [PubMed] [Google Scholar]
- Wang S, Kou C, Liu Y, Li B, Tao Y, D'Arcy C, et al. Rural-urban differences in the prevalence of chronic disease in northeast China. Asia Pac J Public Health. 2015;27: 394–406. doi: 10.1177/1010539514551200 [PubMed] [CrossRef] [Google Scholar]
- Yadav K, Krishnan A. Changing patterns of diet, physical activity and obesity among urban, rural and slum populations in north India. Obesity Reviews. 2008;9: 400–408. doi: 10.1111/j.1467-789X.2008.00505.x [PubMed] [CrossRef] [Google Scholar]
- Yadav S, Arokiasamy P. Understanding epidemiological transition in India. Glob Health Action. 2014;7. doi: 10.3402/gha.v7.23248 [PMC free article] [PubMed] [CrossRef] [Google Scholar

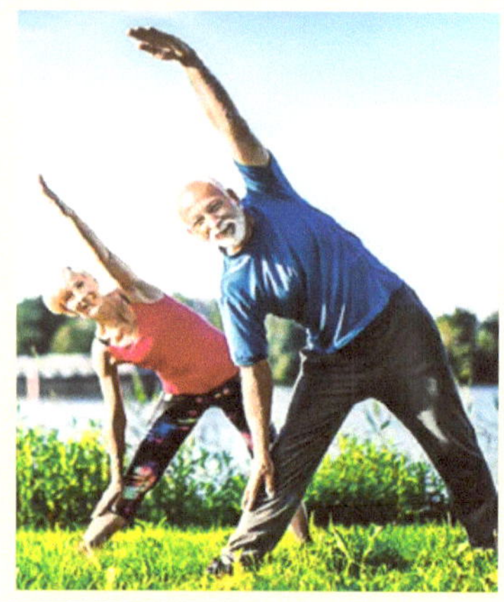

Exercises for Seniors: Effective Ways To Stay Active

The body goes through many changes as it ages. As we age, we tend to have less energy, our muscles will feel weaker, and mobility issues start to surface. According to a 2017 exercise study, regular physical activity can slow down the aging process. Researchers have found that older adults who maintain an active lifestyle live longer and healthier lives.

Balance Exercises for Older Adults

Prioritizing balance helps older adults maintain mobility, independence, and a healthy, engaged lifestyle for longer. Balance training provides both physical and psychological benefits.

Balance exercises for seniors also help improve recovery, promote independence, and reduce the risk of falls by strengthening muscles, tendons, and joints.

One Leg Stance – Stand behind a solid chair and hold on to the back of the chair for support. Lift your right foot and balance on one leg. Hold the pose as long as you can and try to balance on your own. Repeat on the other leg.

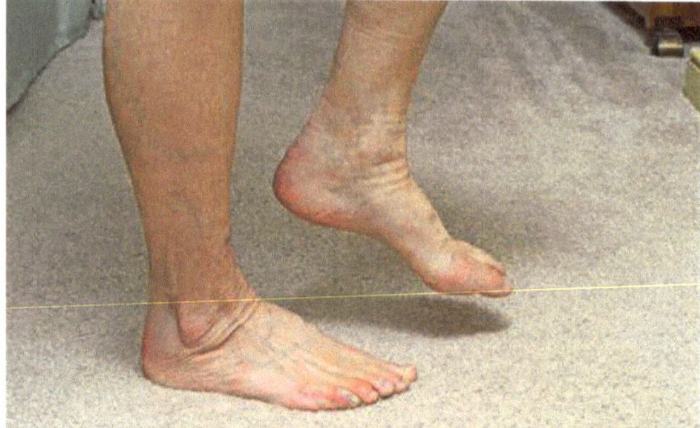

Fig **4.1 one leg stance**

Heel-to-Toe Walk – Stand beside a table or wall for support. Walk slowly, placing your right foot in front of the left, touching the heel on the toe. Take 10 steps forward, turn around, and walk back the same way.

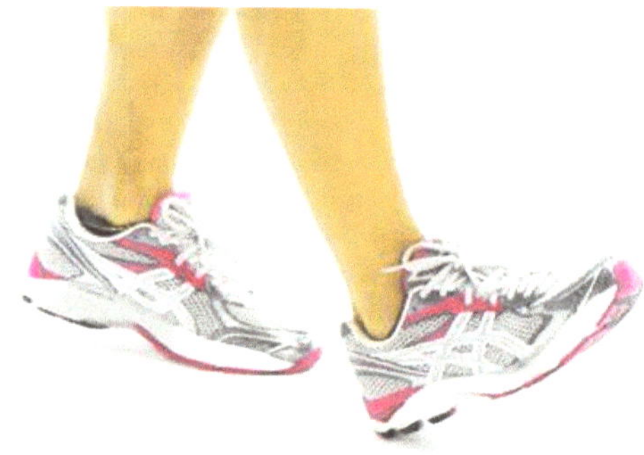

Fig 4.2 **Heel-to-Toe Walk**

Toe Lifts – Hold on to a chair. Slowly stand and place your feet hip width apart. Slowly Raise your heels to stand on your tip toes and then slowly lower yourself back down. Repeat 15 times.

March in Place – Stand next to a steady surface you can hold onto for support. Lift your right knee up and lower it back down. Repeat on the other leg and march in place.

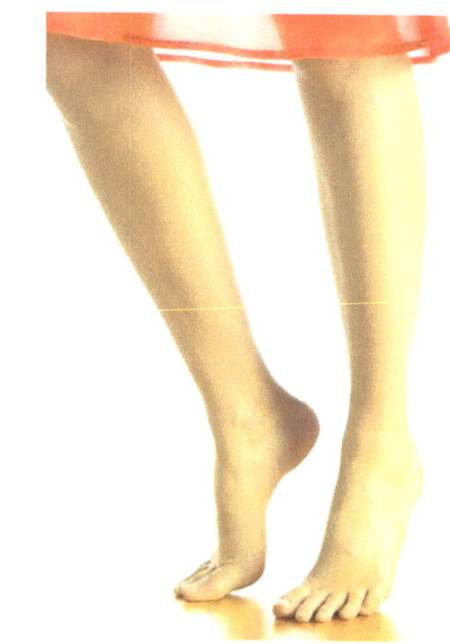

Fig 4.3 **Toe Lifts Walk**

Standing Exercises for Mobility

Standing mobility exercises address multiple components that tend to decline with age – strength, balance, flexibility, bone density, posture, and coordination. Standing exercises engage the major muscle groups in the hips, legs, and abdomen which are important for mobility. Declines in leg strength directly impact the ability to get around.

Hip Circles – Stand up tall and place both hands on the hips. Make a circular motion with your hips clockwise. Repeat in the other direction.

Sit-to-Stand – While sitting on a chair, push off from your knees and slowly stand straight. Complete the rep by sitting back down slowly.

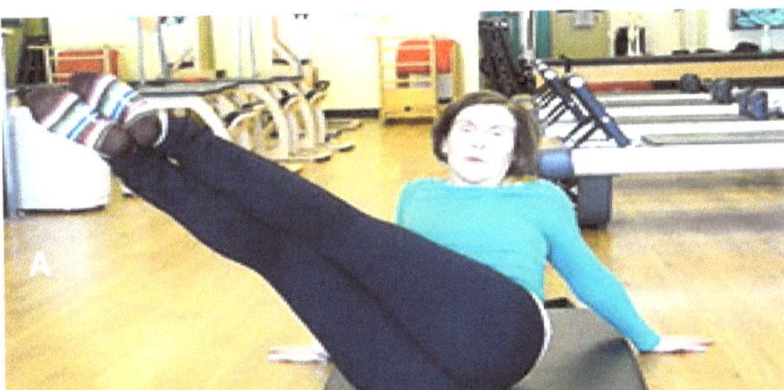

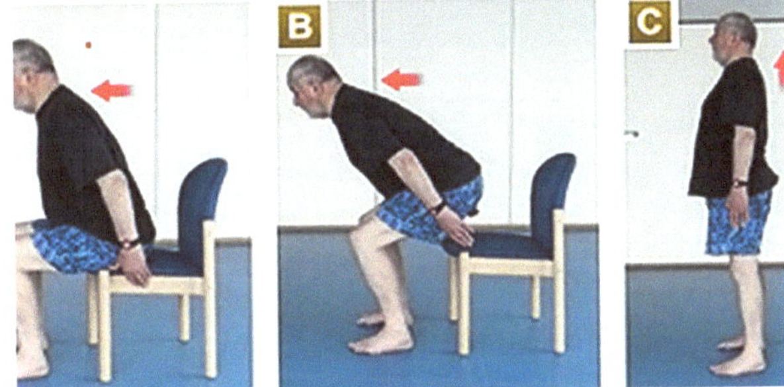

Fig 4.4 Showing (A) Hip Circles (B) Sit to stand

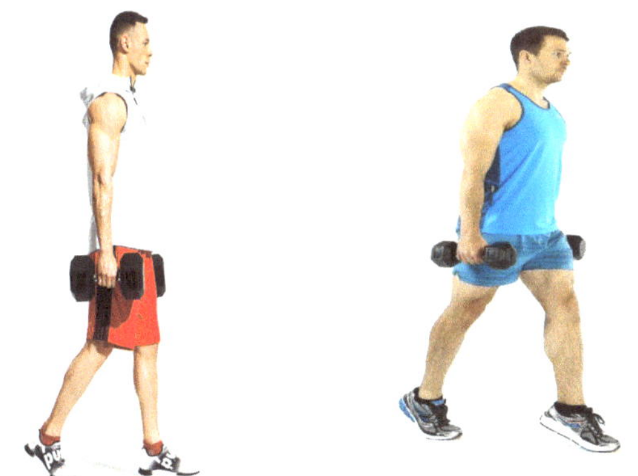

Fig 4.5 Showing (A) (B) Farmer;s walk

Farmer's Walk – While holding small weights in your hands, walk forward slowly. Repeat in the opposite direction.

Hamstring Curl – Hold on to a chair for support. While standing, bend your knee to lift your foot up behind you. Bring it back down and repeat with the other leg. For an additional add ankle weights to this exercise.

Core Stability Exercises for Balance

Training the core muscles with specific stability exercises reaps multiple balance benefits for seniors. These exercises work on trunk control and posture needed to comfortably perform either stationary or mobile activities without losing your balance.

The core muscles of the abdomen, lower back, hips, and pelvis provide foundational support and stability for the body.

A

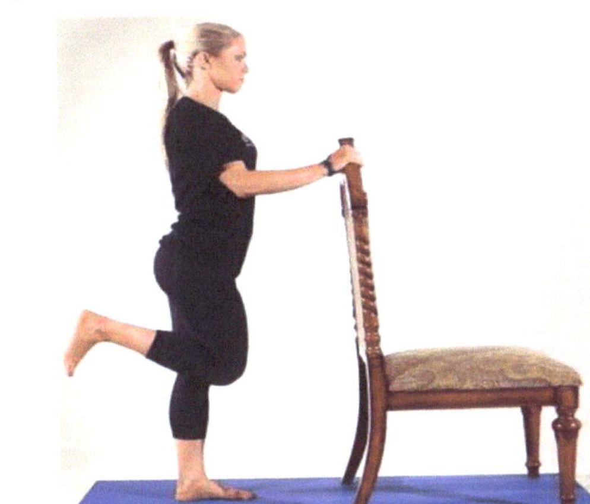

B.

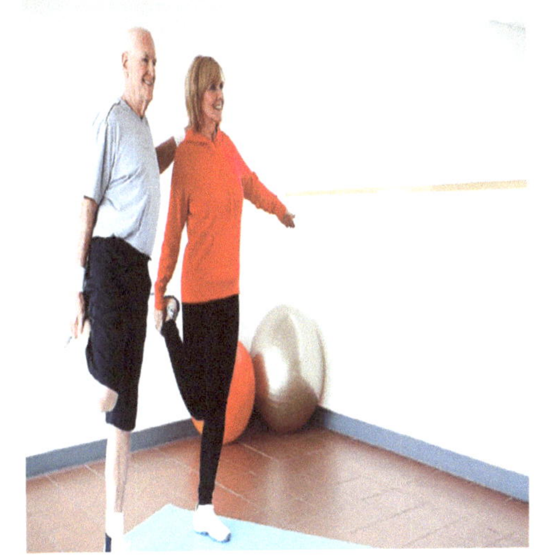

Fig 4.6 Showing (A) Hamsring curl (B) stability exercises

Resistance Band Pull Apart – Using a light resistance band, hold on to each of its ends and pull apart slowly. Repeat 10 times.

Seated Leg Press – While in a seated position, tie a resistance band above the knee area. Slowly open the thighs and close back again. Repeat 10 times.

Bridge – Lie flat on your back and keep the knees bent. Raise your hips up slowly and hold the pose for a few seconds. Lower back down.

Leg Lift – While lying flat on the floor, slowly lift one leg up and hold the pose. Lower back down slowly. Repeat with the other leg.

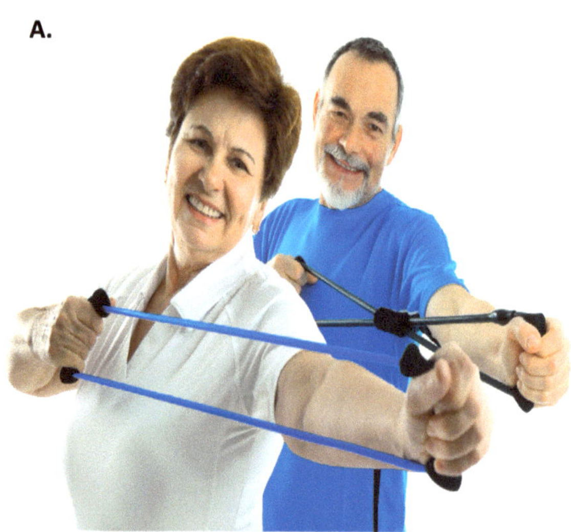

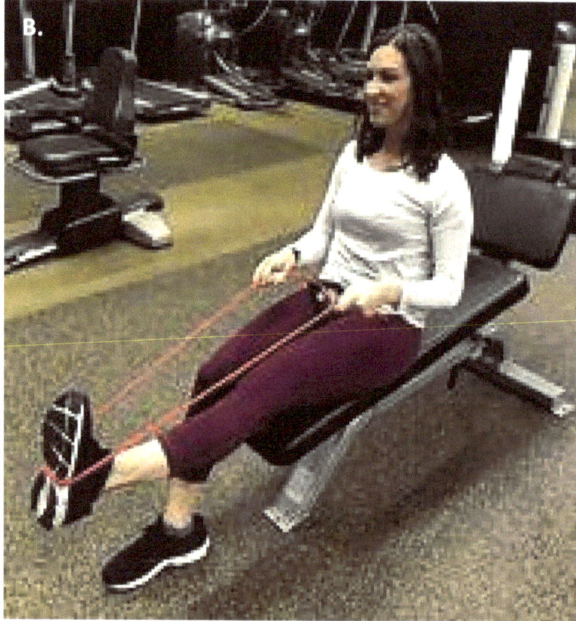

Fig 4.7 Showing (A) band streching (B) Seated Leg Press

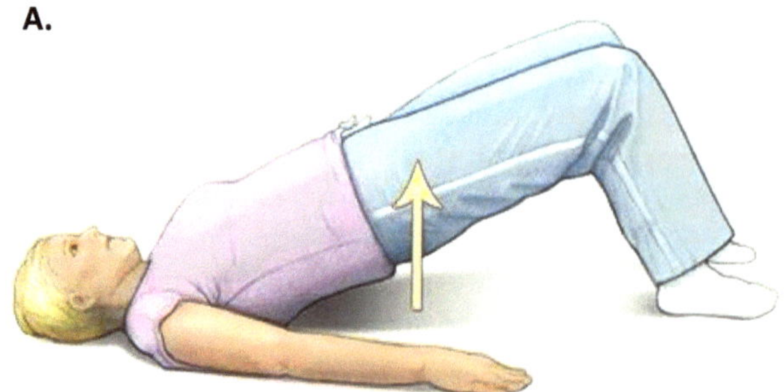

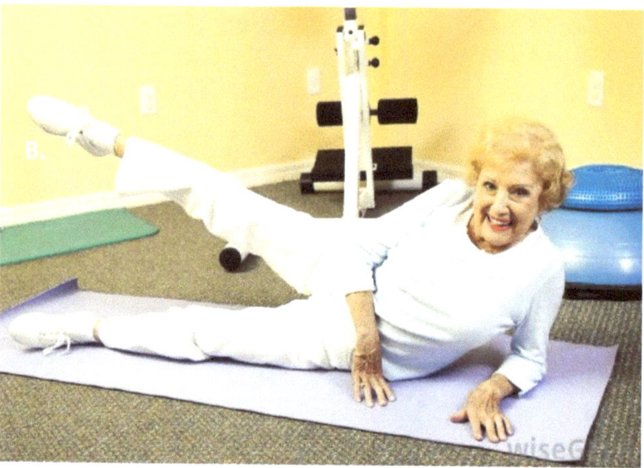

Fig 4.8 Showing (A) Bridge pose (B) Seated Leg lift

Seated Exercises for Seniors

Seated exercises are low impact and gentle on the joints, making them safe and accessible for seniors. They minimize the strain and/or pain that standing puts on the back, hips, knees, etc.

Chair exercises for seniors improve strength, increase flexibility, and provide stability by removing balance challenges.

Seated Knee Extension – While sitting, extend and straighten one leg. Hold the pose for 3 seconds. Lower back down and repeat with the other leg.

Seated Jumping Jacks – Sit up straight close to the edge of the chair. Quickly open your legs out to the side and extend both arms up over the head, like a jumping jack motion. Repeat this 10 times.

Seated Shoulder Rolls – Sit up comfortably with your back straight. Shrug your shoulders up and rotate in a circular motion. Repeat in the other direction.

Seated Tap Dance – While in a seated position, extend one leg and point your toe with one foot. Tap the floor with your toe. Flex your extended leg and tap the floor with your heel. Return to the starting position and repeat on the other leg.

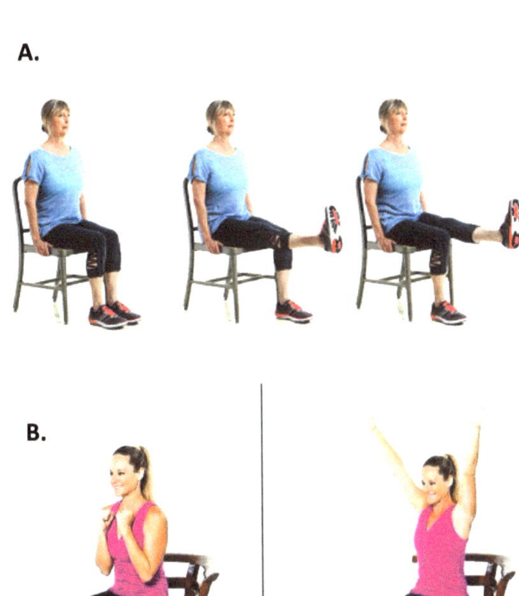

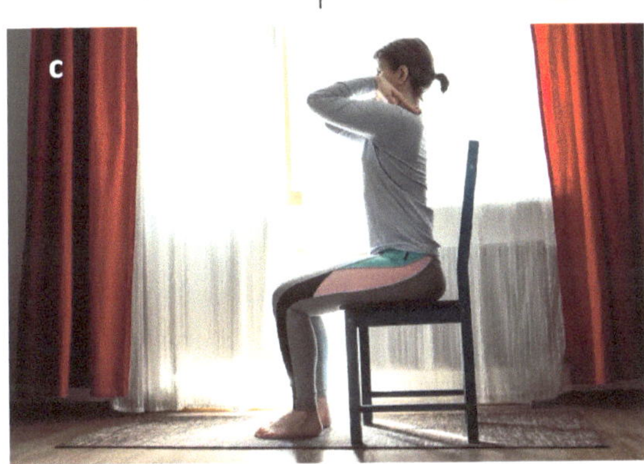

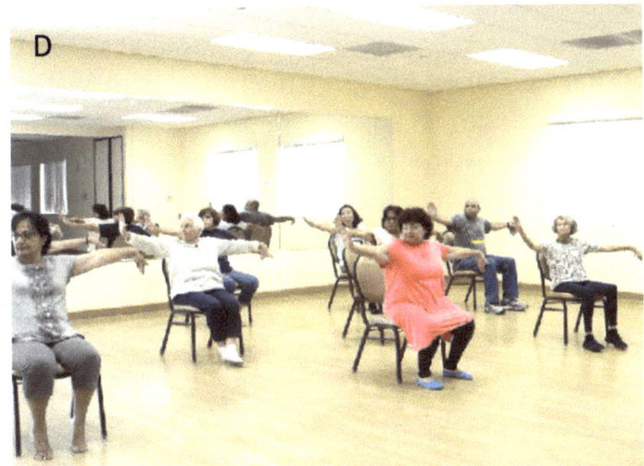

Fig 4.9 Showing (A) Seated Knee Extension (B) Seated Jumping Jacks **(C)** Seated Shoulder Rolls (D) Seated Tap Dance

Seated Dumbbell Exercises for Seniors

Resistance training using light dumbbells can help improve strength, balance, and mobility.

Bicep Curls

•Sit upright with a dumbbell in each hand, arms extended, and palms facing forward.

•Lift the dumbbells to shoulder level by bending your elbows.

•Hold for 2 seconds.

•Lower slowly back to the starting position.

•Complete 3 sets of 12 reps.

Overhead Press

•Hold dumbbells at ear level with elbows bent at 90 degrees and palms forward.

•Fully extend arms to push the dumbbells overhead.

•Slowly lower back to the starting position.

•Complete 3 sets of 10 reps.

Tricep Extension

•Hold a dumbbell overhead with arms fully extended.

•Bend your elbows to lower the dumbbell behind your head, keeping your elbows close to your ears.

•Extend your arms to lift the dumbbell back overhead.

•Complete 3 sets of 15 reps.

Lateral Raises

•Hold a dumbbell in each hand with arms by your sides.

•Slowly lift the dumbbells out to the sides until shoulder level, with elbows slightly bent.

•Lower your arms back to the starting position.

•Complete 3 sets of 12 reps.

Front Raises

•Lift the dumbbells in front of you until shoulder level, keeping elbows slightly bent.

•Lower back to starting position.

•Complete 3 sets of 12 reps.

Leg Lifts

•Place a dumbbell on your thigh for resistance.

•Lift one leg at a time a few inches off the floor.

•Hold for 2 seconds, then lower slowly.

•Complete 3 sets of 15 reps per leg.

Chest Press

•Hold a dumbbell in each hand at chest level with elbows bent.

•Push the dumbbells straight out until arms are fully extended.

•Slowly bring back to starting position.

•Complete 3 sets of 10 reps

Strength Training Exercises

Overhead Press – While seated, extend both arms over your head while holding weights. Slowly bring them back down and repeat.

Arm Curl – Stand tall with your back straight and hold dumbbells in each hand. Lift the weight with one hand, keeping your elbow close to your rib. Slowly bring it back down and repeat with the other arm.

Weighted Row – While seated, lean forward at a 45-degree angle and keep your back flat. Lift the dumbbell on your side and slowly bring it back down, while keeping your angled position. Repeat on the other side.

Dumbbell Squat – Start in a standing position with the weights in each hand. Slowly bend your knees to a squatting position and hold the pose. Straighten back up and repeat.

How Much Exercise is Recommended for Seniors?

According to the CDC, adults aged 65 years and above need at least 150 minutes of moderate physical activity or 75 minutes of vigorous physical activity in one week. To be safe, it is always best to consult with your doctor first.

Seniors Should Avoid These Exercises

• The specific exercises for older adults to avoid will depend on the physical abilities and mobility range of the individual. In general, seniors should avoid these exercises:

- High-Intensity Interval Training
- Sit-ups
- Standard pull-ups
- Deadlifts
- Stair climbs
- Long-distance runs
- Abdominal crunches
- Bench press
- Heavy weights
- Any high-impact exercise

How To Encourage Seniors to Exercise?

It isn't uncommon for older adults to feel reluctant about working out. They may be feeling tired or even fearful to try a new activity. To encourage your loved one to be more active, start with simple exercises that won't be too overwhelming.

Join in and make the workout fun. You can celebrate with progress parties to keep their motivation from stalling out.

How Many Steps Should a 65-Year-old Take per Day?

According to studies, about 7,000 – 8,000 steps are enough for healthy older adults. Those who have chronic conditions and mobility issues may aim for a lower number. What's important is to keep moving as much as possible. If your loved one has difficulty getting out and about on their own, you may consider hiring a private caregiver to provide companionship and supervision

Fun, Easy, and Effective Exercises for Seniors

Keeping up with a regular fitness routine is essential to good health, regardless of your age. Low-impact exercises that build strength and improve balance are the best kinds of exercise for seniors. With a regular routine of mindful workouts, you can enjoy a happier, healthier, and more meaningful life. The best types of exercises for older adults are those that focus on balance, standing, mobility, core stability, and strength. The following is a list of each type of exercise.

- Balance exercises include one-leg balance, heel-to-toe walk, toe lifts, and march-in-place.
- Standing exercises include hip circles, sit-to-stand, farmer's walk, and hamstring curls.
- Core stability exercises include resistance band pulls, seated leg presses, bridges, and leg lifts.
- Seated exercises include seated knee extension, seated jumping jacks, seated shoulder rolls, and seated tap dance.
- Weight exercises include overhead presses, arm curls, weighted rows, and dumbbell squats.

Exercises for Seniors Frequently Asked Questions

Can you build muscle after 65?

Yes, you can build muscle after age 65. Muscles respond differently as the body ages but seniors can still build muscles. The key to building muscle is by doing resistance exercises like lifting weights or using stretchy bands.

What are the best exercises for seniors?

Low-impact exercises like walking, swimming, and yoga are the best kind of workouts for seniors. These activities can effectively condition the body while being gentle on the joints and muscles.

What exercises should seniors avoid?

High-intensity workouts should be skipped, as they can be harmful to fragile bones. Exercises that place too much pressure on joints like deadlifts, squats, and crunches should also be avoided.

Why is exercise important for older adults?

Keeping physically active has many benefits for the mind, body, and soul. Seniors who exercise regularly have been shown to have better cardiovascular health, reduced anxiety, better sleep, and improved well-being.

How do seniors start an exercise program?

Before starting any fitness program, it is best to consult with your doctor first. Start slowly and build up as you go along. Seniors are advised to do 2.5 hours of moderate exercise every week.

Bibliography and Acknowledgement

- Altman DG, Bland JM. How to obtain the p value from a confidence interval. BMJ. 2011;343:d2304. doi: 10.1136/bmj.d2304. [PubMed] [CrossRef] [Google Scholar]
- Anderson D, Seib C, Rasmussen L. Can physical activity prevent physical and cognitive decline in postmenopausal women? A systematic review of the literature. Maturitas. 2014;79:14–33. [PubMed] [Google Scholar
- Bouaziz W, Vogel T, Schmitt E, Kaltenbach G, Geny B, Lang PO. Health benefits of aerobic training programs in adults aged 70 and over: a systematic review. Arch Gerontol Geriatr. 2017;69:110–127. [PubMed] [Google Scholar]
- Burton E, Cavalheri V, Adams R. Effectiveness of exercise programs to reduce falls in older people with dementia living in the community: a systematic review and meta-analysis. Clin Interv Aging. 2015;10:421–434. [PMC free article]
- Cheng P, Tan L, Ning P. Comparative effectiveness of published interventions for elderly fall prevention: a systematic review and network meta-analysis. Int J Environ Res Pub Health. 2018;15:498. doi: 10.3390/ijerph15030498. [PMC free article] [PubMed] [CrossRef] [Google Scholar]
- Chou CH, Hwang CL, Wu YT. Effect of exercise on physical function, daily living activities, and quality of life in the frail older adults: a meta-analysis. Arch Phys Med Rehabil. 2012;93:237–244. [PubMed] [Google Scholar]
- Di Lorito C, Bosco A, Booth V, Goldberg S, Harwood RH, Van der Wardt V. Adherence to exercise and physical activity interventions in older people with mild cognitive impairment and dementia: a systematic review and meta-analysis. Prev Med Rep. 2020;19:101139. doi: 10.1016/j.pmedr.2020.101139.
- Di Lorito C, Bosco A, Pollock K. External validation of the PHYT in Dementia, a theoretical model promoting physical activity in people with dementia. Int J Environ Res Pub Health. 2020;17:1544. doi: 10.3390/ijerph17051544. [PMC free article]
- Fairhall N, Sherrington C, Clemson L, Cameron ID. Do exercise interventions designed to prevent falls affect participation in life roles? A systematic review and meta-analysis. Age Ageing. 2011;40:666–674. [PubMed] [Google Scholar]
- Falck RS, Davis JC, Best JR, Crockett RA, Liu-Ambrose T. Impact of exercise training on physical and cognitive function among older adults: a systematic review and meta-analysis. Neurobiol Aging. 2019;79:119–130. [PubMed] [Google Scholar
- Garcia-Hermoso A, Ramirez-Vélez R, de Asteasu MLS. Safety and effectiveness of long-term exercise interventions in older adults: a systematic review and meta-analysis of randomized controlled trials. Sports Med. 2020;50:1095–1106. [PubMed]
- Hawley H. Older adults' perspectives on home exercise after falls rehabilitation: understanding the importance of promoting healthy, active ageing. Health Educat J. 2009;68:207–218.
- Jung D, Lee J, Lee SM. A meta-analysis of fear of falling treatment programs for the elderly. West J Nurs Res. 2009;31:6–16. [PubMed] [Google Scholar]
- Karr JE, Areshenkoff CN, Rast P, Garcia-Barrera MA. An empirical comparison of the therapeutic benefits of physical exercise and cognitive training on the executive functions of older adults: a meta-analysis of controlled trials. Neuropsychology. 2014;28:829–845.
- Lang PO, Govind S, Aspinall R. Reversing T cell immune-senescence: why, who, and how. Age (Dordr) 2013;35:609–620. [PMC free article] [PubMed] [Google Scholar]
- Marinus N, Hansen D, Feys P, Meesen R, Timmermans A, Spildooren J. The impact of different types of exercise training on peripheral blood brain-derived neurotrophic factor concentrations in older adults: a meta-analysis. Sports Med. 2019;49:1529–1546. [PubMed] [Google Scholar]
- Naseri C, Haines TP, Etherton-Beer C. Reducing falls in older adults recently discharged from hospital: a systematic review and meta-analysis. Age Ageing. 2018;47:512–519. [PMC free article] [PubMed] [Google Scholar]
- Perri MG, Martin AD, Leermakers EA, Sears SF, Notelovitz M. Effects of group- vs. home-based exercise in the treatment of obesity. J Consult Clin Psychol. 1997;65:278–285. [PubMed] [Google Scholar]
- Robertson MC, Campbell AJ, Gardner MM, Devlin N. Preventing injuries in older people by preventing falls: a meta-analysis of individual‐level data. J Am Geriatr Soc. 2002;50:905–911. [PubMed] [Google Scholar]
- Sexton BP, Taylor NF. To sit or not to sit? A systematic review and meta‐analysis of seated exercise for older adults. Australas J Ageing. 2019;38:15–27. [PubMed] [Google Scholar]
- Taylor LM, Kerse N, Frakking T, Maddison R. Active video games for improving physical performance measures in older people: a meta-analysis. J Geriatr Phys Ther. 2018;41:108–123. [PMC free article] [PubMed] [Google Scholar]
- Van Abbema R, De Greef M, Crajé C, Krijnen W, Hobbelen H, Van Der Schans C. What type, or combination of exercise can improve preferred gait speed in older adults? A meta-analysis. BMC Geriatr. 2015;15:72. doi: 10.1186/s12877-015-0061-9. [PMC free article] [PubMed] [CrossRef] [Google Scholar
- Wu WW, Kwong E, Lan XY, Jiang XY. The effect of a meditative movement intervention on quality of sleep in the elderly: a systematic review and meta-analysis. J Altern Complement Med. 2015;21:509–519. [PubMed] [Google Scholar]
- Yamamoto S, Hotta K, Ota E, Mori R, Matsunaga A. Effects of resistance training on muscle strength, exercise capacity, and mobility in middle-aged and elderly patients with coronary artery disease: a meta-analysis. J Cardiol. 2016;68:125–134. [PubMed] [Google Scholar]
- Yusif S, Soar J, Hafeez-Baig A. Older people, assistive technologies, and the barriers to adoption: a systematic review. Int J Med Inform. 2016;94:112–116. [PubMed] [Google Scholar]
- Zhang Y, Zhang Y, Du S, Wang Q, Xia H, Sun R. Exercise interventions for improving physical function, daily living activities and quality of life in community-dwelling frail older adults: a systematicreview and meta-analysis of randomized controlled trials. Geriatr Nurs. 2020;41:261–273. [PubMed] [Google Scholar]
- Zhao R, Bu W, Chen X. The efficacy and safety of exercise for prevention of fall-related injuries in older people with different health conditions, and differing intervention protocols: a meta-analysis of randomized controlled trials. BMC Geriatr. 2019;19:341. doi: 10.1186/s12877-019-1359-9. [PMC free article] [PubMed] [CrossRef] [Google Scholar]

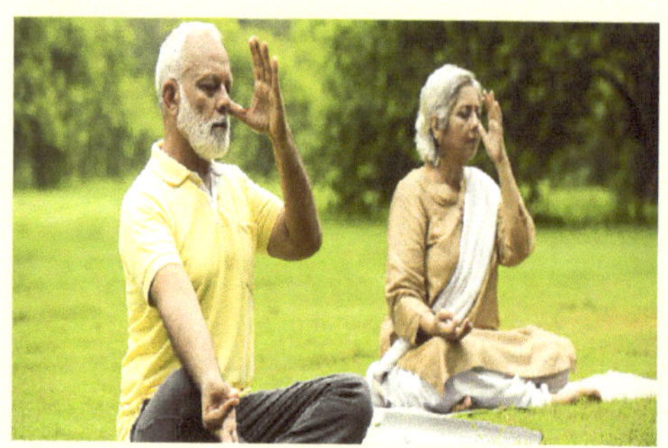

Yoga Practices By Seniors

Yoga is truly for everyone. The flexible and inflexible. The athletic and the stationary. The young the old. One of the best things about yoga is this unique feature: it can be adapted to suit anyone with any needs or challenges. When it come to exercise for seniors, there may be no better choice than yoga. Because of its gentle and adaptive nature, yoga makes the perfect wellness routine for seniors of any age. It's no surprise that as we age, certain aspects of our bodies may become impaired. Some of us have trouble with joints or bones, cardiovascular issues, trouble standing or sitting, or other general ailments. Yoga poses can be adapted to suit all of these physical challenges, all while helping to improve the health and quality of life of the student. Many seniors are looking for a gentle exercise routine to pick up to help stay active and prevent illness and injury later on. Yoga is that ideal activity that can keep seniors healthy long into their golden years. Let's look at ten yoga poses that are key for maintaining health for seniors.

Yoga for Seniors: How to Get Started (And Why You Should)

You're never too old to reap the rewards of yoga. For seniors who are looking for a safe, effective way to enhance their physical health and overall wellness, the stretching, breathing, and meditation practices of yoga can be a great solution. In fact, as you will see, doing yoga regularly can result in a host of benefits for older adults, from greater flexibility and improved balance to lower stress and better sleep.

It's no wonder, then, that yoga is becoming increasingly popular among seniors. The 2016 Yoga in America Study found that nearly 14 million Americans over the age of 50 practiced yoga that year. That was a significant jump from the four million who did so in 2012.

This article outlines the many benefits of senior yoga and describes several of the best types of yoga for older men and women (including the increasingly popular discipline of chair yoga). It also offers information about basic poses and explains what you should do before you begin any yoga routine. And it even provides examples of helpful books, videos, and DVDs as well as tips on how to find appropriate classes.

The Benefits of Yoga for Older Adults

Yoga cultivates a mind-body connection, combining stretching and strengthening postures with deep breathing and relaxation. Despite its roots in Eastern philosophy, yoga as practiced in the West is generally focused on physical fitness. It still has a spiritual aspect, but it is not overtly religious. People of all faiths and belief systems can benefit from participating in yoga.

Because the poses (called asanas) can easily be modified or adapted to suit an individual's needs, yoga is safe for seniors of all fitness or ability levels. In fact, it can be an excellent way to keep your body strong and healthy without the joint stress that comes from other activities like weightlifting or jogging. And it's never too late to begin: You can start yoga at any age. (Just be sure to clear it with your doctor before you get going.)

Here are some of the benefits of yoga for seniors:

- **Better balance:** Many yoga poses for seniors focus on strengthening the abdominal muscles and improving your core stability. That can help you become steadier on your feet and reduce your risk of falls.
- **Improved flexibility:** Yoga movements can be fantastic stretching exercises for seniors. Holding a pose for several breaths encourages your muscles and connective tissues to relax and loosen, which helps to increase your range of motion. In fact, research in the International Journal of Yoga Therapy has shown that regularly engaging in yoga can dramatically boost the overall flexibility of older adults.
- **Enhanced breathing:** The breathing control practices of yoga (known as pranayama) can expand your lung capacity and improve your pulmonary health. A study published in the Journal of Human Kinetics found that elderly women who practiced yoga three times a week for 12 weeks saw a significant improvement in their respiratory function

• **Stronger bones:** If you're worried about brittle bones and osteoporosis, try yoga. For older women and men, a consistent yoga routine that includes weight-bearing postures can help bolster bone strength. Some promising research has suggested that doing yoga can actually improve bone density in postmenopausal women.

• **Reduced anxiety and stress:** Through meditation and mindful breathing, yoga encourages you to focus on the present and find a sense of peace. Research has demonstrated that that can lower levels of the stress hormone cortisol and help ease symptoms of anxiety and depression. In a National Institutes of Health survey, more than 85 percent of people who engaged in yoga said they experienced reduced stress as a result.

• **Better sleep:** Yoga can help alleviate sleep disturbances, which are common complaints among seniors. In a study published in Alternative Therapies in Health and Medicine, adults over age 60 who struggled with insomnia participated in yoga classes twice a week and underwent daily sessions at home. After three months, the group reported significant improvements in both the duration and overall quality of their sleep.

• **Reconnecting with your body:** Life's stressors and events have a way of separating us from ourselves. Hormonal and other physical changes can make our bodies feel more foreign over time, and a sense of disconnection can set in between mind and body. Yoga offers the potential to work on your mind, body, and spirit at the same time, and for you to integrate those changes in your daily life.

Improving your flexibility, both in how you move and in how you think, can open doors to exciting possibilities. Whether the end goal is to love yourself more, feel more in-tune with your health, venture into the dating world, strengthen your spirituality, or something else, the benefits are worth exploring.

The Best Types of Yoga for Senior Citizens

Whether you're aiming to get stronger and more flexible or you just want to decompress and still your mind, yoga can help. But with the dozens of different styles that exist, it can be tough to figure out which type is most appropriate for you. Remember that a key consideration is your physical condition and fitness level. Always consult your healthcare provider before beginning any new exercise regimen. Here are eight types of yoga that may offer what you need:

• **Hatha:** Not really a specific style, hatha is a generic term which encompasses all forms of yoga that concentrate on physical postures.

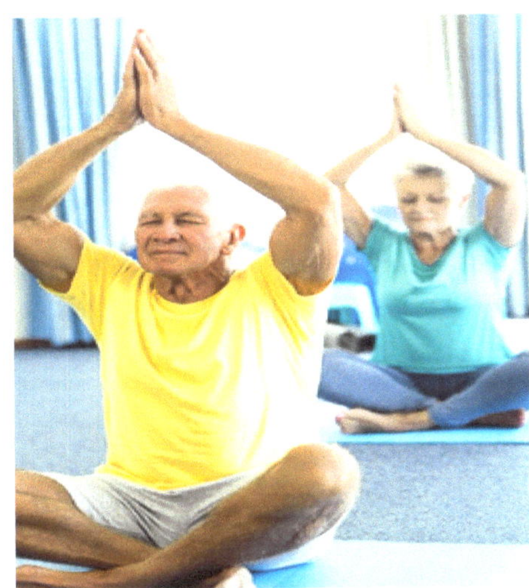

Fig 5.1 Yoga is being practiced by seniors

But in most cases, classes advertised as hatha yoga feature a slow-paced series of sitting and standing poses. They are typically about stretching and breathing, not boosting your heart rate or getting your leg up behind your head. That's why many people believe that hatha is the best type of yoga for beginners.

• **Iyengar:** Iyengar yoga is methodical and precise, with a strong emphasis on proper form. Practitioners are encouraged to use props like bolsters, straps, blocks, and incline boards to help them get into the correct alignment. Because the props allow for all kinds of modifications, this is a good style of yoga for seniors with arthritis or other chronic conditions.

• **Restorative:** Restorative yoga is a slow, meditative form of yoga that is designed to release tension passively, without stretching. Props are used to totally support the body, and poses are held for a long time, sometimes up to 10 minutes. Restorative is the best type of yoga for seniors who want to cultivate relaxation and contentment. It's not uncommon for people to fall asleep in class.

• **Yin:** Like restorative yoga, yin yoga is slow and focuses on holding poses for a long time. The difference between yin and restorative yoga is that restorative involves no active stretch, whereas in yin you work on stretching your deep connective tissues. Doing yin yoga regularly can help relieve stiffness and enhance flexibility.

• **Vinyasa:** This is a general term for yoga styles that involve matching breathing with a series of continuous movements that flow from one to another. Pacing can vary, but routines are often very fluid and quick. Vinyasa emphasizes the transitions between postures as much as the poses themselves. Some people liken it to dancing. Vinyasa yoga is hard in the sense that it tends to be physically vigorous, but seniors who are reasonably fit may enjoy the challenge.

- **Ashtanga:** Fast-paced and physically challenging, ashtanga comprises a predetermined set of poses that are performed the same way every time. It's an intense, acrobatic activity that boosts your heart rate and circulation, which is why some people say that ashtanga is the best type of yoga for weight loss. While it is not generally recommended for beginners, some older adults find it to be greatly beneficial.
- **Bikram:** In Bikram yoga, rooms are typically heated to more than 100 degrees and have 40-percent humidity. That guarantees you will sweat buckets as you spend 90 minutes going through the sequence of 26 poses and two breathing techniques. The idea is to strengthen muscles and flush out body toxins. However, overheating is a real risk. If you have low blood pressure symptoms, high blood pressure, or some sort of heart condition, Bikram is not for you.
- **Kundalini:** Known as the "yoga of awareness," kundalini can be appealing to seniors who are keenly interested in the spiritual as well as the physical components of yoga. It combines physical postures, breathing exercises, meditation, and chanting.

How to Prepare for Yoga

Yoga offers some of the best strength and flexibility exercises for seniors. But as with any physical regimen, it's important to make sure you're prepared. Here are a few tips to help you get ready:

1. Evaluate your physical condition.

While people of any age can get started in yoga, some movements are not advisable for folks with certain medical issues. For instance, people with glaucoma should avoid inverted or head-down positions because such poses can increase pressure on the eyes. That's why it's crucial to talk to your doctor (and your instructor) before you try even a simple yoga routine

2. Gather your gear.

You need comfortable, stretchy clothing for yoga. Fitted clothes work best, especially for tops, since you will be bending into different positions and you don't want your shirt falling into your eyes. Leggings or jogging pants along with a fitted T-shirt or tank top are good choices. You won't generally need special footwear because yoga is typically performed barefoot. However, non-slip socks or even sneakers can be worn if you're concerned about losing your footing.

You will also need a yoga mat. Some studios provide these at no charge, but others expect you to bring your own and many people prefer to have their own for hygienic reasons. Look for one that is long enough to support your whole body when you lie down and sticky enough that you won't slip when you try to hold a pose. You may also want to consider the material: Cheaper mats tend to be made of PVC, but if eco-friendliness is important to you, focus on mats made of rubber, cotton, or jute.

Most mats are one-eighth of an inch thick, but some are slightly thinner or thicker. Thicker mats offer more support for sensitive joints, but they can make standing balance poses more difficult; they are also bulkier and harder to carry around. Portability won't matter if you only practice at home, but it might be an issue if you plan to tote your mat to and from a studio or community center.

3. Seek out a qualified teacher.

It's important to find a trained instructor who understands the unique challenges faced by the 55-plus crowd. Yoga Alliance maintains a voluntary registry of yoga teachers throughout the U.S. who meet certain standards. Also, Yoga for Seniors offers a directory of instructors who have undergone special training to enable them to adapt yoga programs specifically for older adults.

Ask potential teachers how long they've been leading classes and whether they have any experience teaching seniors or people with health issues. If possible, observe an actual class to get a sense of the teacher's techniques. And once you choose an instructor, be sure to tell him or her about any physical limitations you have, such as arthritis, balance problems, back pain, or high blood pressure.

4. Start slow.

You can become more flexible for yoga by easing into it. For instance, if your goal is to be able to bend over and touch your toes, start by putting your hands on your thighs. Take a few deep breaths, then reach down to your knees. Pause again and take some more deep breaths before reaching down to the middle of your shin, and so on. The point is to avoid overstretching.Be sure to get enough rest after each pose, and never rush into new postures. It's best not to add any new movements until your body has fully adjusted to your routine. Always remember that yoga is not about keeping up with the people around you. Just focus on going at your own pace.

A yoga posture should never hurt. You may feel challenged, but you should not get to the point of feeling strained. If you can't do a certain pose comfortably, ask your teacher for a modified version.

Almost every yoga pose can be altered to accommodate a wide range of physical needs. And don't hesitate to use props like straps, blocks, walls, or chairs for additional support.

Easily Practiced yoga poses by Seniors

1.Tadasana — Mountain Pose

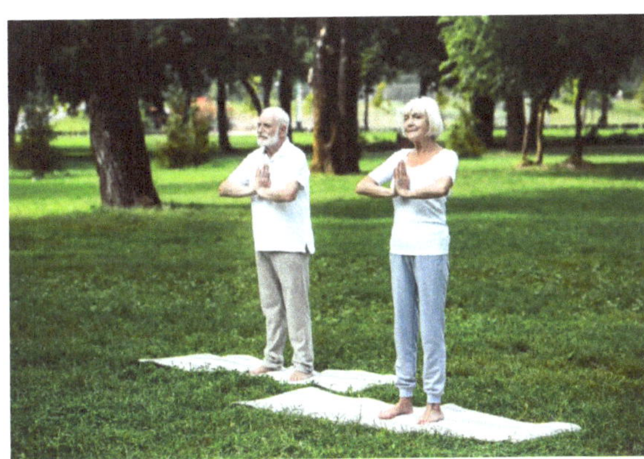

Fig,5,2 Stand tall with your feet together, keep your shoulders back, neck firm and straight, and tuck the chin slightly. Rest your arms by your side with palms facing in front of you. Engage your thigh muscles, lift your kneecaps, and envision a straight line connecting your pelvis to the top of your head. Connect to the ground beneath your feet.

2. Vrksasana — Tree Pose

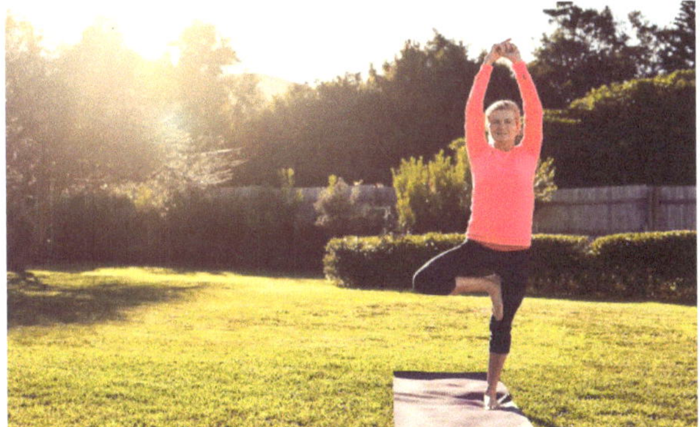

Fig,5,3 Stand tall, with feet firmly on the ground in Mountain pose. Slightly shift your weight on to the left foot and lift the right foot slightly. Depending on your flexibility and state of balance, you can lift the right foot to the ankle, shin, or thigh. Keep your pelvis centered over the left foot to maintain balance and keep your gaze straight ahead. Bring your hands to prayer position in front of the heart. Breathe deeply while focusing your attention to the heart and chest. Take 5-10 breaths, slowly release your foot and return to mountain pose. Repeat with the opposite side.

3. Virasana — Hero Pose

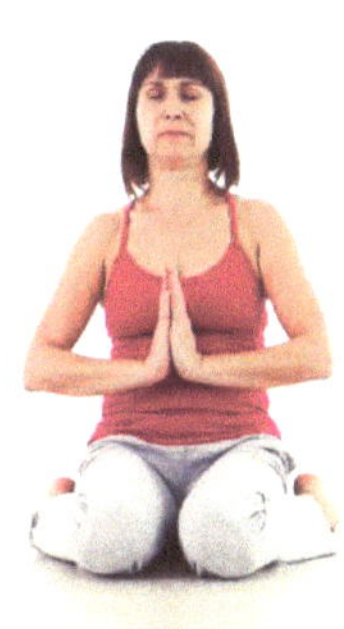

Fig, 5.4 Gently sit on your mat with your legs bent underneath, buttocks resting on feet. With your thighs perpendicular to the floor and inner knees touching, slide your feet out to the sides of your hips and keep them flat against the floor. On an exhale, sit back but lean your torso slightly forward. With your thighs perpendicular to the floor and inner knees together, slide your feet out to the sides of your hips and keep them flat against the floor. On an exhale, sit back but lean your torso slightly forward. If you suffer from knee problems, you may benefit from using a bolster or blanket underneath the buttocks to reduce the strain on the knees.

4. Marjaryasana — Cat-Cow Pose

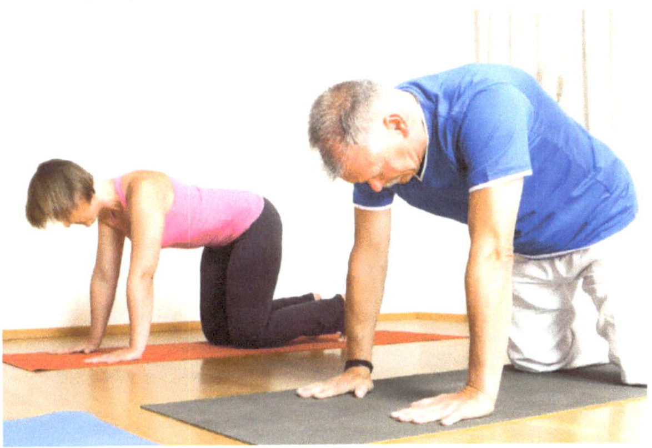

Fig 5.6 Begin on your mat on all fours. Bend your knees bent directly below your hips and plant your palms firmly on the ground, resting right below your shoulders. Inhale and look up to the sky while gently bending your back. If you have back pain, bend only to feel a stretch, not pain or straining. Exhale and bring your back up, roll your shoulders, tuck your head down, and feel the spine open into Cow pose. Repeat several times, taking slow and easy breaths.

5.Adho Mukha Svanasana-Downward Facing Dog Pose

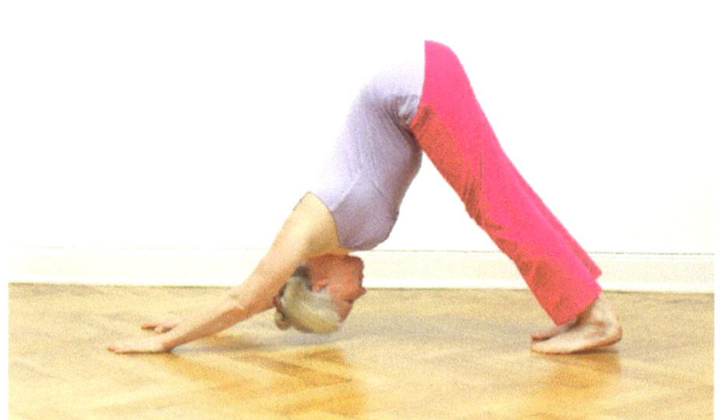

Fig 5.7 Come to the floors on hands and knees in a tabletop position. Use a blanket to comfort the knees if this is uncomfortable. With your hands and toes firmly planted on the ground, stretch the knees to come to a V-shape, into Downward Dog position. Start with the knees slightly bent and heels off the ground, then exhale and slowly straighten the legs bringing the feet fully to the ground if possible. Feel free to bend the knees and stretch the feet and ankles.Rest here for a few breath cycles.

6.Baddha Konasana – Cobbler's Pose

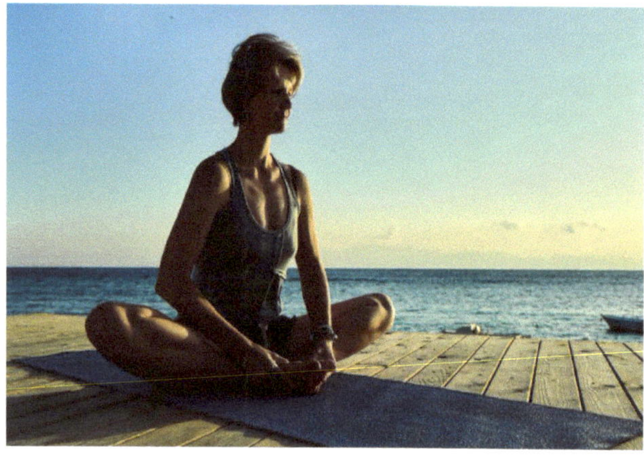

Fig 5.8 Sit on your mat and bend your knees to bring the soles of your feet together. The knees will fall to the sides, like a butterfly. Bring the knees closer into the body until you reach a stretching, yet comfortable position. Be careful not to overstrain the knees. Press your feet together, potentially clasping them with your hands. Sit up with a tall spine and keep your shoulder blades down. Rest here for several full breath cycles.

7.Salamba Bhujangasana — Sphinx Pose

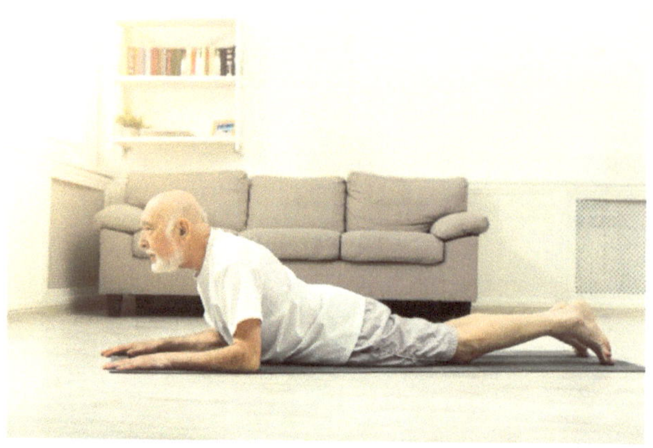

Fig 5.9 Start by laying face-down on your mat, with your arms by your side and your legs together. Point your toes back towards the wall behind you to activate the leg muscles. Move your arms so that your elbows are below your shoulders and your forearms straight out in front of you. Inhale and lift the chest and head to sphinx pose. Engage (but try not to clench too hard) the buttocks and legs. Draw the belly in slightly to reach the spine. Take 5-10 breaths, then on an exhale, lower your chest back down slowly, turn your head to one side to rest on the floor, and rest for a few breaths. Repeat 2-3 times or as long as is comfortable.

8.Viparita Karani — Legs Up The Wall Pose

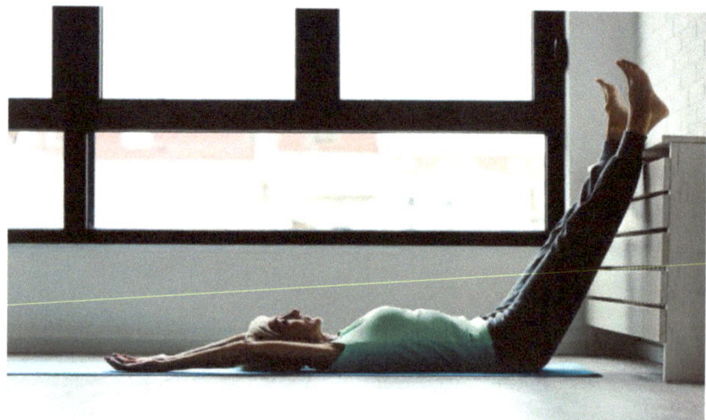

Fig 5.10 Start by sitting on the floor near a wall. Swing your legs up to land on the wall ahead of you. Move your buttocks to the wall so that you are as close to it as possible and lay back so your back is resting on the floor. Extend your legs up the wall either straight up or in a relaxed 'V' position. Rest your arms by your sides with palms facing upwards, out to your sides in a T, or on your lower bell. Rest here for about five minutes.

9.Balasana — Child's Pose

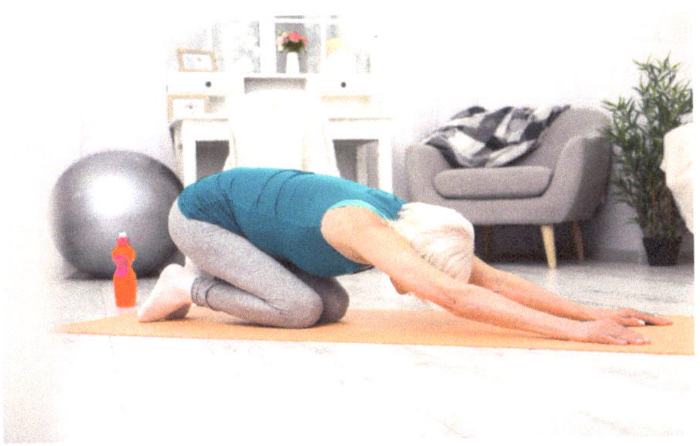

Fig 5.11 Child's pose is a fantastic resting position. Begin this pose by kneeling on the floor with your knees spread slightly wider than your hips. Let your bottom rest on your heels. Exhale and slowly lower your torso forward to rest in between your thighs. Rest your forehead on the floor ahead of you and place your arms down by your sides. Take several deep breaths here for a few minutes.

10.Savasana — Supported Corpse Pose

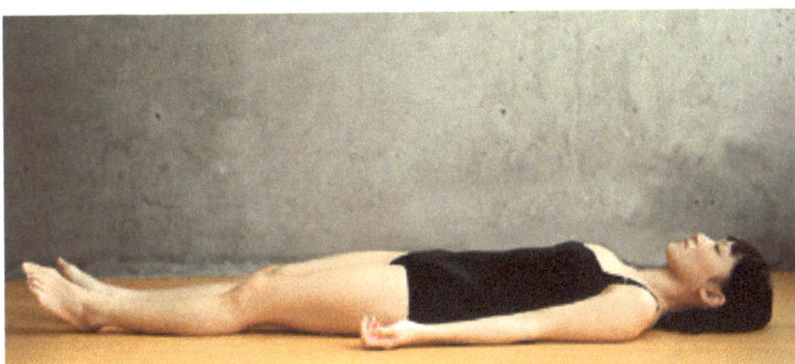

Fig 5.12 Place a rolled towel or blanket on your mat and lay down on top of it. Position it so that your upper back, neck, and head are fully supported. This will allow you to completely relax. Rest your arms by your side with palms up. Feel the chest open and relax into the pose. Take several deep breaths here and rest for as long as you need.

11.Anulom Vilom Pranayama

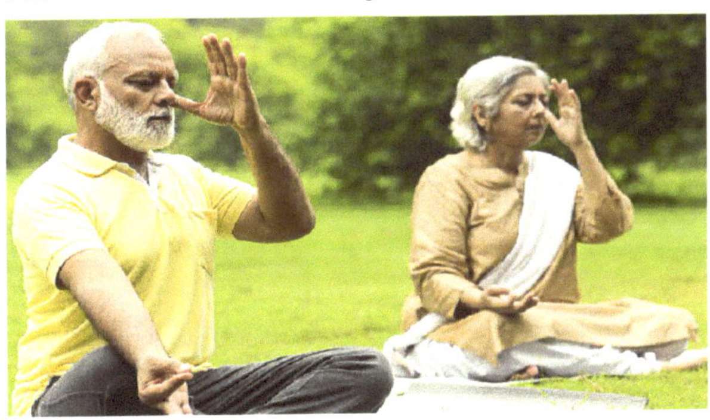

Fig 5.13 Elders performing Anulom Vilom Pranayama

How to Do Anulom Vilom Pranayama?

Sit straight in any meditative pose. Place the thumb of the right hand on the side of the right nostril to block that part. (Your hand should be in Vayu Mudra) Breathe slowly from the left nostril for 2.5 seconds and release in 2.5 seconds. (Keep in mind to start it always from the left nostril).Repeat the same process by blocking the left nostril and breathing and releasing through the right nostril. One round of alternative breathing is of 5 minutes and it is done 1 time in 10 seconds. If you are not having any disease or illness, then you can practice it for 15 minutes but if you are suffering from any specific disease, try to do it for 30 minutes daily.

In yoga, the left nostril is termed Chandra Nadi, Ida Nadi, and Ganga Nadi while the right nostril is termed Surya Nadi, Pingala Nadi, and Yamuna Nadi. Sushumana Nadi is between Ida Nadi and Pingala Nadi. With Anulom Vilom Pranayama, all three Nadis or Energy channels get purified

Benefits of Anulom Vilom Pranayama

Even just 15 minutes of Anulom Vilom Pranayama provides a plethora of benefits. Do it regularly and observed how your body is changing for betterment. Some of the known and proven benefits of Anulom Vilom Pranayama are –

- It cures hypertension.
- It is beneficial for Heart issues.
- It improves the brain by making sharp memory and high IQ level.
- It purifies Nadis (Energy Channels).
- It activates Chakras or Energy Centres.
- It provides an individual with good control over the body, mind, thoughts, emotions, feelings, and actions.
- It cures problems like migraine and epilepsy.
- It manages anger issues.
- It overcomes stress and depression.
- It gives relief to autoimmune diseases.
- It is good for the eyes.
- It makes you free from diseases.

Precautions of Anulom Vilom Pranayama

Well, yoga is not a practice which has many precautions. As it is not just a practice of the body but that of mind and soul too, it improvises your whole well-being. The same goes with Anulom Vilom Pranayama. Anulom Vilom Pranayama can be done by anyone irrespective of age and gender.

- Never do Anulom Vilom Pranayama after a heavy diet.
- Never try to hold your breath forcefully.
- If you are having congestion, never practice Anulom Vilom

Chair Yoga for Seniors

Staying active as you get older has many benefits for your body and mind. Physical activity lowers your risk of disease, lessens pain, improves mood, and enhances cognitive function. Yoga is an effective and accessible exercise for people of all ages. It is low-impact, and combines strengthening and stretching movements with breathing exercises. That's good news, especially as the global population continues to age. But 35% of adults over the age of 70 experience mobility issues that can make a traditional yoga practice out of reach. Fortunately, you can perform many yoga poses using a chair for support and reap just as many benefits. Chair yoga includes the same elements of traditional yoga, including physical poses (asanas), meditation (dyana), and breathing techniques (pranayama). But the gentle practice modifies standard yoga poses so that you can do them while sitting in a chair. Or you can use a chair to keep you steady while performing standing postures.

What is chair yoga?

Chair yoga is a modified form of yoga that allows you to practice traditional yoga poses while sitting on or standing with the support of a chair. These modifications make yoga more accessible and more gentle for people with limited mobility or balance. Like traditional yoga, chair yoga helps build flexibility, strength, and balance. And it can also promote relaxation through breath. Almost any type of yoga pose — from twists to backbends — can be modified using a chair. This allows people of all abilities to reap the benefits of yoga.

Chair yoga benefits

Chair yoga is a safe and accessible version of traditional yoga for older adults or anyone with mobility challenges.

- **Chair yoga can offer a low-impact workout:** Low-impact exercise is easier on the body. And it's a good exercise option if you have age-related changes in your joints and muscles. You can still get a good workout without injuring yourself or exacerbating old injuries.
- **Boost muscle strength:** Pumping iron isn't the only way to build muscle. This 2016 study shows that yoga is as good as traditional strength training for improving functional fitness. Keep your muscles engaged throughout chair yoga poses. Slowly work your way up to more challenging poses to build strength.
- **Enhance flexibility and joint health:** Yoga is one of the best exercises to keep your muscles flexible and your joints mobile as you age. Maintaining flexibility and mobility helps you stay independent and prevents life-threatening falls.
- **Improve balance:** Poor balance is one of the main reasons for falls in older adults. You can use chair yoga to build a foundation of balance. For example, you can progress by performing the seated yoga poses (as shown below) while standing with the support of a chair. This is one way to slowly improve your balance.
- **Provide a mood boost:** As a mind-body exercise, yoga is well-known for its ability to enhance mood. Yoga offers stress relief, and improves mental and emotional well-being. It also helps with sleep, which is crucial to maintaining a positive mood.
- **Help with chronic conditions:** Yoga may be an effective supplement to regular medical treatment. It can help treat chronic conditions like heart disease, stroke, and chronic obstructive pulmonary disease (COPD), according to a 2015 research review.
- **Relieve aches and pains:** The stretching and strengthening movements of yoga have been shown to improve symptoms of fibromyalgia, low back pain, and neck pain.

Chair yoga exercises

While traditional yoga combines standing and seated poses, chair yoga helps make the poses more accessible. If you are able to stand, you can use a chair for support during standing yoga poses. You can combine those with the following seated poses that fully support your body. Remember to talk to your primary care provider first, and stick with postures that are right for your body and abilities in the present moment.

A Closer Look at These Chair Yoga Exercises:

Unless you have some experience with chair yoga, you probably need more than a graphic to perform the exercises above. Proper technique is important for your personal safety, and to make sure you're getting the most out of these exercises. Read more about the exercises below for a closer look at these essential **Chair yoga poses.**

1. Overhead Stretch

Begin in a seated position, facing forward with your arms down by your sides. Take a long, deep breath in and slowly stretch your arms upward to the ceiling. Hold this position for a moment, and bring your arms back downward with a long exhale. Throughout this exercise, make sure your core is engaged and your back is as straight as possible.

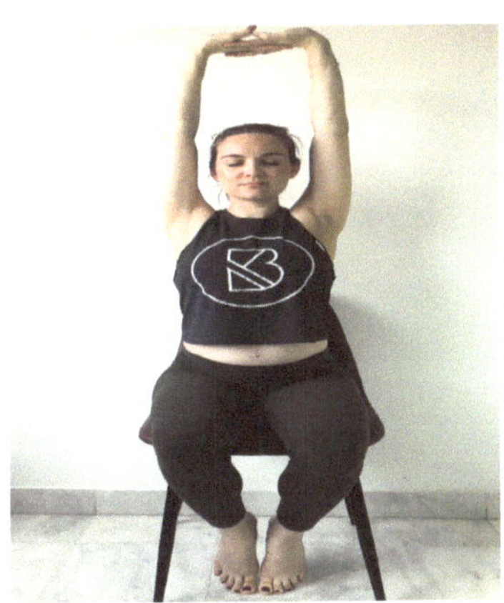

Fig 5.14 Overhead Stretch pose

2.Neck Stretch

Sit up straight in your chair, and do not let your back touch the back of your chair. Extend your neck slowly upward so you feel the crown of your head rising towards the ceiling. While holding the base of your chair with your right hand, slowly reach upwards with your left hand to hold your left temple. Take a deep breath, and upon exhalation, gently dip your left ear towards your left shoulder without bending your back or raising your right shoulder. Take several slow breaths in and out in this position, before alternating this stretch to the opposite side.

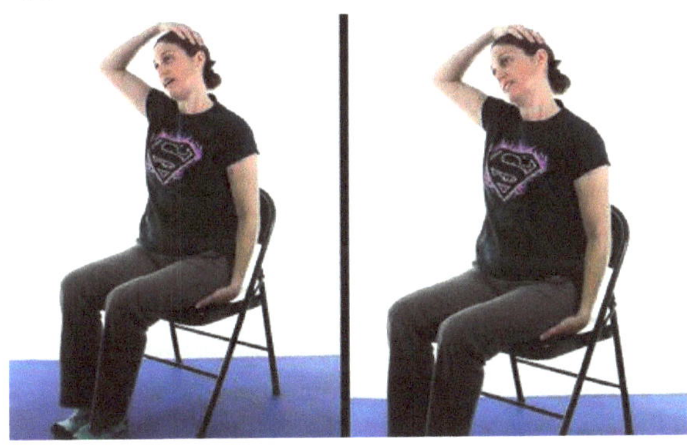

Fig 5.15 Neck Stretch pose

3. Reverse arm hold

Begin this pose in a seated position with your back straight and apart from the back of the chair. While you inhale deeply, reach your arms straight out to your sides at a low and wide angle. Exhale slowly and reach your hands behind your back, bending your elbows slightly. Arch your back slightly to feel the stretch in your shoulders, and take several breaths in and out.

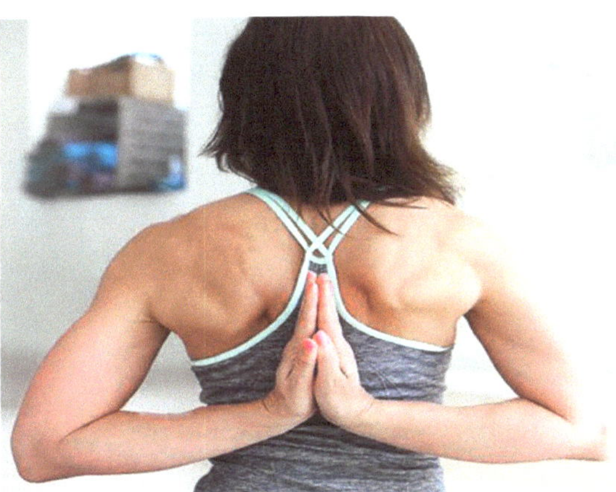

Fig 5.16 Reverse arm hold pose

4. Chair pigeon(Chair Kapotasana)

Sit upright with your back away from the back of the chair and facing forward. Gently raise your left ankle to rest on top of your right knee or thigh. If you have trouble bringing your ankle to your knee, feel free to use your hand to assist. Inhale deeply, flex your left foot slightly, and bend forward upon exhale. After several deep breaths in the forward position, return to sitting up straight. Gently switch sides, so your right ankle is resting upon your left thigh or knee, and repeat the above steps

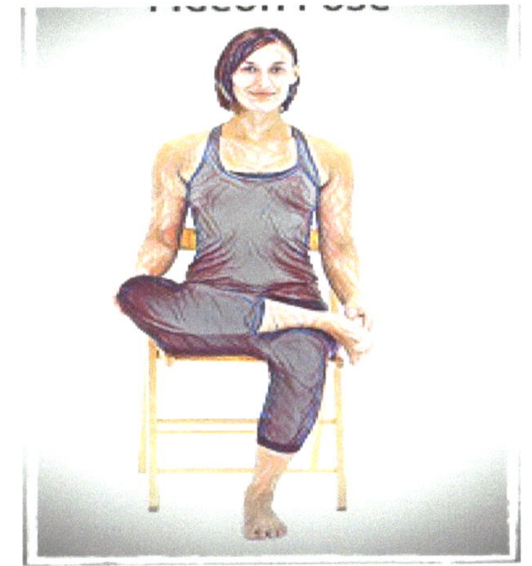

Fig 5.17 Chair pigeon pose

5..Seated forward bend (Paschimottanasana)

Begin this exercise sitting up straight with your knees touching and your feet on the floor. Take a deep breath in. Upon exhaling, slowly bend forward, feeling your back extend one vertebrae at a time. Lean forward as far as you can without feeling strain or discomfort. Hold this position for several deep breaths before returning to an upright position.

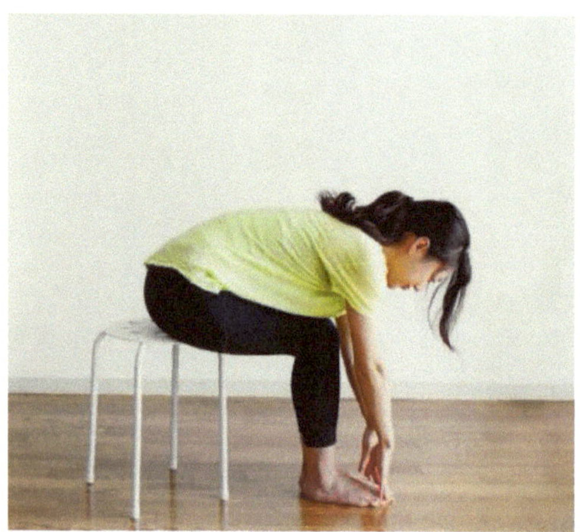

Fig 5.18 Seated forward bend pose

6. Eagle arms

Sit upright in your chair and stretch your arms straight out in front of you. Cross your left arm over your right arm, and bend your elbows to bring your forearms together. Interlace your fingers and raise your elbows slightly, arching your back a bit. Hold this position for several deep breaths. Upon completion, switch to your right arm over your left arm.

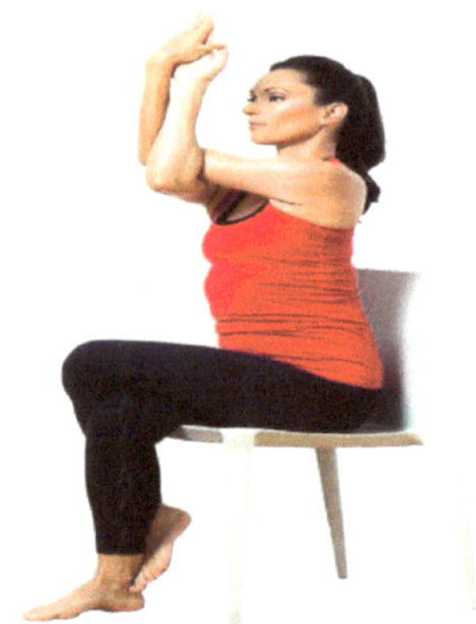

Fig 5.19 Eagle arms pose in the chair pose

7. Chair warrior

Begin this pose facing forward with your arms down by your side at a wide and low angle, or with one leg across the chair with your torso turned forward (if you're flexible enough for this position). Take a deep breath and slowly raise your arms straight above your head. Hold this pose for several breaths before lowering your arms back down to your sides. If you began this pose with your leg across the chair, switch to the opposite leg across the chair and perform this pose again.

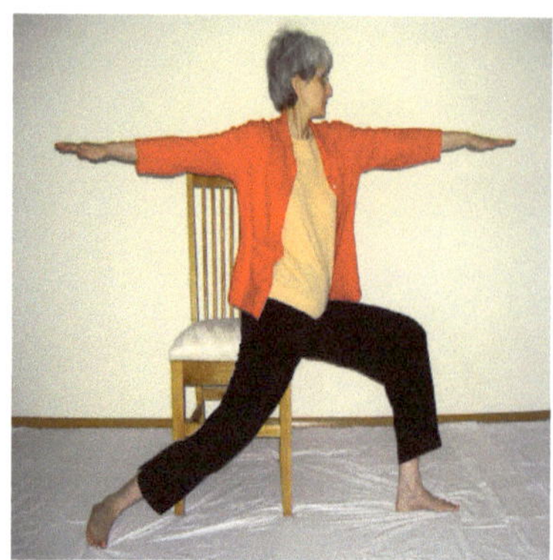

Fig 5.20 Chair warrior pose

8. Cat-cow stretch

Sit at the edge of your chair with your back as straight as it can be and your core muscles engaged. Inhale and gently arch your back as far as is comfortable for the "cow" portion of the stretch, holding the position for three to five breaths. Then bring your back to its original position, and invert the stretch for the "cat" position. Your shoulders will be directly above your hips, but your back will curve into a forward arch. Hold this position for several breaths before returning to your original seated position.

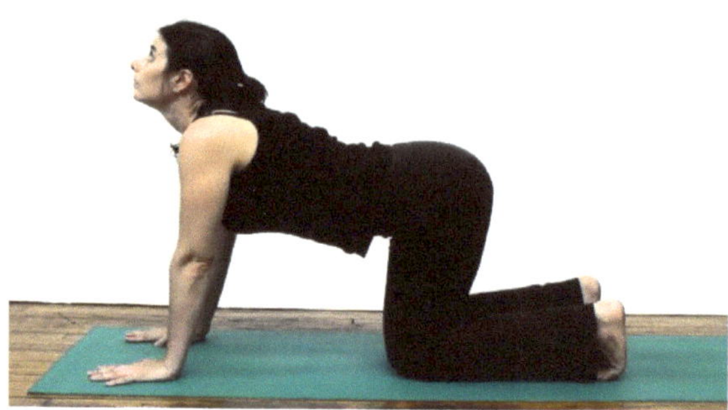

Fig 5.21 Cat-cow stretch pose

9. Chair spinal twist

Begin this pose sitting sideways in your chair, with your knees over the right side of the chair and the back of the chair next to your right arm. Make sure your back is straight, and your body is apart from the back of the chair. Hold the back of the chair with both hands, inhale deeply, and slowly turn your body toward the back of the chair while exhaling. Hold this position for several breaths before returning to the original position. After this pose is complete, switch to the other side of the chair, so your knees are over the left side of the chair and the back of the chair is next to your left arm.

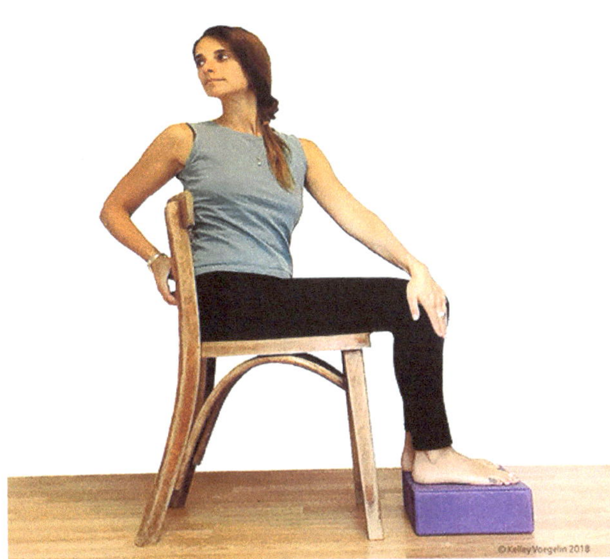

Fig 5.22 Chair spinal twist pose

10. Seated mountain

Start this pose sitting on the front half of your chair with a straight back and an engaged core. Bend your knees at 90-degree angles with your knees above your ankles and a small space between your knees. Inhale slowly and roll your shoulders downward upon exhaling. Activate your abdominal muscles and hold your arms down at your sides. Hold the pose for several deep breaths.

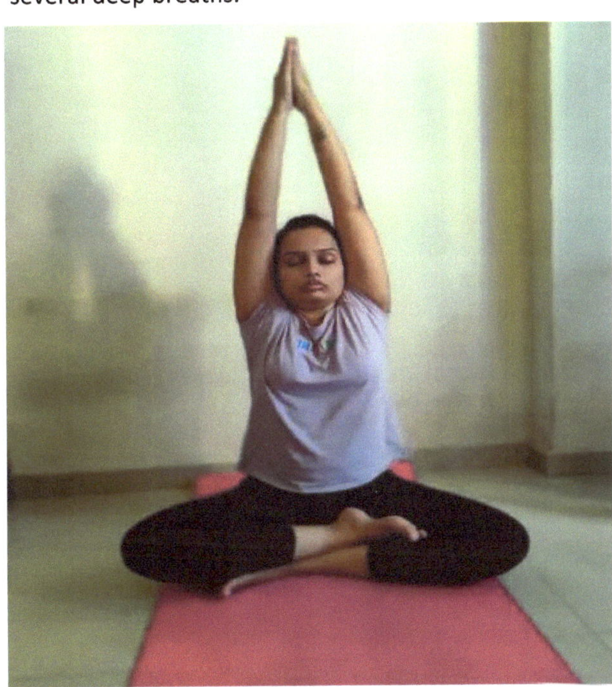

Fig 5.23 Seated mountain pose

11. A simple chair yoga meditation

How to Do Chair Yoga Meditation

A chair is a perfect place to meditate if you sit properly. Place your feet flat on the floor hip-width apart, anchor your sitz bones, and roll your shoulders down and back. Your spine should be nice and tall. If we slouch, our breath is diminished.

Once you find a nice, tall, comfortable seat, you can close your eyes and rest your hands on your lap. I like to turn my palms up and join the thumb and forefinger. When our palms are open, we are receptive, and it also helps flip the lungs open.

The mudra of thumb and forefinger is just a nice gesture to remind us we are stopping to do something important and more formal than just sitting. Once you are set, start to observe your breath.

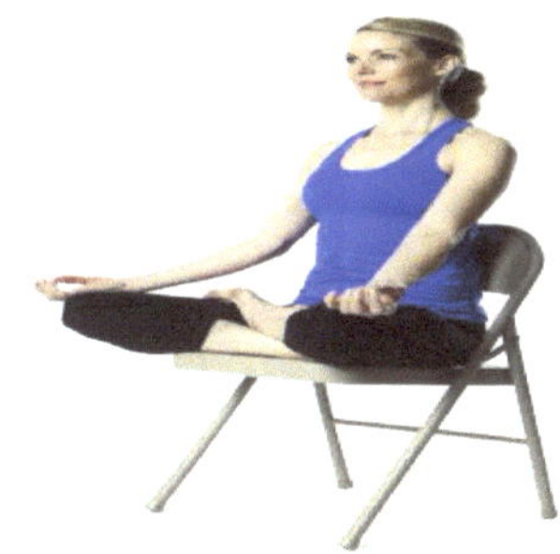

Fig 5.24 A simple chair yoga meditation pose

12.Chair camel pose

Camel is a backbending posture that stretches the front of your body, including your abdominals and chest. It also strengthens the back muscles.

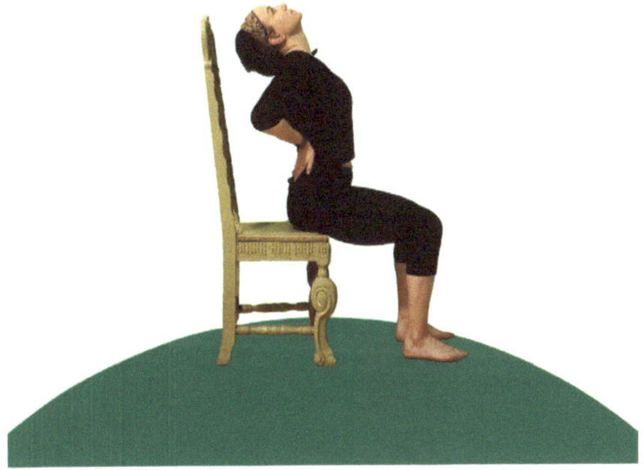

Fig 5.25 Chair camel pose

PART 1 Summary in Chair poses yoga for seniors

1. Ujjayi Breathing

A great starter pose. Sit up tall at the edge of your seat and place your hands on your waist. Take a deep breath in through the nose, expanding through your sides and abdomen, then exhale slowly.

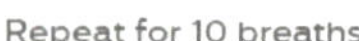
Repeat for 10 breaths.

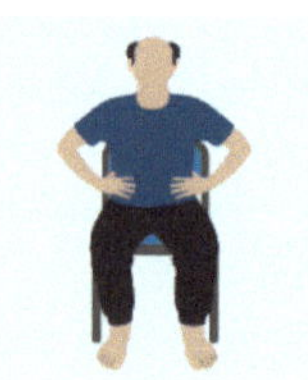

2. Cat/Cow

This pose helps to relieve back and neck tension. Inhale and arch your back to look up at the ceiling. Exhale, pulling your abdominals in and rounding your back as you bend forward.

Repeat this 5 times.

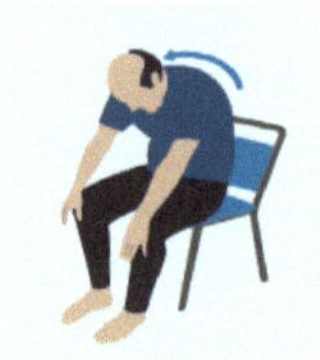

3. Circles

To release and relax the hip muscles, circle your hips clockwise 5 times while seated without moving your upper body, then counterclockwise 5 times.

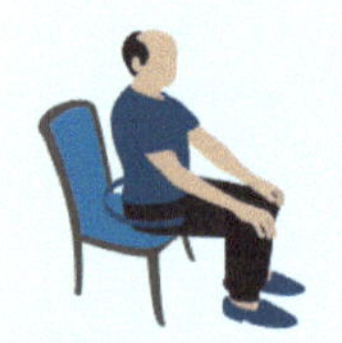

4. Sun Salutation Arms

Lengthens the spine, releases tension in the shoulders and neck. Sitting tall, breathe in and lift your arms up, pressing your palms overhead. On an exhale, float the arms back down to your sides.

Repeat 5 times.

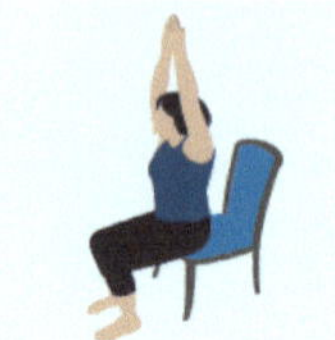

5. Sun Salutations with Twists

Repeat the previous exercise, adding a twist as you exhale.

Repeat 5 times on each side, holding the last twist for 5 seconds.

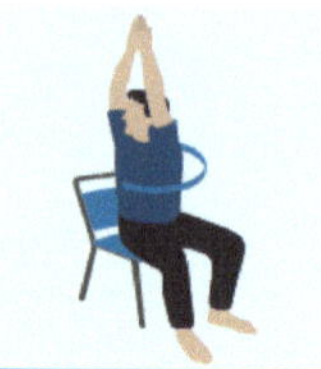

6. High Altar Side Leans

Stretches spine and shoulders. Lift your arms and interlace your fingers in front of you. Turn your palms to the ceiling as you straighten your arms above your head.

Lean to the right for 3 breaths, then to the left for 3 more.

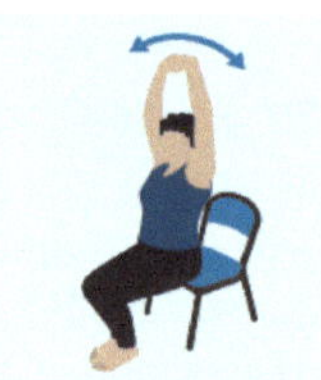

PART 11 Summary in Chair poses yoga for seniors

7. Eagle Arms

Banishes shoulder aches. Stretch your arms out to each side, bring one arm under the other at shoulder height and bend your arms at the elbows with palms together.

Hold for 5 breaths, unwind and repeat with opposite arms.

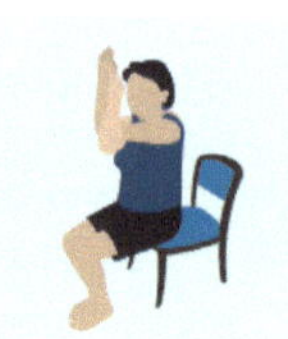

8. Assisted Neck Stretches

The neck is a major stress area. Take your right arm and drape it over your head until your palm reaches your left ear. Let your head fall to your right shoulder, and hold for 5 breaths.

Repeat on the opposite side.

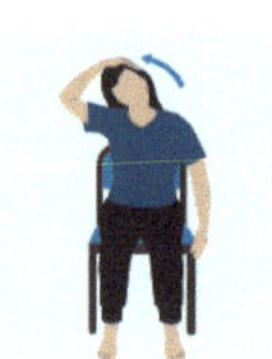

9. Ankle to Knee

The hip area is also a stress spot. To loosen things up, sit up straight, bend your right knee and place your right ankle over your left knee. For a deeper stretch, lean forward.

Hold for 5 breaths, then repeat on the opposite side.

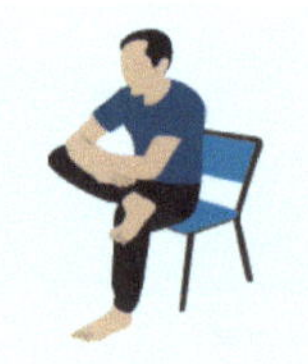

10. Goddess with a Twist

Another great hip stretch: Open legs wide and point toes out. Place your right arm inside your right leg, reaching for the floor. Lift your left arm toward the ceiling and look up to the palm.

Hold for 5 breaths, then repeat on the opposite side.

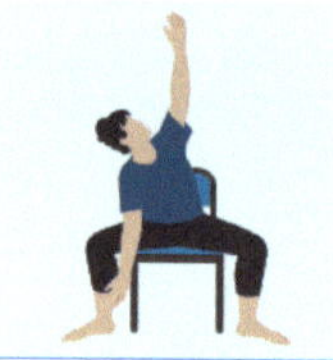

11. Warrior 2

This gives you a full-body stretch. Sit tall at the edge of your seat. Bend your right knee to the side and stretch your left leg out behind you as you press your outer heel down.

Hold for 5 breaths, then repeat on the opposite side.

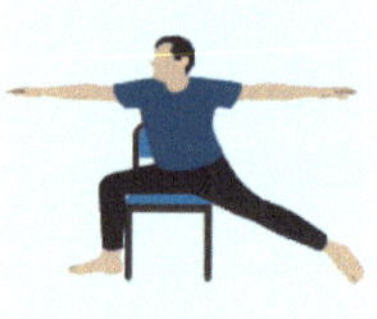

12. Forward Fold

To finish, let blood flow to the brain. Sit tall and straight, then fold down over your legs, letting your head, neck and body hang limp.

Hold for as long as you want before rolling back up to a sitting position.

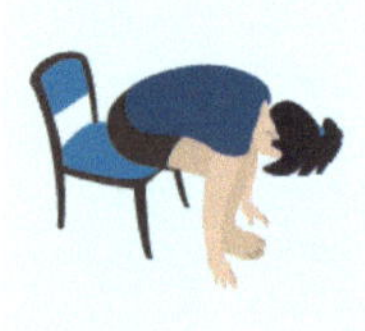

Bibliography and Acknowledgement

- Bergen G, Stevens MR, Burns ER. Falls and fall injuries among adults aged > 65 Years-United States, 2014. MMWR Morb Mortal Wkly Rep. 2016; 65: 993-998.
- Bone health and osteoporosis: A report of the surgeon general. Final report. Rockville: US. Department of Health and Human Services. 2004.
- Brenes GA, Divers J, Miller ME, Anderson A, Hargis G, Danhauer SC. Comparison of cognitive -
- Carson K, Krucoff C. Relax into yoga for seniors: A six-week program for strength, balance, flexibility and pain relief. Oakland: New Harbinger Publications; 2016.
- Cauley JA. Defining ethnic and racial differences in osteoporosis and fragility fractures. Clin Orthop Relat Res. 2011; 469: 1891-1899.
- Chu P, Gotink RA, Yeh GY, Goldie SJ, Hunink MM. The effectiveness of yoga in modifying risk factors for cardiovascular disease and metabolic syndrome: A systematic review and meta-analysis of randomized controlled trials. Eur J Prev Cardiol. 2016; 23: 291-307.
- Chu P, Gotink RA, Yeh GY, Goldie SJ, Hunink MM. The effectiveness of yoga in modifying risk factors for cardiovascular disease and metabolic syndrome: A systematic review and meta-analysis of randomized controlled trials. Eur J Prev Cardiol. 2016; 23: 291-307.
- Clarke BL, Khosla S. Physiology of bone loss. Radiol Cli. 2010; 48: 483-495.
  Cramer H, Quinker D, Schumann D, Wardle J, Dobos G, Lauche R. Adverse effects of yoga: A national cross-sectional survey. BMC Complement Altern Med. 2019; 19: 190.
- Dhalwani NN, Fahami R, Sathanapally H, Seidu S, Davies MJ, Khunti K. Association between polypharmacy and falls in older adults: A longitudinal study from England. BMJ Open 2017; 7: e016358.
- Gothe N. P., & McAuley E. (2016). Yoga is as good as stretching–strengthening exercises in improving functional fitness outcomes: Results from a randomized controlled trial. The Journals of Gerontology. Series A, Biological Sciences and Medical Sciences, 71(3), 406–411. 10.1093/gerona/glv127
  Hamrick I, Mross P, Christopher N, Smith PD.
- Yoga's effect on falls in rural, older adults. Complement Ther Med. 2017; 35: 57-63.
  Krucoff C, Carson K, Peterson M, Shipp K, Krucoff
- M.Teaching yoga to seniors: Essential considerations to enhance safety and reduce risk in a uniquely vulnerable age group. J Altern Complement Med. 2010; 16: 899-905.
- Melnyck B., & Morrison-Beedy D. (2019). Intervention research: Designing, conducting, analyzing, and funding (2nd ed.). Springer.
- Noradechanunt C., Worsley A., & Groeller H. (2017). Thai yoga improves physical function and well-being in older adults: A randomised controlled trial. Journal of Science and Medicine in Sport, 20, 494–501. 10.1016/j.jsams.2016.10.007 PMID:27866841 death in hip fracture patients aged 65 or older: A population-based study. BMC Musculoskelet Disord. 2011; 12: 1-6.
- Panula J, Pihlajamäki H, Mattila VM, Jaatinen P, Vahlberg T, Aarnio P, et al. Mortality and causePanday K, Gona A, Humphrey MB. Medication-induced osteoporosis: Screening and treatment strategies. Ther Adv Musculoskelet Dis. 2014; 6: 185-202.
- Shvedko A., Whittaker A. C., Thompson J. L., & Grieg C. A. (2017). Physical activity interventions for treatment of social isolation, loneliness or low social support in older adults. Psychology of Sport and Exercise, 34, 128–137. 10.1016/j.psychsport.2017.10.003
- Sparling P. B., Howard B. J., Dunstan D. W., & Owen N. (2015). Recommendations for physical activity in older adults. BMJ, 350, h100 10.1136/bmj.h100 PMID:25608694
- Stephens I. Medical yoga therapy. Children. 2017; 4: 12. 8.2016 Yoga in America study [Internet]. New York: Ipsos Public Affairs; 2016. Available from: Study-Comprehensive-RESULTS.pdf. 9.65
- Schultz AB, Andersson GB, Hadersperk K, Ö rtengren R, Nordin M, Björk R. Analysis and measurement of lumbar trunk loads in tasks involving bends and twists. J Biomech. 1982; 15: 669-675.
- Suls J. Anger and the heart: Perspectives on cardiac risk, mechanisms and interventions. Prog Cardiovasc Dis. 2013; 55: 538-547.
- Swain TA, McGwin G. Yoga-related injuries in the United States from 2001 to 2014. Orthop J Sports Med. 2016; 4: 2325967116671703.
- Szanton S. L., & Gill J. M. (2010). Facilitating resilience using a society-to-cells framework: A theory of nursing essentials applied to research and practice. Advances in Nursing Science, 33(4), 329–343. 10.1097/ANS.0b013e3181fb2ea2 PMID:21068554
- Tolahunase M, Sagar R, Dada R. Impact of yoga and meditation on cellular aging in apparently healthy individuals: A prospective, open-label single-arm exploratory study. Oxid Med Cell Longev. 2017; 2017: 7928981. trial. Depress Anxiety. 2020; 37: 1194-1207.
- Tulloch A., Bombell H., Dean C., & Tiedemann A. (2018). Yoga-based exercise improves health-related quality of life and mental well-being in older people: A systematic review of randomised controlled trials. Age and Ageing, 47, 537–544. 10.1093/ageing/afy044 PMID:29584813 Crossref MedlineGoogle Scholar
- Vollbehr NK, Bartels-Velthuis AA, Nauta MH, Castelein S, Steenhuis LA, Hoenders HR, et al. Hatha yoga for acute, chronic and/or treatment-resistant mood and anxiety disorders: A systematic review and meta-analysis. PLoS One. 2018; 13: e0204925.
- World Health Organization. (2019). Decade of healthy aging 2020–2030.https://www.who.int/docs/default-source/documents/decade-of-health-ageing/decade-ageing-proposal-en.pdf?Status=Temp&sfvrsn=b0a7b5b1_12 >Google Scholar
- World Health Organization. (2021). Ageing and health. https://www.who.int/news-room/fact-sheets/detail/ageing-and-health>Google Scholar
- Xia N, Li H. Loneliness, social isolation, and cardiovascular health. Antioxid Redox Signal. 2018; 28: 837-851.

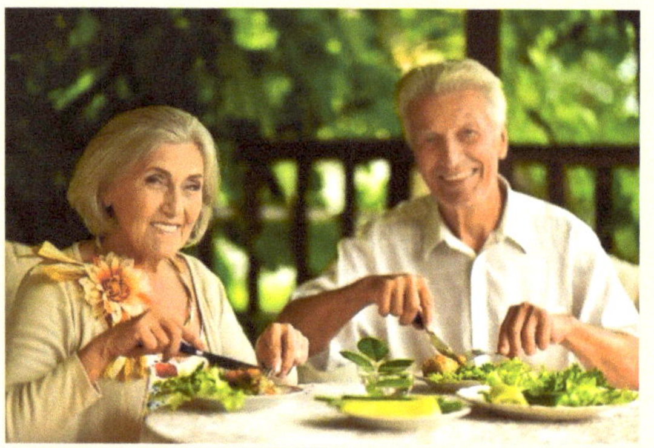

Diet Plans For Older Adults And Senior Citizens

Research into food preferences in older adults and seniors considers how people's dietary experiences change with ageing, and helps people understand how taste, nutrition, and food choices can change throughout one's lifetime; particularly when people approach the age of 70, or beyond. Influencing variables can include: social and cultural environment, gender and/or personal habits, and also physical and mental health. Scientific studies have been performed to explain why people like or dislike certain foods and what factors may affect these preferences

Research in this area is usually done in order to examine the variables that cause the elderly to change their food preferences; an example is the Elderly Nutrition Program (ENP). The ENP was implemented in 1972 to explore how food preferences varied depending on biological sex and ethnic groups, the goal being to improve the quality of meal programs. Meals and preferences for 13 food groups, including fresh fruit, chicken, soup, salad, vegetables, potatoes, meat, sandwiches, pasta, canned fruit, legumes, deli meats, and ethnic foods, are being assessed in order to gain a general impression of people's dietary habits and food preferences. After adjusting for variables, older male subjects were found to be significantly more likely to prefer deli meats, meat, legumes, canned fruit, and ethnic foods compared to females. In addition, compared with African Americans, the study found that "Caucasians demonstrated higher percentages of preference for 9 of 13 food groups including pasta, meat, and fresh fruit", and recommended that "... To improve the quality of the ENP, and to increase dietary compliance of the older adults to the programs, the nutritional services require a strategic meal plan that solicits and incorporates older adults' food preferences"

Influences on food preference

There are multiple factors in an elderly person's life that can affect food preferences. Aspects like their environment, mental and physical health, and lifestyle choices can all contribute to the individual taste and/or habits of elderly people.

An article about Influences on Cognitive Function in Older Adults (Neuropsychology, November 2014) states that "the nutritional status of older adults relates to their quality of life, ability to live independently, and their risk for developing costly chronic illnesses. An aging adult's nutritional well-being can be affected by multiple socio-environmental factors, including access to healthy and affordable foods, congregate meal sites, and nutritious selections at restaurants. The Academy of Nutrition and Dietetics, American Society for Nutrition, and the Society for Nutrition Education have identified an older adult's access to a balanced diet to be critical for the prevention of disease and promotion of nutritional wellness so that quality of life and independence can be maintained throughout the aging process and excessive health care costs can be reduced"

Younger vs. older adults

A person's taste buds, needs for certain vitamins and other nutrients, and their desire for different types of food can change throughout that person's life. 50 young adults and 48 elderly adults participated in a study by the Monell Chemical Senses Center. "Young" subjects ranged from 18 to 35 years of age, and "elderly" subjects were defined as 65 years of age or older. There were more females than males in the study, but there were approximately equal proportions of males and females in the two age groups.

The study observed that younger females had stronger cravings for sweets than elderly females. Possible causes considered for this difference were the younger female test subjects' menstrual cycles and the fact that elderly women no longer go through menopause. The study also postulated that "... Ninety-one percent (91%) of the cycle-associated cravings were said to occur in the second half of the cycle (between ovulation and the start of menstruation)" These physical changes can be considered when assessing why an older person might not be getting the nutrition they need. As taste buds change with age, certain foods might not be seen as appetizing. For example, a study done by Dr. Phyllis B. Grzegorczyk concluded that as people age, their sense for tasting salty foods slowly goes away

Male vs. female

There are differences in food preferences between the sexes. In a study conducted by the ENP, preferences of male and female subjects were identified in the following 13 individual food groups: fresh fruit, chicken, soup, salad, vegetables, potatoes, meat, sandwiches, pasta, canned fruit, legumes, deli meats, and ethnic groups.

Through this study, it was apparent that older males were "significantly more likely to prefer deli meats, meat, legumes, canned fruit, and ethnic foods compared to females"

Another study by the Monell Chemical Senses Center concluded that females had significantly more cravings for sweets and for chocolate than males; and the study results suggested that males had more cravings or preferences for entrées than sweets.

Personal Health

Physical health:- Some older people avoid certain foods or are unwilling to modify their diets due to oral health problems. These issues, such as ill-fitting dentures (false teeth) or gum disease, are correlated with significant differences in dietary quality, which is a measure of the quality of the diet using a total of eight recommendations regarding the consumption of foods and nutrients from the National Academy of Sciences (NAS). Approaches to minimize food avoidance and promote changes to the diets of people with eating difficulties due to oral health conditions are needed desperately, because without being able to chew or take in food properly, their health is affected dramatically, and their food preferences are limited greatly (too soft or liquids only). Due to varying factors in older adults' physical and mental well-being, eating choices can become more restricted. Many elderly people are forced into eating softer foods, foods that incorporate fiber and protein, drinking calcium-packed liquids, and so on.Six of the leading causes of death for older adults, including cardiovascular disease, cancer, chronic lower respiratory disease, stroke, Alzheimer's disease, and diabetes mellitus, have nutrition-related causes and/ or respond favorably to nutrition interventions. These six illnesses can implement certain restrictions and heavily influence the diet of elderly persons.

Declines in physical health, such as conditions like arthritis, can also cause deterioration in diet due to difficulties in preparing and eating food. At the 2010 "Providing Healthy and Safe Foods As We Age" conference sponsored by the Institute of Medicine, Dr. Katherine Tucker noted that the elderly are less active and have lower metabolic rates, with a consequent reduced need to eat. In addition, they tend to have existing diseases and/or take medications that interfere with nutrient absorption. Based on their research dietary requirements, one study developed a modified food pyramid for adults over There is not enough evidence to confidently recommend the use of any form of carbohydrate in preventing or reducing cognitive decline in older adults with normal cognition or mild cognitive impairment. More evidence is needed to evaluate memory improvement and find nutritional issues due to carbohydrates.

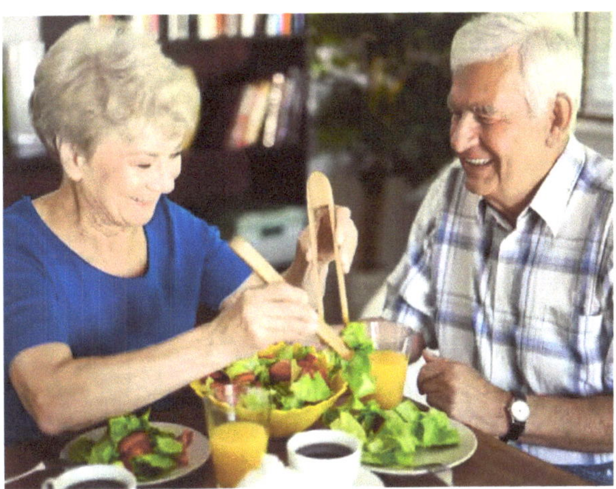

Fig 6.1 . Food preference of elderly

Some older people avoid certain foods or are unwilling to modify their diets due to oral health problems. These issues, such as ill-fitting dentures (false teeth) or gum disease, are correlated with significant differences in dietary quality, which is a measure of the quality of the diet using a total of eight recommendations regarding the consumption of foods and nutrients from the National Academy of Sciences (NAS). Approaches to minimize food avoidance and promote changes to the diets of people with eating difficulties due to oral health conditions are needed desperately, because without being able to chew or take in food properly, their health is affected dramatically, and their food preferences are limited greatly (too soft or liquids only) Due to varying factors in older adults' physical and mental well-being, eating choices can become more restricted. Many elderly people are forced into eating softer foods, foods that incorporate fiber and protein, drinking calcium-packed liquids, and so on. Six of the leading causes of death for older adults, including cardiovascular disease, cancer, chronic lower respiratory disease, stroke, Alzheimer's disease, and diabetes mellitus, have nutrition-related causes and/ or respond favorably to nutrition interventions. These six illnesses can implement certain restrictions and heavily influence the diet of elderly persons. Declines in physical health, such as conditions like arthritis, can also cause deterioration in diet due to difficulties in preparing and eating food At the 2010 "Providing Healthy and Safe Foods As We Age" conference sponsored by the Institute of Medicine, Dr. Katherine Tucker noted that the elderly are less active and have lower metabolic rates, with a consequent reduced need to eat. In addition, they tend to have existing diseases and/or take medications that interfere with nutrient absorption. Based on their research dietary requirements, one study developed a modified food pyramid for adults over 70. There is not enough evidence to confidently recommend the use of any form of carbohydrate in preventing or reducing cognitive decline in older adults with normal cognition or mild cognitive impairment . More evidence is needed to evaluate memory improvement and find nutritional issues due to carbohydrates.

Mental health:- The impact of certain diseases can also impact the quality of the food in the elderly population, especially those that are in care facilities. Certain risk factors include conditions that impair cognitive function, such as dementia. When a person falls victim to a condition that limits mental capacity, mortality risk can rise if due care is not implemented As a result of certain mental health conditions and/or diseases—like Alzheimer's disease —a person's food preferences might become affected. With certain diseases, individuals can develop specific preferences or distaste for various types of food that were not present before onset. For example, people with Alzheimer's disease may experience many big and small changes as a result of their symptoms. One change identified by Suszynski in "How Dementia Tampers with Taste Buds" is within the taste buds of a patient with dementia, which contain the receptors for taste. Since the experience of flavor is significantly altered, people with dementia can often change their eating habits and take on entirely new food preferences. In this study, the researchers found that these dementia patients had trouble identifying flavors and appeared to have lost the ability to remember tastes, therefore leading to a theory that dementia caused the patients to lose their knowledge of flavors Psychological conditions can also affect elderly eating habits. For instance, the length of widowhood may affect nutrition. Depression in elderly people is also associated with a risk of malnutrition.

Lifestyle choices:- Elderly people, like all people, have different lifestyle choices involved in their eating habits. Dietary choices are often a result of personal beliefs and preferences. A survey based on self-reporting found that many rural elderly Iowans adopted eating habits that provided inadequate levels of some key nutrients, and most did not take supplements to correct the deficiencies In contrast, a restaurant study found that the impact of a lifestyle of health and sustainability on healthy food choices is much stronger for senior diners than for non-senior diners Other research has found that adults, regardless of age, will tend to increase fruit and vegetable consumption following a diagnosis of breast, prostate, or colorectal cancer.

Social Environment and Conditioning:-The environment can greatly impact the food preferences of older adults. Those around 75 years old and older are more likely to suffer from limited mobility due to health conditions and often rely on others for food shopping and preparation. In some areas, homebound seniors receive one meal per day (several fresh and frozen meals may be included in a single delivery) from communities[clarification needed] that offer congregate[clarification needed] meals, or meals served in community settings such as senior centers,churches,orseniorhousingcommunitiesThesec ongregate meal programs are encouraged[by whom?] to offer these elderly people a meal at least five times per week. Impeded access to transportation may also be an issue for elderly persons, especially in rural areas where there is less public transportation. This can vary greatly with geographic location; for instance, an Iowa-based study failed to find problems in purchasing food among the elderly in rural open country and towns, as those without their own transportation relied on family, friends, and senior services A separate study found a slight difference in urban areas with[clarification needed] elderly who did not own a car . Aside from transportation, the kind and quality of available food can also shape food choices if a person lives in a so-called "food desert". Social network type can also affect individuals' food choices in our elderly population. For example, one study showed that someone with a larger social network and lower economic status is more likely to have proper nutrition than someone who has a smaller social network and higher economic status Health and social aid can be instrumental in introducing positive change for those at risk.

Best Time for Breakfast, Lunch and Dinner According to Ayurveda

In Ayurveda, an ancient Indian system of medicine and wellness, the timing of meals is considered crucial for maintaining overall health and well-being. According to Ayurvedic principles, the best time to eat is when our digestive fire, known as Agni, is at its strongest By aligning our meals with the natural rhythms of the day, we can optimize digestion, and absorption of nutrients, and support our body's natural healing processes

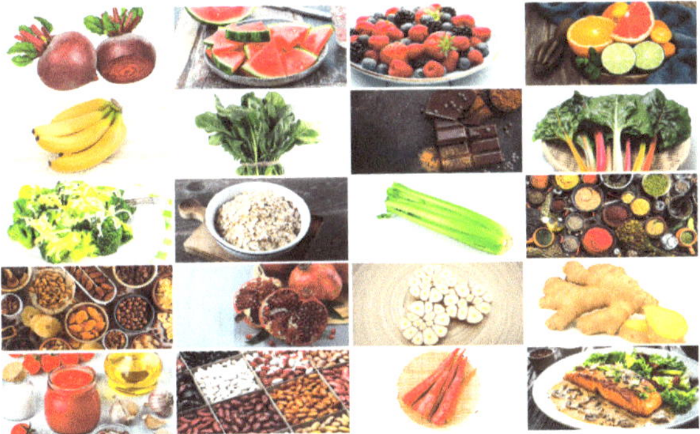

Fig 6.2 The various types of foods available to be taken in a 3 times meal plan

Ayurveda emphasizes the importance of not only what we eat but also when we eat. It recognizes that our bodies have different needs at different times of the day, and by aligning our meals accordingly, we can support optimal digestion, energy levels, and overall well-being.

The Concept of Agni in Ayurveda

Agni, often referred to as the digestive fire, is a central concept in Ayurveda. It represents the transformative power of digestion and metabolism. According to Ayurvedic principles, Agni is strongest during specific times of the day, and eating during these periods enhances digestion and nutrient absorption.

Morning: The Ideal Time for Breakfast

In Ayurveda, breakfast is considered an essential meal, providing nourishment and setting the tone for the day. It is recommended to have breakfast shortly after waking up, ideally within one to two hours. This helps kick-start Agni and provides the necessary energy and nutrients to fuel the body and mind for the day ahead.

Midday: Nourishing Lunch for Sustained Energy

Lunch is considered the most important meal of the day in Ayurveda. It should be consumed when the sun is at its peak, around midday. This is when our digestive fire is naturally strongest, allowing for efficient digestion and assimilation of nutrients. A balanced lunch with a variety of whole foods, including grains, vegetables, legumes, and healthy fats, provides sustained energy throughout the day.

Afternoon: Light and Digestible Snacks

During the afternoon, our digestive fire begins to decrease. It is recommended to have light and easily digestible snacks if hunger arises between meals. Opt for fresh fruits, nuts, seeds, or herbal teas to satiate your appetite without burdening the digestive system.

Evening: Dinner and the Importance of Early Supper

Dinner should ideally be consumed during the early evening, at least two to three hours before bedtime. Ayurveda advises against having heavy meals late at night when our Agni is naturally weaker. A lighter dinner consisting of soups, steamed vegetables, and lean proteins is recommended to promote easy digestion and sound sleep.

Nighttime: Avoiding Late-Night Eating

Ayurveda strongly discourages late-night eating. When we eat close to bedtime, our digestive system is already winding down, making it difficult for the body to process and assimilate food properly. Late-night snacking can disrupt sleep, lead to indigestion, and contribute to weight gain. It is advisable to allow for at least two to three hours of fasting before bedtime.

Conclusion

In Ayurveda, the best time to eat is when our Agni, or digestive fire, is at its strongest. By aligning our meals with the natural rhythms of the day, we can optimize digestion, absorption of nutrients, and overall well-being.

Following the recommended eating times according to Ayurveda can contribute to improved energy levels, balanced weight, and a healthy digestive system.

Frequently Asked Questions

1. Q: Can I skip breakfast if I'm not hungry in the morning?

A: While Ayurveda encourages having breakfast, it's important to listen to your body. If you don't feel hungry in the morning, you can start with a light meal or have brunch instead.

2. Q: What should I eat for dinner according to Ayurveda?

A: Ayurveda recommends a lighter dinner consisting of soups, steamed vegetables, and lean proteins to support digestion and promote restful sleep.

3. Q: Is it okay to have snacks before bedtime?

A: It's generally advised to avoid eating close to bedtime. However, if you feel the need for a snack, opt for light and easily digestible options like herbal teas, fresh fruits, or a handful of nuts.

4. Q: How long should I wait after dinner before going to bed?

A: It is recommended to allow at least two to three hours of fasting after dinner before going to bed to facilitate proper digestion and promote quality sleep.

5. Q: Can I have a heavy lunch instead of dinner?

A: While lunch should be a substantial meal, it's important to have a balanced dinner as well. Having a heavy lunch and a lighter dinner ensures sustained energy throughout the day and supports optimal digestion.

By understanding the concept of Agni and aligning our eating habits with the natural rhythms of the day, we can promote optimal digestion, energy levels, and overall well-being. Remember to listen to your body's cues, choose wholesome and nourishing foods, and cultivate a mindful approach to eating for a harmonious and balanced life.

When Should You Eat Breakfast, Lunch, and Dinner? A Guide to Balanced Eating

Three balanced meals a day, plenty of exercise, and a good eight hours of sleep are crucial to maintaining a healthy lifestyle in today's fast-paced world. Moreover, people are becoming increasingly health-conscious and following various meal plans to stay fit.

While you must be mindful of what you eat, the timing of your meals also significantly impacts your overall well-being. So, when should you eat breakfast, lunch, and dinner?

Ideally, you should eat breakfast at 7:11 am, lunch at 12:38 pm, and dinner at 6:14 pm. But let's face it; it's not possible to always have your meals at these specific times. Instead, there's an optimal time for each meal to help establish a balanced eating routine. Let's dig in to know more about this.

Breakfast: To Kickstart Your Day

How often have you heard, 'Breakfast is the most important meal of the day?' They don't say it without a reason. The day's first meal will fuel your body with nutrients and energy to get you through the rest of the day positively.

Experts recommend eating breakfast within an hour of waking up to jumpstart your metabolism and provide energy for the day. It also allows your body to completely digest the food and rest for a few hours before the second meal of the day.

This early meal will replenish your blood glucose levels that may have depleted during the night.

Ideally, a balanced breakfast includes a combination of protein, complex carbohydrates, and healthy fats. Items like eggs, whole-grain cereals, fruits, and nuts make a filling and nutritious first meal.

It's best to have breakfast about 12 hours after your last meal; this is especially important if you want to lose weight.

Listen to your body's hunger cues instead of strictly adhering to set meal times. If you're not hungry for breakfast right away, it's absolutely fine if you wait until you feel hungry

What Happens if You Skip Breakfast?

As paradoxical as it may seem, skipping breakfast leads to weight gain instead of weight loss. This could be mainly because when you skip breakfast, you get so hungry that you overeat later in the day, possibly during lunchtime.

However, it's a totally different scene if you're practicing intermittent fasting. This is the 16/8 method, where you eat during an 8-hour window and fast for 16 hours.

The eating window stretches from lunchtime until dinner, meaning you skip breakfast daily. In such cases, intermittent fasting helps effectively reduce calorie intake, improves metabolic health, and increases weight loss.

Skipping breakfast or intermittent fasting may not suit everyone, and the effects vary individually. While it may benefit some positively, others may experience a drop in blood sugar, headaches, dizziness, and lack of concentration.

Lunch: To Keep You Going

Lunchtime is crucial in providing sustenance and replenishing energy for the afternoon.

You should have lunch around midday, ideally between 12 pm – 2 pm, or approximately 4 – 5 hours after breakfast. This gives your body sufficient time to fully digest the breakfast while also helping maintain stable blood sugar levels.

Have you felt yourself slouch around mid-noon? There are two reasons for this – you had an extremely filling lunch, or you skipped your lunch.

Having a well-rounded lunch on time prevents this energy slump and also prevents you from overeating later in the day.

However, remember that lunch isn't about eating as much as you can until you have to pop open your pant's top button for breathing space.

A balanced lunch is one that includes plenty of vegetables, complex carbohydrates (legumes, whole grains), and lean proteins (tofu, fish, chicken). Add healthy fats using olive oil or avocado oil to feel satiated for longer.

If you're into losing weight, it's essential to understand that lunchtime appears to have the least impact on weight loss. And for some, it's the biggest meal of the day.

Moreover, those who habitually eat a late lunch (after 3 pm) tend to lose less weight than those who have an early lunch (before 3 pm).

Have you been longingly eyeing something unhealthy and wondering when you should have it? Lunchtime is an excellent time to have it, but only in small quantities, just to satisfy your cravings.

Read about the best lunch foods that can help you reach your weight loss goals.

What Happens if You Skip Lunch?

How often have you skipped lunch because you've been really busy or distracted? Do you recall how you felt on those days?

Skipping lunch will result in problems later in the day; your body will be depleted of energy, and you'll experience drowsiness or brain fog. That's not all; it can also cause increased hunger pangs, irritability, and low blood sugar.

More often than not, when you skip lunch, you tend to consume a majority of calories in the evening, possibly excess, uncontrollable night eating too.

On the other hand, if you aren't with a large appetite around lunchtime, you could always reduce your lunch portions rather than skipping lunch altogether.

Dinner: To Maintain a Balance

Dinner, the last substantial meal of the day, must be had neither too early nor too late. The best time to have dinner will largely depend on your schedule.

Studies show that having a late dinner or eating late into the night is linked with increased risks of obesity and metabolic issues like hyperglycemia and dyslipidemia.

Ideally, you must consume dinner at least two hours before bedtime to aid digestion.

Having your dinner about 2 – 3 hours before bedtime allows your body time to digest the meal sufficiently before you go to sleep. This, in turn, minimizes any discomfort or disrupted sleep patterns. If you eat too close to bedtime, it could lead to indigestion or disturbed sleep, followed by bloating the next morning.

Your dinner must be lighter than lunch and easily digestible. Try to include lean proteins like fish, poultry, or plant-based alternatives and some colorful vegetables.

Limiting your intake of high-fat foods and refined carbohydrates for dinner is best.

What Happens if You Skip Dinner?

For those with normal metabolisms, skipping dinner or having it late in the afternoon is absolutely fine. It'll help optimize digestion and aid in the absorption of nutrients.

However, if you're with chronic health conditions like diabetes, it would be best to discuss this with your doctor before you make any changes to your food schedules.

Remember, skipping dinner is like going through an overnight fast until morning. Don't jump into this routine until you're certain about your hunger cues, and feel confident that you'll do just fine without dinner.

How About Snacks?

Now that you've understood when should you eat breakfast, lunch, and dinner, the question about snacks is probably popping into your mind.

Snacking throughout the day helps maintain steady energy levels, regulates appetite, and prevents overeating during meals.

While reaching out for those unhealthy, processed foods is easy, you must choose healthy snacks that won't sabotage your overall nutrition goals. Fresh fruits, celery sticks with peanut butter or hummus, yogurt, nuts, or raw vegetables make nutrient-rich snack options.

Incorporating healthy snacks between meals will help

maintain stable blood sugar levels and curb excessive hunger. Generally, it's best to allow at least 2 – 3 hours after a meal (allowing for complete digestion) before having a snack.

If your snack is more about munching on something when you're bored or feeling low instead of actual hunger, you're adding excess calories that can lead to unwanted weight gain. Make that snack a combination of protein with fiber for a healthier option.

Important Considerations

The timings of meals may vary depending on individual schedules, preferences, and cultural norms.Some people may benefit from intermittent fasting or adjusting their meal timing based on their needs or health conditions. Consult with a healthcare professional or registered dietitian to determine the best approach for you.

If you thought skipping meals aids in weight loss, you might want to reconsider that strategy. When you skip meals or eat irregularly, you're bound to face negative health consequences like weight gain, poor digestion, and decreased energy levels.

Regardless of the mealtimes, you must practice portion control for a balanced diet. Heed to your body's hunger and feeling of fullness to avoid overeating.

Finally, practice mindful eating rather than gobbling down your food in a rush or when distracted by a screen. Eat slowly and pay more attention to the flavors and textures of the foods; savor every mouthful. Note: When you eat with distractions, you tend to eat faster and twice more than you usually would, yet, you'll end up feeling less full.

Summing It Up

While research has come up with an answer to 'When should you eat breakfast, lunch, and dinner?', it's best to understand your internal clock and decide wisely.

Breakfast should be about an hour after waking up, lunch 4 – 5 hours after breakfast, and dinner 2-3 hours before bedtime.

What you eat helps nourish your body, and when you eat determines your weight, metabolic rate, and sleep cycle. Remember, skipping meals is not a healthy way to lose weight.

Whether you're a fitness enthusiast or looking to shed a few pounds, perfectly timed breakfasts, lunches, and dinners will help you unlock your body's potential.

7 Day Meal Plan for the Elderly:

Good nutrition is crucial at every stage of life, but it becomes even more important as we age. For the elderly, a well-thought-out meal plan can be the difference between merely aging and aging well. This plan is designed to support weight maintenance, prevent malnutrition, and cater to the unique dietary needs of older adults.

As a Registered Dietitian, my goal is to provide a 7-day meal plan for the elderly that is not only nutritious but also enjoyable and easy to follow. It focuses on high-quality proteins, energy-sustaining carbohydrates, and essential fats, all of which are key to maintaining health and vitality in the later years.

This meal plan is more than just a list of foods; it's a guide to healthy aging. By incorporating a variety of nutrient-dense foods, I aim to support the overall well-being of the elderly, ensuring they get the most out of their meals every day.

Nutrition plays a pivotal role in how we age, influencing everything from our physical health to our cognitive function. With this plan, we address the nutritional needs that are critical for the elderly, making each meal an opportunity to nourish the body and mind.

Understanding Nutritional Needs of the Elderly

As we age, our bodies undergo various changes that affect our nutritional requirements. Elderly individuals need fewer calories due to a slower metabolism and possibly less physical activity, but their need for certain nutrients may increase. This balance is crucial for maintaining health and preventing chronic diseases.

Protein is essential for preserving muscle mass, which tends to decline with age. Research suggests the elderly need 1.2 grams/kg body weight daily of protein.

If you want some ideas for more protein, look at High Protein Foods for the Elderly: Why They Need More!

Carbohydrates should be sourced from whole grains, fruits, and vegetables to ensure a steady energy supply and adequate fiber intake. But the goal should be between 25-38 grams of fiber per day for men and women.

Fats should come from healthy sources like olive oil and avocados, supporting brain health and reducing inflammation. Other good fats that also provide protein can be from dairy products. Opt for full fat dairy options if weight loss is a problem.

Vitamins and minerals deserve special attention in an

elderly diet. Calcium and vitamin D are vital for bone health. Calcium daily goals are about 500 mg/day and Vitamin D is between 600IU to 1000 IU per day.

While B vitamins are important for energy metabolism and cognitive function. Ensuring a diet rich in these nutrients can help mitigate the risk of age-related conditions.

Hydration is another key aspect often overlooked. Older adults may not feel thirsty as often, leading to inadequate fluid intake. Regular consumption of water, herbal teas, and other hydrating fluids is essential to prevent dehydration and its associated risks.

Principles of a Healthy Meal Plan for the Elderly

Creating a meal plan for the elderly requires a focus on nutrient density and meal variety. Every meal and snack should pack a nutritional punch, offering vitamins, minerals, fiber, and hydration to meet the body's needs. It's about choosing foods that offer the most nutritional benefits that can add the best calories and protein in smaller amounts. The reason behind this goal is weight is a protective factor as we age. A higher body mass index (BMI) between 23.0-29.9 has a lower risk of early mortality.

The foundation of a healthy meal plan includes plenty of fruits and vegetables, lean proteins, whole grains, and healthy fats. These components ensure a balanced diet that supports all bodily functions. Fruits and vegetables, for example, are high in vitamins and antioxidants, which are crucial for immune health and chronic disease prevention.

Incorporating foods that the elderly enjoy and can easily consume is also important. Soft-cooked vegetables, moist proteins, and smoothies can make eating not only more manageable but also more enjoyable. Adapting meals to individual dietary needs and preferences encourages better nutrition intake and overall satisfaction with meals. Lastly, regular, balanced meals and snacks throughout the day help maintain energy levels and prevent blood sugar spikes. Planning for snacks between meals can also ensure that nutritional needs are met, especially for those with smaller appetites. This approach to eating supports sustained energy and health in the elderly.

Day-by-Day Meal Plan Overview

Meal planning can be overwhelming trying to fit all the nutrition goals into one day. Instead try to reach these goals in 1 week instead. This is why a 7 day meal plan for the elderly can help! Here is a brief breakdown of how to meet overall nutrition goals in 7 days.

Day 1: Focus on Heart Health

Start the week with meals rich in omega-3 fatty acids, fiber, and antioxidants. Breakfast might include oatmeal topped with walnuts and berries, while lunch and dinner focus on leafy greens, whole grains, and fatty fish like salmon. These foods support cardiovascular health and help reduce inflammation.

Day 2: Bone Health and Strength

Incorporate calcium and vitamin D-rich foods to support bone density. A breakfast of fortified yogurt with sliced almonds, a lunch featuring leafy green salads, and a dinner with dairy or fortified plant milk can provide these essential nutrients. Snacks like cheese or almond butter on whole grain toast also contribute to bone health.

Day 3: Brain Function and Cognitive Health

Meals rich in antioxidants and healthy fats, such as avocados, nuts, and seeds, support brain health. Start with a smoothie made from spinach, blueberries, and flaxseed oil. For lunch and dinner, include lean proteins and whole grains to fuel cognitive function and memory.

Day 4: Skin and Hair Vitality

Focus on foods high in vitamins C and E, zinc, and selenium. Breakfast could be a citrus fruit salad, while lunch and dinner feature lean proteins and vegetables like bell peppers and tomatoes, known for their skin-supporting nutrients. Snacks might include sunflower seeds or a small piece of dark chocolate.

Day 5: Eye Health and Vision Support

Incorporate foods rich in lutein and zeaxanthin, such as kale, spinach, and eggs. A spinach omelet for breakfast, a kale salad for lunch, and a dinner featuring eggs or fish with a side of sweet potatoes can support eye health.

Day 6: Digestive Health

Focus on fiber-rich foods to support gut health. Begin with a breakfast of whole grain toast with avocado, followed by a lunch of lentil soup, and a dinner that includes a variety of cooked vegetables and whole grains. Snacks like fruits or vegetable sticks with hummus can add extra fiber.

Day 7: Immune System Boost

End the week with a focus on foods rich in vitamins A, C, and zinc. Breakfast could include pumpkin or carrot pancakes, lunch a chicken and vegetable soup, and dinner a stir-fry with beef and a variety of colorful vegetables. Snacks might be citrus fruits or nuts, both good for the immune system

15 Best Breakfast, Lunch & Dinner Meals for Seniors

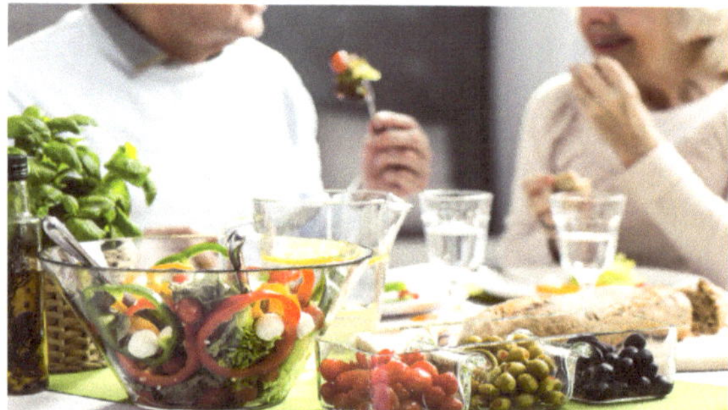

Fig 6.3 Senior citizens are taking their breakfast

Senior living should bring more time to focus on enjoying life, family and relaxation. While good nutrition is important for any age, it is essential for getting the most out of our twilight years. A well-balanced diet for the elderly contributes to better health, more energy and a fulfilling day-to-day life. For healthy people over the age of 70, nutritionists recommend eating foods rich in nutrients, increasing the amount of fibre in their diets, and drinking plenty of water to avoid dehydration.

Here is a list of simple and healthy meal ideas tailored to the nutritional needs of senior citizens. While you should discuss the particulars of your diet or the diet of the elderly person in your life with a doctor or retirement facility professional, this list covers some fundamentals for healthy senior meals for every meal of the day.

1. Breakfast Meals for Seniors

Too many people make a habit of skipping "the most important meal of the day," and this includes seniors. Because older people generally eat less in a single sitting, spreading a senior's daily caloric intake out over the day is all the more important. Breakfast offers an opportunity to introduce necessary foods high in fibre and fruits that are great for overall digestive health.

Breakfast is especially important to people on medications that can only be taken on a full stomach. As with all meals, seniors should drink plenty of liquids, taking water, juice or tea throughout the day.

Hard-boiled eggs and Poached egg are frequently included in many meals for seniors. Pair this simple breakfast staple with some fresh fruit and a slice of whole grain toast for a balanced meal. A breakfast classic, served here without the unhealthy cream sauce or heavy cheeses of an Eggs Benedict. . Eggs are rich in bone-building Vitamin D, brain-boosting choline, and the amino acid tryptophan, which helps to regulate mood. Egg yolk contains iron which improves energy. Its protein promotes tissue growth, helping the body's natural ability to heal and repair itself. Poaching preserves many of the health benefits that eggs have to offer for seniors

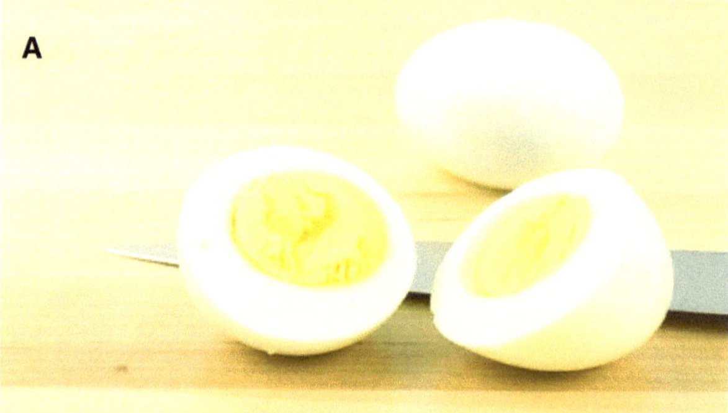

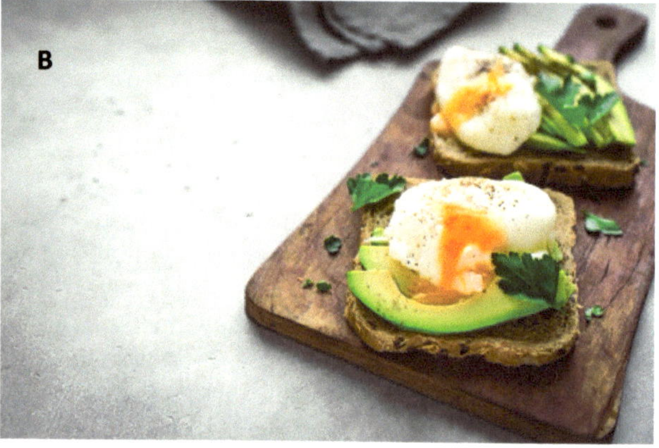

Fig 6.4 Showing (A) hard-boiled and (B) poached eggs

Hot oatmeal with fruit. High in fibre and delicious, warm oatmeal should be augmented with fresh berries, apples, or even yogurt. For an added treat, enjoy with a hint of Canadian maple syrup.

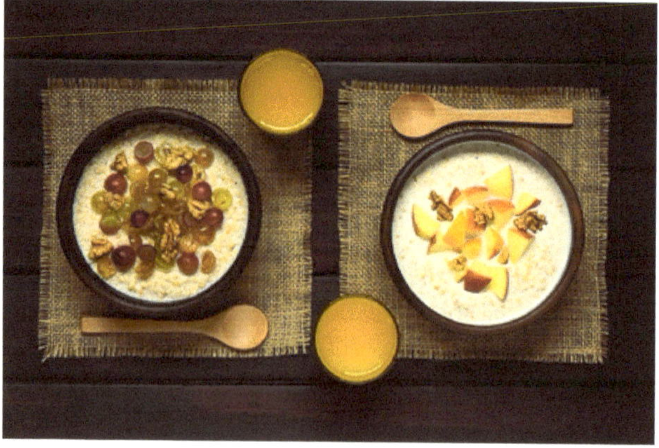

Fig 6.5 Showing hot oatmeal with fruit

Whole grain pancakes/waffles:- It's no secret that pancakes and waffles a re made from the same basic batter. However, what goes into the base batter really matters for senior health. Whole grains like barley, buckwheat, bulgur, millet, high-protein quinoa, steel-cut whole oats, and whole wheat make excellent batter choices. Using whole grains instead of traditional flour makes this tasty breakfast food high in essential fatty acids and proteins. It can also lower inflammation. Add chia seeds to mix for additional nutrients.

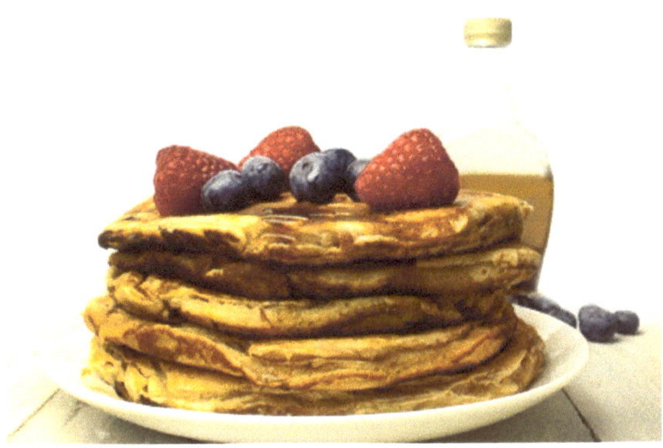

Fig 6.6 Showing Whole grain pancakes/waffles

Avocado toast. This trendy and tasty brunch item is popular among the younger generation, and for good reason! Did you know that avocado contains more potassium than bananas? It's true. Avocados are rich in nutrients, heart-healthy fats, and fiber. They have also been demonstrated to lower cholesterol and triglycerides, promoting better overall health. Served sliced over whole grain toast they taste incredible! For the full experience, combine with a small serving of tasty greens like spinach, arugula or kale.

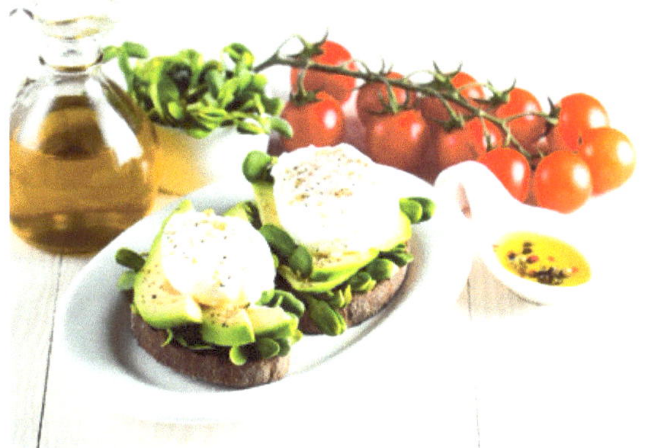

Fig 6.7 Showing Avocado toast.

Toast:- With whole wheat or whole grain bread and a spread of traditional peanut butter spread peanut butter, almond butter, or whole nut butter, toast is provides healthy fat and a little extra protein. Avoid butter, margarine, and sugary hazelnut-based spreads. Add fresh fruit.

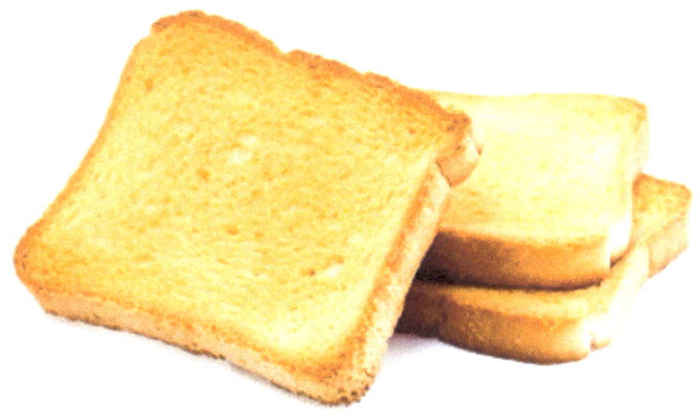

Fig 6.8 Showing whole wheat or whole grain bread toast

2. Lunch Meals for Seniors

According to the USDA, seniors should consume two and a half cups of fresh vegetables every day, and lunch is a great opportunity to build a vegetable-rich diet. A healthy lunch for seniors should combine plenty of vegetables, a source of protein from lean meat, eggs, legumes or fish, and hearty grains like whole grain pasta, brown rice or whole grain bread. For added nutrients, add spinach, kale and carrots to any lunch.

Meat and barley soup :-Soups are among the healthiest meals for seniors. Packed with vegetables, healthy grains and the savoury protein from beef, this classic soup makes for a hearty and comforting

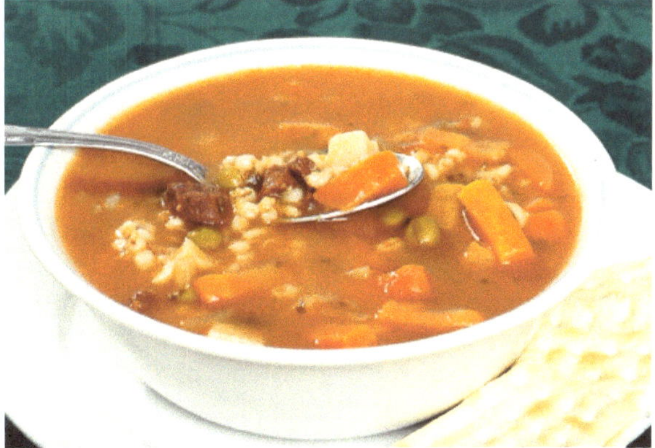

Fig 6.9 Showing Meat and barley soup

Tuna salad sandwich:-A lunch time favourite made up of tuna, light or low-fat mayonnaise, chopped celery, spinach and heart-healthy whole grain bread. Add a side of chopped baby carrots and tomatoes for extra nutrients.

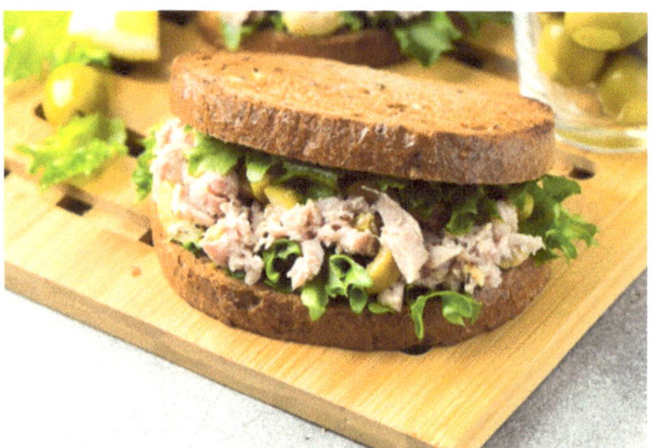

Fig 6.10 Showing Tuna salad sandwich

Grilled Chicken and Cashew Salad:-Many healthy salads combine vegetables, protein, and great taste. The grilled chicken and cashews in this salad doubles its protein content. Using a mixture of spinach, kale and romaine lettuce provides additional vitamins and minerals.

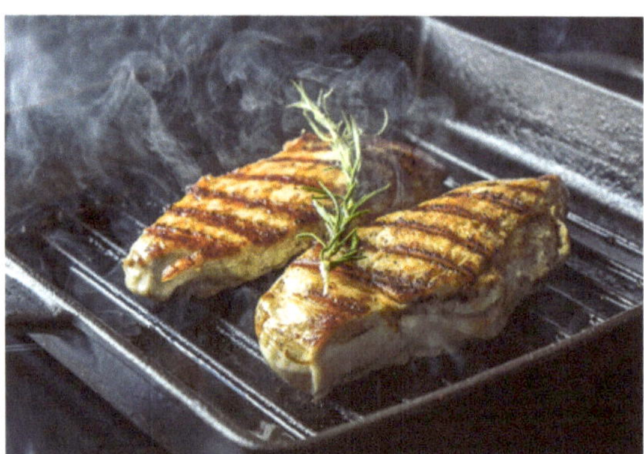

Fig 6.11 Showing Grilled Chicken andC ashew Salad

3. Dinner Meals for Seniors

Many seniors prefer to eat a light meal earlier in the evening or late afternoon. It is important that this meal complete the rest of the daily recommended servings of vegetables, grains and protein that seniors need. Doctors recommend using extra virgin olive oil and avocado oil for cooking instead of canola oil, butter or lard. Any of these delicious dishes can be improved with the addition of a side of boiled or steamed seasonal vegetables and a nutritious side salad or soup.

Baked or grilled salmon:-In addition to being a great source of protein, antioxidants and Vitamin B, salmon is rich in omega-3 fatty acids which help reduce the risk for heart disease and stroke, and boosts both mood and the effectiveness of anti-inflammatory drugs.

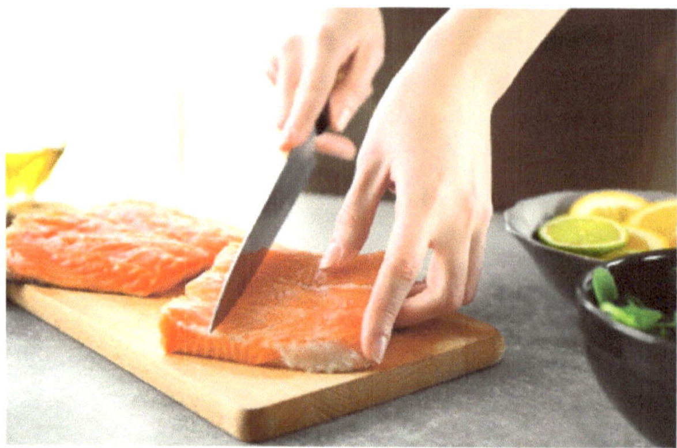

Fig 6.12 Showing Baked or grilled salmon.

Spaghetti and meat balls:-The health benefits of this Italian-American original are enhanced by adding veggies like zucchini, carrots, kale, spinach, and celery. Use whole grain noodles instead of fatty white flour pasta.

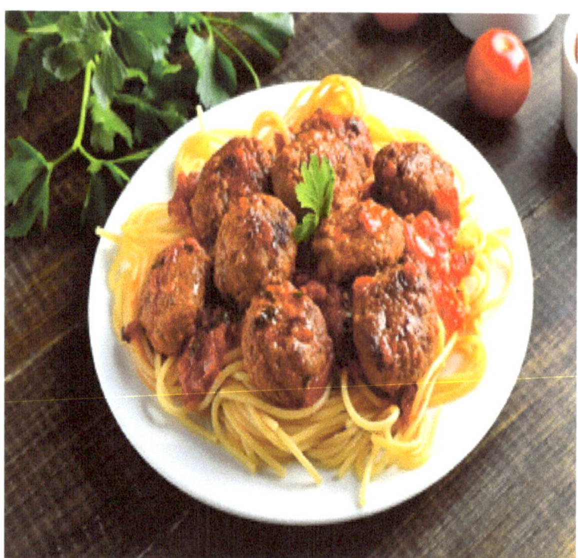

Fig 6.13 Showing Spaghetti and meat balls

Chicken and vegetable mini-pot pies:-This is a nostalgic entrée that mixes whole grains, vegetables, and protein. It's an unexpected choice when it comes to meals for seniors, so many will find this food a delightful surprise.

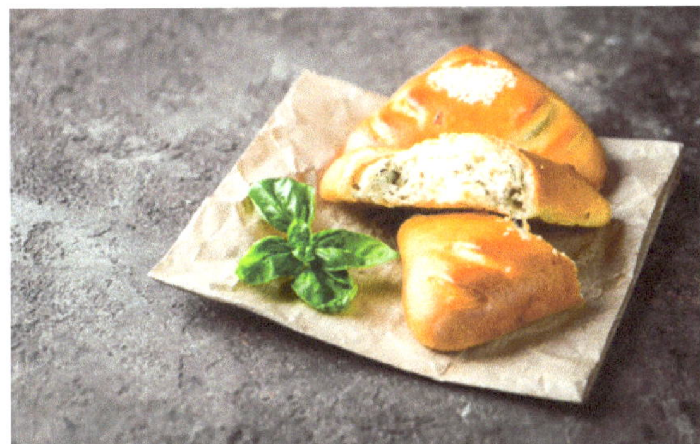

Fig 6.14 Showing Chickenand vegetable mini-pot pies:

Beans and brown rice:-These meals for seniors are made with black, pinto or white beans and served with brown rice, or whole grains like oats

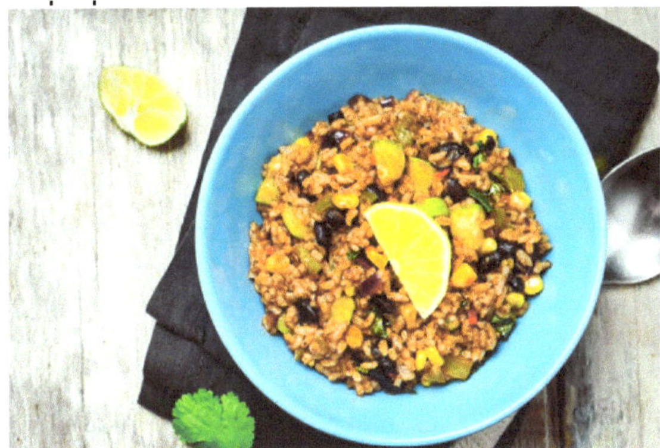

Fig 6.15 Showing Beans and brown rice.

4. Snacks and Desserts for Seniors

Some nutritious snacks for seniors include dried fruits, soft nuts, yogurt, high-fiber crackers with hummus dip, and chopped bell pepper with guacamole

Seasonalfreshfruit :-Whether served individually or in a fruit salad, seniors need to eat plenty of fruits as part of the healthy meals for seniors.

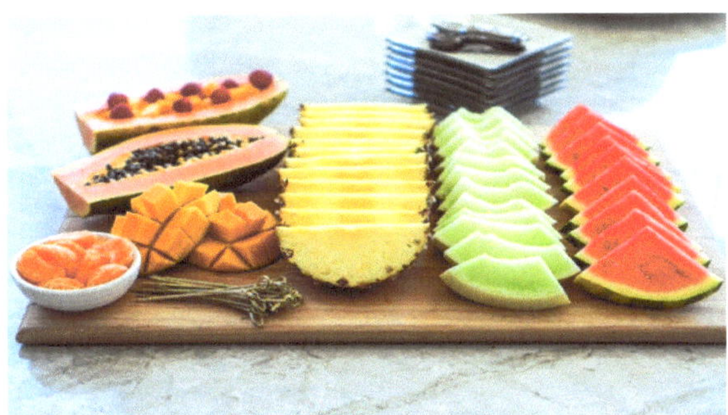

Fig 6.16 Showing Seasonal fresh fruit

Greek Yogurt:- Greek yogurt is great for seniors because it is a great source that helps control blood pressure and keeps bowels working. When you mix in nuts and fruits, you create a healthy mix of fat, vitamins and minerals

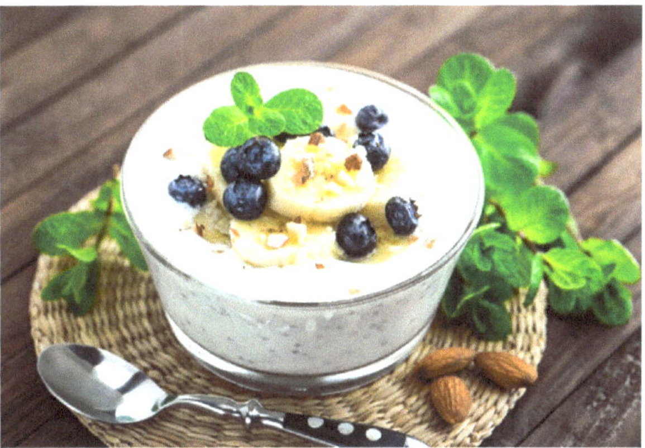

Fig 6.17 Showing Greek Yogurt

7-Day Meal Plan for the Elderly

As we age, our dietary needs change, and it becomes crucial to consume nutrient-dense foods that are easy to digest. However, planning meals for the elderly can be challenging as they may have specific dietary restrictions and health conditions that require attention.

In this blog post, I'll provide a 7-day meal plan for the elderly, taking into consideration their nutritional requirements, dietary restrictions, and taste preferences

Day 1: Breakfast

For breakfast, you can start with oatmeal or yogurt topped with berries and honey. Add a slice of whole-grain toast and a boiled egg on the side. Serve with a glass of orange juice or low-fat milk.

Day 1: Lunch

For lunch, you can prepare a chicken salad with mixed greens, cherry tomatoes, avocado, and a vinaigrette dressing. Serve with a slice of whole-grain bread or a handful of whole-grain crackers.

Day 1: Dinner

For dinner, you can make a baked salmon filet with roasted vegetables and brown rice. Alternatively, you can prepare a vegetarian lasagna with plenty of colorful vegetables and a side salad.

Day 2: Breakfast

For breakfast, you can make a smoothie with frozen berries, bananas, and almond milk. Add a tablespoon of chia seeds for an extra boost of fiber and nutrients. Serve with a slice of whole-grain toast and a boiled egg on the side.

Day 2: Lunch

For lunch, you can prepare a turkey and avocado wrap with whole-grain tortillas, sliced turkey breast, avocado, lettuce, and tomato. Serve with a side of vegetable soup or a small green salad.

Day 2: Dinner

For dinner, you can make a beef stir-fry with plenty of colorful vegetables and brown rice. Alternatively, you can prepare a lentil soup with plenty of spices and herbs.

Day 3: Breakfast

For breakfast, you can prepare scrambled eggs with spinach and mushrooms. Add a slice of whole-grain toast and a small bowl of fresh fruit on the side.

Day 3: Lunch

For lunch, you can prepare a tuna salad with mixed greens, cherry tomatoes, olives, and a vinaigrette dressing. Serve with a slice of whole-grain bread or a handful of whole-grain crackers.

Day 3: Dinner

For dinner, you can make a baked chicken breast with roasted vegetables and quinoa. Alternatively, you can prepare a vegetable stir-fry with tofu or tempeh.

Day 4: Breakfast

For breakfast, you can make a bowl of Greek yogurt topped with fresh fruit, nuts, and honey. Add a slice of whole-grain toast on the side and a glass of orange juice or low-fat milk.

Day 4: Lunch

For lunch, you can prepare a ham and cheese sandwich with whole-grain bread, sliced ham, Swiss cheese, lettuce, and tomato. Serve with a side of vegetable soup or a small green salad.

Day 4: Dinner

For dinner, you can make a grilled shrimp skewer with mixed vegetables and quinoa. Alternatively, you can prepare a vegetable curry with plenty of spices and herbs.

Day 5: Breakfast

For breakfast, you can prepare a smoothie with banana, peanut butter, and almond milk. Add a tablespoon of flaxseed for an extra boost of fiber and nutrients. Serve with a slice of whole-grain toast and a boiled egg on the side.

Day 5: Lunch

For lunch, you can prepare a roast beef and Swiss cheese sandwich with whole-grain bread, sliced roast beef, Swiss cheese, lettuce, and tomato. Serve with a side of vegetable soup or a small green salad.

Day 5: Dinner

For dinner, you can make a baked cod filet with mixed vegetables and brown rice. Alternatively, you can prepare a lentil and vegetable stew with plenty of herbs and spices

Day 6: Breakfast

For breakfast, you can make a bowl of oatmeal topped with chopped nuts, dried fruit, and a drizzle of honey. Add a glass of low-fat milk or almond milk on the side.

Day 6: Lunch

For lunch, you can prepare a grilled cheese sandwich with whole-grain bread and a side of tomato soup. Alternatively, you can make a vegetable and chicken stir-fry with brown rice.

Day 6: Dinner

For dinner, you can make a turkey meatloaf with roasted vegetables and mashed sweet potatoes. Alternatively, you can prepare a vegetarian chili with plenty of beans, vegetables, and spices.

Day 7: Breakfast

For breakfast, you can make a veggie omelet with mixed vegetables and cheese. Serve with a slice of whole-grain toast and a small bowl of fresh fruit on the side.

Day 7: Lunch

For lunch, you can prepare a tuna melt sandwich with whole-grain bread, canned tuna, cheddar cheese, and sliced tomatoes. Serve with a side of vegetable soup or a small green salad.

Day 7: Dinner

For dinner, you can make grilled chicken breast with mixed vegetables and quinoa. Alternatively, you can prepare a vegetable and bean soup with plenty of herbs and spices.

Frequently asked questions (FAQs)

Is this meal plan suitable for seniors with dietary restrictions?

Yes, the meal plan is customizable to accommodate dietary restrictions and preferences.

Can I prepare these meals in advance?

Yes, many of the meals can be prepared ahead of time and stored in the fridge or freezer for convenience.

Are these meals easy to digest for elderly individuals with digestive issues?

Yes, the meals are designed to be nutrient-dense and easy to digest for elderly individuals with digestive issues.

Will these meals provide enough nutrients for seniors?

Yes, the meals are designed to provide essential nutrients for seniors, including protein, fiber, vitamins, and minerals.

Can I substitute ingredients if I don't have certain items on hand?

Yes, you can substitute ingredients as needed to fit your preferences and dietary restrictions.

Is this meal plan affordable for seniors on a budget?

Yes, the meal plan uses affordable and accessible ingredients and is designed to be cost-effective.

Can I use this meal plan for elderly individuals with specific health conditions?

It's always best to consult with a healthcare professional or registered dietitian to ensure the meal plan is suitable for the individual's specific health conditions.

Can I modify the portion sizes of the meals based on the appetite of the elderly person?

Yes, you can modify the portion sizes of the meals to fit the appetite of the individual.

Can I find all the ingredients for these meals at my local grocery store?

Yes, the ingredients used in the meal plan are common and can be found at most local grocery stores.

Table 6.1 **A sample Diet plan schedule**

Day	Breakfast	Lunch	Dinner
1	Oatmeal with nuts and fruit	Tuna salad with whole-grain crackers and veggies	Grilled chicken breast wi sweet potatoes and gree
2	Greek yogurt with berries and granola	Lentil soup with whole-grain bread and salad	Baked salmon with quin steamed asparagus
3	Scrambled eggs with whole-wheat toast and fruit	Chicken and vegetable stir-fry with brown rice	Beef stew with whole-gr. steamed broccoli
4	Smoothie with spinach, banana, and peanut butter	Turkey sandwich with vegetable soup	Baked pork chop with ba and mixed vegetables
5	Cottage cheese with fruit and whole-grain crackers	Baked sweet potato with black beans and avocado	Grilled shrimp with whol and roasted tomatoes
6	Whole-grain waffles with yogurt and fruit	Vegetable omelet with whole-grain toast and salad	Vegetarian chili with corn steamed green beans
7	Omelet with spinach, mushrooms, and whole-grain toast	Baked chicken with sweet potato fries and green salad	Grilled steak with roaste and brown rice

Diabetes diet: Create your healthy-eating plan

A diabetes diet is a healthy-eating plan that helps control blood sugar. Use this guide to get started, from meal planning to counting carbohydrates.

The plate method

The American Diabetes Association offers a simple method of meal planning. It focuses on eating more vegetables. Follow these steps when preparing your plate:

Fill half of your plate with nonstarchy vegetables, such as spinach, carrots and tomatoes.

Fill a quarter of your plate with a lean protein, such as tuna, lean pork or chicken.

Fill the last quarter with a carbohydrate, such as brown rice or a starchy vegetable, such as green peas.Include "good" fats such as nuts or avocados in small amounts.Add a serving of fruit or dairy and a drink of water or unsweetened tea or coffee.

Diabetes & Chronic Kidney Disease Foods

Close-up of diet plan

Your dietitian can give you lots of tasty ideas for healthy meals.

Below are just a few examples of foods a person with both diabetes and CKD can eat. Your dietitian can give you lots more suggestions and help you find recipes for tasty meals:

Fruits: berries, grapes, cherries, apples, plums

Veggies: cauliflower, onions, eggplant, turnips

Proteins:lean meats (poultry, fish), eggs, unsalted seafood

Carbs:white bread, bagels, sandwich buns, unsalted crackers, pasta

Drinks: water, clear diet sodas, unsweetened tea

Here's one way your CKD diet and diabetes diet can work together: If you drink orange juice to treat low blood sugar, switch to kidney-friendly apple or grape juice. You'll get the same blood-sugar boost with a lot less potassium

Menus for heart-healthy eating:

Cut the fat and salt

Heart-healthy eating doesn't have to be difficult. Use these menus to get started on a heart-healthy diet.

Do you want to follow a heart-healthy diet, but aren't sure where to start? One way to begin is to create a daily meal plan. The plan should include plenty of lean protein, vegetables, fruits and whole grains. Limit high-fat foods such as red meat, cheese and baked goods. Also limit foods that are high in sodium such as sandwiches, pizza, soup and processed foods. Cut back on foods and drinks with added sugar too.

Below are two days' worth of heart-healthy menus. Use them as examples of heart-healthy eating.

Breakfast

1 cup cooked oatmeal, sprinkled with 1 tablespoon chopped walnuts and 1 teaspoon cinnamon

1 banana

1 cup skim milk

Lunch

1 cup low-fat (1% or lower), plain yogurt with 1 teaspoon ground flaxseed

1 cup peach halves, canned in juice

5 Melba toast crackers

1 cup raw broccoli and cauliflower

2 tablespoons low-fat cream cheese, plain or vegetable flavor (as a spread for crackers or vegetable dip)

Sparkling water

Dinner

4 ounces salmon

1/2 cup green beans with 1 tablespoon toasted almonds

2 cups mixed salad greens

1/2 cup cherry tomatoes

2 tablespoons low-fat salad dressing

1 tablespoon sunflower seeds

1 cup skim milk

1 small orange

Snack

1 cup skim milk

1/4 cup raisins or dried fruit, no added sugar

20 dark chocolate chips

Day 1 nutrient analysis

Calories 1,688

Total fat 46 g

Saturated fat 12 g

Monounsaturated fat 13 g

Polyunsaturated fat 17 g

Meals for Elderly with No Teeth

As we age, we are more likely to encounter dental problems. So much so, that 68% of adults aged 65 years or older have periodontitis in the United States. Periodontitis is also known as gum disease and can lead to mouth pain and tooth loss.

Dentures are a common substitute when teeth are lost; however, dentures can be costly, don't work as efficiently as natural teeth, and some find wearing them to be uncomfortable.

Because of this, there is a strong link between dental health and nutrition. We need to be making appropriate meals for elderly with no teeth an important part of maintaining overall health.

Nutrition Needs for Meals for Elderly with No Teeth

Many foods contain specific nutrient benefits. For example, we often associate milk with calcium and vitamin D, meat with protein, and orange juice with vitamin C.. However, the foods that are more difficult to eat without teeth, are often those with high nutrient value, such as meats and raw vegetables.

To ensure that meals for elderly with no teeth contain adequate nutrients, including protein and fiber, we need to make sure that food substitutions or alterations contain similar nutrient values.

Specific Nutrients of Importance

Seniors may need certain nutrients, or more of specific nutrients to keep up with their health while aging.

Turning Regular Foods Into Easy to Chew Foods

Now that we are aware of what foods to avoid, we can take a look at how to prepare appropriate nutritious, appealing, and varied meals for elderly with no teeth.

Fruits and Vegetables

Vegetables can be made softer by steaming or boiling. Fruits should be soft enough to break into pieces with a spoon. Fibrous parts of fruit should be removed, such as apple skins and the white fibers in an orange.

Fruits that can not be found in soft form can be blended into a delicious smoothie for breakfast. Different colored fruits and vegetables are rich in different nutrients, so the more colorful your plate is, the more varied the nutrients!

Meat, Fish, and Protein

Meats can be cooked until tender, or slow-cooked with sauce added. Ground meats such as ground turkey, beef, and pork are often easier to chew. Fish when steamed or baked are generally soft enough and require minimal chewing.

Grains and Dairy

A lot of grain and dairy foods do not need any changes to be appropriate in meals for elderly with no teeth. Many grains such as rice, oatmeal, pasta, and lightly toasted bread are all soft in their natural form

Breakfast Meals for Elderly with No Teeth

- Scrambled eggs with lightly toasted multi-grain bread, milk, and canned fruit cup
- Oatmeal or cream of wheat topped with blueberries and milk
- Breakfast smoothie made with frozen berries, spinach, milk or milk alternative, ground flax seeds, and Greek yogurt
- Eggs Benedict served with orange juice
- Lightly toasted multigrain bread topped with creamy nut butter and a banana
- French toast topped with berries and whipped cream, serve with milk
- Omelet with cheese and soft/cooked vegetables

Lunch Meals for Elderly with no Teeth

- Meat (very tender) stew with potatoes and vegetables
- Grilled cheese on multigrain bread, served with a side of soft-fruit
- Tomato soup and lightly toasted sandwich that includes meat or a nut butter
- Tuna pasta salad with cooked peas or other soft vegetables
- Macaroni and cheese served with 100% juice
- Quiche with cheese, spinach, and feta
- Lentil and vegetable soup

Dinner Meals for Elderly with No Teeth

- Cheese ravioli and tomato sauce
- Shepard's pie
- Salmon, rice, and steamed broccoli with butter
- Slow-cooked roast beef shredded with gravy, garlic mashed potatoes, and steamed green beans
- Pulled pork on a bun, served with cut-up steamed carrots
- Cheesy mashed potatoes served with very tender Salisbury steak and creamed corn
- Fish cakes, served with dipping sauce and a side of soft vegetables

Conclusion

Meals for elderly with no teeth can be tasty, easy to chew, and still meet nutrient needs. With variety and a few extra steps to steam longer, add a sauce, or make a substitution, meals can continue to be an enjoyable, appetizing experience.

Bibliography and Acknowledgement

- A.K. KantDietary patterns and health outcomesJ. Am. Diet. Assoc.(2004)
- A.L. Anderson et al. Dietary patterns and survival of older adultsJ. Am. Diet. Assoc.(2011)
- C. Palacios et al.Is vitamin D deficiency a major global public health problem? J. Steroid Biochem. Mol. Biol.(2014)
- D.E. King et al.Trends in dietary fiber intake in the United States 1999–2008J. Acad. Nutr. Diet.(2012)
- E.M. Inelmen et al.Differences in dietary patterns between older and younger obese and overweight outpatientsJ. Nutr. Health Aging(2008)
- Gopinath et al.Adherence to dietary guidelines positively affects quality of life and functional status of older adults J. Acad. Nutr. Diet.(2014)
- H.A. Hiza et al.Diet quality of Americans differs by age sex, race/ethnicity, income, and education levelJ. Acad. Nutr. Diet.(2013)
- J.A. Zimmerman et al.Nutritional control of agingExp. Gerontol.(2003)
  J.C. GallagherVitamin D and agingEndocrinol. Metab. Clin. North Am.(2013)
- K. Zhu et al.Adequacy and change in nutrient and food intakes with aging in a seven-year cohort study in elderly womenJ. Nutr. Health Aging(2010)
- L.A. Berner et al.Characterization of dietary protein among older adults in the United States: amount animal sources, and meal patternsJ. Acad. Nutr. Diet.(2013)
- M. Asp et al.Physical mobility, physical activity, and obesity among elderly: findings from a large population-based Swedish surveyPublic Health(2017)
- N.E. Deutz et al. Protein intake and exercise for optimal muscle function with aging: recommendations from the ESPEN Expert GroupClin. Nutr.(2014)
- P. Wakimoto et al.Dietary intake, dietary patterns, and changes with age: an epidemiological perspectiveJ. Gerontol. A. Biol. Sci. Med. Sci.(200
- R. Johnston et al.Eating and aging. Trends in dietary intake among older Americans from 1977 to 2010J. Nutr. Health Aging(2014)
- S.E. Power et al.Food and nutrient intake of Irish community-dwelling elderly subjects: who is at nutritional risk?J. Nutr. Health Aging(2014)
- S.K. Jyvakorpi et al.High proportions of older people with normal nutritional status have poor protein intake and low diet qualityArch. Gerontol. Geriatr. (2016)
- S.M. Solon-Biet et al.The ratio of macronutrients not caloric intake, dictates cardiometabolic health, aging, and longevity in ad libitum-fed miceCell Metab.(2014)
- W. Leslie et al.Aging, nutritional status and healthHealthcare(2015)
- Y. Boirie et al.Nutrition and protein energy homeostasis in elderlyMech. Ageing Dev.(2014)
- Zhou, A.; Selvanayagam, J.B.; Hyppönen, E. Non-linear Mendelian randomization analyses support a role for vitamin D deficiency in cardiovascular disease risk. Eur. Heart J. 2022, 43, 1731–1739. [Google Scholar] [CrossRef]

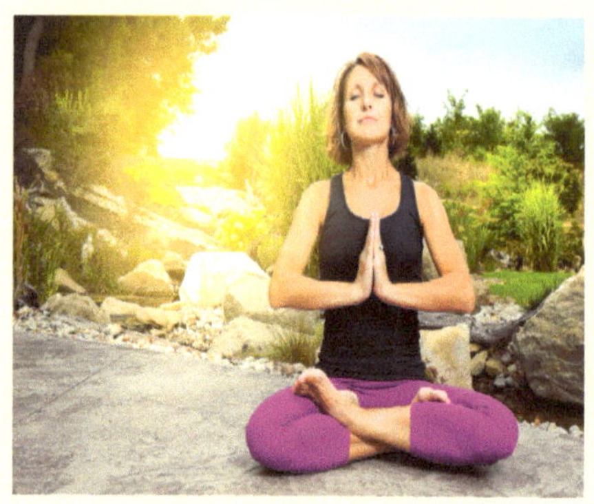

Ayurvedic Guidelines Of The Daily Routines And Healthy Aging

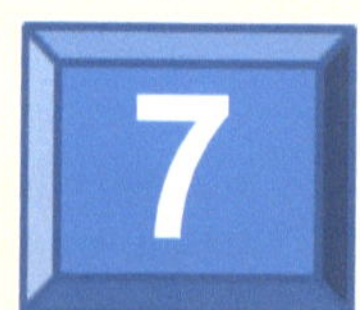

PART 1. DAILY ROUTINES

A daily routine is absolutely necessary to bring radical change in body, mind, and consciousness. Routine helps to establish balance in one's constitution. It also regularizes a person's biological clock, aids digestion, absorption and assimilation, and generates self-esteem, discipline, peace, happiness, and longevity.

1. Wake Up Early in the Morning

It is good to wake up before the sun rises, when there are loving (sattvic) qualities in nature that bring peace of mind and freshness to the senses. Sunrise varies according to the seasons, but on average vata people should get up about 6 a.m., pitta people by 5:30 a.m., and kapha by 4:30 a.m. Right after waking, look at your hands for a few moments, then gently move them over your face and chest down to the waist. This cleans the aura.

2. Say a Prayer before Leaving the Bed

"Dear God, you are inside of me, within my very breath, within each bird, each mighty mountain.
Your sweet touch reaches everything and I am well protected. Thank you God for this beautiful day before me. May joy, love, peace and compassion be part of my life and all those around me on this day. I am healing and I am healed." After this prayer touch the ground with your right hand, then the same hand to the forehead, with great love and respect to Mother Earth.

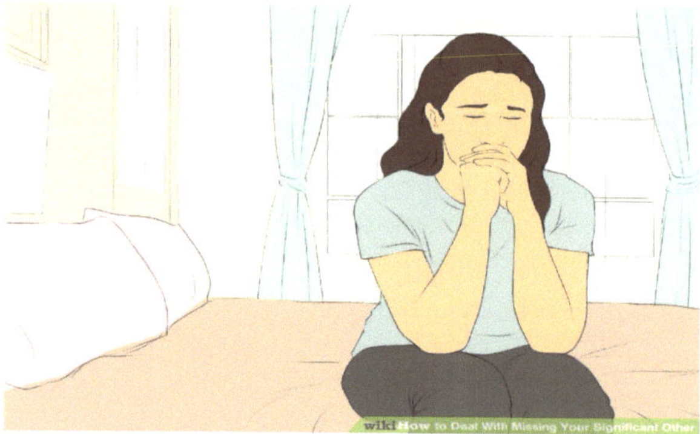

Fig. 7.1 A young lady is saying a prayer before leaving bed.

3. Clean the Face, Mouth, and Eyes

Splash your face with cold water and rinse out your mouth. Wash your eyes with cool water (or one of the eye washes mentioned below) and massage the eyelids by gently rubbing them. Blink your eyes 7 times and rotate your eyes in all directions. Dry your face with a clean towel.

Tridoshic eyewash: try triphala eyewash -¼ tsp. in 1 cup water, boil for 10 minutes, cool and strain.

Pitta eyewash: use cool water or rose water from organic rose petals – most commercial rose water has chemicals in it that will sting the eyes.

Kapha eyewash: try diluted cranberry juice, 3-5 drops in a teaspoon of distilled water.

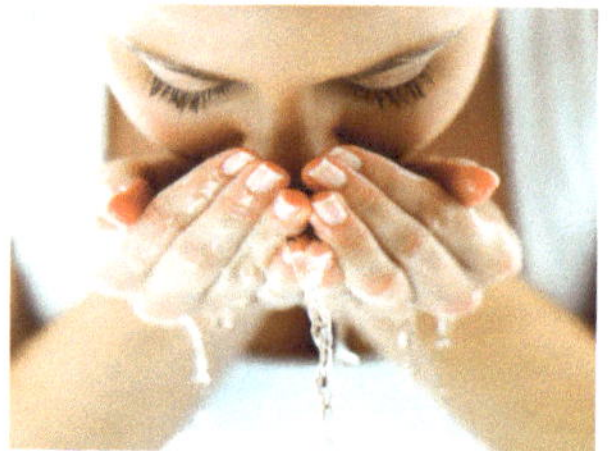

Face wash

Netra basti

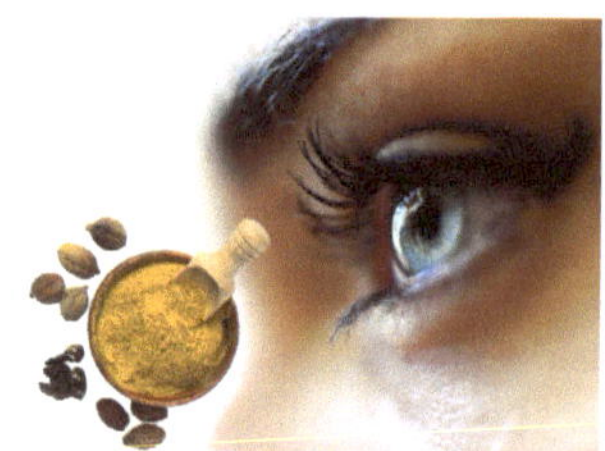

Triphala eye wash

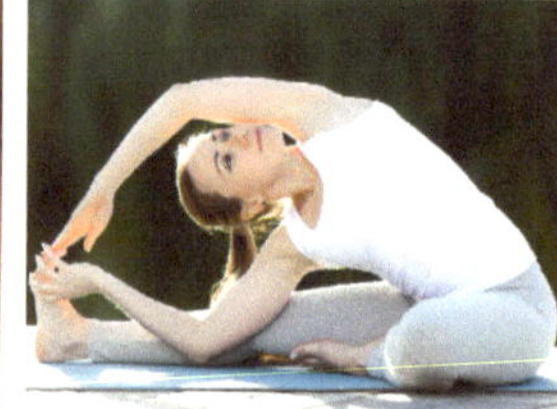

Practice Netra Vyayam

Fig 7.2 A young lady is washing her face, doing netra wash with oil,triphala eye wash and netra yogic eye exercises

4. Drink Water in the Morning

Then drink a glass of room temperature water, preferably from a pure copper cup filled the night before. This washes the GI track, flushes the kidneys, and stimulates peristalsis. It is not a good idea to start the day with tea or coffee, as this drains kidney energy, stresses the adrenals, causes constipation, and is habit-forming.

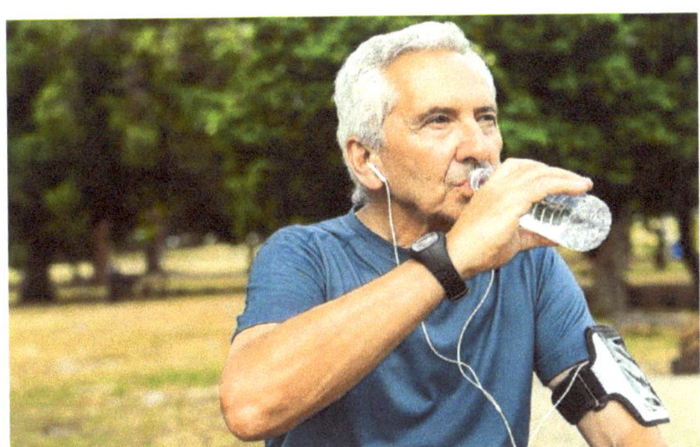

Fig. 7.3 Elderly person is drinking water in the morning

5. Evacuation

Sit, or better squat, on the toilet and have a bowel movement. Improper digestion of the previous night's meal or lack of sound sleep can prevent this. However the water, followed by sitting on the toilet at a set time each day, helps to regulate bowel movements. Alternate nostril breathing may also help. After evacuation wash the anal orifice with warm water, then the hands with soap.

6. Scrape your Tongue

Gently scrape the tongue from the back forward, until you have scraped the whole surface for 7-14 strokes. This stimulates the internal organs, helps digestion, and removes dead bacteria. Ideally, vata can use a gold scraper, pitta a silver one, and kapha copper. Stainless steel can be used by all people.

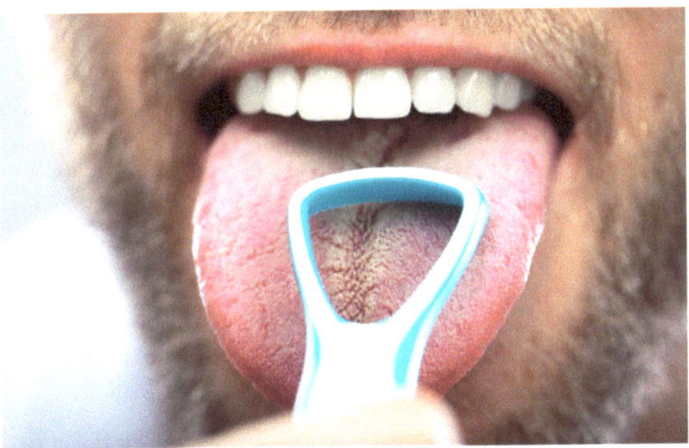

Fig.7.4 Gently scrape the tongue from the back forward,

7. Clean your Teeth

Always use a soft toothbrush and an astringent, pungent, and bitter toothpaste or powder. The traditional Indian toothbrush is a neem stick, which dislodges fine food particles from between teeth and makes strong, healthy gums. Licorice root sticks are also used. Roasted almond shell powder can be used for vata and kapha, and ground neem for pitta.

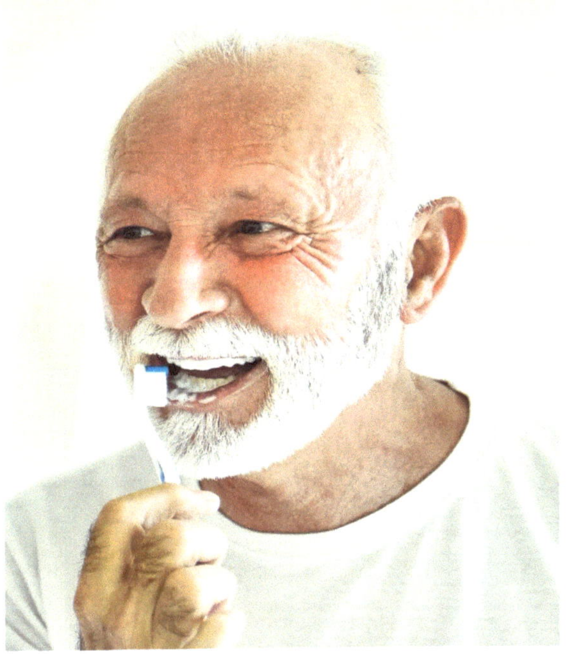

Fig. 7.5 Elderly person is cleaning his teeth in the morning

8. Gargling

To strengthen teeth, gums, and jaw, improve the voice and remove wrinkles from cheeks, gargle twice a day with warm sesame oil. Hold the oil in your mouth, swish it around vigorously, then spit it out and gently massage the gums with a finger.

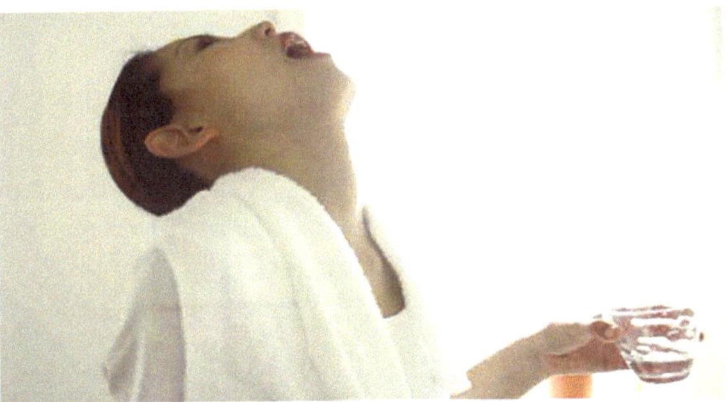

Fig. 7.6 Person is gargling twice a day with warm sesame oil.

9. Chewing

Chewing a handful of sesame seeds helps receding gums and strengthens teeth. Alternatively, chew 3-5 dried dates and an inch of dried coconut meat. Chewing in the morning stimulates the liver and the stomach and improves digestive fire. After chewing, brush the teeth again without using toothpaste or powder

10. Nasal Drops (Nasya)

Putting 3 to 5 drops of warm ghee or oil into each nostril in the morning helps to lubricate the nose, clean the sinuses, and improve voice, vision, and mental clarity. Our nose is the door to the brain, so nose drops nourish prana and bring intelligence.

1.**For vata:** sesame oil, ghee, or vacha (calamus) oil.
2.**For pitta**: brahmi ghee, sunflower or coconut oil.
3.**For kapha:** vacha (calamus root) oil.

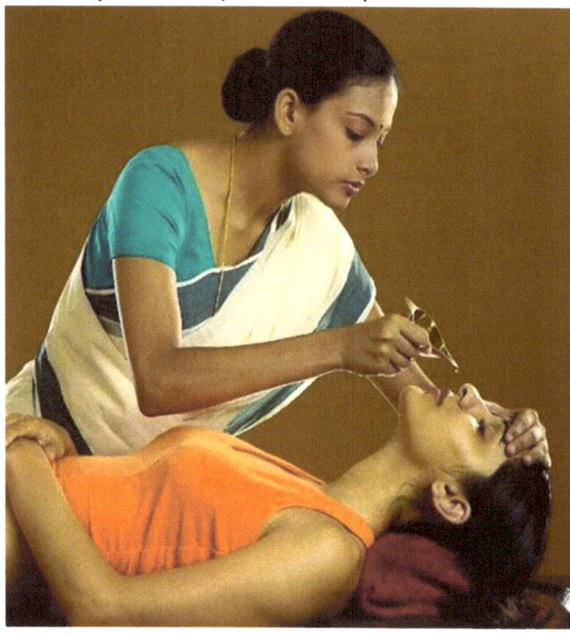

Fig. 7.7 Nurse is putting 3 to 5 drops of warm oil into each nostril in the morning

11. Oil Drops in the Ears (Karana purana)

Conditions such as ringing in the ears, excess ear wax, poor hearing, lockjaw, and TMJ, are all due to vata in the ears. Putting 5 drops of warm sesame oil in each ear can help these disorders.

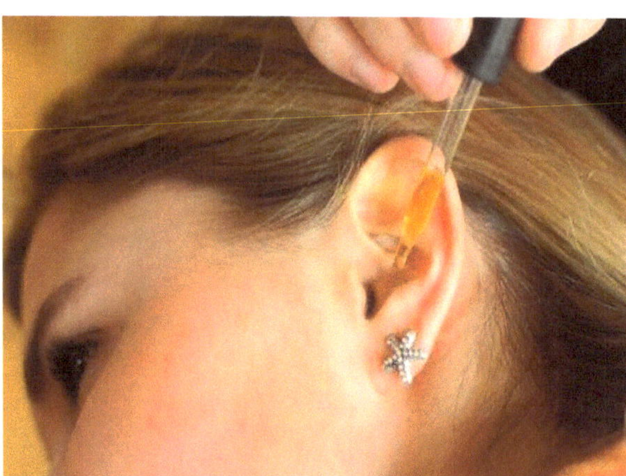

Fig. 7.8 Nurse is Putting 5 drops of warm sesame oil in each ear

12. Apply Oil to the Head & Body (Abhyanga)

Rub warm oil over the head and body. Gentle, daily oil massage of the scalp can bring happiness, as well as prevent headache, baldness, graying, and receding hairline. Oiling your body before bedtime will help induce sound sleep and keep the skin soft.

1.For **vata** use warm sesame oil.
2.For **pitta** use warm sunflower or coconut oil.
3.For **kapha** use warm sunflower or mustard oil.

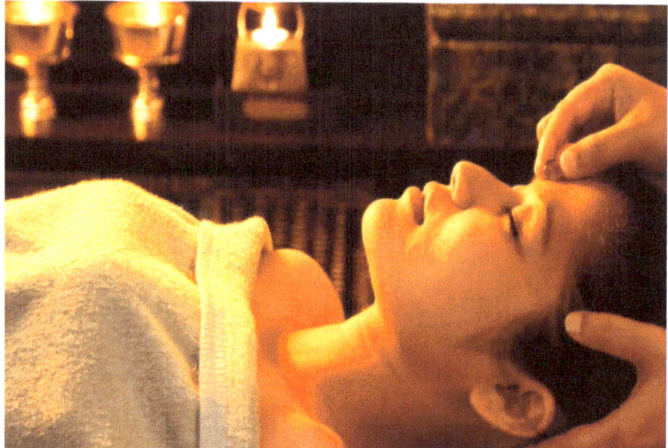

Fig. 7.9 Applying Oil to the Head & Body (Abhyanga

13. Bathing

Bathing is cleansing and refreshing. It removes sweat, dirt, and fatigue, brings energy to the body, clarity to the mind, and holiness to your life.

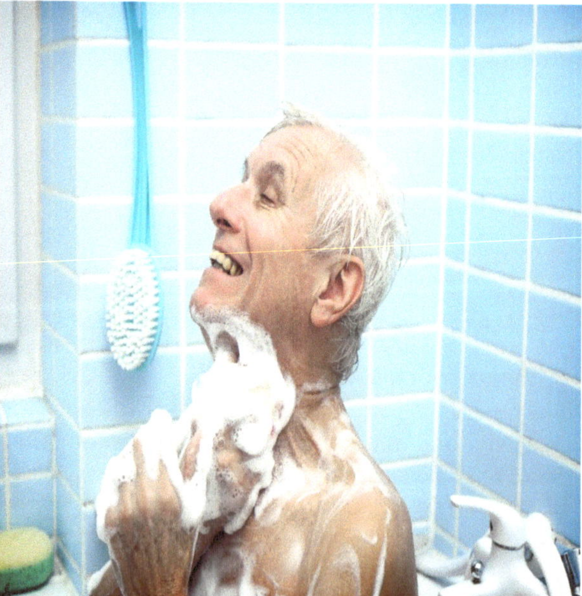

Fig. 7.10 old person is taking bath in his bath room.

14. Dressing

Wearing clean clothes brings beauty and virtue.

15. Use of Perfumes

Using natural scents, essential oils, or perfumes brings freshness, charm, and joy. It gives vitality to the body and improves self-esteem.

1.For vata the best scent to use is hina or amber.
2.For pitta try using khus, sandalwood, or jasmine.
3.For kapha use either amber or musk.

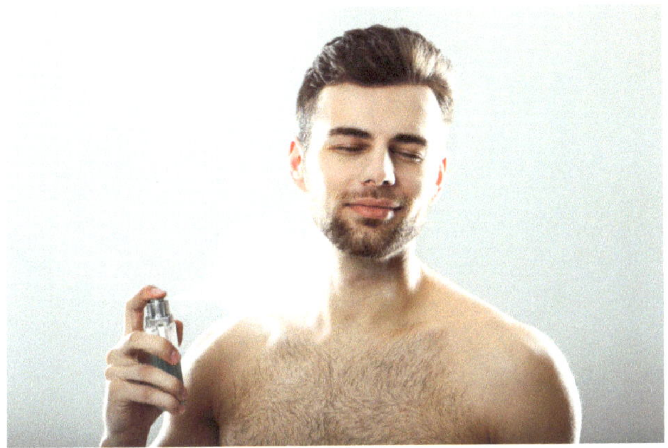

Fig. 7.11 young person is applying perfume over his body.

16. Exercise

Regular exercise, especially yoga, improves circulation, strength, and endurance. It helps one relax and have sound sleep, and improves digestion and elimination. Exercise daily to half of your capacity, which is until sweat forms on the forehead, armpits, and spine.

1.**Vata:** Sun salutation x 12, done slowly; Leg lifting; Camel; Cobra; Cat; Cow. Slow, gentle exercise.
2.**Pitta:** Moon salutation x 16, moderately fast; Fish; Boat; Bow. Calming exercise.
3.**Kapha:** Sun salutation x 12, done rapidly; Bridge; Peacock; Palm tree; Lion. Vigorous exercise.

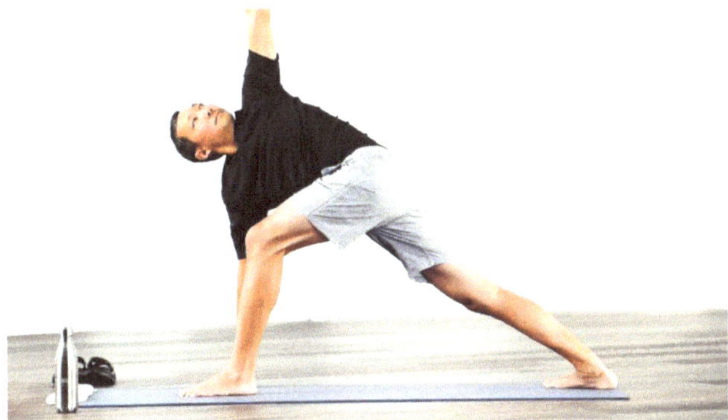

Fig.7.12 person is doing regular yoga, exercise, improves circulation, strength, and endurance.

17. Pranayama

After exercise, sit quietly and do some deep breathing exercises as follows:

- 12 alternate nostril breaths for vata;
- 16 cooling shitali breaths (curling up your tongue lengthwise and breathing through it) for pitta;
- 100 bhastrika (short, fast breaths) for kapha.

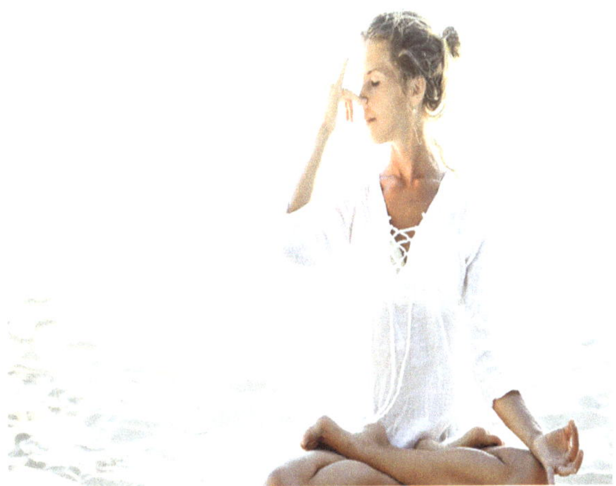

Fig.7.13 Young lady is doing Pranayama for healthy living.

18. Meditation

It is important to meditate morning and evening for at least 15 minutes. Meditate in the way you are accustomed, or try the "Empty Bowl Meditation". Meditation brings balance and peace into your life

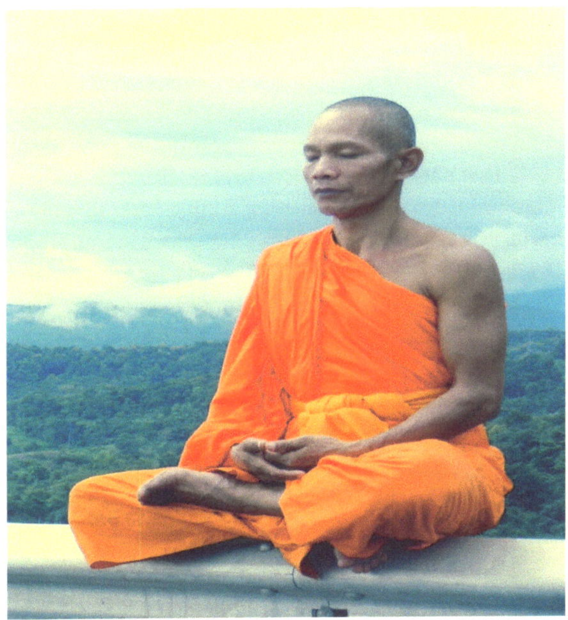

Fig.7.14 A sadhu is practicing meditation in achieving mental peace

PART 11. AYURVEDA AND HEALTHY AGING

The world's population is aging, most people will live beyond 60 and by 2050, about a fourth of the world is likely to be older than 60 (WHO). Society often glorifies youth and ageism is a challenge but the fact is we will all grow old. Aging is a transition that should be celebrated for adding serenity and wisdom. How best can we be active and healthy in our golden years?

Common, costly, and preventable health problems that aging adults face (CDC) include chronic diseases like heart disease, stroke, cancer, Type 2 diabetes, obesity, and arthritis. Mental health, cognitive decline, falls, the health of sense organs and joints, and staying connected with the community are other challenges.

Ayurveda and aging

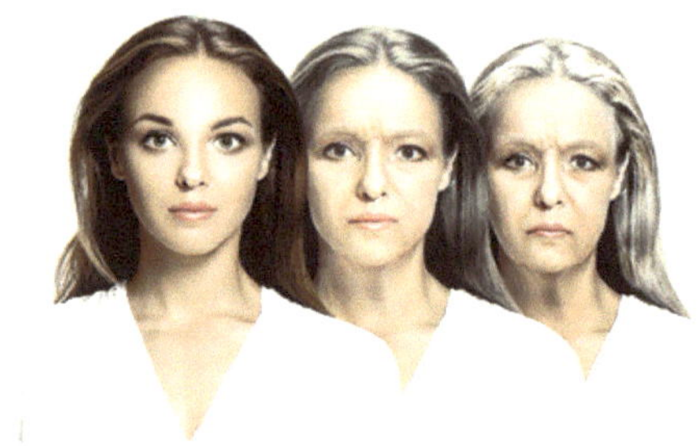

Fig. 7.15 Awomen is aging gracefully

Ayurveda defines Jara or aging as a natural phenomenon, inevitable as the seasons, hunger, or thirst. The difference is that it is degenerative. Of the Doshas (energy principals), Kapha dominates during childhood, Pitta during youth, and aging post 50 or 60 is the Vata stage of life. Health depends on the status of Doshas and can bring about early depletion and aging or delay the process and make it smoother. Diseases are hastened by wrong nutrition and lifestyle choices and misuse of senses.

Ayurveda aids natural, holistic, healthy aging and helps prevent and manage chronic disorders. A study found using preventive Ayurveda techniques during late youth and middle-age can reduce health issues in the elderly and increase longevity. I find Ayurvedic strategies for healthy aging to be similar to those of 'Blue Zone' areas of high longevity like Okinawa in Japan

Principles for healthy aging

Ayurveda focuses on,

- **Balancing Vata** - Unbalanced Vata (Dosha of air and ether) causes dryness, degeneration, feeling cold, joint disorders, reduced bone density, and digestive and sleep disturbances. These increase in fall and early winter. Find tips on balancing Vata here.
- Enhancing Ojas- Ojas is the body's strength and vitality that is responsible for our immunity and mental resistance against stress.
- Employing Rasayana or rejuvenating, anti-aging strategies, herbs, and therapies.

Tips for aging gracefully

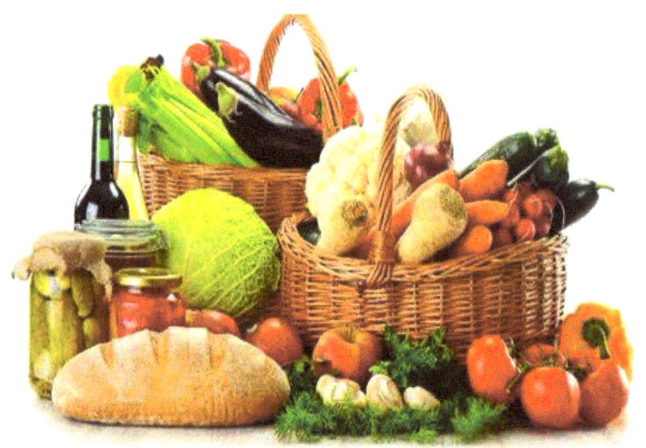

Fig. 7.16 Role of diet in aging gracefully

1.Nutrition and Metabolism – A regulated Agni (digestive and metabolic fire) has a profound impact on healthy aging. Nurture this by eating easy to digest appropriately spiced fresh food at regular meal timings; avoid skipping meals, overeating, eating late, or having incompatible, junk, or processed food. Make lunch the biggest meal of the day and favor foods high in antioxidants, fruits, vegetables, whole grains, legumes, and nuts incorporating all six tastes (read more here). Reduce caffeine and have herbal teas instead. Try periodic cleansing which detoxifies the system and kicks in cellular regeneration or autophagy.

2.Sleep is rejuvenating – Poor sleep disrupts circadian rhythms and can trigger depression, chronic inflammation, and metabolic disorders like diabetes, obesity, and cardiovascular diseases. Meditation and simple Ayurvedic principles are great sleep aids.

3.Follow a routine - Researchers have found that following circadian rhythms improves longevity. Ayurveda accords high importance to a routine with Dinacharya (daily rhythms) and Ritucharya (seasonal guidelines) for healthy aging. Stay grounded but avoid inertia with creative hobbies and learn new things that challenge the mind.

4.Oleation – Snehana or oleation in Sanskrit also means self-love and helps combat Vata-triggered dryness,

•Abhyanga (Massage) – Self-massage with warm oil improves circulation, skin and joint health, balances Doshas, and is recommended for CNS conditions and stress reduction.

•Internal oil/hydration – Make sure to add healthy fats, ghee, and oils in your diet and hydrate enough.

5.Yoga and Exercise :-Yoga improves flexibility, joint health, bladder control, digestive disturbances like constipation, sleep, and mental health. Researchers at Duke found that long-term yoga practitioners (who practiced 45 minutes 3-4 a week) had protective effects on the aging brain and greater gray matter in parts related to emotional regulation and stress. For women, the transition to menopause can be eased by Ayurveda and Yoga (read more here). Similarly, moderate physical exercise in older people helps retain cognitive abilities longer.

6.Meditation:- Ayurveda recommends meditation to protect and enhance Ojas. There are multiple studies about how meditation delays the process of aging through stress reduction, physical and mental benefits, improved cognitive function, enhanced neuroplasticity, and offsetting age-related cortical thinning of the brain.

7.Panchakarma:-Panchakarma is a powerful rejuvenating, detoxifying treatment in Ayurveda, individualized to help chronic and degenerative disorders. It aids circulation, cerebral blood flow, lymphatic drainage and helps prevent the recurrence of ailments. Panchakarma involves a pretreatment, primary treatment, and most importantly, posttreatment rejuvenation with herbs, dietary, and lifestyle changes.

8.Rasayana herbs: Formulations like Chyawanprash (named after Sage Chyawana who is said taken Chyawanprash to restore vitality after marrying a young damsel), Shakti Drops, Triphala and Amruth are immune-boosting daily tonics (Nitya Rasayanas). However, Ayurveda is personalized; do consult an Ayurvedic Practitioner before taking herbs.

Triphala Recipe (as a Daily Tonic) - 3.5 ounces of Triphala made into a paste with water can be applied over a clean iron vessel or plate and left to dry for 24 hours. Scrape the paste, store it in a clean, dry container else it can spoil. This can be stored for 1-2 months, made again, and taken for a year. Have 1-2 teaspoons daily in the morning on an empty stomach with 1 tsp honey (if tolerated well) and water. Take 1 teaspoon of ghee or sesame oil in your diet in the evening. If Triphala is taken in the night, consume ghee/sesame oil while having the next day's breakfast.

9. Protect Sense Organs: Attend to senses organs in your daily regimen through practices like splashing

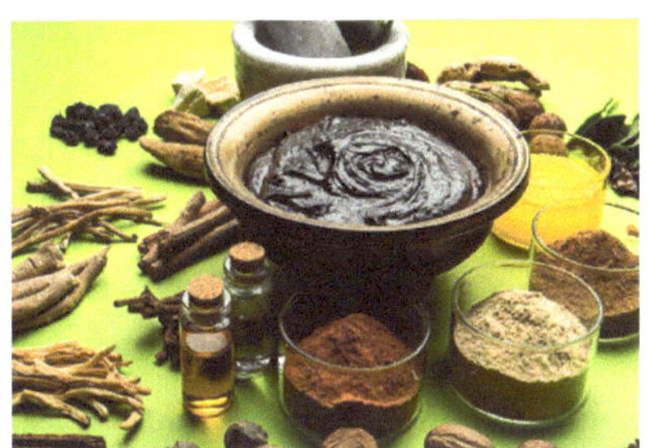

Fig. 7.17 Rasayana herbs in aging

the eyes with water, an eye-care routine, tongue cleaning, oil pulling, and oiling ears and nostrils (Nasya). Avoid sensory overload and schedule media breaks. A radical rejuvenation concept in Ayurveda is intramural-rejuvenation (kutipravesika) where a person is treated inside a special cottage in isolation. This is practiced in limited settings now and I believe Silent Retreats work on a somewhat similar principle of rejuvenation!

10. Ayurveda and Skin Health: Amongst visible signs of aging are sparse and falling hair, wrinkles, pigmentation, and sagging skin, and some of us wear them as trophies of a life well spent! However, self-care is always advised. Ashish Pandya, VP Education, Shankara Naturals beautifully enunciates "Ayurveda defines beauty as inner beauty (health), outer beauty and lasting beauty (enduring health). Aging gracefully is about attending to all these levels."

Here are some tips,

•For **Vata** skin, susceptible to wrinkles and premature aging, opt for products that nourish and rehydrate. Favor warm oil self-massage and natural moisturizers.

•For **Pitta** skin, use sunscreens and good facial/body oils. Avoid tanning treatments that expose sensitive skin to steam or heat for an extended time.

•For **Kapha** skin, cleanse with a gentle exfoliant, try a light, warm oil-massage, and a suitable moisturizer.

11. Stay connected – Loneliness is the bane of our society that needs addressing.

Foster social connections with your community or spiritual group.

• Connect with yourself through nature walks, meditation, and creative pursuits

• Connect with a higher purpose (Brahmacharya), one of the pillars of health in Ayurveda that lends resilience.

• Sadvritta is a code of ethics focused on social values and service that strengthen our mental fabric. A 50-year study involving high school graduates found increased longevity in those who performed selfless service. An added bonus is the community we build through service activities.

Bibliography and Acknowledgement

1. Ashtanga Hridayam of Vagbhata, Pandit Hari Sadashiv Sastri Paradkar,Sutrasthana, Ch 2,verse1. Varanasi: Chaukhamba Sanskrit Sansthan; 2010.p. 23.

2. Sushrut Samhita of Dalhan and Gayadas edited by Keval Krushna Thakaral, Sutrasthana, ch 15 verse 41.Varanasi Chaukhamba Orientaliya 2014,p.179.

3. Ashtanga Hridayam of Vagbhata, Saroj Hindi Vyakhya,Sutrasthana, Ch 1 verse 14, Chaukhamba Sanskrit Prakashana Delhi; 2009.p. 11.

4. Ashtanga Hridayam of Vagbhata, Saroj Hindi Vya khy a,Su tra stha na, Ch 1 2 ver se 3 4-44, Chaukhamba Sanskrit Prakashana Delhi; 2009.p. 197-198.

5. Sushrut Samhita of Dalhan and Gayadas edited by Keval Krushna Thakaral, Sutrasthana, ch 21 verse 36.Varanasi Chaukhamba Orientaliya 2014,p.260.

6. Ashtanga Hridayam of Vagbhata, Saroj Hindi Vyakhya,Sutrasthana, Ch 2 verse 1, Chaukhamba Sanskrit Prakashana Delhi; 2009.p. 27.

7. Ashtanga Hridayam of Vagbhata, Saroj Hindi Vy a k h y a , S u t r a s t h a n a , C h 1 v e r s e 1 , haukhambaSanskrit Prakashana Delhi; 2009.p.27

8. Ashtanga Hridayam of Vagbhata, Saroj Hindi Vyakhya,Sutrasthana, Ch 1 verse 2-3, Chaukhamba Sanskrit Prakashana Delhi; 2009.p. 28.

9. Rajeshwar dutt Shastri, commented by Tarashankar Mishra, Swasthavrittasamuchchya, 11th edition, published by AkhileshwarduttaMishara, Assi, Varanasi, UP, 1985, page no. 8-40.

10. CharakSamhita of Agnivesha, Ayurved Dipika Commentry edited by Yadavji Trikamji , Sutrasthana 5 verse 71-73 Chaukhamba Surbharti Prakashan, Varanasi, 2008, page no 42.

11. CharakSamhita of Agnivesha, Ayurved Dipika Commentry edited by Yadavji Trikamji , Sutrasthan 5 verse 74-75 Chaukhamba Surbharti Prakashan, Varanasi, 2008, page no 42.

12. CharakSamhita of Agnivesha, Ayurved Dipika Commentry edited by Yadavji Trikamji , Sutrasthan
5 verse 14-19 page no Chaukhamba Surbharti Prakashan, Varanasi, 2008, 38- 39.

13. CharakSamhita of Agnivesha, Ayurved Dipika Commentry edited by Yadavji Trikamji , Sutrasthana 5 verse 20-56 Chaukhamba Surbharti Prakashan, Varanasi, 2008, page no 39-41.

14. CharakSamhita of Agnivesha, Ayurved Dipika Commentry edited by Yadavji Trikamji , Sutrasthan 5vers 56-71 Chaukhamba Surbharti Prakashan, Varanasi, 2008, page no 41-42.

15. CharakSamhita of Agnivesha, Ayurved Dipika Commentry edited by Yadavji Trikamji , Sutrasthana 5 verse 76-80 Chaukhamba Surbharti Prakashan, Varanasi, 2008, page no 42.

16. Ashtanghridyayam of Vagbhata, Saroj Hindi Vy a k h y a , Su t r a s t h a n a , C h 2 v e r s e 1 6 - 1 7 , Chaukhamba Sanskrit Prakashana Delhi; 2009.p. 34.

17. Susruta, Susruta Samhita, Ayurveda tatva sandipika Hindi Commentry by Kaviraj.Ambika dutt Shastri, Chikitsasthan,Chaukhamba Sanskrit Samsthana, Varanasi, 2001, page 105-110.

18. Vagbhata, Astanga Samgraha, Hindi Commentry by
Kaviraj Atridev Gupta, Sutrasthana Ch 1 verse 1 Chaukhamba Krushnadasa Academy, Varanasi, 2016,p.19.

19 Vagbhat, Astanga Samgraha, Hindi Commentry by Kaviraj Atridev Gupta, Sutrasthana Ch 1 verse 1 Chaukhamba Krushnadasa Academy, Varanasi, 2016,p.19.

20 The awakening cortisol response: methodological issues and significance. Stress. Clow A, Thorn L, Evans P, Hucklebridge F. 2004 Mar 1;7(1):29-37.

21 Cortisol and immunity. Medical hypotheses. Jefferies WM. 1991 Mar 1;34(3):198-208.

22 A Decent Science Behind the Brahma Muhurta Gupta R, Shukla O, ShrivastavaV, P. .IJAHM, 2017 Nov-Dec.;7(6):3005-9)

23.Ashtang hridyayam of Vagbhata, Saroj Hindi Vyakhya,Sutrasthana, Ch 7 verse 65, Chaukhamba Sanskrit Prakashana Delhi; 2009.p. 130.

24.Ashtang hridyayam of Vagbhata, Saroj Hindi Vya khya ,Sut r ast h ana, Ch 4 v erse 12-- 1 3Chaukhamba Sanskrit Prakashana Delhi; 2009.p. 58.

25.Ashtang hridyayam of Vagbhata, Saroj Hindi Vyakhya,Sutrasthana, Ch 1 verse 8, Chaukhamba Sanskrit Prakashana Delhi; 2009.p. 7-8.

26.Ashtang hridyayam of Vagbhata, Saroj Hindi Vyakhya,Sutrasthana, Ch 4 verse 2-7, Chaukhamba Sanskrit Prakashana Delhi; 2009.p. 57-58.

27 Charak Samhita of Agnivesha, Ayurved Dipika Commentry edited by Yadavji Trikamji , Sutrasthan 5 verse 71 Chaukhamba Surbharti Prakashan, Varanasi, 2008, page no 42.

28 Ashtang hridyayam of Vagbhata, Saroj Hindi Vyakhya,Sutrasthana, Ch 2 verse 2, Chaukhamba Sanskrit Prakashana Delhi; 2009.p. 28.

29.Ashtang hridyayam of Vagbhata, Saroj Hindi Vyakhya,Sutrasthana, Ch 2 verse 2, Chaukhamba Sanskrit Prakashana Delhi; 2009.p. 28.

30. Are all additives of toothpastes rational?Mani A, Thawani V; Journal of Mahatma Gandhi Institute of Medical Sciences. 2019 Jul 1;24(2):71.a

31.Charak Samhita of Agnivesha, Ayurved Dipika Commentry edited by Yadavji Trikamji , Sutrasthana 5 verse 74-75 Chaukhamba Surbharti Prakashan, Varanasi, 2008, page no 42.

32 Ohmori M, Baba R, Miyazaki A, Sato H, Katano S, Sawaki A, Tanabe S, Masatuki N, Yasukawa T, Hasegawa A, Imade S. P19 A study for the effect of tongue cleaning. Oral Diseases. 2005 Mar; 11:111-2.

33 CharakSamhita of Agnivesha, Ayurved Dipika Commentry edited by Yadavji Trikamji , Sutrasthan 5verse78-80 Chaukhamba Surbharti Prakashan, Varanasi, 2008, page no 42.

34. Effect of Oil Pulling with Sesame Oil on Plaque-induced Gingivitis: A Microbiological Study. Saravanan, D, Ramkumar, S., &Vineetha, K. (1970); Journal of Oro-facial Research, 3(3), 175– 180.

35 Efficacy of oil pulling with sesame oil in comparison with other oils and chlorhexidine for oral health: a systematic review.Jeevan S, Sindhu R, Manipal S, Prabu D, Mohan R, Bharathwaj VV; . Journal of Pharmaceutical Sciences and Research. 2019 Nov 1;11(11):3573-8

36 Griessl T, Zechel-Gran S, Olejniczak S, Weigel M, Hain T, Domann E. High-resolution taxonomic examination of the oral microbiome after oil pulling with standardized sunflower seed oil and healthy par tic ipants: A p ilot stu dy. Cl inic al O ral Investigations. 2021 May;25(5):2689-703.

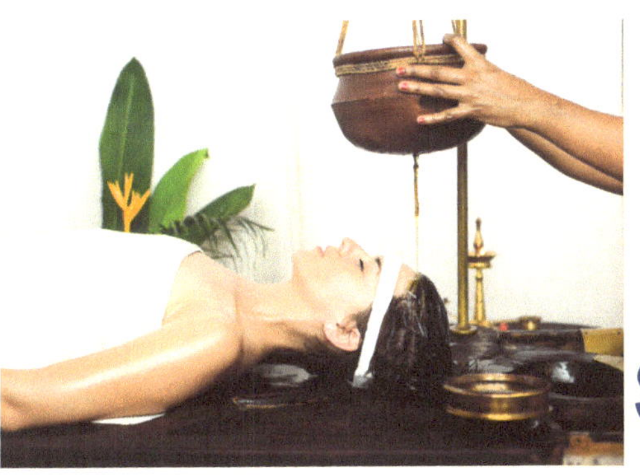

Ayurveda And The Science Of Aging

Aging has been defined as the total sum of physiological changes that progressively leads to the death of the individual. It is also defined as the intrinsic, inevitable, and irreversible age-associated loss of viability that render us more susceptible to a number of diseases and death or a progressive functional decline of physiological function and a decrease in fecundity with age. Undoubtedly, human aging is associated with a wide range of physiological and cellular changes that limit our normal functions and make us more susceptible to death. Aging has two main components, Chronological Aging which refers to the actual age of the person in terms of years, months, and days. This component of aging is unstoppable, unchangeable and irreversible. Physiological/Biological aging is the second component and refers to an individual's development and changes based on certain cellular or molecular parameters. This involves looking at the individuals as they are and as they function, and not when they are born . Thus, biological aging is a set of processes that triggers deterioration of health and ultimately to death as a function of chronological age. Unlike chronological aging, biological aging can be reversed or delayed . Other terms that constitute aging include:

Lifespan: It is the period of time during which we are alive. Lifespan also includes the years spent in poor health as there are several age-associated health conditions that lack proper treatment or cure . Morbidity: The period of ill health during an individual's lifespan is referred to as morbidity. Although our lifespans have increased significantly due to better nutrition and modern medicine, middle-aged and elderly people suffer many years of ill health before they die. Age-associated diseases include heart disease, stroke, diabetes, osteoporosis, and other chronic problems resulting in the individual being in a state of morbid condition .

Healthspan: Health span is equal to the lifespan devoid of the amount of time an individual spends in ill health (Lifespan–morbidity). This is the period in an individual's life during which the person is generally healthy and free from serious or chronic illness. Thus, healthspan refers to how long an individual lives a disease-free healthy life .

Therefore, biological aging in terms of healthspan is a result of complex structural and functional changes across molecules, cells, tissues and whole body systems. Its manifestation is influenced by several factors including genomic instability, telomere attrition, epigenetic alterations, loss of proteostasis, deregulated nutrient sensing, mitochondrial dysfunction, cellular senescence, stem cell exhaustion, and altered intra-and intercellular communication. Since aging is accompanied by impairment of normal physiological functioning of cells, tissue, organs and bodily systems that increases the risk of death, some in the aging field consider aging itself to be a deadly disease .

There is no one single cause or trigger of the aging phenomenon as there are many different and often conflicting theories of aging. At the cellular level, changes that contribute to aging include reduction in stem cell proliferation in a number of tissues, accumulation of toxic protein aggregates and free radicals, accumulation of senescent cells that trigger inflammation and impairment in mitochondrial function. At the genomic level, accumulation of mutations in DNA together with faulty DNA repair processes and telomere shortening are all associated with early signs of aging. Several researchers believe that a combination of several of these factors may contribute to overall aging . Theories of aging include but are not limited to

1.Genetic theory of aging,
2.Damage or Error theory,
3.Dilman's Neuroendocrine theory,
4.DNA damage theory,
5.Free radical damage theory,
6.Gene mutations,
7.Cell divisions/telomere shortening,

8.Cellular senescence

9.Antagonistic Pleiotropy

Some of these causes may appear non-specific with regard to suitable interventions, because it is unclear which among them is more amenable to pharmacological intervention in order to reverse the aging process.

Factors that promote biological aging

While aging in itself is inevitable, there are ways to reduce or delay the pathological effects of aging. This involves looking at strategies to combat aging both at the cellular and/or genomic level and to see if any of the above mentioned triggers of aging are amenable to suitable drug interventions. Researchers propose at least seven highly intertwined processes that promote aging, thus providing a format for the identification of program mediators and therapeutic candidates. Deciphering these factors that are also responsible for age-associated diseases will be helpful in drug discovery efforts to decelerate aging . Among these factors, one that has inspired a lot of excitement is metabolism, and researchers have been trying to understand why caloric restriction extends the life span in mice and other animals . Metabolizing fewer calories could result in reduced oxidative damage or alternatively, absence of nutrients may trigger certain defense mechanisms that protect the body from decaying. Researchers have managed to identify several molecular pathways that govern metabolism. Modification of these pathways or their specific products through proper drug-based interventions, could one day mimic the life expanding effects of caloric restriction in humans without compromising on the food intake .

Another factor that is being thoroughly explored is the fallout from long term chronic inflammation. While several age-associated diseases involve the inflammatory process, long lived healthy individuals including centenarians are generally free from age-associated inflammatory diseases .

Interventionsn targeted to reduce chronic inflammation are being examined closely for their life enhancing effects . Inflammation cannot be completely shut down as our bodies need the short term adaptive inflammatory process to fight infections and ward off short term stress . Thus, we need to better understand the inflammatory process at a molecular level to see if drugs can be developed that specifically target the aberrant pathways.In addition, extension of lifespan in humans could also be achieved by lowering the rate of free radical , induced-oxidative damage to tissues, replacementand/or rejuvenation of damaged tissues and cellsreversal of harmful epigenetic changes, or enhancing the telomerase activity . Several experts are also developing strategies to combat multiple age-associated diseases at the same time .

Aging is a major risk factor for most chronic diseases and researchers agree that if we can address the issue of aging itself, we could potentially delay and diminish age-associated diseases all at once . Researchers are looking at slowing down aging with the premise that a drug targeting the aging process will not only slow down aging but will also delay age-associated pathologies and diseases . This approach is very attractive as researchers do not need to discover drugs to combat specific age-associated conditions like cancer, diabetes or dementia, but instead treat the aging process itself .

Therapies for a successful healthspan

1. **The free-radical theory of aging** suggests that antioxidant supplements, such as vitamin C, vitamin E, Q10, lipoic acid, carnosine, and N-acetylcysteine, might extend human life. However, despite several studies, it is not clear if β-carotene supplements and high doses of vitamin E extend life span or increase mortality rates .

2. **Resveratrol is a sirtuin** stimulant that has been shown to extend life in animal models, but the effect of resveratrol on lifespan in humans is unclear .

3. **The anti-diabetes drug metformin h**as shown to extend the life of animals and the US-FDA has permitted a clinical trial to see if the life-extending benefits replicate in humans. If metformin turns out to be successful in delaying the aging process, a person taking metformin would be young at 90 .

4. **Drugs like acarbose (**a common drug prescribed for Type 2 diabetes), and anti-inflammatory drugs such as masoprocol and basic aspirin extend lifespan in mice, but these drugs can have multiple effects, and their mechanism of action is not clear. The fact that they tackle chronic inflammation could just be one piece of the puzzle, not the whole solution .

5. **The most promising drug** to combat aging has been rapamycin, an immunosuppressant often used in organ transplants. In addition to life span extension, rapamycin has an unbelievably wide range of effects in mice ranging from preventing Alzheimer's and cardiovascular disease to reducing cancer

6. **Non-drug therapies** that extend lifespan include calorie restriction (CR). CR also retards age-related chronic diseases in a variety of species, including rats, mice, fish, flies, worms, and yeast. The mechanism through which this occurs is unclear

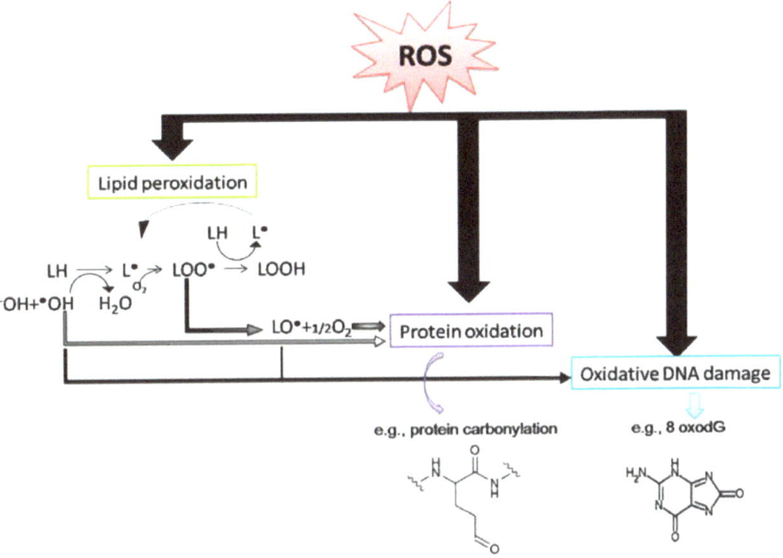

Fig.8.1 General mechanism of oxidative damage to biomolecules. Oxidative damage to lipids yields lipid peroxidation products, mainly localized at the cellular membrane, which results in a loss of membrane properties/function. Their reactive end products can induce damage to other molecules, such as proteins and DNA. In nuclear and mitochondrial DNA, 8-oxo-7,8-dihydro-2′-deoxyguanosine (8-oxodG) is one of the predominant forms of free radical-induced oxidative lesions (Valavanidis et al., 2009). Potential outcomes include dysfunction of the affected biomolecules and interference with signaling pathways. Adapted from (Thanan et al., 2014).

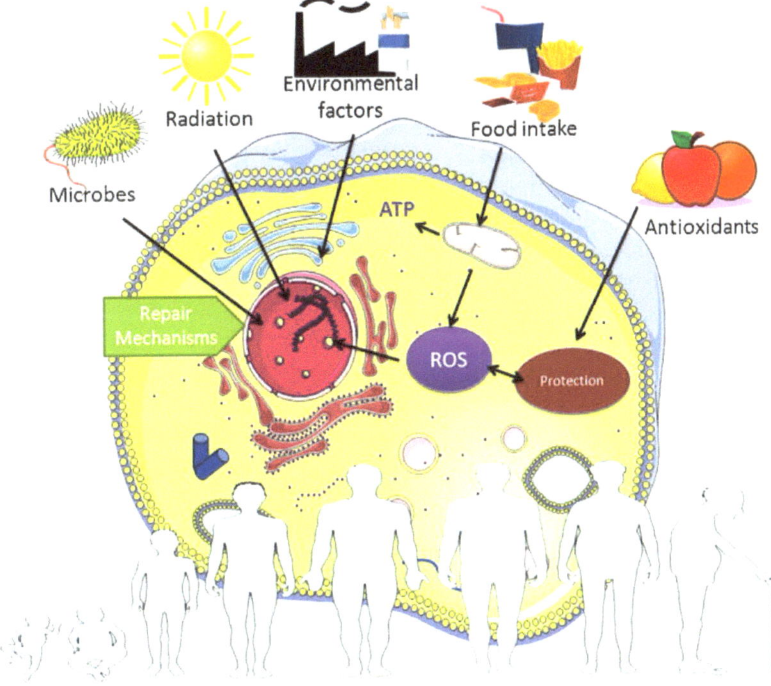

Fig.8.2 The cumulative effect of ROS over time. ROS accumulation, oxidative stress and the imbalance of the normal redox state increases exponentially with age, accompanied by a marked decline of the cell repair machinery. Note that, despite only depicting the general stress response pathways, a typical Golgi pathway has yet to be described. Nonetheless, multiple stress factors may influence gene expression in the nucleus and cell homeostasis via alterations in the function of the Golgi apparatus (Kourtis and Tavernarakis, 2011). The figure was partly created using Servier medical art image bank (Servier, France).

Therapeutic cloning, body part replacement and stem cell research could one day provide a way to generate cells, body parts, or even entire bodies that do not decay . Researchers have succeeded in growing artificial body parts in the lab, including nose, ears, tear ducts, bladders and blood vessels from human stem cells. The use of human stem cells for the purpose of cultivating organs, that can be transplanted into people, is another attractive approach to combat age-associated organ decay .

Ayurveda and science of aging

Jara also called as Vardhakya (aging) is defined as that which has become old by the act of wearing out. According to Ayurveda, Jara/aging is not a disease but a natural phenomenon like hunger, thirst or sleep. In thetheoryofnaturaldestructions(Swabhavoparamavada), Charaka describes that there is a causative factor for the manifestation of a being but there is no cause for the cessation of this manifestation, since death following birth is a state of natural flow . The term Jara denotes four entities: Nityaga which signifies continuation of consciousness, Dhari which denotes the factor(s) that prevent the body from Jara/aging, Jeevitam which represents the act of keeping alive and Anubandha that denotes transmigration of the body . Accordingly, Jara/ aging is influenced by factors affecting Shareera (physical), Indriya (emotional), Satwa (psychiclevel), Agni (metabolism)andBala/Ojas(immunity).Inaddition, Parinama (cellular transformation), Sharira vriddhikara bhavas (genotypic and phenotypic characteristics) and Garbhahinivrittikara bhava (pregnancy-induced fetal development and changes) also affect an individual's aging process . Jara is accompanied by the process of decay and manifests in the form of various degenerative changes. Although these changes are natural **(Kalaja Vriddhavastha-**natural aging), they are not pleasant . Everyone is aware that a person who has taken birth must grow and finally die, but nobody wants to grow old and certainly no one wishes to die. Humans in general consider aging and age-associated diseases as unnatural even though our choices and actions are responsible for the rapid biological aging. Misusing the five senses (pancha tanmatras) and bringing in disharmonious impressions through the five sense organs (pancha jnanendriyas), making incorrect choices that promote unhealthy transformation of the body and mind (Parinama), all trigger the disease process resulting in mental and physical suffering . Mental and physical ill-health weakens dhatusamya (homeostasis), resulting in Akalaja vriddhavastha (pathological aging) . Ayurveda takes a holistic approach toward the maintenance of dhatusamya, a state of equilibrium of normal anatomical, biological,physiological, mental and spiritual well-being . Hence a balanced state (sama) of tissue (dhatu), energy systems (Dosha), heat of transformation (Agni) and metabolic wastes (mala) constitute homeostasis in Ayurveda that leads to healthy aging (Sukhayu/Kalaja Vriddhavastha) . Some of the most important factors that affect Jara/healthy aging include:

Kala Parinama (time and transformation) is one the most important and potent factors that influences Jara or aging as it includes all creation in itself . Kala Parinama refers to the physical and mental transformation that occurs as a function of time and as we age. Being out of harmony with the rhythms and cycles of nature can trigger unhealthy transformation and disharmonious changes, making the body vulnerable to disease and rapid aging . Kala influences a human from conception till death and this time period is called Ayush (lifespan). Ayurveda divides Ayush into Vaya (various stages of life)— childhood (Bala-up to the age 16 years), adolescent/ teenage (vivardhamana, 16–20 years of age), youth (youvana, 20–30 years), matured individual (sampoornata, 30–40 years), aged individual (parihani, 40–60 years) and older adults (last stage of life-Jirna or Vriddhavastha) . Owing to the influence of Kala, various changes occur in the body during these stages of life and hence the lifestyle adopted during each stage of this growth has a profound influence on the aging process.

Prakruti refers to the biological constitution (anatomical, physiological and psychological) of an individual. The Prakruti which is unique to each individual reflects the baseline characteristics of the individual including metabolism, mental makeup, immunity, inherent strength and weakness and proclivities . Thus, Prakruti determines an individual's capacity for transformation at the physical, mental and emotional levels owing to the interactions with internal and external stimuli all of which affect the aging process .

Doshas or biological energy systems determine the longevity at the cellular level. **Vata,** which is closely related to pranic life energy, governs all life functions and biological activity and is the energy of movement. **Pitta** governs digestion and metabolism. Kapha controls anabolism and is the energy of movement. Pitta governs digestion and metabolism. **Kapha** controls anabolism and is the energy of building and lubrication that provides the body with physical form, structure, and the smooth functioning of all its parts.Health and disease is a direct reflection of the status and interaction of the Doshas in the body that in turn provokes or delays the aging process . Proper diet, exercise and a harmonious lifestyle can create a balance among these Doshas ensuring a healthy healthspan .

Subtle Doshas are subtle counterparts of Doshas and an elaboration of the mental and emotional aspects of the physical Doshas that also influence the Jara/aging process. The subtle counterparts of the biological **Vata, Pitta and Kapha** Doshas are Prana (subtlelifeenergy), Ojas (subtleimmunity)and tejas (subtle vitality/subtle fire or energy) that are necessary for smooth longevity . Prana controls breath, sensory perceptions and the thought process and thus is responsible for mind-body coordination. **Teja**s represents the digestion and transformation of sensory impressions, intelligence, thoughts, perception and awareness that results in a suitable action. **Oja**s represents robustness, strength and vitality and is responsible for the auto-immune system and mental resistance against stress. The lifespan and healthspan of an individual has a direct correlation with the person's status and integration of prana, tejas and Ojas .

Ahara (diet) is another important factor that influences aging/Jara. A poor or defective diet (GramyaAhara) together with disharmonious lifestyle triggers the vitiation of any or all three Doshas, leading to pathological changes and reduced lifespan . Poor dietary practices include among others, improper timing of food intake, eating meals late at night, incorrect choices of food, consuming stale, processed or highly refined food, cold foods, eating in a noisy environment, and eating in a stressed mental state. An over-abundance of calories and the highly refined foods together with poor eating practices may lead to increased inflammation, reduced control of infection, increased rates of cancer, increased risk for allergic disease and reduced immunity (Ojas). These changes coupled with altered enthusiasm, insomnia, and lethargy can result in failure to live out the complete lifespan

Achara (routines) refers to the physiological machinery that controls the circadian rhythm or the 24-h body clock and is another component that has an important role in the aging process. According to Ayurveda, the health of all living beings is governed by an internal clock that runs on a 24-h, light–dark cycle in conjunction with the sun and earth's movement. Ayurveda provides several guidelines about the operations of the body clock in terms of time and season-based routines called day routines (dinacharya), night routines (ratricharya) and seasonal routines (ritucharya) . These guidelines include optimal times to arise and sleep, breathing routines, elimination, bath, massage, exercise, diet, study, travel, and other pursuits. Ayurveda recommends healthy and harmonious lifestyle routines to sustain and maintain the synchronicity of the circadian rhythm that results in good health, vitality and immunity, all of which delay biological aging Modern medicine recognizes these internal clocks as the circadian rhythms that are intimately tied to our health, well-being and the aging process. In humans, these biological clocks or circadian rhythms anticipate various activities throughout the day, from waking up to sleeping and eating. In addition, these clocks regulate hormone levels, body temperature, and metabolism.

Jatharagni (digestive fire) not only regulates the digestion, absorption and assimilation of food but also has a profound influence on the lifespan and healthspan of an individual. Jatharagni is the root of all the digestive fires in the body . Jatharagni serves as the central digestive fire and is the representation for all metabolic functions in the body. This includes the digestive function, cellular metabolism, sense perception, thought function and transformation of mental and emotional impressions . If Jatharagni is too weak, the digestion of food is compromised resulting in malabsorption and accumulation of toxins (ama). If Jatharagni is too strong, it burns out the associated tissues resulting in tissue degeneration. Thus, the state of Jatharagni influences the aging process

Ayurvedic recommendations for a successful healthspan

Unlike the modern medicine approach of seeking pills and supplements or replacing body parts to extend the healthspan of the individual, Ayurveda relies on a comprehensive program that includes dietary, lifestyle, behavioral and psychological intervention for extension of healthspan. The rationale for such a broad therapeutic intervention is to restore the normal balance and functioning of all the systems simultaneously at the level of the body, mind and emotions. The entire approach is a customized and individualized approach that covers the scope of all treatment procedures to enhance the healthspan of the individual and includes the following:

Diet and conscious eating

The philosophy of conscious eating (Ahara Vihara) is emphasized in the Ayurvedic texts. According to Ayurveda, our personality is determined by what, when, where and how we eat. Ayurveda insists that conscious eating favors optimal digestion that directly and swiftly corrects imbalances and, in doing so, prevents diseases, ends suffering and delays the aging process. Ayurveda recommends the

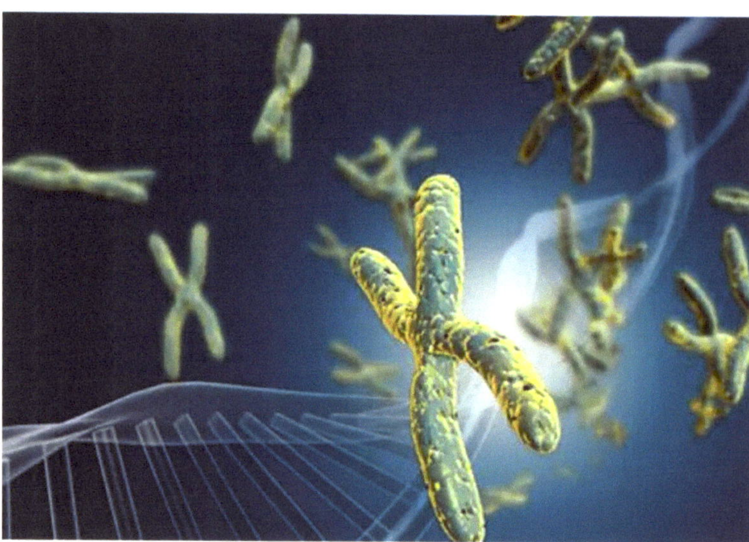

Fig.8.3 **Signs of aging appear deeper than just your skin and hair. Did you know you can see it in your DNA? That's right, your own genetic makeup indicates your age through the ends of your chromosomes, known as telomeres. These telomeres shorten as you age, which is associated with easier sickness and worse chances of survival. You can keep them longer by the way you live. Better diet and some activities can protect your DNA from the influence of aging, leading to a longer life.**

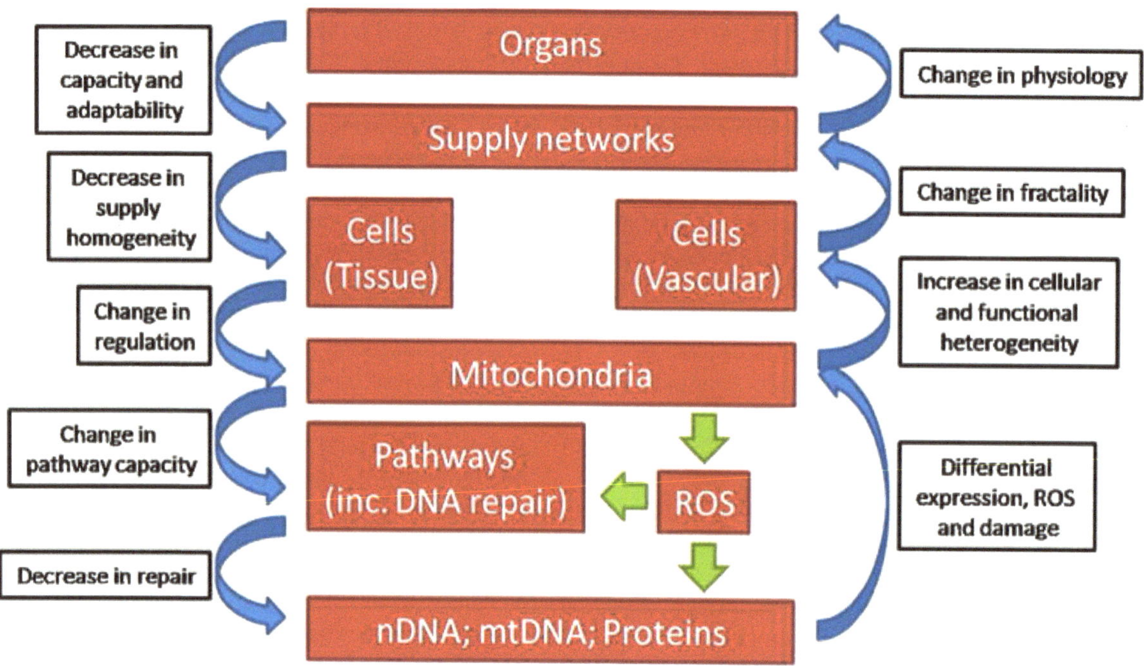

Fig.8.4 An integrated physiological view of the functional and structural changes observed during aging. Multiple feedback loops exist at both the genomic and the organ levels, suggesting that aging is an accelerated process, countered only by the robustness of each level. Adapted from (Kriete et al., 2006)

importance of eating a wholesome, constitution-specific diet and being in tune with nature while eating, as it influences and impacts our digestion, metabolism and lifespan . In realizing the close connection to nature through eating, the relationship with food becomes a sacred experience. The sun represents the fire element and in the physical body this is reflected as the process of transformation of the food by the heat of the digestive juices (Jatharagni) . Thus, when the sun is at its peak, digestion is stronger and optimal. Ayurveda recommends eating the largest meal during the midday hours and smaller meals in the morning and evening to prevent the metabolism from going awry.

Nutritionists and other researchers are also realizing the importance of relationship between the timing of feeding, metabolism, weight regulation and aging . In an interesting case study demonstrating a relationship between the timing of feeding and weight regulation, 420 individuals were grouped into early eaters (lunch before 1500 h) and late eaters (lunch after 1500 h) . Late lunch eaters lost less weight and displayed a slower weight-loss rate during the 20 weeks of treatment suggesting that eating late may influence the success of weight-loss therapy . While the strength of the study was its relatively large sample size and numerous biomarkers and genetic indicators, the work was mostly observational and requires further interventional studies to demonstrate the causality of this observation. Thus, time-bound meals may not only prevent weight gain and onset of other digestive related problems, but also enhances the healthspan of the individual .

In addition to the timing of food intake, the quality of food consumed and its impact on growth, metabolism and development of an individual, is also of considerable interest to health care professionals . Furthermore, nutritionists are also closely looking at maternal diet and its impact on fetal growth and metabolism. While maternal undernutrition is a major factor contributing to adverse pregnancy, over indulgence of poor quality food during pregnancy is also a contributing factor for adverse metabolic outcomes in the offspring later in life . Several research studies have now revealed a strong link between in utero nutrition and disease outcomes later in life termed as "maternal nutrition–offspring metabolic disease cycle". According to these studies, prepregnancy maternal nutrition affects fetal metabolism and growth, child growth during the preschool years and increases risk for metabolic disease in adult life . In a retrospective study involving 174 women, researchers concluded that women receiving poor diets had a greater incidence and recurrcnce of fetal neural tube defects than women eating a nourishing diet.

In addition, dietary counselling was effective in reducing the incidence of fetal neural-tube defects . One mechanism that links poor maternal diet to metabolic diseases is diet-induced differential regulation of microRNA. Researchers who sought out to understand why a poor maternal diet increases the risk of developing diabetes in the offspring, found that miR-483-3p was produced at higher levels in individuals who had experienced a poor diet in their mother's wombs than those who were better nourished . High levels of miR-483-3p resulted in the suppression of a protein called GDF3. GDF3 is responsible for fat metabolism and low levels of GDF3 are associated with low birth weight and metabolic deficits . Thus, poor quality foods and irregular eating habits are posing new challenges to which our bodies poorly adapt resulting in unforeseen health problems, confirming the importance of proper diet and nutrition at all stages of life to ensure a disease-free lifespan.

Sleep

Sleep (Nidra) is one of the main pillars of good health in Ayurveda, and is as important as diet in sustaining a quality healthspan . Sleep can be influenced by age, lifestyle, daily routines, diet and environment . Ayurveda cautions that poor sleep patterns can be debilitating as it triggers age-associated pathological conditions that can hasten the aging process. Research studies indicate that insufficient sleep can disrupt circadian rhythms that results in negative health outcomes, including obesity, cardiovascular disease, and cognitive impairment . In a study involving 26 participants, researchers exposed the subjects to 1 week of insufficient sleep (sleep-restriction) followed by 1 week of sufficient sleep . Following each condition, whole-blood RNA samples were collected from each participant for transcriptome analysis. The analysis revealed that 711 genes were differentially regulated by insufficient sleep. Genes affected by insufficient sleep were predominantly associated with circadian rhythms, sleep homeostasis, chromatin modification, inflammation, immune and stress responses, oxidative stress and metabolism .Poor sleep quality not only disrupts the circadian rhythms but also triggers metabolic diseases including diabetes, obesity, and cardiovascular disease. In a large, well-conducted meta-analysis study, researchers systematically combined the results of cohort studies that investigated an association between sleep duration, incidence of type 2 diabetes and death from any cause .. Most of the participants were over 60 when they participated in the study, and the different studies varied in length between four and 25 years. The major conclusion from this study was that poor sleep quality predicted the risk of development of type 2 diabetes. In addition, sleeping less than 6 h a night was associated with an increased risk of early death . These studies not only highlight the close connection between sleep, circadian rhythm and metabolism but confirm the Ayurvedic concept of sleep being a pillar of life that endows the body with strength, complexion and healthy growth that continues throughout life. The research findings are in agreement with Ayurvedic's emphasis on good quality sleep as a staple of optimal health and longevity.

Regular routines

For health and optimum healthspan, Ayurveda recommends a set of daily routines (morning, noon and night) of self-care. These guidelines include time of waking and sleeping, elimination, hygiene, massage, mindfulness practices, diet, work, and travel all during the course of the day and night. The routine calls for optimal times to awake, sleep, oral care, care of eyes, nose, ears and skin. Routines also include cleansing procedures, bowel habits, yoga, breath practices and massage. These daily observances were encouraged in order to maintain the synchronicity of circadian rhythms with time of the day, night and seasons (dinacharya, ratricharya & ritucharya respectively) and to help ward off all acute or chronic conditions that have a deleterious influence on the aging process . These Ayurvedic concepts of daily routines have had major implications for health research and helped establish a growing field of science called chronobiology. Scientists are only now beginning to understand the importance of routines, biological clocks and circadian rhythms and their role in aging, well-being and morbidity. Researchers studying chronobiology have noticed that increased longevity and improved health can be achieved by time-bound routines. Furthermore, disturbances in the circadian rhythm can trigger fatigue, disorientation, insomnia and increased susceptibility to cancer . Similarly, frequent long distance travels, shift work, jet lag, eating late in the night or sleep disorders destabilize the close coordination between the biological clock, circadian rhythms and the environment that has a serious impact on overall health and lifespan .

Panchakarma

Periodical detoxification, purification, and rejuvenation therapies classified as panchakarma therapies in Ayurveda, are highly recommended as they provide the strength and nourishment to the deeper tissues (Dhatus) and pacifies age-associated health issues. Oleation and fomentation therapies are important as they neutralize the Vata-triggered coldness and dryness that accompany aging. Panchakarma therapies ensure rapid blood circulation, continuous cerebral blood flow and efflux of toxic matter through increased lymphatic drainage .A recent study on the cellular effects of panchakarma revealed changes in several metabolites across many pathways . The study involved 65 healthy male and female subjects who participated in a 6-day panchakarma-based Ayurvedic intervention that also included herbs, vegetarian diet, meditation, yoga, and massage . Significant reductions in 12 phosphatidylcholines and other metabolites including amino acids, biogenic amines, acylcarnitines, glycerophospholipids and sphingolipids were observed in the panchakarma group compared to the control group. The significant alterations in plasma metabolites are consistent with metabolic changes in the gut microbiota and host metabolism that promote general health and well-being . Similar studies with a larger sample size, longer follow-up period and suitable outcome measures are warranted to confirm the broad ranging effects of panchakarma therapies in delaying the aging process

Abhyanga

Regular oil massage (Abhyanga) with warm oil that is often infused with the individual's constitution-specific herbs is beneficial for maintaining good health and to delay age-associated pathological changes. Abhyanga can be incorporated as a daily routine as it restores the balance of the Doshas and enhances well-being and longevity . Abhyanga is also recommended for CNS conditions including brain-related injuries, dementia and mental stress. Significant brain functional activation changes together with increased cerebral blood flow were observed in participants who received oil massage. Massage reduced the levels of stress-related hormones with a concomitant increase in circulating lymphocytes and regional cerebral blood flow . Researchers are of the opinion that application of medicated oil followed by a gentle massage could relax the tight junctions between endothelial cells in the CNS vessels and facilitate the entry of solutes and other components into the CNS. In another pilot study involving 20 healthy subjects (10 male and 10 female) that underwent a 1-h Abhyanga, subjects showed clinically significant reduction in subjective stress experience. Furthermore, a significant reduction in heart rate in all subjects and lowered blood pressure in prehypertensive subjects were also observed . Further studies with a large sample size involving normal adults and adults with age-associated pathologies are needed to confirm the impact of oil massage in delaying the aging process and reversing age-associated pathological changes.Mindfulness practices A daily practice of yoga, meditation and pranayama (breath practices) helps to delay the aging process. The results from a meta-analysis study clearly show that the above mentioned yogic practices enhance muscular strength and body flexibility, improve respiratory and cardiovascular function, promote recovery from addiction, reduce stress, anxiety, depression, and chronic pain, improve sleep patterns, and enhance overall well-being and quality of life . These combined practices facilitate the transport of oxygenated blood to various organs and body tissues, eliminates waste, and improves proper coordination of the body, mind and emotions. These practices sustain equanimity of the physical, mental and emotional body, thereby fostering a longer health span .

Sadvritta

Sadvritta could be defined as moral reasoning, code of ethics or good conduct and is required to guide daily living and maintain a balanced state of mental and physical life. It includes guiding principles of proper conduct that helps to reflect on the importance of an individual's life extending beyond the single individual. Sadvritta allows the individual to examine one's values, interpersonal and social behavior. Cultivating these ethical regimens help to strengthen mental health and sustain the balance between an individual's mind and body . Selfless service/action that is rendered without any personal expectation for the service provided is one of those ethical regimens. Selfless service requires for an individual to perform any service without any expectation, and also remain unaffected by the results of such service . The individual also needs to cultivate a loving attitude towards the selfless task irrespective of the outcome.In a longitudinal >50 year study involving high school graduates, researchers caught up with over 3000 individuals and found that those individuals who had performed selfless service regularly lived longer compared to those who did not render any selfless service . Additionally, participants who volunteered only for compassionate reasons achieved the most health benefits compared to those who performed the service purely for personal gain or self-growth. The researchers concluded that while selfless service provided a longer health span and reduced mortality rates, those same benefits were lost if the main motive for performing selfless service was for personal gain or self-growth . The findings of the research study confirm the Ayurvedic concept of Sadvritta and suggest that ethical regimens and good conduct stabilize body-mind function, help to ward off mental disorders, and helps to overcome life's challenges that accompany the aging process

Conclusion

While there are various steps to manage the aging process, the modern medicine approach is different from the Ayurvedic approach. While neither approach is superior or inferior, the paramount difference lies in how both these sciences address the aging process. A subset of researchers consider aging itself to be a disease because, 1) aging is associated with an accumulation of cellular and molecular changes that impair normal physiology, 2) impairment of normal physiological functioning of cells, tissue, organs and bodily systems, in turn triggers age-associated diseases, and 3) aging itself is a risk factor for other diseases . Anti-aging approaches would therefore require an ideal disease-free physiological state at a certain age and a "to-do" list of drug interventions to keep the individual as close to that ideal state as possible. If aging is viewed as a disease as some researchers do, than the most logical approach would be to overcome the aging process with drugs like metformin, resveratrol, masoprocol, rapamycin and others. However, a drug approach de-emphasizes the enormous potential of disease prevention through lifestyle changes as the entire aging process is viewed in mechanistic and reductionistic terms that involve manipulating a specific pathway or molecules with powerful drugs . In contrast, a systems approach is designed to address multiple pathogenic mechanisms and optimizing the therapeutics for each of those targets . The past few decades of genetic and biochemical research have revealed an extensive network of molecular interactions involved in the aging process, suggesting that a systems approach or a network-based therapeutics approach, rather than a single target-based approach, may be feasible and potentially more effective for delaying or reversing the aging process.

Ayurveda considers aging as a natural and inevitable process and offers time-tested therapies for healthy aging. Ayurveda professes the principles of harmonious living and being in tune with nature, universal consciousness, environment, and individual constitution. Healthy aging would therefore require for the individual to bring in harmonious impressions, incorporate healthy lifestyle practices and routines that promote good health and well-being, and encourage healthy transformation of the body and mind through harmonious choices and actions. Unfortunately, lack of systematic safety and efficacy studies or proof-of-concept trials have relegated these Ayurvedic concepts of aging to a conceptual model. Thus, it is imperative that these concepts are revisited and re-examined to generate best research .

Bibliography and Acknowledgement

- Agrawal A.K., Yadav C.R., Meena M.S. Physiological aspects of agni. Ayu. 2010;31:395–398. [PMC free article] [PubMed] [Google Scholar]
- Ahn A.C., Tewari M., Poon C.S., Phillips R.S. The limits of reductionism in medicine: could systems biology offer an alternative? PLoS Med. 2006;3:e208. [PMC free article] [PubMed] [Google Scholar
- Baghel M.S. Need of new research methodology for ayurveda. Ayu. 2011;32:3–4. [PMC free article] [PubMed] [Google Scholar]
- Balasubramanian P., Howell P.R., Anderson R.M. Aging and caloric restriction research: a biological perspective with translational potential. EBioMedicine. 2017;21:37–44. [PMC free article] [PubMed] [Google Scholar]
- Caplan A.L. Death as an unnatural process. Why is it wrong to seek a cure for aging? EMBO Rep. 2005;6:S72–S75. [PMC free article] [PubMed] [Google Scholar]
- Cappuccio F.P., D'Elia L., Strazzullo P., Miller M.A. Quantity and quality of sleep and incidence of type 2 diabetes: a systematic review and meta-analysis. Diabetes Care. 2010;33:414–420. [PMC free article] [PubMed] [Google Scholar]
- Datta H.S., Mitra S.K., Paramesh R., Patwardhan B. Theories and management of aging: modern and ayurveda perspectives. Evid Based Complement Altern Med. 2011;2011
- Devi D., Srivastava R., Dwivedi B.K. A critical review of concept of aging in ayurveda. Ayu. 2010;31:516–519. [PMC free article] [PubMed] [Google Scholar]
- Ferland-McCollough D., Fernandez-Twinn D.S., Cannell I.G., David H., Warner M., Vaag A.A. Programming of adipose tissue miR-483-3p and GDF-3 expression by maternal diet in type 2 diabetes. Cell Death Differ. 2012;19:1003–1012.
- Finkel T. The metabolic regulation of aging. Nat Med. 2015;21:1416–1423. [PubMed] [Google Scholar]
- Gaillard R. Maternal obesity during pregnancy and cardiovascular development and disease in the offspring. Eur J Epidemiol. 2015;30:1141–1152. [PMC free article] [PubMed] [Google Scholar]
- Halpern M. vol. 14. Lotus Press; 2011. pp. 169–188. (Healing your life-lessons on the path of ayurveda-the healing rhythms of daily life). [Google Scholar]
- Izpisua Belmonte J.C. Human organs from animal bodies. Sci Am. 2016;315:32–37. [PubMed] [Google Scholar]
- Jia L., Zhang W., Chen X. Common methods of biological age estimation. Clin Interv Aging. 2017;12:759–772.
- Keir S.T. Effect of massage therapy on stress levels and quality of life in brain tumor patients–observations from a pilot study. Support Care Cancer. 2011;19:711–715.
- Larsson S.C., Kaluza J., Wolk A. Combined impact of healthy lifestyle factors on lifespan: two prospective cohorts. J Intern Med. 2017;282:209–219. [PubMed] [Google Scholar]
- Manikrao G.P., Tulsiram S.A., Anantarao K.V., Kumar A.P., Lal M.K. Comprehensive review of gramya ahara. Int Res J Pharm. 2012;3:69–71. [Google Scholar]
- Newman J.C., Milman S., Hashmi S.K., Austad S.N., Kirkland J.L., Halter J.B. Strategies and challenges in clinical trials targeting human aging. J Gerontol A Biol Sci Med Sci. 2016;71:1424–1434. [PMC free article]
- Ouchi Y., Kanno T., Okada H., Yoshikawa E., Shinke T., Nagasawa S. Changes in cerebral blood flow under the prone condition with and without massage. Neurosci Lett. 2006;407:131–135. [PubMed] [Google Scholar]
- Panickar K.S., Jewell D.E. The beneficial role of anti-inflammatory dietary ingredients in attenuating markers of chronic low-grade inflammation in aging. Horm Mol Biol Clin Invest. 2015;23:59–70. [PubMed] [Google Scholar]
- Pan H., Finkel T. Key proteins and pathways that regulate lifespan. J Biol Chem. 2017;292:6452–6460. [PMC free article] [PubMed] [Google Scholar
- Rakesh N.V. SADVRITTA: a key for the stress management. PunarnaV. 2015;2 [Google Scholar]
- Sadowska-Bartosz I., Bartosz G. Effect of antioxidants supplementation on aging and longevity. Biomed Res Int. 2014;2014 [PMC free article] [PubMed] [Google Scholar]
- Salminen A., Ojala J., Kaarniranta K., Kauppinen A. Mitochondrial dysfunction and oxidative stress activate inflammasomes: impact on the aging process and age-related diseases. Cell Mol Life Sci. 2012;69:2999–3013. [PubMed] [Google Scholar]
- Samarakoon S.M., Chandola H.M., Ravishankar B. Effect of dietary, social, and lifestyle determinants of accelerated aging and its common clinical presentation: a survey study. Ayu. 2011;32:315–321. [PMC free article] [PubMed] [Google Scholar]
- Singh K. Yogic life style and geriatric care–a review article. Int Ayurvedic Med J. 2017;5:263–268. [Google Scholar]
- Tawalare K.A., Nanote K.D., Gawai V.U., Gotmare A.Y. Contribution of ayurveda in foundation of basic tenets of bioethics. Ayu. 2014;35:366–370. [PMC free article] [PubMed] [Google Scholar]
- Van Regenmortel M.H. Reductionism and complexity in molecular biology. Scientists now have the tools to unravel biological and overcome the limitations of reductionism. EMBO Rep. 2004;5:1016–1020. [PMC free article] [PubMed] [Google Scholar]
- Vinaya P.N. The dynamics of degeneration: a conceptual view from ayurveda. Int J Res Ayurveda Pharm. 2015;6:182–184. [Google Scholar]
- Vivek A. An ayurvedic insight towards ageing with its preventive measures. Int J Res Ayur Pharm. 2013;4:31–33. [Google Scholar]
- Watson N.F., Badr M.S., Belenky G., Bliwise D.L., Buxton O.M., Buysse D. Joint consensus statement of the American academy of sleep medicine and sleep research society on the recommended amount of sleep for a healthy adult: methodology and discussion. Sleep. 2015;38:1161–1183. [PMC free article] [PubMed] [Google Scholar]
- Weinert B.T., Timiras P.S. Invited review: theories of aging. J Appl Physiol. 1985;2003(95):1706–1716.
- Woodyard C. Exploring the therapeutic effects of yoga and its ability to increase quality of life. Int J Yoga. 2011;4:49–54. [PMC free article] [PubMed] [Google Scholar]
- Yoon I.Y., Kripke D.F., Elliott J.A., Youngstedt S.D., Rex K.M., Hauger R.L. Age-related changes of circadian rhythms and sleep-wake cycles. J Am Geriatr Soc. 2003;51:1085–1091.
- Zhavoronkov A., Bhullar B. Classifying aging as a disease in the context of ICD-11. Front Genet. 2015;6:326. [PMC free article] [PubMed] [Google Scholar]

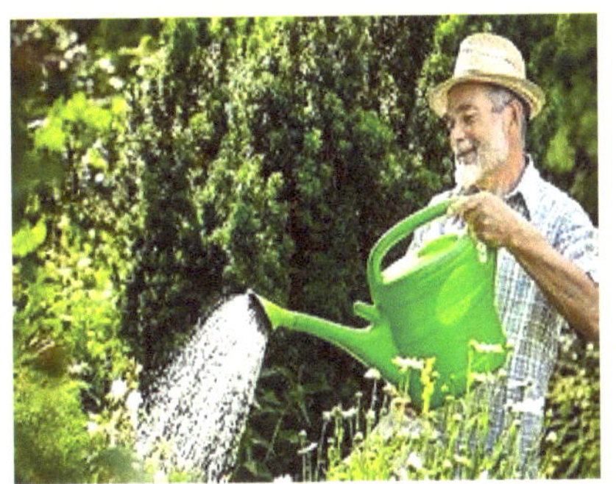

Chores That Are Safe For Seniors To Help Keep Them Active

As people grow older, their physical and cognitive abilities begin to decline. They may no longer be able to safely complete certain activities to maintain the home, from clearing the gutter to cleaning the bathroom. However, seniors can safely perform the following chores to stay active.Household chores are a necessary and important part of maintaining a home. Older adults, however, may be challenged physically or cognitively in completing some of them. Arthritic fingers can make scrubbing the bathtub a near-impossibility. Similarly, cooking is exhausting for seniors with fatigue. Basic tasks like these are among the many chores that are required for the proper upkeep of a home. Since the majority of older adults prefer to age in place, caregivers must determine which chores they can handle safely. Plus, seniors' well-being is enriched when they complete household tasks.

How does completing chores benefit the elderly?

Older adults are likely to have spent a lifetime performing ordinary chores to keep the household clean and well-managed. But as they age, they may no longer be able to do some of these tasks. As a result, these seniors begin to experience low self-esteem and a loss of energy.

Caregivers who assign their elderly loved ones a range of non-risky household chores give them an opportunity to feel greater self-worth and value. Aging people who perform a set of regular chores feel more confident and live with greater purpose.Furthermore, seniors' brains benefit from the light physical activity of doing chores. Greater brain volume, especially in the hippocampus (which plays a large role in memory and learning) and frontal lobe (which is involved in cognition), is observed in these active older adults. Completing chores is believed to have the same effects on heart and blood vessels as engaging in light aerobic exercise. Seniors who actively perform chores are less sedentary (being sedentary adversely effects brain health). New neural connections also form when seniors organize their chores.

What chores can seniors safely perform?

The safest chores for seniors are those that are low-impact and that do not require significant physical exertion. Caregivers are advised to assign their elderly care recipients, especially those with mobility issues, chores that can be done either seated or standing.

1. Folding Laundry

Rudimentary household chores include laundry. Folding laundry, a basic task, is ideal for older adults who have difficulty standing for prolonged periods. The light activity of folding dinner napkins or clothing can be done seated and is recommended for seniors with balance issues.

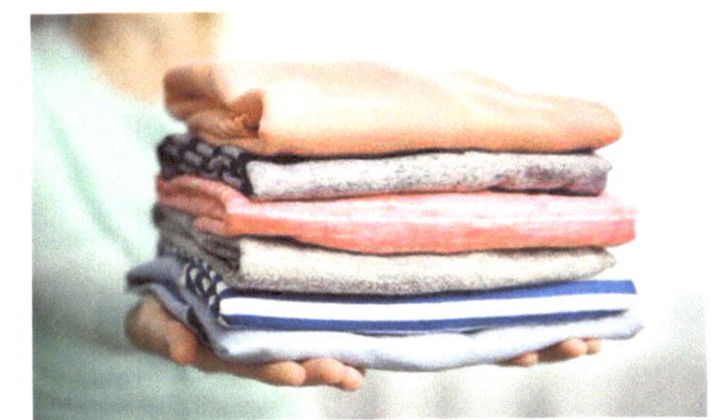

Fig.9.1 Folding laundry, a basic task, is ideal for older adults

2. Dusting and Vacuuming

Dusting keeps seniors active. Seniors should use a damp cloth when dusting to avoid breathing in dust particles. Vacuuming is another light chore that can be safely done when the vacuum is held close to the body; this prevents a strain on the senior's back and shoulders

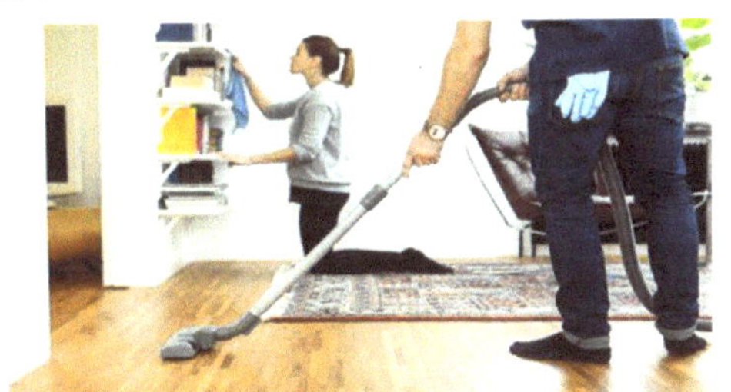

Fig.9.2 Dusting keeps seniors active.

3. Kitchen Help

Invite the aging loved one into the kitchen to help prepare food. Seniors can knead bread, which is not only a safe activity but provides a vigorous workout. Kneading is a good exercise for the hands and fingers and keeps their motor skills in top shape.

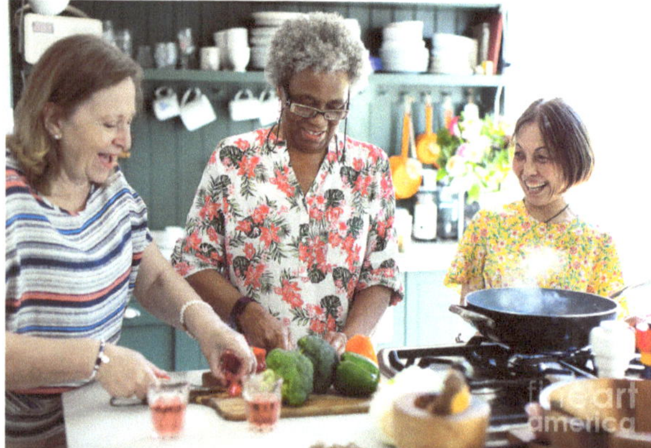

Fig.9.3 Elders should enter into the kitchen to help prepare food.

4. Dog Walks

The family dog must be walked daily, and an aging loved one can be the right person to handle this task. Walking is a gentle exercise that builds strength in the senior's leg muscles. Strong leg muscles in turn protect the elderly from falls.

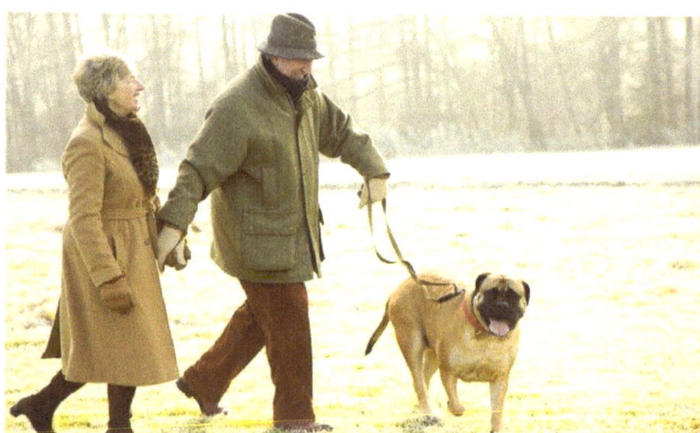

Fig.9.4 Elder one can be the right person to handle dog walking task

5. Gardening

Gardening provides numerous health benefits. Exposure to sunshine and breathing in fresh air do wonders for an individual's health. Give an elderly care recipient the task of watering the garden or the lawn. While they are outside, ensure they remain adequately hydrated and wear sun protection

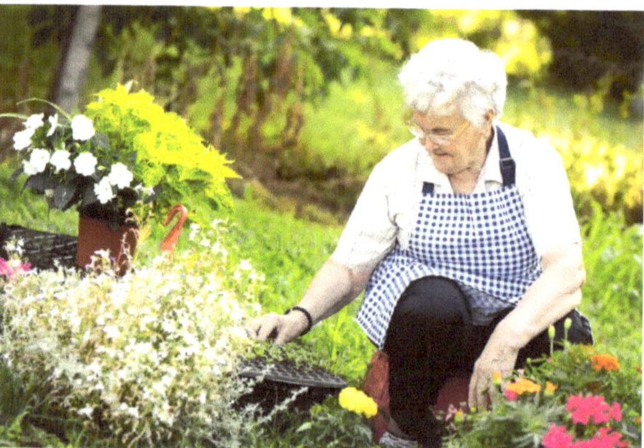

Fig.9.5 Elder can choose gardening for gentle exercise

6. Mowing the Lawn

Older adults who boast physical fitness may be ideal candidates for mowing the lawn. Using a push mower requires physical stamina, but almost anyone can manage the task of cutting the grass with a riding lawn mower. Caregivers must exercise caution as the senior performs this activity.

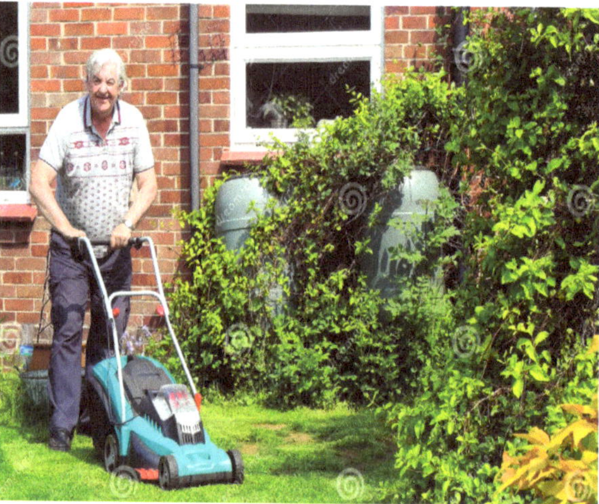

Fig.9.6 Older adults who boast physical fitness may be ideal candidates for mowing the lawn.

Juliano-Villani recommends picking simple tasks together that seniors can manage, such as:

- Getting dressed and combing their hair.
- Making themselves coffee or breakfast.
- Making a weekly call to a friend or relative to check in.
- Making a grocery list and shopping.
- Doing some deep breathing, chair yoga or mindfulness exercises.

What chores are unsafe for seniors?

Many seniors have hopes of growing old while maintaining their independence in their homes; however, completing chores may become difficult for some seniors as they age. Seniors may find that they are not able to clean as well as they once could. Chronic aches and pains may cause them to move slowly, and some chores can become extremely dangerous, especially for those with arthritis or other mobility issues.

Standing on ladders to dust, or bending to reach under or around furniture, becomes a dangerous and sometimes impossible feat to complete. Fortunately, modifications can be made around the home to minimize dangers to seniors while completing chores.Studies have shown that home injuries are one of the biggest causes of adult hospitalization, especially for the elderly.

- Some household chores are unsafe for seniors to handle alone. Tasks that require climbing a ladder can be perilous for older people. Cleaning windows or changing light bulbs are examples of risky activities. If the senior must do these tasks, ensure they are accompanied.
- Cleaning the bathroom is likewise not advised for older adults. Aging skin is thinner and more fragile; the elderly are susceptible to rashes, skin irritations and chemical burns when they work with chemical cleaning products. Plus, a high level of physical exertion is required to bend and scrub.
- Do not allow them to perform home repairs, which can be dangerous. If a chore is expected to extend for hours and cause exhaustion, hire a professional to do the job. Lifting heavy objects should be prohibited in the aging population as it can intensify chronic pain or cause injury.
- Older adults may need extra support to age in place. Help with household chores that seniors cannot or are not advised to handle on their own can be obtained from reputable elder care agencies, like Assisting Hands Home Care. We promote the overall health of seniors in our care.
- Professional caregivers are instrumental in keeping the senior's home hygienic and comfortable. We perform light housekeeping tasks and remove clutter; our efforts prevent trips and falls. Grocery shopping, meal preparation, medication reminders, and transportation are included in our care services.
- Social engagement is vital to the health of older people, and our pleasant companionship keeps them active and stimulated.

Bibliography and Acknowledgement

- Adams JS (1965). Inequity in social exchange In Berkowitz L (Ed.), Advances in experimental social psychology (Vol. 2, pp. 267–299). New York: Academic Press. [Google Scholar]
- Barrett AE, & Raphael A (2017). Housework and Sex in Midlife Marriages: An Examination of Three Perspectives on the Association. Social Forces, 96(3), 1325–1350. [Google Scholar]
- Chen E, & Matthews KA (2001). Cognitive appraisal biases: An approach to understanding the relation between socioeconomic status and cardiovascular reactivity in children. Annals of Behavioral Medicine, 23(2), 101–111. [PubMed] [Google Scholar]
- Friedman EM (2011). Sleep quality, social well-being, gender, and inflammation: An integrative analysis in a national sample. Annals of the New York Academy of Sciences, 1231(1), 23–34. [PMC free article] [PubMed] [Google Scholar]
- Geist C, & Tabler J (2018). Somebody has to DUST! Gender, health, and housework in older couples. Journal of Women & Aging, 30(1), 38–48. [PubMed] [Google Scholar]
- Hochschild A (1989). The second shift: Working parents and the revolution at home. New York, NY: Viking Press. [Google Scholar]
- Kluwer ES, Heesink JA, & Van de Vliert E (1996). Marital Conflict About the Division of Household Labor and Paid Work. Journal of Marriage and Family, 58, 958–969. [Google Scholar]
- Lachance-Grzela M, & Bouchard G (2010). Why do women do the lion's share of housework? A decade of research. Sex Roles, 63(11–12), 767–780. [Google Scholar]
- Mezick EJ, Wing RR, & McCaffery JM (2014). Associations of self-reported and actigraphy-assessed sleep characteristics with body mass index and waist circumference in adults: moderation by gender. Sleep Medicine, 15(1), 64–70. [PMC free article] [PubMed] [Google Scholar]
- Newkirk K, Perry-Jenkins M, & Sayer AG (2017). Division of household and childcare labor and relationship conflict among low-income new parents. Sex Roles, 76, 319–333. [PMC free article] [PubMed] [Google Scholar]
- Ryan RM, & Deci EL (2001). On happiness and human potentials: A review of research on hedonic and eudaimonic well-being. Annual Review of Psychology, 52(1), 141–166. [PubMed] [Google Scholar
- Seeman TE, Crimmins E, Huang MH, Singer B, Bucur A, Gruenewald T,& Reuben DB (2004). Cumulative biological risk and socio-economic differences in mortality:
- MacArthur Studies of Successful Aging. Social Science & Medicine, 58(10), 1985–1997. [PubMed] [Google Scholar]
- Thompson L (1991). Family Work: Women's Sense of Fairness. Journal of Family Issues, 12(2), 181–196. [Google Scholar]
- Wong JD, & Almeida DM (2012). The effects of employment status and daily stressors on time spent on daily household chores in middle-aged and older adults. The Gerontologist, 53(1), 81–91. [PMC free article] [PubMed] [Google Scholar]
- Wood W, & Eagly AH (2002). A cross-cultural analysis of the behavior of women and men: implications for the origins of sex differences. Psychological Bulletin, 128(5), 699–727. [PubMed] [Google Scholar]

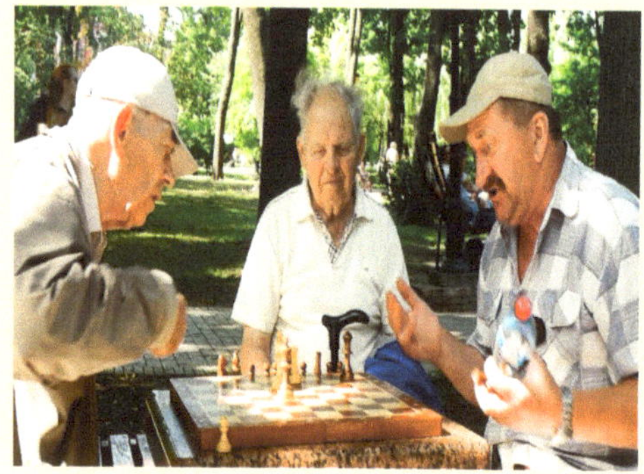

What To Do After Retirement ?

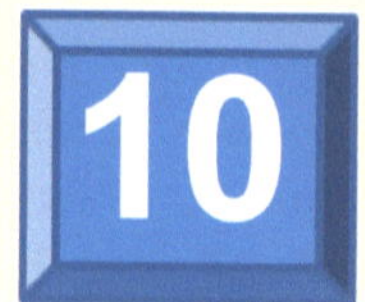

Retiring from the workforce can be a chance to reconnect with your greatest passions and most important goals—it all depends on what you choose to do in your retirement. You can try new experiences, develop new skills, and devote more time to the people and hobbies you love. It's all up to you.

As a retiree, you no longer have to deal with work-related deadlines; you are free to have fun and do what you want, on your own terms. Plus, even though your income might be lower than it was when you were working full-time, you can take advantage of a huge array of senior discounts, and you may be free of certain financial burdens like a mortgage, student loans, and credit card debt. In fact, a Merrill Lynch survey revealed that people feel happier, more relaxed, and less anxious in retirement than at any other time in their adult lives. During a person's working years, leisure often means relaxing and getting away from structure. But in retirement, it's more about engaging in activity and connecting with people. So we've identified a wide range of activities that can help keep you physically active, mentally stimulated, and engaged in opportunities for socialization and fulfillment.

But remember: Retirement is all about freedom and choice. These ideas are just a starting point—use them as inspiration for charting your own path!

Common Goals of Retirees

Without the restrictions of full-time work, how do you envision spending your hours? In the Merrill Lynch survey of adults over age 50, 95 percent of respondents said they would rather focus on having more enjoyable experiences than on buying more stuff. And financial constraints had little impact on most retirees' ability to enjoy life. In fact, more than 88 percent of retirees across all income levels said they had increased flexibility and freedom to do the things they wanted to do.

Here's what the Merrill Lynch survey respondents were looking to accomplish through their everyday activities:

- Get or stay health: 83 percent
- Relax: 72 percent
- Connect with family: 58 percent
- Have fun: 57 percent
- Make or expand social connections: 56 percent
- Learn: 47 percent
- Grow spiritually: 43 percent
- Give back: 41 percent

Fun Things to Do in Retirement

When you retire, you suddenly find yourself with all the time in the world. So, what are you going to do with it? Here are 24 awesome ideas:

1.Travel

Satisfy your wanderlust! With no limits on your vacation time, you can get out and explore the world. Retirees have the flexibility to go on extended holidays and take advantage of last-minute deals. Many enjoy regular trips dedicated to biking, golf, shopping, or the arts. Some stick to domestic destinations, while others go further afield to explore places like the Caribbean, Europe, and Latin America.

In a survey of more than 1,300 American retirees, author Wes Moss found that the happiest ones took an average of 2.4 vacations each year. Here's more good news: A study in Applied Research in Quality of Life has shown that simply planning a trip can boost happiness levels because you are anticipating the good times to come.

Here are a few senior travel ideas to consider:

•Rent or buy a trailer or motorhome and hit the open road. Make a goal of dipping a toe in each ocean, driving the entire length of Route 66, or visiting every national park in the country. If you're over 62, you can get a lifetime federal parks pass for only $80; in some cases, the pass also gives you significant discounts on camping and boat launch fees.

•Become a campground host. Many campgrounds and RV parks provide free campsites and amenities in exchange for help with tasks like collecting fees, enforcing rules, and tidying the grounds. Campground hosting jobs might last for a few weeks or for an entire season; they are often volunteer positions, but some provide a small stipend. This can be a great way to travel for less cost.

• Trade houses. Exchange houses with like-minded travelers and take advantage of completely free holiday accommodations. House swapping provides an immersive experience and lets you live like a local. Whether you're looking for a weekend getaway in a nearby region or an extended vacation abroad, you can find options to suit you. Websites like Home Exchange 50plus and HomeExchange.com cater to older adults; membership fees vary.

• Take a cruise. Do you dream of a vacation at sea? Cruises are popular among retirees because they offer an almost-all-inclusive experience that lets you see different places every day. In fact, an AARP study found that 37 percent of baby boomers who traveled internationally did so on a cruise ship. And cruising may be more affordable than you think: Major lines like Carnival and Royal Caribbean offer discounts on some sailings for travelers over the age of 55.

Get an education

Retirement could be the perfect time to get that degree you've always wanted or just learn more about a subject that fascinates you. Every state offers options for free or discounted college tuition for older adults, although age requirements vary.

If you're more interested in gaining knowledge than acquiring formal credentials, you may want to check out one of the lifelong learning programs sponsored by the Bernard Osher Foundation. Programs are aimed at adults over 50 and are offered through colleges and universities across the country. Courses are fairly inexpensive (some cost as little as $35), but they do not come with college credit.

Plus, there are plenty of ways to expand your mind without spending any money. Listen to a podcast or TED talk. Visit museums and science centers—many have free admission on certain days or for seniors in general. Or consider massive open online courses (MOOCs) that offer free college-level training in a huge range of areas, including web design, game development, communication, chemistry, music, art, economics, psychology, and more.

Indulge in a hobby (or three)

Hobbies give you something interesting and fun to do, either on your own or as part of a group. Expand on hobbies you enjoyed during your working years or pursue new nterests. Research conducted by Wes Moss found that the happiest retirees regularly participated in three to four hobbies. The possible activities are endless, but here is a sample of ideas that may appeal to you:

- Gardening
- Sailing
- Dancing
- Baking or cake decorating
- Antique collecting
- Reading
- Model building
- Bird watching
- Singing
- Horseback riding
- Walking or hiking
- Wine making
- Furniture restoring
- Pottery making

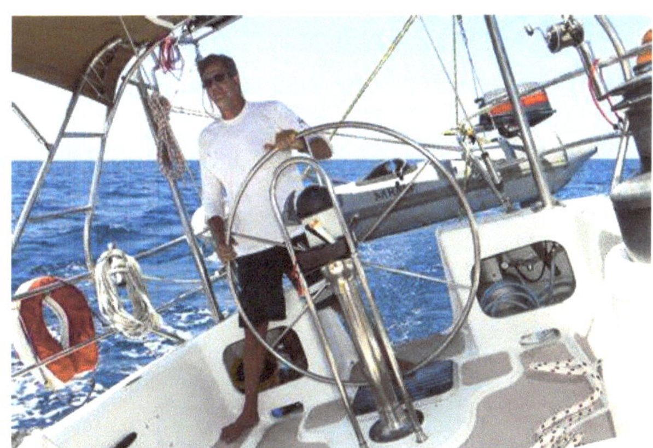

Fig.10.1 Boat sailing by retired person.

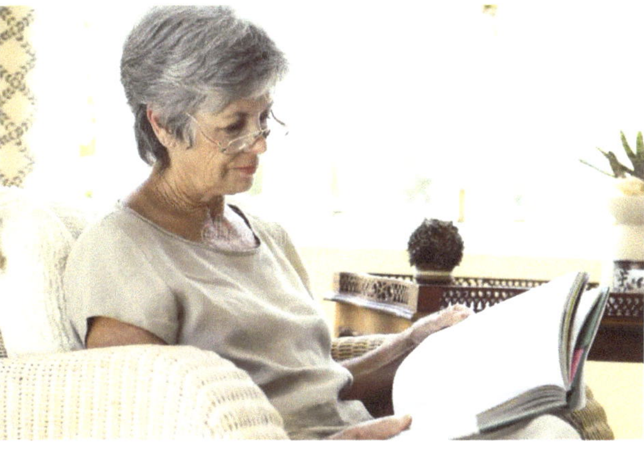

Fig.10.2 Reading a book by retired person.

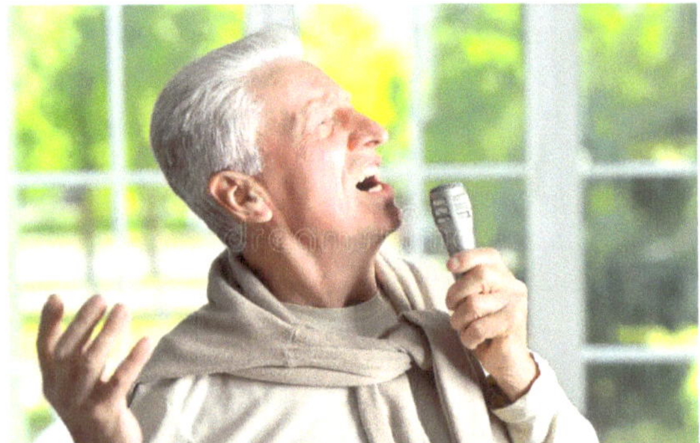
Fig.10.3 Singing a melodious song by retired person.

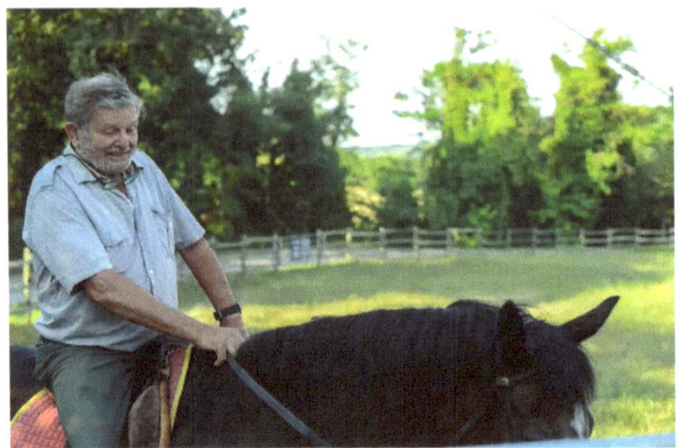
Fig.10.4 Horse back riding by retired person.

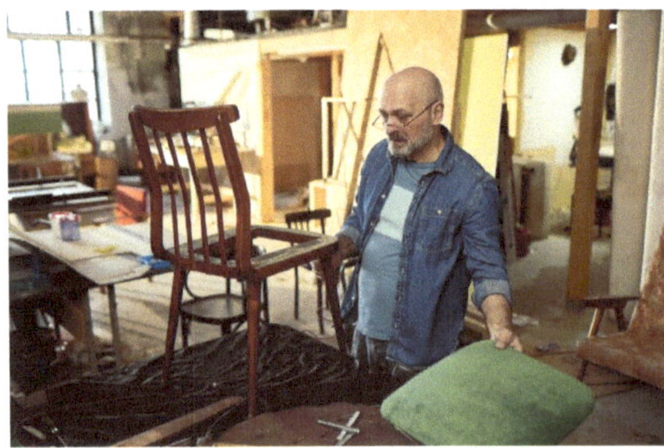
Fig.11.5 Furniture restoring by retired person.

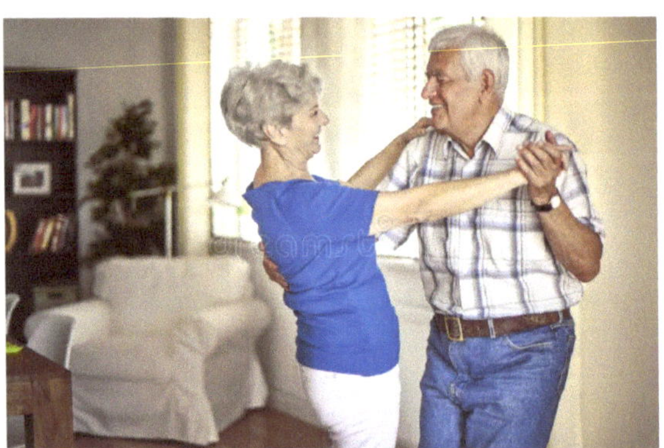
Fig.10.6 Couple dancing by retired person.

Donate your time

Volunteering gives you a sense of purpose and lets you contribute to a greater good. Almost one-quarter of retirees volunteer on a regular basis, according to the Transamerica Center for Retirement Studies. Identify the types of organizations you're interested in and see if they can use your abilities. You could work with Meals on Wheels, teach English to immigrants, become a Scout leader, or build a house with Habitat for Humanity. Check out VolunteerMatch to research opportunities in your area. (Or consider opportunities overseas: There is no age limit for joining the Peace Corps!)

Other places that could potentially use your help include:

- **Libraries**: Sort books, plan special events and fundraisers, or deliver library materials to home-bound adults.
- **Hospices:** Support patients by visiting with them, reading to them, or taking walks with them.
- **Seniors' centers**: Greet patrons at the front desk, teach a computer class, or help out in the kitchen.
- **Theaters:** Hand out playbills and show people to their seats (and possibly see a show for free).
- **Churches or other houses of worship:** Organize and lead community outreach initiatives or youth programs.
- **Museums:** Lead tours and answer questions from the public about exhibits.
- **Animal shelters:** Feed and groom animals, clean cages, or walk dogs.
- **Food banks:** Receive shipments, sort food items, and prepare packages.
- **Veterans homes:** Help with craft activities, play music with residents, or escort veterans to appointments.

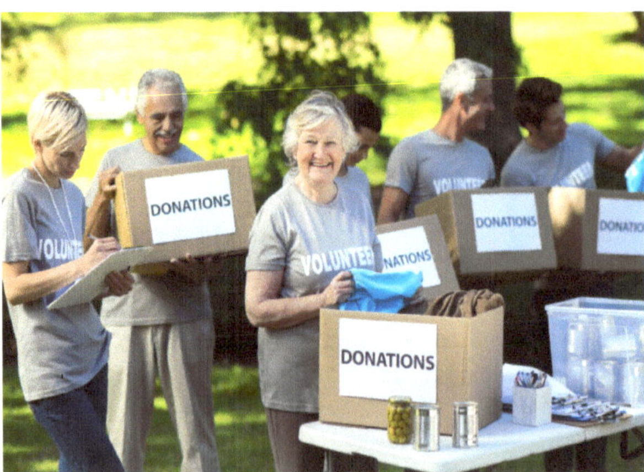

Fig.10.7 Retired persons helping in donation to senior citzens

Get involved in a sport

Being physically active comes with a whole host of health benefits: You can improve your flexibility, boost your immune system, and keep your heart and lungs healthy. Playing sports is also an easy way to meet new people and have fun. Bocce, pickleball, bowling, golf, tennis, and water aerobics are just some of the sports that are popular among retirees. You could join a team for older adults or use your athletic expertise to coach younger people.And just because you're retired doesn't mean you have to give up serious competition.The National Senior Games Association sponsors an Olympic-style competition for the 50-plus crowd that features 20 sports, including cycling, archery, horseshoes, power walking, volleyball, shuffleboard, badminton, and table tennis. Participants must qualify at the state level before going on to the national games

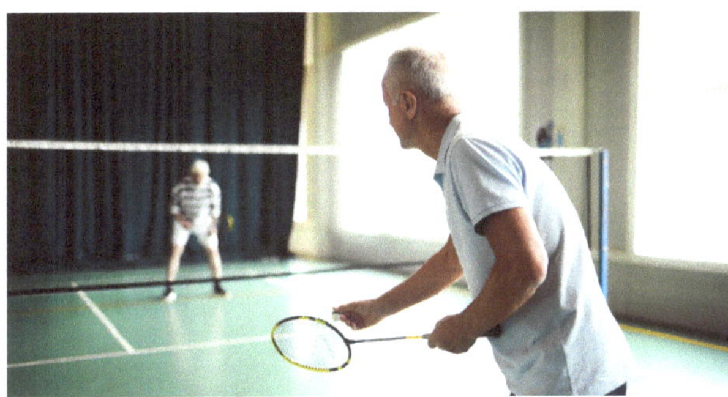

Fig.10.8 Badminton competition among senior citzens

Set new fitness goals

You can keep fit and stay active even if you're not the sporty type. Participating in an exercise class for seniors is a good way to stay accountable for your fitness goals. Low-impact activities like swimming, biking, and tai chi are excellent ways to boost your endurance, strength, flexibility, and balance. Join a gym, train for a marathon, take up yoga for seniors, or become part of a walking group. As an added bonus, being more active over the course of the day will help you get a better sleep at night

Mentor others

Sharing your expertise can be a very fulfilling way to give back. Becoming a mentor to a young person lets you act as both a teacher and a coach and make a positive difference in a kid's life. Plus, research in The Journals of Gerontology Series A: Biological Sciences and Medical Sciences has demonstrated that older adults who mentor young people are three times as happy as those who don't. According to a Harvard Business Review article, mentors also show improved cognitive functioning. Here are a few ways you can get involved:

- Experience Corps
- The National Mentoring Partnership
- Big Brothers Big Sisters of America

Of course, there are many additional ways to help others benefit from your knowledge and experience. Teach a course at your local community center or library. Offer tutoring services to high school or college students.

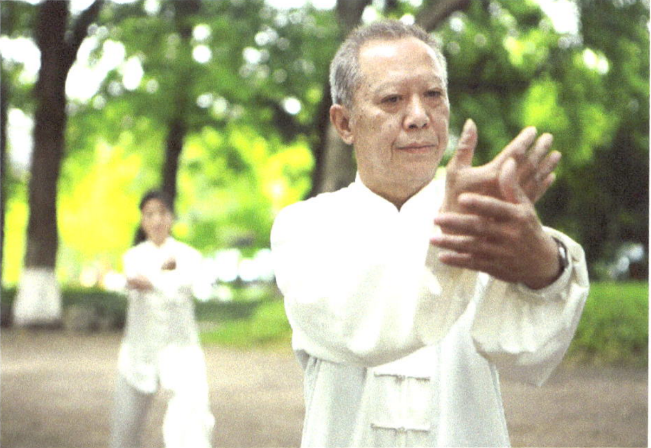

Fig.10.9 Senior citizen is teaching tai chi exercise to others for prevention of heart disease.

Join (or start) a club

Meeting with other people who share your interests is a fantastic way to make new friends and expand your knowledge. Check with your local seniors' center to see what types of groups are active in your area. Clubs centered around books, films, walking, gardening, and quilting are common. If you can't find a group that's focused on your particular interest, think about starting your own.

Be social

Human beings are social animals. Now that you no longer have to go to work every day, you have plenty of time to focus on deepening your social connections. Doing so is not just enjoyable, it's also good for your health. Research in the American Journal of Epidemiology and Ageing Research Reviews suggests that maintaining strong social ties can boost your overall cognitive health and lower your risk of developing conditions like heart disease and dementia.

So arrange regular get-togethers with other retirees. Plan wine-tasting parties or movie nights. Spend quality time with grandkids or other family members. Or reconnect with old friends on Facebook or at school reunions.

Start dating (singles and couples)

Most people who have been happily married or together long-term know that a strong relationship takes maintenance. But some of the regular maintenance you and your partner do must be fun activities that remind you of what you like and love about each other. Planning fun dates with your partner is one of the best ways to keep that spark alive that initially drew you to each other.

And what about the single seniors? Research from Harvard University projects that over the next twenty years, single-person households among the 80+ age group will more than double, from 4.7 million households in 2018 to over ten million in 2038. There are many reasons for this growth, including getting divorced or separating, having a partner with dementia or other issues debilitating enough to require full-time care in a facility, or experiencing the death of a partner.

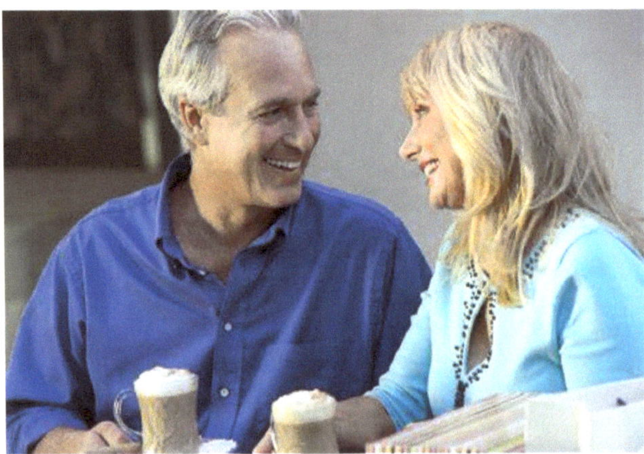

Fig.10.10 Senior citizen is dating to another one to counter loneliness which is a big concern among them

Loneliness is already a big concern for today's seniors, so for those who prefer a partnership, it may be time to take the leap into meeting new people.

Single seniors also have a lot to potentially gain by meeting and going on small adventures with potential love interests. Not only do you get out of the house, but you also can enrich your life with experiences, meet new people, practice your dating confidence, and potentially meet that special someone you want to spend the rest of your life with. Speed dating for seniors can be a safe, fun, and low-pressure way to get started. And if meeting people more organically "in the wild" is intimidating, online dating services for seniors are available to help make those connections easily.

Work part-time

Want to keep one foot in the work world? Almost 70 percent of newly retired people get part-time jobs, according to the Merrill Lynch survey. Many seniors find that such an arrangement gives them an opportunity to use their existing skills (or develop new ones) while earning a little extra money. You have the freedom to pursue any field that interests you without worrying about climbing the corporate ladder. And research by IZA World of Labor found that people who continued to work beyond retirement age had high levels of well-being and life satisfaction.

Learn a new skill

Pushing yourself to learn something new is not only enjoyable, it also keeps the brain agile. Attending formal classes and workshops is one option, but depending on what you want to learn, you could also explore free online videos that demonstrate the techniques you're looking to master. Consider learning how to:

- Speak a new language
- Play a musical instrument
- Drive an 18-wheeler
- Scuba dive
- Cook a different type of cuisine

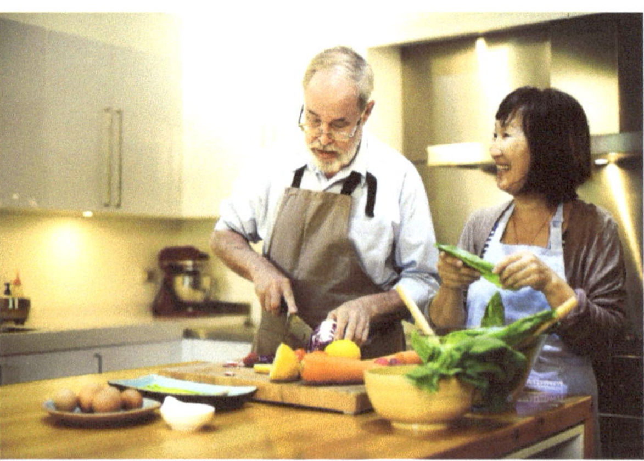

Fig.10.11 Retirees can earn extra money in homemade cooking. If you know how to cook you can take advantage of the fashion of healthy foods and share your love for the culinary arts making lunches for office workers who do not have time to prepare their own lunches.

Foster a pet

Open your home to a shelter or rescue pet and give an animal a brighter future. You could care for sick or injured dogs or cats and help them adjust to life in a home. The idea is to provide a loving and stable environment for the animals until a permanent home can be found for them. This is a great way to get the benefits of animal companionship without the high price tag. (Most fostering organizations, such as Dogs Without Borders, cover the cost of food, toys, and medical care.)

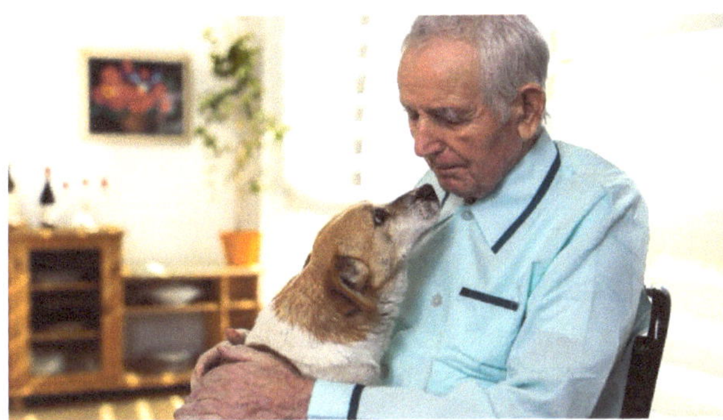

Fig.10.12 Senior citizen has given a shelter to an ailing dog.

Make crafts

Work with your hands to produce something unique and original! You could explore projects involving knitting, woodworking, painting, photography, scrapbooking, jewelry making, and more. Craft stores and community colleges frequently offer inexpensive workshops where you can learn about new crafts and join up with other people who share your interests. You might even be able to take advantage of programs at studios that give you access to professional-grade tools and materials for a small fee

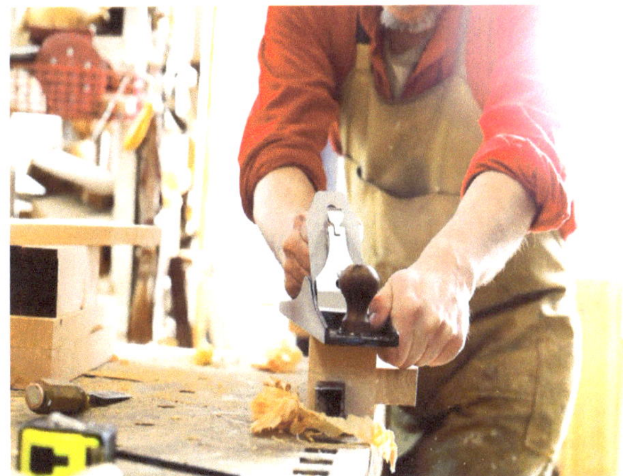

Fig.10.13 Senior citizen is learning woodcrafting after retirement

Play games

Games can be an awesome way to challenge your brain and have fun either by yourself or with others. Get together with neighbors, friends, or family members to play board games, card games, dice games, and more. Attend bingo nights or join a chess club. You could even explore the world of online or video games.

Start a small business

Now that you're not focused on making a living, you have the chance to develop and sell any product or service you like. Many retirees draw on their years of experience to become freelance advisors or consultants. You could also consider generating additional income by:

- Selling crafts through an Etsy shop
- Offering homemade cakes or jams at a farmers' market
- Babysitting for families in your area
- Walking dogs or looking after pets
- Fixing computers

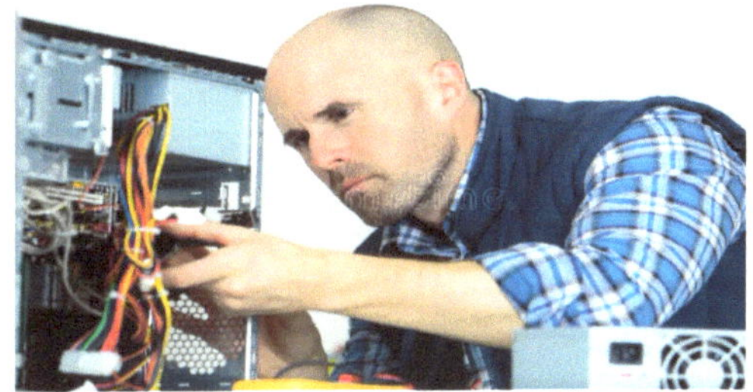

Fig.10.14 Senior citizen is repairing computer after retirement

Go to summer camp

A growing number of specialized camps are giving older adults the opportunity to partake in canoeing, ziplining, archery, river rafting, ropes courses, climbing walls, and camp fires. Adapted activities are available for those with physical challenges. You won't be roughing it quite the same way as when you were younger. (Most camps offer comfortable accommodations, often in air-conditioned lodges with private bathrooms.) Some camps allow couples to bunk together, while others separate male and female campers. Costs vary from around $500 to more than $1,400 for a week-long stay, which includes all your meals and activities. Here are a few options to check out:

- Camp Chief Ouray
- City of Sacramento Senior Summer Camp

Horses and Canoes: Summer Camp in the Ozarks With Your Family (open to seniors along with their adult children and grandchildren over age 10)
CampIsabellaFreedman

Improve your home

Why not undertake projects to make your home more beautiful, convenient, or secure? You could build a fence, convert a child's old room into a home office or exercise space, update your walls, cabinets, or other décor with a fresh coat of paint, or boost your home's curb appeal with simple additions like shutters, window boxes, or solar spotlights.

Explore your family history

Delve into your roots and discover where you came from. This could involve sorting through family photos or amassing a collection of stories that have been passed down through the generations. You can use websites like MyHeritage and Ancestry to build a family tree and track down details about your ancestors, although you will need a paid subscription to access the full range of resources; prices range from $80 to $200 per year. Or check out the list of free genealogy resources for each state at Family History Daily.

Write

With more time to think and reflect, you might realize you have special stories or know-how that could be shared with the world. Many retirees enjoy penning memoirs, novels, cookbooks, how-to guides, poems, or theatrical plays. You could start a blog dedicated to travel, cooking, music, or the retirement experience in general. Or write strictly for yourself: Keeping a personal journal can be a great way to document memories, relieve stress, and work through your emotions.

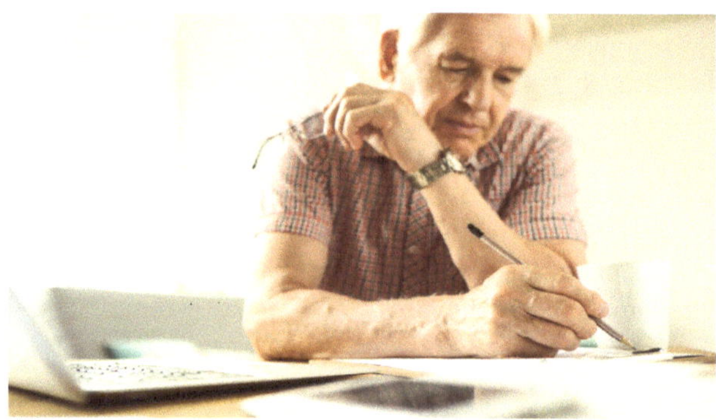

Fig.10.15 Senior citizen is writing a book after retirement

Organize a charity drive

Make a real difference in your community by leading a project to help others. Enlist family, friends, club members, former colleagues, and anyone else who can contribute to your efforts. Talk to local charities to see what's needed most. You might consider collecting clothing for disaster victims, raising money for a special needs group, or gathering toys for sick children.

Get involved in the political scene

Do you have an activist bent? There's no better time than retirement to take a greater interest in the issues affecting your city, your state, or the country in general. You could become a poll worker, volunteer on election campaigns, organize rallies, collect signatures on petitions, attend town hall meetings, or even run for local office.

Enjoy events that interest you

Get in tune with the special events going on in your community so that you can take in whatever strikes your fancy: theater shows, concerts, sports competitions, monster truck rallies, film festivals, etc. Many such events offer special pricing for seniors.

Just Take it Easy

Not every moment of your retirement needs to be packed with activities. Everyone needs a little downtime now and then, so don't feel guilty about watching a bit of TV or taking a nap if that's what you feel like. After all, you've earned this time—if you want to relax and do absolutely nothing, go for it.

Top Games for Seniors and the Elderly

Get ready to play! It's time to learn about the best games for seniors so that you can reap the benefits of having fun. After all, joy, amusement, and mental stimulation are necessary for every senior's overall well-being. And we all have days when we just want to spend a little time doing something engaging.

Games provide convenient ways to have fun, alone or in a group. They eradicate boredom, relieve stress, and make parties and other social engagements easier, more enjoyable, and less intimidating.

They also help exercise our brains. For some people, playing certain games might benefit things like mood, memory, concentration, reasoning, and imagination. Games might be especially helpful for your brain if they require you to learn something new.

Plus, countless games can be modified for seniors or elderly people with physical or cognitive limitations. For example, it's easy to find or create games with large type, which is good for older people with vision problems. And if time or attention spans are a concern, many games can be played and completed in less than 30 minutes.

The variety of senior-friendly games that are now available is astonishing. To help you narrow down the possibilities, we've provided some of the best examples within seven main categories:

- Puzzle, tile, and board games
- Video games
- Card games
- Dice games
- Word and number games
- Indoor games for large groups
- Outdoor games

Puzzle, Tile, and Board Games

Tabletop games are fantastic for social gatherings. That's why many seniors turn to this form of entertainment, especially when they want to encourage friends or family members to visit. Plus, a study in BMJ Open suggests that playing board games might help slow cognitive decline or reduce depression in elderly people. And since board games are generally played sitting down, they are good for seniors with limited mobility.

The best board games for seniors are fun, absorbing, and challenging (without being too complicated). They are also great for multi-generational play. Here are some popular examples:

1. **Qwirkle:** Mix and match tiles with different shapes and colors, scoring points by completing or adding to lines of the same shapes or colors.
2. **Dixit:** Out-bluff your opponents while using your imagination to match stories to beautifully illustrated cards.
3. **Ticket to Ride:** Claim as many North American railway routes as possible by collecting illustrated train cards and reaching more cities than your opponents within a short time.
4. **Rummikub:** Be the first to play all your numbered tiles by placing them in consecutive sequences or groups of the same numbers or colors.
5. **Sorry! Sliders:** Slide your pawns into home or take out your opponents' pawns in this twist on the classic Sorry! game that ditches the cards in favor of a mini-shuffleboard type of experience.
6. **Ubongo:** Race against other players as you try to solve puzzles of interlocking geometric shapes to grow your treasure of gems.
7. **Jenga:** Beware of gravity as you try not to be the one who pulls out the wooden block that makes the whole tower come crashing down.
8. **Bugs** in the Kitchen: Set the path and lure the little scuttling bug into your trap before anyone else.
9. Cranium: Be the first one to circle the board by successfully solving puzzles and other challenges that will have you acting, guessing, sculpting, sketching, and humming.
10. **Backgammon:** Beat your opponent by getting lucky, planning your moves, and being the first to get each of your 15 checkers off the board
11. **Chess:** Use your most creative strategies to protect your king while outwitting your opponent and putting his or her king into checkmate.
12. **Mahjong:** Be the first player to build a winning combination of tiles based on rummy-like groupings of symbols and characters.
13. **Checkers:** Capture and remove all 12 of your opponent's game pieces before he or she can do the same to you.
14. **Dominos:** Play all of your domino tiles before the other players by laying them down end-to-end with matching tiles that have already been played.

Video Games for Seniors

According to a 2019 article from Entertainment Software Association, 25 percent of men and 22 percent of women between the ages of 55 and 64 have been video game players (aka "gamers") for more than 25 years. AARP states that 45 percent of all 50-plus adults play video games. And almost half of those gamers play video games every day. So there seems to be a lot to love about this type of entertainment, regardless of your age.

Video games offer a form of visual and auditory engagement that most other kinds of games can't match. Many of them provide truly thrilling experiences as well as opportunities to connect with other players (of all ages). They are downright fun.

But here's something you should know: Some electronic game developers claim that their "brain training" products can improve your brain health and cognitive performance. However, their marketing is often misleading.

The science behind brain-training games is controversial at best. Many of the world's top psychologists and neuroscientists say there is little or no solid evidence to support claims that certain kinds of video games can improve a senior's mental faculties.The truth is that "brain games" may not boost your cognitive abilities for everyday life or prevent or slow down brain-related diseases. Rather, by playing a game repeatedly, you'll get better at the particular tasks for that game (and possibly other tasks that are very closely related to them). But you won't necessarily get better at doing unrelated tasks in the "real world" outside of the game.

If you really want to improve your brain health, you're better off exercising, getting good sleep, and learning new thingsThat said, if a video game is completely new to you, then your brain may benefit from the challenge of learning how to play it. And you can't overlook the pure enjoyment factor. After all, having fun should be your top reason for playing any video game.

According to AARP, the most popular types of video games among older adults are card, tile, puzzle, and logic games. But many seniors also enjoy strategy, role-playing, and action-oriented games. So try out several different kinds and see what you enjoy.

Most seniors play video games on their laptops or desktop computers. But you can also play games on a smartphone, digital tablet, handheld game console, or TV game console (such as the Nintendo Switch, Sony PlayStation, or Microsoft Xbox). Games for computers and mobile devices can often be downloaded for free or played online at no cost. Here are some electronic games that are especially worth checking out:

1. **Match-three puzzle games** like Bejeweled, Candy Crush Saga, and Gummy Drop involve switching around colorful shapes to form three-of-a-kind matches within a time limit or fixed number of moves, then moving to the next level. They are typically played on a mobile phone or tablet.

2. **Snipperclips Plus:** Solve all kinds of creative puzzles in this funny game for the Nintendo Switch by interacting with various objects and cutting paper characters into different shapes.

3. **Puyo Puyo Tetris:** Quickly rotate and position falling blobs of color or shaped blocks so that they land in places that will help complete a puzzle in this game for the Nintendo Switch.

4. **Words With Friends 2:** Challenge your friends or family to a crossword-style mobile game that's similar to Scrabble.

5. **AARP's free online games:** Play a huge variety of card, puzzle, word, strategy, sports, and arcade games directly in your web browser.

6. **Gametable's free online games:** Enjoy easy-to-play games like checkers and tic-tac-toe on your computer or mobile device without any distracting ads.

Card Games

When it comes to portability, it's hard to beat a deck of cards. After all, card games don't require any electricity. In most cases, aside from cards, you only need a flat surface (and sometimes a paper and pen). Generation after generation has celebrated card games for their ability to facilitate pressure-free social gatherings, relaxing recreation, and memorable conversations. Whether you play games of chance or strategy (or both), you'll likely have tons of fun. You can make these games even more accessible by purchasing oversized playing cards, decks with large print, playing card holders, or an automatic card shuffler.Here are some of the most popular card games among seniors:

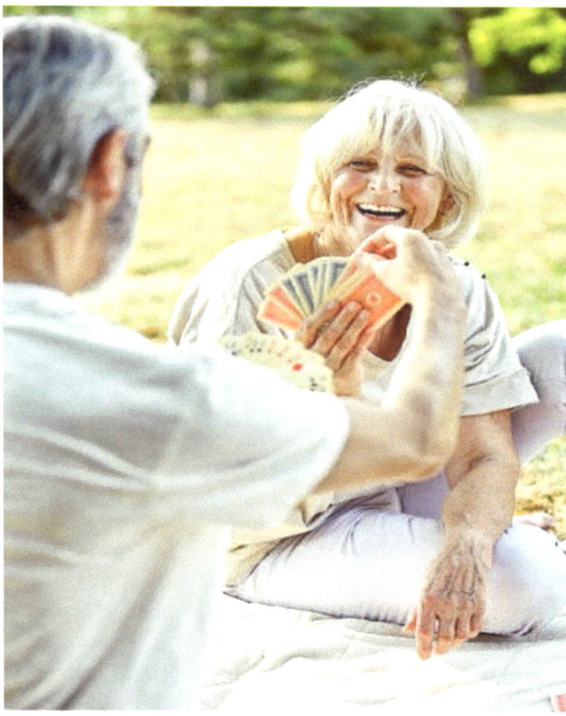

Fig.10.16 Senior citizen is playing card game after retirement

1. **Gin Rummy:** Get all your playing cards into sequences (i.e., cards in a consecutive order according to their rank) and/or groups of the same rank before your opponent does.

2. **Bridge:** Choose a playing partner and work together to defeat another team by making "bids" and winning "tricks."

3. **Canasta:** Play this rummy-style game with a partner, scoring points by collecting sets of cards with the same rank.

4. **Cribbage:** Use a special cribbage board (optional) to keep score as you try to win by being the first player to reach 121 points.

5. **Spades:** Partner up with somebody and play together as you "bid" on the strength of your hands and get as close as you can to that estimate when winning "tricks."

6. **Crazy Eights:** Get rid of all your cards before the other players by laying down eights or cards of a specified suit.

7.**Pinochle:** Exchange and collect various combinations of playing cards to score as many points as possible per an opening "bid".

8. **Euchre:** Team up with a partner and win at least three out of five "tricks" in this fast-moving game that is similar to bridge.

9. UNO: Be the first player to get rid of all your cards by matching them, one by one, to the upturned color or number cards on the top of the deck when it's your turn.

10. Phase 10: Complete 10 hands of rummy-style play, each requiring you to collect a different grouping of cards or risk being left behind.

11. No Thanks!: Try to get the lowest score by constantly weighing the potential consequences of picking up a particular card or playing one of your chips.

Dice Games

Sometimes, the only things you need to have fun are a few dice, a pad of paper, and a pencil. Like cards, dice are ultra-portable. And dice games just as much enjoyment and social bonding. Plus, there's something uniquely satisfying about rolling the dice and watching them all land exactly as you had hoped. Try popular dice games like:

1. Bunco: Win a game of Bunco by earning as many points as you can by rolling numbers.

2. Mexico: Be the last player standing by avoiding the lowest roll in each round.

3. Liar's Dice: Outlast your opponents by successfully deceiving them and recognizing when they are bluffing you.

4. Farkle: Race your opponents to a predetermined scoring level by constantly deciding between taking a risk or playing it safe.

5. Yahtzee: Defeat your competition by rolling the highest-scoring combinations.

6. Can't Stop: Beat the other players by taking risks, getting lucky, and avoiding the trap of being too much of a gambler for your own good.

Word and Number Games

Many seniors enjoy keeping their math or language skills sharp by playing fun games or solving satisfying puzzles related to words or numbers. Great options are available for playing solo or as part of a group. Consider these examples:

1. **Crossword Puzzles:** Solve clues to fill out a grid of squares with interconnected words and phrases.

2. **Word Search:** Discover and circle all the hidden words in a grid of letters.

3. **Sudoku:** Fill out a partially completed grid of numbers so that each row, column, and sub-grid contains all of the numbers from one to nine.

4. **Kakuro:** Fill out each white square of the puzzle with a number from one to nine so that the sums of the entries in each row or column match the associated clues.

5. Scrabble: Outscore your opponents by strategically forming new words or adding to existing ones on a crossword-style board.

6. **Boggle**: Shake a tray of 16 letter dice and spot more words in the randomized grid of letters than your opponent does before the time runs out.

7.Scattergories: Partner up and defeat the other teams by coming up with creative answers that all match a specific category, contain the same first letter, and won't be thought of by your opponents.

8. Balderdash: Fool the other players by making them believe your fake answers or definitions represent the truth about obscure words, people, and movies.

Indoor Games for Large Groups

Many nursing homes and assisted living communities regularly organize fun games that large groups of residents can participate in. The best activities directors try to keep things fresh by changing things up frequently. Most games in this category are homemade and require only time and creativity to pull together. You can put your own spin on any of them. Plus, many of them can be used as fun party games for seniors or elderly residents celebrating birthdays or other milestones. Use the following examples as inspiration:

1. Bingo: Be the first player to match five numbers in a row (or another pattern) in this popular game of chance.

2. Smile Toss: Prepare to laugh when playing this great balloon game for seniors. Draw a smiley face on a balloon. Sit in a circle with the other players. Have someone be in charge of playing some recorded music and stopping it randomly. As the music plays, pass the balloon around the circle to each other. If you're left holding the balloon when the music stops, you must try not to smile for at least 10 seconds. If you do smile, you'll have to leave the circle. The last person remaining wins the game.

3. The Best (or Worst) Advice My Parents Ever Gave Me: Choose someone to be the judge. Pass out slips of paper and have everyone write down the best advice they ever received from their mom or dad. Have the judge collect all the answers, read them out loud, and select the top three. Then, get each of those three winners to write down the worst advice they ever received from their parents. Have the judge collect them, read them aloud, and select the final winner.

4. Fact or Fiction?: Get some books about strange or funny facts, such as 1,227 Quite Interesting Facts to

Blow Your Socks Off or Mind = Blown: Amazing Facts About This Weird, Hilarious, Insane World. Select five weird facts from the books, make up five other fake facts, and randomly number them from one to 10. Pass out a sheet of paper to each player that is numbered from one to 10. One by one, read each strange (or fake) fact out loud and ask the players to write down whether it is fact or fiction. To determine the winner(s), collect the sheets and find out who had the most correct guesses.

5. The Price Is Right: Go to the store and buy four common, lower-priced items as well as four mid- to higher-priced items to use as prizes, being sure to write down their prices. Put everyone's name in a bowl. Draw four names to become the first contestants. Showcase your first item and have them each guess its price. The person closest to the actual price without going over is the winner of that round. Draw another name from the bowl to replace that winner. Continue the process for the other common items until you have four winners. Then, have each of the four winners guess the total of the four higher-priced items to determine the final winner of those prizes.

6. **Photo Puzzle Race:** Get large color prints on heavy stock of various photos, preferably of the people who will be playing the game. Cut each of the photo prints into relatively small puzzle pieces. Divide players into teams and have them compete to see which team can solve its puzzle the fastest.

7. **Name That Tune:** Choose a selection of songs that will create feelings of nostalgia for the seniors who will be playing the game. Gather everyone together a day ahead of time to listen to each song and learn the artists and song titles. On game day, start playing one of the songs, pausing the music after a few seconds. See if anyone can guess what it is. Keep playing and pausing the song until someone makes a correct guess. Do the same thing for the remaining songs. Give prizes to each of the winners.

8. Year of Invention: Collect 10 everyday objects and find out when they were first invented. Put them all on a table, numbered from one to 10. Hand out sheets of paper numbered the same way and have each player write down the year they think each object was invented. (Make sure that nobody has access to an Internet-enabled device.) Score each player's sheet: six points for correctly guessing the exact year, three points for being within 50 years,

, or one point fobeing within 100 years. The player with the highest point total wins the game.

Outdoor Games

Don't overlook the benefits of physical games. For seniors with good or decent mobility, getting outside can provide opportunities for enjoyable exercise that boosts overall health and well-being. For instance, many older adults who are in good shape enjoy playing tennis games. But you don't necessarily have to do something quite so active. Here are several other popular outdoor games:

1. Shuffleboard: Win by sliding your colored disks into the highest scoring zones and strategically knocking out your opponent's disks.

2. Pickleball: Outscore your opponent by using a solid paddle to hit a lightweight ball over a net while avoiding tennis-like faults.

3. Bocce: Roll more of your balls closer to the target than your opponent.

4. Water Balloon Toss: Partner with someone else and beat other teams by tossing a water balloon back and forth to each other over an increasing distance without breaking it.

5. Croquet: Be the first one to hit your balls against the center peg by knocking them through a six-hoop course in the proper sequence.

6. Beach Ball Volley: Team up with someone else and try to keep a beach ball in the air longer than any other team as you volley it back and forth to each other over a distance that keeps growing.

7. **Lawn Bowling**: Roll special balls designed to curve along their path, choosing your shots carefully to get your balls closer to the jack than your opponent's.

8. **Horseshoes:** Outscore your competition by tossing your horseshoes and getting them to land closer to the stake than your opponent's.

9. **Badminton:** Win points by hitting a shuttlecock over a net with a special racquet, forcing the opposing player(s) to miss the shuttlecock or hit it out of bounds or into the net.

10. **Flying Disc** Target Toss: Be the first to score 21 points by hitting various targets with a Frisbee-like disc.

11. **Bean Bag** Toss: Score 21 points before your opponents by getting your bean bags to land in the hole or within a designated target area.

Bibliography and Acknowledgement

- Adams GA, Rau BL. Job seeking among retirees seeking bridge employment. Pers Psychol. 2004;57(3):719–744. doi: 10.1111/j.1744-6570.2004.00005.x. [CrossRef] [Google Scholar]
- Atchley RC. A continuity theory of normal aging. The Gerontologist. 1989;29(2):183–190. doi: 10.1093/geront/29.2.183. [PubMed] [CrossRef] [Google Scholar]
- Beehr TA, Bennett MM, Shultz KS, Adams GA. Examining retirement from a multi-level perspective. In: Shultz KS, Adams GA, editors. Aging and work in the 21st century. Mahwah: Erlbaum; 2007. pp. 277–302. [Google Scholar]
  Braun V, Clarke V. Using thematic analysis in psychology. Qual Res Psychol. 2006;3(2):77–101.
- Cahill KE, Giandrea MD, Quinn JF. Retirement patterns from career employment. The Gerontologist. 2006;46(4):514–523. doi: 10.1093/geront/46.4.514. [PubMed] [CrossRef] [Google Scholar]
- Centraal Bureau voor de Statistiek: [Increasing pension age for the ninth year] 2016. https://www.cbs.nl/nl-nl/nieuws/2016/09/pensioenleeftijd-voor-negende-jaar-omhoog.
- Centraal Bureau voor de Statistiek: [Labor participation; the elderly] 2016. Centraal Bureau voor de Statistiek: [Prognosis population; key figures 2006–2050]. 2016.
- Colcombe, S. J., Erickson, K. I., Scalf, P. E., Kim, J. S., Prakash, R., McAuley, E., et al. (2006). Aerobic exercise training increases brain volume in aging humans. J. Gerontol. A Biol. Sci. Med. Sci. 61, 1166–1170. doi: 10.1093/gerona/61.11.1166
- de Wind A, Geuskens GA, Reeuwijk KG, Westerman MJ, Ybema JF, Burdorf A, et al. Pathways through which health influences early retirement: a qualitative study. BMC Public Health. 2013;13(1):1. doi: 10.1186/1471-2458-13-1. [PMC free article] [PubMed] [CrossRef] [Google Scholar]
- Dingemans E, Henkens K, Solinge H. Working Beyond Retirement in Europe: An Investigation of Individual and Societal Determinants Using Share. Netspar Discus Pap. 2016;6.
- Giandrea MD, Cahill KE, Quinn JF. Bridge jobs: a comparison across cohorts. Res Aging. 2009;31(5):549–576. doi: 10.1177/0164027509337195. [CrossRef] [Google Scholar]
- James BD, Wilson RS, Barnes LL, Bennett DA. Late-Life Social Activity and Cognitive Decline in Old Age. Journal of the International Neuropsychological Society [Internet]. 2011;17:998–1005. Available from: https://
- Kim S, Feldman DC. Working in retirement: The antecedents of bridge employment and its consequences for quality of life in retirement. Acad Manag J. 2000;43(6):1195–1210. doi: 10.2307/1556345. [CrossRef] [Google Scholar]
- Kitzinger J. Qualitative research: Introducing focus groups. Br Med J. 1995;311:299–302. doi: 10.1136/bmj.311.7000.299. [PMC free article] [PubMed] [CrossRef] [Google Scholar]
- Kromer B, Howard D. Labor force participation and work status of people 65 years and older. Census Bureau: United States; 2013. [Google Scholar]
- Liu, H., Yang, Y., Xia, Y., Zhu, W., Leak, R. K., Wei, Z., Wang, J., & Hu, X. (2017). Aging of cerebral white matter. Ageing research reviews, 34, 64–76. https://doi.org/10.1016/j.arr.2016.11.006
- Lusardi A, Michell OS. Baby boomer retirement security: the roles of planning, financial literacy, and housing wealth. J Monet Econ. 2007;54(1):205–224. doi: 10.1016/j.jmoneco.2006.12.001. [CrossRef] [Google Scholar
- McMichael AJ. Standardized mortality ratios and the 'healthy worker effect': scratching beneath the surface. Int J Occup Environ Med.1976;18(3):165–168.doi: 10.1097/00043764-197603000-00009.[PubMed] [CrossRef] [Google Scholar]
- Patton MQ. Qualitative research and evaluation methods. 4. Thousand Oaks: Sage Publications Inc; 2015. [Google Scholar
- Reeuwijk KG, de Wind A, Westerman MJ, Ybema JF, van der Beek AJ, Geuskens GA. 'All those things together made me retire': qualitative study on early retirement among Dutch employees. BMC Public Health. 2013;13:516. doi: 10.1186/1471-2458-13-516. [PMC free article] [PubMed] [CrossRef] [Google Scholar]
- Stuckey, H. L., & Nobel, J. (2010). The connection between art, healing, and public health: a review of current literature. American journal of public health, 100(2), 254–263. https://doi.org/10.2105/AJPH.2008.156497
- Tong A, Sainsbury P, Craig J. Consolidated criteria for reporting qualitative research (COREQ): a 32-item checklist for interviews and focus groups. Int J Qual Health Care. 2007;19(6):349–357. doi: 10.1093/intqhc/mzm042. [PubMed] [CrossRef] [Google Scholar
- Tong A, Sainsbury P, Craig J. Consolidated criteria for reporting qualitative research (COREQ): a 32-item checklist for interviews and focus groups. Int J Qual Health Care. 2007;19(6):349–357. doi: 10.1093/intqhc/mzm042. [PubMed] [CrossRef] [Google Scholar]
- Tu J-C, Yang C-H, Liang C-Y, Chen H-Y. Exploring the Impact of Puzzle Games for the Elderly from Experiential Learning. Thinking Skills and Creativity. 2022;45:101107.
  Ulrich LB, Brott PE. Older workers and bridge employment: Redefining retirement. J Employ Couns. 2005;42(4):159.
- Virtanen M, Oksanen T, Batty GD, Ala-Mursula L, Salo P, Elovainio M, et al. Extending employment beyond the pensionable age: a cohort study of the influence of chronic diseases, health risk factors, and working conditions. PLoS One. 2014;9(2) doi: 10.1371/journal.pone.0088695.
- Wheaton F, Crimmins EM. The Demography of Aging and Retirement. In: Wang M, editor. The Oxford Handbook of retirement. New York: Oxford University Press; 2013. pp. 22–41. [Google Scholar]
- •Ybema JF, Geuskens GA, van den Heuvel SG, de Wind A, Leijten FR, Joling C, et al. Study on Transitions in Employment, Ability and Motivation (STREAM): The design of a four-year longitudinal cohort study among 15,118 persons aged 45 to 64 years. Br J Med Med Res. 2014;4(6):1383.

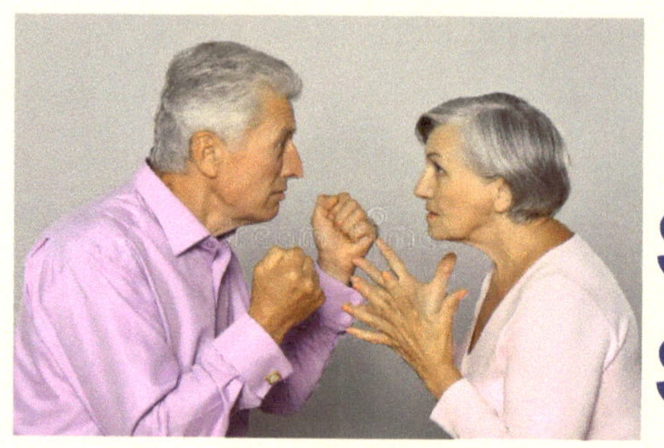

Self-Defense For Senior Citizens

Everyone deserves to feel secure. That's why self-defense for seniors is such an important topic. As people age, their bodies tend to get slower and weaker, which can make them vulnerable to attacks by criminals. Fortunately, there are a variety of good tactics that older adults can learn in order to protect themselves.

The sad reality is that some people do prey on seniors. A U.S. Department of Justice report noted that between 2003 and 2013, 93 percent of all crimes against people over age 65 were property crimes such as burglary and theft. And even though seniors and the elderly experience lower rates of violent crime than those in other age groups, the report showed that over the same time period, the rate of violent crime against people over 65 increased by 27 percent. This article will help you understand different types of self-defense training that are available (including martial arts and cane self-defense) and how such training can benefit your health and well-being. You'll learn about steps you can take to avoid becoming a target and discover basic techniques for defending yourself if you do end up in a dangerous situation. You'll also read about important factors to consider before turning to a firearm for your defense.

Benefits of Self-Defense Training

Age and physical limitations do not have to prevent you from learning how to protect yourself. Whether you study basic self-defense techniques or pursue advanced martial arts training, knowing that you're capable of defending yourself can be a great confidence booster. And when you feel (and look) confident, you show the world that you are not weak or vulnerable. That can potentially deter would-be aggressors and keep you from having to defend yourself at all.

Self-defense training teaches you how to stay aware of your surroundings and focus on your safety. You will learn to recognize where potential attackers could be lurking and where you could go to escape. You will also learn how to prepare for the unexpected and how to quickly disable an assailant if necessary. With practice, you can develop the reactions that are required to protect yourself in an emergency.Such training also brings a host of physical benefits: You can improve your balance, coordination, stamina, strength, and flexibility. Even if you never have to use the techniques you learn in class, the exercise you get through self-defense training can have a positive impact on your overall health.

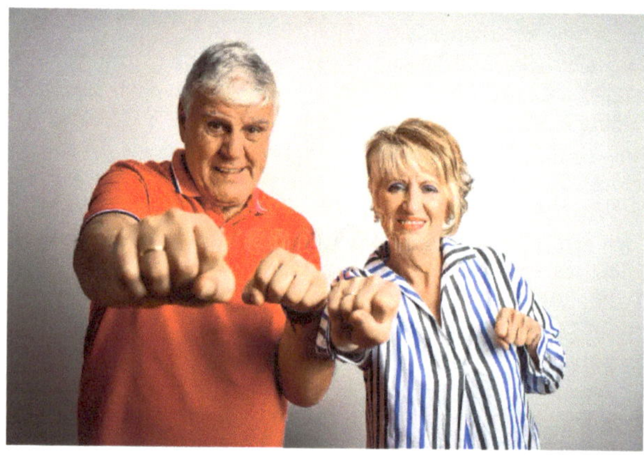

Fig.11.1 Senior citizens are learning techniques of self defence

Safety Tips: How to Avoid Being Targeted

Prevention should always be your primary objective. After all, the best way to stay safe is to not get into dicey situations in the first place.

Did you know that your body language and mannerisms can give off signals that make you more likely to be a target for criminals? In one famous study, researchers recorded more than 60 people walking along a busy New York City street. Then, they showed the video to a group of prison inmates who had been convicted of assaulting strangers. The prisoners were asked to identify the people on the video who would make the most desirable targets.

The inmates were remarkably consistent in their choices. It turned out that age, size, and gender were not the deciding factors. Instead, the criminals selected victims who dragged their feet and moved awkwardly, who were slumped over, and who kept their eyes on the ground. Those people were perceived as being easy to overpower.

If you can exhibit confidence and self-assurance, a potential attacker may decide you're not the easy mark he or she was hoping for. To avoid appearing vulnerable, try following these tips:

- Be alert and aware of your surroundings. Developing the habit of scanning the area around you will help you spot potential threats and allow you to avoid them.
- Stand straight and keep your chin up and your shoulders back. A hunched posture and a lowered gaze will make you seem fearful and timid.
- Walk smoothly and fluidly to convey confidence. If possible, keep the same pace as the pedestrians around you.
- Make brief eye contact with the people around you to demonstrate that you are aware of them (but don't stare or act aggressively). If a potential assailant knows you have seen him or her, the advantage of surprise disappears.
- Don't talk on your phone or stare at a map while out walking. Doing so indicates that you aren't paying attention to what's going on around you. Plan your route before you leave your home, hotel, or other point of origin; if you need assistance, step into a store and ask a clerk to help you.
- Don't let a potential attacker distract you. If a stranger asks you for the time, don't stop and look down at your watch. Instead, keep walking and raise your watch up to your eye level in order to keep the person in your line of sight.
- Stick to well-lit and populated areas at night. It's also a good idea to keep a mini flashlight and whistle on your key ring and keep the keys in your hand (with one key sticking out between your fingers) while you're walking.
- Don't draw attention to yourself. Keep valuables out of sight and don't wear expensive clothes or flashy jewelry. If you use a purse, carry it close to you and don't let it dangle too far from your body. You might even want to conceal your purse under your jacket or coat

Basic Techniques to Fend Off an Attack

Even if you do your best to prevent becoming a target of crime, you still might end up in a dangerous situation. So it's important to know how to stay safe and defend yourself.

Always remember that self-preservation is the ultimate goal. So if a thief demands your money or personal property, especially if he or she is wielding a weapon, give it to him or her. *Nothing in your pockets or purse is worth more than your life.*If you have no easy way to escape, it's far better to just give the mugger what he or she wants so that he or she will leave you alone. If you're able to do so, keep a safe distance from the thief by tossing your valuables in his or her direction rather than handing them over at close range.

Sometimes, however, a physical confrontation is unavoidable. You typically have just a few seconds to make a move, so you need to be prepared. These tips can help you better protect yourself if you end up in such a situation:

1.Make noise.

Shout, blow a whistle, or activate a personal alarm. Emergency whistles or alarms that fit in your pocket or attach to your keychain can be effective ways of scaring off attackers who are seeking easy prey. (Some personal alarms are so loud that they can be heard up to 300 feet away.) Such devices can also let bystanders know that you need help.

2.Use whatever you have on hand.

It could be anything from car keys to canned goods. Throw dirt in the attacker's eyes if possible. Swinging a cane at an assailant can also be very effective; in fact, there is an entire discipline devoted to cane self-defense for seniors.

Pepper spray causes extremely painful burning of the eyes and nose and will temporarily blind your attacker. Some pepper sprays also contain UV dyes that will mark the attacker even if he or she tries to wash it off, which is useful if police later need to confirm that the person was involved in the incident.

All states allow pepper spray to be used for self-defense, but some states and cities restrict a spray's size or strength, so be sure to check the regulations in your area.

Stun guns are non-lethal tools that use a high-voltage charge to immobilize an assailant. Many are designed to look like cameras, cell phones, flashlights, or other ordinary items, and they can be easily carried in a pocket or handbag. They are legal to own in most states, but some states require permits or place other restrictions on their use. In a few states (and cities), stun guns are illegal. It's important to research the laws that apply where you live.

A firearm can also be an effective weapon, but you need to be extremely cautious about using one. Learn more about factors to consider before getting a gun

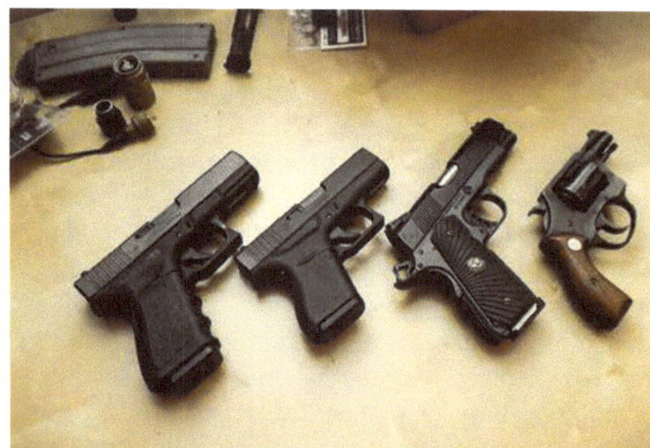

Fig.11.2 Best Home-Defense Firearms

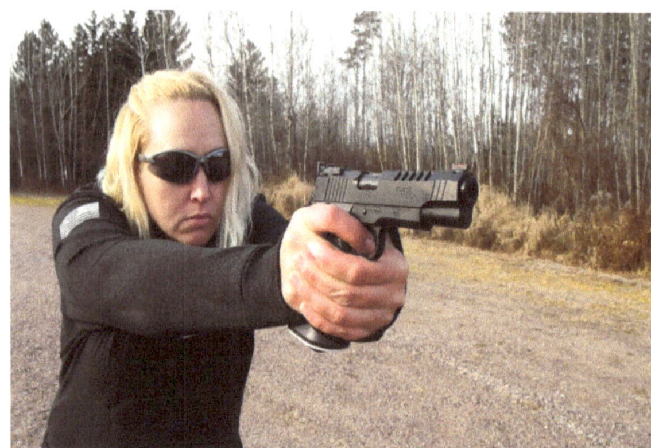

Fig.11.3 vStun guns for self defence

3.Aim for the most vulnerable areas.

Even if your attacker is bigger and stronger than you, he or she still has weak areas that you can exploit. Sensitive pressure points include the eyes, nose, neck, groin, and knees. The one you should target depends on how agile you are, how close the attacker is, and what position he or she is in relative to you. For instance, if he or she is a leg's length away from you, try kicking the side of his or her knee (or whacking it with a cane). That will throw him or her off balance and may allow you to escape. You might also choose to kick or knee the attacker in the groin.

If the assailant is very close, the best move is to jab your fingers, knuckles, or keys into his or her eyes. It doesn't take much pressure on the eyes to cause extreme pain, and it may incapacitate your attacker long enough for you to get away. If your arms are pinned down, try stomping on the assailant's foot as hard as you can. That might make him or her release at least one of your arms, and then you can go for the eyes.

Martial Arts for Seniors of All Ability Levels

Studying martial arts regularly can be an empowering way for seniors to learn how to defend

Studying martial arts regularly can be an empowering way for seniors to learn how to defend themselves. It can also help boost their stamina, coordination, range of motion, and mental acuity. In addition, students learn respect and self-discipline. This type of training allows people of all ages and ability levels to realize their maximum potential.

There are hundreds of martial arts, which means it can be difficult to choose the most appropriate one. The best martial art for seniors is the one that aligns with their capabilities. So before beginning any training regimen, be sure to assess your physical abilities. You don't want to overdo things and injure yourself. It's important to begin slowly, then gradually build up your skill level. (If you have some sort of physical limitation, talk to the instructor. He or she should be able to adapt the exercises and techniques to suit your needs.)

It's often said that tai chi is the best martial art for beginners because it involves slow, gentle movements with low impact. Most tai chi for seniors classes focus on health and meditation as opposed to self-defense, but they can show you how to move your body and can act as a good bridge to other disciplines.

Here are a few types of defensive martial arts that may be good options for seniors:

1. **Judo**

Judo focuses on using an adversary's strength against him or her. It lets you disable an opponent by throwing him or her to the ground, then subduing him or her through pins, holds, and locks. You need a certain amount of dexterity, since the throwing and grappling can be demanding. Some instructors can adapt their classes so that seniors avoid moves that are too strenuous or uncomfortable.

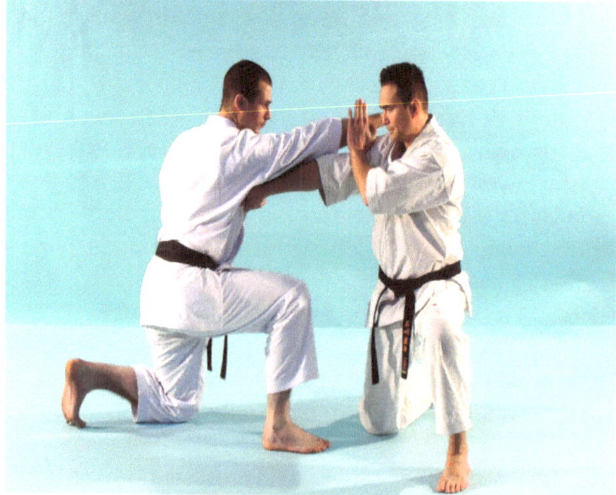

Fig.11.4 Senior is learning judo. technique for self defence

2. Aikido

Aikido is ideal for older adults as well as people with disabilities. Like judo, aikido is based on turning an attacker's strength and power against him or her. By redirecting the force of an attack, a less physically equipped adult can overcome a younger and stronger opponent. Aikido does not generally involve punches and kicks. It can also teach you how to fall properly in order to avoid getting injured.

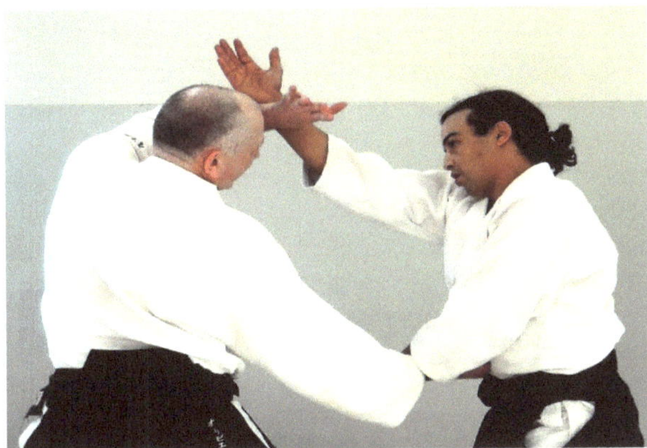

Fig.11.5 Senior is learning Aikido technique for self defence

3.Jiu-Jitsu

Another soft art based on defending oneself against a more powerful opponent, jiu-jitsu concentrates on manipulation and balance rather than counterforce. While it does incorporate some striking, most of its movements involve throws and joint locks. You will be taught how to dodge attacks and escape from holds. It's about leverage and technique as opposed to size and strength

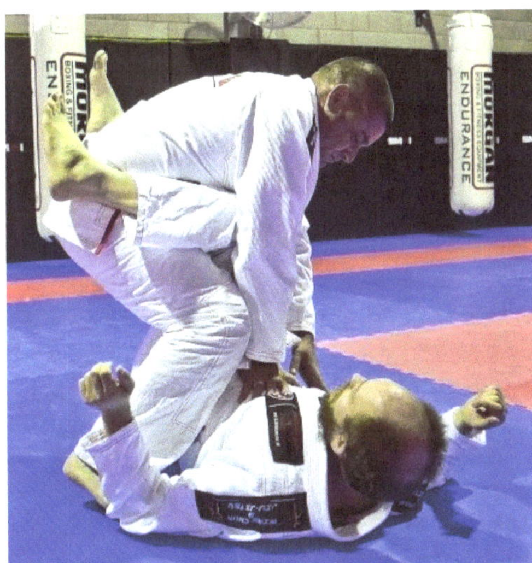

Fig.11.6 Senior is learning Jiu-Jitsu technique for self defence

4. Wing Chun

This form of kung fu uses open-handed strikes and low kicks. Because it focuses on precision and posture rather than raw power, wing chun can be excellent training for older adults. It's a low-impact activity that does not involve jumping or acrobatics, so it's easier on the knees than some other forms of martial arts.

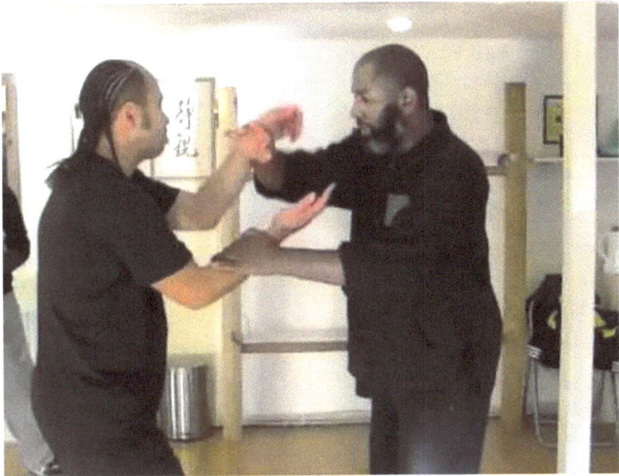

Fig.11.7 Senior is learning Wing Chun technique for self defence

5. Krav Maga

Many people believe that Krav Maga is the best martial art for self-defense. Developed by the Israeli military, Krav Maga is really more of a street combat system than a martial art. There are no sporting applications; the whole focus is on surviving an attack. You learn to neutralize an assailant quickly using simple, natural movements (including groin kicks and eye gouges, which are not permitted in other types of martial arts). The techniques are highly efficient and can be used by people of any age, since they do not rely on strength, speed, or flexibility

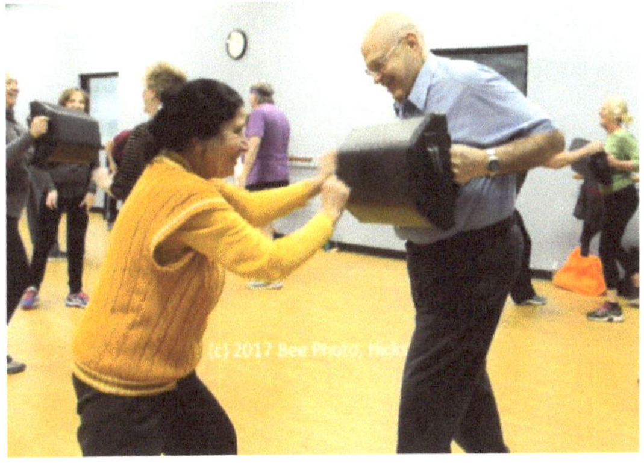

Fig.11.8 Senior is learning Krav Maga technique for self defence

Cane Fu: A Growing Trend

Why not transform a common mobility aid into an effective tool for self-defense? A discipline known as "cane fu" teaches seniors to fight back against attackers using an ordinary walking stick. Defense experts point out that unlike weapons such as pepper spray or stun guns, a cane can be taken anywhere and is always ready for action. Often perceived as a symbol of weakness, a cane can instead be an excellent way to inflict pain and neutralize aggressors.

Some techniques include swinging the cane in circles, hooking an assailant's neck or foot, and striking the knee, nose, or throat. The video below, from Cane Masters International founder Mark Shuey, illustrates some basic methods of self-defense using a cane:

And this video, also from Mark Shuey, demonstrates cane self-defense techniques that can be used by an individual in a wheelchair:

If you're choosing a cane with an eye on self-defense, it's important to get the right kind. Any high-quality walking stick will work, but some are better designed for defending yourself from attackers. For instance, a cane with a wide crook will allow you to hook or trap an assailant. Wooden canes are heavier than metal or fibreglass ones, which means they have more impact on an attacker; however, they also require more strength to wield. You'll want to make sure you choose a cane that you can handle comfortably.

Some canes are optimized for defensive use and are sometimes known as combat canes. Legal in all states (so long as they don't conceal another weapon such as a blade or firearm), such canes cost more than simple walking sticks but offer greater potential as self-defense tools. For example, a cane with a series of notches along the length of the shaft will concentrate the force of a strike on the raised area of each notch and cause considerably more pain when you strike an attacker.

Cane-fighting classes are becoming increasingly available through senior centers, retirement communities, and police departments. Some are offered free of charge. Ask around to see what the options are in your community.

Self-Defense Classes for Seniors

Taking a formal self-defense class offers plenty of advantages. For one thing, being part of a group can help you stay motivatedIt's also easier to practice your techniques on real live people. Plus, you can get help from the instructor or your fellow students if you find that you're having difficulty.Locate classes by contacting your local senior center,YMCA, public library, or police department. Fullpower International also offers workshops on self-defense for the elderly throughout a handful of states.

In addition, check out martial arts schools in your area. Most offer self-defense classes (especially for women), and a growing number of them are gearing such classes toward the specific needs of seniors.

When considering any class, be sure to get answers to the following questions:

•What are the instructor's credentials? Does he or she have any experience with street attacks?

•Can the techniques be adapted to students with physical challenges?

•Does the program teach situational awareness as well as techniques for talking down an attacker?

•How long is the training? (Unlike martial arts programs, which are meant to be ongoing, self-defense classes should be able to cover the basics in a fairly short amount of time.)

•What is the cost? (Some organizations offer classes for free.)

•Is it possible to observe a class before deciding to participate in one?

What to Consider Before Getting a Gun

For some older adults, having a gun for self-protection can alleviate anxiety and make them feel like they are in a better position to defend themselves against an aggressor. In fact, statistics show that one-third of American adults over the age of 50 own a gun. That's a higher percentage than any other age group.

However, many self-defense experts advise against carrying a gun, as it can easily be used against you in an attack. Also, many seniors have issues like poor eyesight or weak fine motor skills that can make it difficult to operate a gun safely.

If you're thinking about getting a firearm, here are some important factors to consider:

- Are you willing to fire it?
- Do you understand your state's gun laws?
- Can you physically handle such a weapon?
- Are you willing to get firearms training? This is the best way to ensure you will be able to handle and shoot a gun properly and safely.

Be Confident in Your Abilities

Self-defense for seniors can take many forms. Whether you choose to take up martial arts, learn cane fu, or take a basic self-defense class, you'll be better prepared to protect yourself from attacks and escape from aggressors.

Bibliography and Acknowledgement

- Amiri-Khorasani M, Osman NAA, Yusof A. Acute effect of static and dynamic stretching on hip dynamic range of motion during instep kicking in professional soccer players. J Strength Cond Res. 2011;25(6):1647–1652. [PubMed] [Google Scholar]
- Arkkukangas M, Karin Strömqvist B, Ekholm A, Tonkonogi M. A 10-week judo-based exercise programme improves physical functions such as balance, strength and falling techniques in working age adults. BMC Public Health. 2021;21:1–8.[PMCfreearticle][PubMed][GoogleScholar
- Australian Institute of Health and Welfare. Australia's health 2018. Canberra: AIHW; 2018. [Google Scholar
- Brudnak MA, Dundero D, Van Hecke FM. Are the 'hard' martial arts, such as the korean martial art, taekwondo, of benefit to senior citizens? Medical Hypotheses. 2002;59(4):485–491.[PubMed][GoogleScholar]
- Canadian Agency for Drugs and Technologies in Health. Grey matters: A practical tool for searching health-relatedgreyliterature.2021[GoogleScholar]
- Ciaccioni S, Capranica L, Forte R, Pesce C, Condello G. Effects of a 4-month judo program on gait performance in older adults. J Sports Med Phys Fit. 2020;60(5):685–692.[PubMed][GoogleScholar]
- de Souza F, Felipe Nunes L, Márcia Mendonça Marcos de S, Schuelter-Trevisol F, Daisson José T. Effectiveness of martial arts exercise on anthropometric and body composition parameters of overweight and obese subjects: A systematic review and meta-analysis. BMC Public Health.2020;20:1–12. [PMC free article] [PubMed] [Google Scholar]
- Douris P, Chinan A, Gomez M, Aw A, Steffens D, Weiss S. Fitness levels of middle aged martial art practitioners. Br J Sports Med. 2004;38(2):143–147. [PMC free article] [PubMed][GoogleScholar]
- Fong SSM, Tsang WWN. Relationship between the duration of taekwondo training and lower limb muscle strength in adolescents. Hong Kong Physiother J. 2012;30(1):25–28.[GoogleScholar]
- Guo Y, Shi H, Yu D, Qiu P. Health benefits of traditional chinese sports and physical activity for older adults: A systematic review of evidence. J Sport Health Sci. 2016;5(3):270–280. [PMC free article] [PubMed] [Google Scholar]
- Johnson NF, Hutchinson C, Hargett K, Kosik K, Gribble P. Bend don't break: Stretching improves scores on a battery of fall assessment tools in older adults. J Sport Rehabil. 2020;30(1):78–84. [PubMed] [Google Scholar]
- Kehler DS, Theou O. The impact of physical activity and sedentary behaviors on frailty levels. Mech Ageing Dev. 2019;180:29–41. [PubMed] [Google Scholar]
- Langhammer B, Stanghelle JK. Functional fitness in elderly norwegians measured with the senior fitness test. Adv Physiother. 2011;13(4):137–144. [Google Scholar]
- Muanjai P, Srijunto W, Namsawang J. Immediate effects of high-intensity interval training with punching, kicking, or stretching exercise on physical function in healthy young and older adults. J Exerc Physiol Online. 2021;5:10–22. [Google Scholar]
- Navalta JW, Stone WJ, Lyons TS. Ethical issues relating to scientific discovery in exercise science. Int J Exerc Sci. 2019;12:1–8. [PMC free article] [PubMed] [Google Scholar]
- Okely AD, Kontsevaya A, Ng J, Abdeta C. 2020 who guidelines on physical activity and sedentary behavior. J Sport Health Sci. 2021 [PMC free article] [PubMed] [Google Scholar]
- Origua Rios S, Marks J, Estevan I, Barnett LM. Health benefits of hard martial arts in adults: A systematic review. J Sports Sci. 2018;36(14):1614–1622. [PubMed] [Google Scholar]
- Osho O, Owoeye O, Armijo-Olivo S. Adherence and attrition in fall prevention exercise programs for community-dwelling older adults: A systematic review and meta-analysis. J Aging Phys Act. 2018;26(2):304–326. [PubMed] [Google Scholar]
- Page MJ, Moher D, Bossuyt PM, Boutron I, Hoffmann TC, Mulrow CD, Shamseer L, Tetzlaff JM, Akl EA, Brennan SE, Chou R, Glanville J, Grimshaw JM, Hrobjartsson A, Lalu MM, Li T, Loder EW, Mayo-Wilson E, McDonald S, McGuinness LA, Stewart LA, Thomas J, Tricco AC, Welch VA, Whiting P, McKenzie JE. Prisma 2020 explanation and elaboration: Updated guidance and exemplars for reporting systematic reviews. BMJ. 2021;372:n160. [PMC free article] [PubMed] [Google Scholar]
- Peterson MD, Rhea MR, Sen A, Gordon PM. Resistance exercise for muscular strength in older adults: A meta-analysis. Ageing Res Rev. 2010;9(3):226–237. [PMC free article] [PubMed] [Google Scholar]
- Pons van Dijk G, Leffers P, Lodder J. The effectiveness of hard martial arts in people over forty: An attempted systematic review. Societies. 2014;4(2):161–179. [Google Scholar]
- Pons Van Dijk G, Lenssen A, Leffers P, Kingma H, Lodder J. Taekwondo training improves balance in volunteers over 40. Front Aging Neurosci. 2013 [PMC free article] [PubMed] [Google Scholar]
- Pothier K, Vrinceanu T, Intzandt B, Bosquet L, Karelis AD, Lussier M, Vu TTM, Nigam A, Li KZH, Berryman N, Bherer L. A comparison of physical exercise and cognitive training interventions to improve determinants of functional mobility in healthy older adults. Exp Gerontol. 2021;149:111331. [PubMed] [Google Scholar]
- Rikli RE, Jones CJ. Senior fitness test manual. Champaign, IL: Human Kinetics; 2013. [Google Scholar]
- Vigorito C, Giallauria F. Effects of exercise on cardiovascular performance in the elderly. Front Physiol. 2014;5:51. [PMC free article] [PubMed] [Google Scholar]
- Voigt M, Klausen K. Changes in muscle strength and speed of an unloaded movement after various training programmes. Eur J Appl Physiol. 1990;60:370–376. [PubMed] [Google
- Wong RMY, Chong KC, Law SW, Ho WT, Li J, Chui CS, Chow SKH, Cheung WH. The effectiveness of exercises on fall and fracture prevention amongst community elderlies: A systematic review and meta-analysis. J Orthop Translat. 2020;24:58–65. [PMC free article] [PubMed] [Google Scholar]
- Zhao Y, Chung PK, Tong TK. Effectiveness of a balance-focused exercise program for enhancing functional fitness of older adults at risk of falling: A randomised controlled trial. Geriatr Nurs. 2017;38(6):491–497.

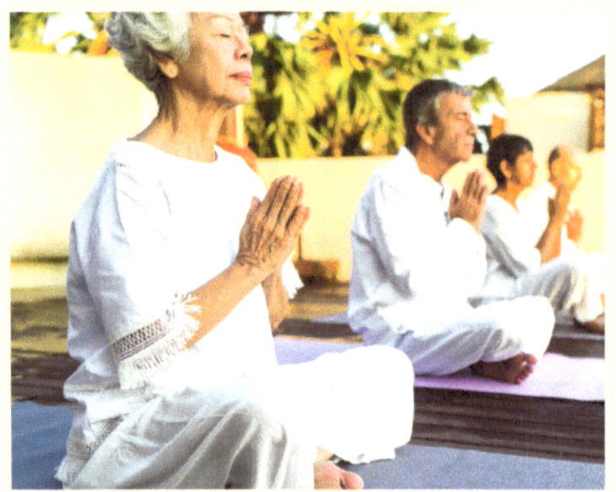

Spirituality and Aging

A lot of people believe that spirituality and aging go hand in hand. And they're probably right (at least when it comes to most of today's seniors). After all, getting older tends to deepen a person's longing for the very things that a spiritual life can provide—things like a sense of comfort, meaning, purpose, and connection.

That's why seniors who want to age well often choose to focus more of their attention on their spiritual needs and aspirations. It's a way to renew their outlook on life, become more attuned to their place in the world, and benefit from the potentially restorative nature of life-affirming spiritual practices. In short, having faith or a feeling of interconnectedness can make a person's heart sing. And that's something everyone deserves, regardless of age.

What Is Spirituality?

Everyone answers this question a little differently. That's because spirituality tends to be a very personal matter. For some people, spirituality is defined by their belief in God or their practice of a particular religion. For other people, it's defined by certain kinds of deeply felt emotion, and it may or may not involve belief in a higher power, belief in a supernatural realm, or a devotion to any single philosophy or set of beliefs.

At its core, spirituality is an aspect of human life that frequently involves a search for answers to fundamental questions about our existence, such as:

- Why are we here?
- What is our purpose?
- What happens after we die?
- Can we transcend the material world?
- How should we live our lives?
- What matters most?
- Is each of us alone, or are we all connected?

When people talk about their spirit, they are often referring to the hard-to-describe force that animates the core of their inner being. By extension, anything that enlivens our spirit or helps us attune to it can be described as spiritual. That's whymany people say that they've had spiritual experiences when they've been deeply moved by certain activities, events, personal interactions, or moments of profound insight or inspiration.

Although beliefs and opinions vary substantially, a lot of people see a clear distinction between spirituality and religion. In fact, religion is often said to be just one possible path to spirituality. Despite some overlap, other distinctions can also be made.

Spirituality is often perceived or described as:

- A broad, subjective, and unifying concept
- Informal and non-denominational
- Highly personal and not dogmatic
- Feeling-oriented
- An inward experience

Religion is often perceived or described as:

- Well-defined and highly structured
- Formal and denominational
- Focused on community, rituals, and specific doctrines
- Behavior-oriented
- An outward experience with inward benefits

Does Spirituality Become More Important As You Age?

For many people, spirituality does become more important. But it's a highly individualized experience. No two people are the same. We all have distinct needs, perceptions, personalities, and life histories. Some seniors see aging itself as a spiritual journey, whereas others turn to spiritual development as a way to find more richness, meaning, inner strength, or comfort in their lives as they reflect on the past and think about what's still to come.

Many factors can affect a senior's desire to explore more of his or her spirituality. For example, a senior or elderly American may be drawn closer to spirituality or religious faith because of factors like:

- **Retirement:** This stage of life often comes with big changes to our daily activities, the roles we play, and the way we see ourselves. Although it is often an exciting and fulfilling time, it can also feel unfamiliar. That's particularly true for people who retire from full-time careers or who no longer spend the bulk of their time raising or supporting a family.

•Grieving: As we get older, more of our friends and family members are likely to pass away. As a result, we may go through the grieving process more frequently than when we were younger. Faith or spirituality can provide us with extra stability as we cope with the loss of our loved ones and reflect on what they've meant to us.

•Decreased independence: Another reason why aging and spirituality are so closely linked is that many of us experience some physical decline during our later years. We may need assistance with certain aspects of everyday living, which can make us feel embarrassed or uncomfortable. We may even wonder who we've become if the way we perceive ourselves doesn't match reality. Spirituality can help us bridge that gap.

•Increased time to reflect: One of the gifts of getting older is that we often have more time each day to ponder the mysteries of life and reflect on everything we've done so far. We get to review our achievements as well as our setbacks while beginning to recognize a meaningful narrative that ties it all together. We may even start to see deeper connections between our life and the lives of people from past or future generations. In fact, one major aspect of the spirituality of aging is that, upon extra reflection, our perspective may shift in surprisingly profound and positive ways.

•A growing awareness of one's own mortality: Many of us fear passing away. We don't know what the experience will be like or whether our spirit (or soul) will continue to live on. Will our consciousness remain intact? What will happen to the loved ones we leave behind? Have we created a meaningful legacy that will live on? What will we be remembered for? Spirituality or religious faith can help us make peace with our mortality.

As part of their experiences with aging and spirituality, seniors may adopt new habits or ways of living. For example, many spiritually inclined seniors:

- Place more focus on their inner lives than on external expectations
- Speak from their hearts more frequently
- Put more effort into making meaningful connections with other people
- Develop more patience and attentiveness
- Seek more opportunities for silence and solitude
- Change their perception of time by living more in the moment
- Allow more time for reflection, sharing, and loving

Can You Be an Atheist and Spiritual at the Same Time?

That depends on your individual perspective. Many people of faith think that a spiritual life requires belief in God or a supreme being. But atheists, by definition, do not believe in the existence of a literal God. However, many atheists do consider themselves to be spiritual, just not in a way that conforms to how some religious people tend to think of spirituality.

For "spiritual atheists," meaning, connection, purpose, and morality are not derived from religious doctrines or ideas about the supernatural. Instead, they are derived from everyday experiences, observations, philosophical reflection, logical reasoning, and from what we continue to learn about the physical universe through science. All of those things are compatible with a definition of spirituality that's based on profound emotion and a search for answers about the biggest mysteries of life.

Simply put, many atheists feel a deep sense of connection to the world and have a desire and willingness to improve themselves and help their fellow human beings. It's all part of their own search for meaning in a constantly changing universe.

When Does a Senior Need Spiritual Care?

A person's well-being is defined by much more than just his or her physical health. People also have mental and spiritual needs. That's why many seniors with mental or physical conditions benefit from holistic care and counseling that addresses their spirituality. In fact, some older adults experience faster or more complete healing from injuries, emotional grief, or other afflictions when they have the support of a chaplain or spiritual counselor. And, of course, spiritual guidance can provide a sense of peace, comfort, and courage when a person is battling a terminal illness or nearing death. Other positive outcomes of receiving spiritual care can include:

- Improved confidence and self-esteem
- Restored relationships
- A more hopeful outlook
- A higher sense of purpose and meaning
- A greater sense of personal dignity

For seniors who devoutly practice certain religions, faith-specific spiritual care is frequently very important.

After all, they may want to observe specific rituals or follow other practices related to aspects like their diet. Faith-specific care is often especially vital when a devoutly religious person is close to passing away.

What Are the Best Spiritual Activities for Seniors?

As an older American, you can do all kinds of things to get more in tune with your spiritual core. And by doing activities that promote a deeper sense of connection, wholeness, meaning, and purpose, you can awaken new perceptions that renew your outlook and give you inner strength for the rest of your human journey.

Every religion offers spiritual practices that are designed to bring you closer to a sense of the divine. They include activities like praying, chanting, fasting, taking part in rituals, celebrating special milestones, and many other practices. But you don't necessarily need to follow any particular religious practices in order to enliven your spirituality. Anything that you love doing, that makes you feel whole or truly alive, or that gives you a feeling of deeper connection to the world can be considered a spiritual activity. For example, consider pursuits such as:

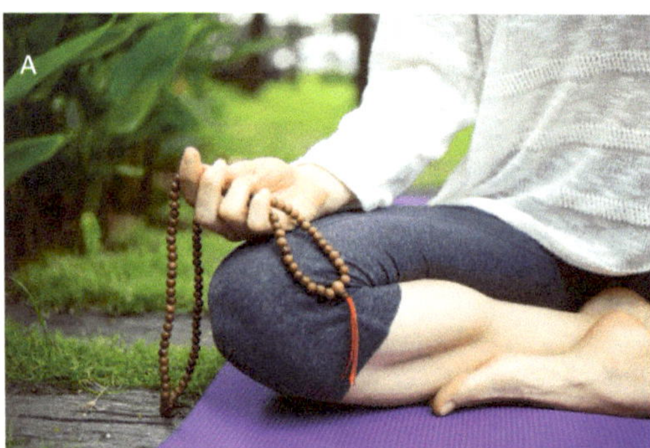

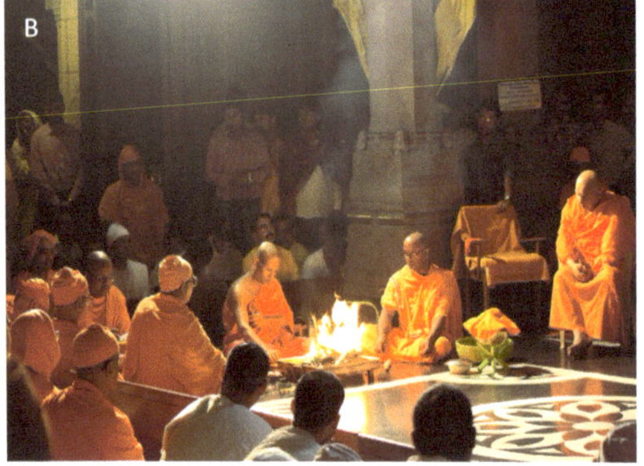

Fig 12.1 A & B Hindu spirtual activities

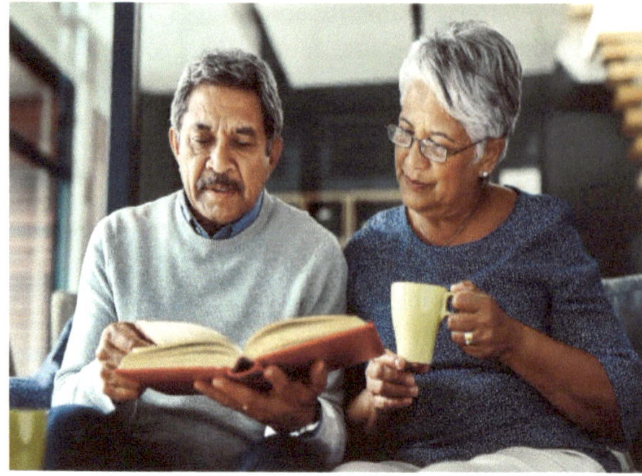

Fig 12.2 Eldely Couple is reading the bible

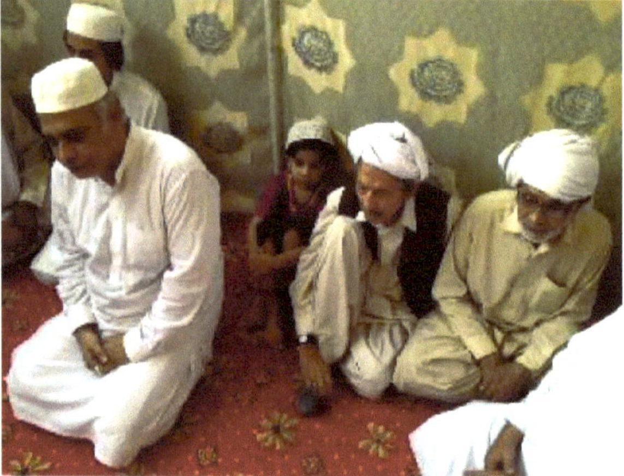

Fig 12.3 Eldely muslims performing their prayers to "Allaha:

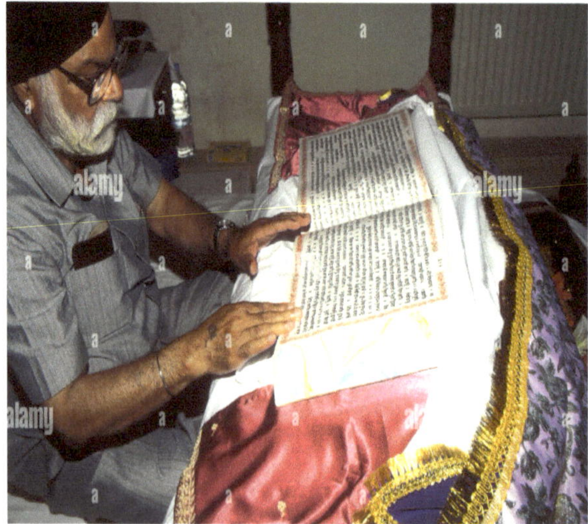

Fig 12.4 Elderly sikh is reading Gurugranth sahib as a part of religeous activity

•Volunteering: Providing your time and efforts to a worthy cause can generate many positive emotions that feel deeply rooted in your spiritual core.

•Spending time with nature: The world is full of natural wonders—big and small—that can help you sustain an inspiring enchantment with life. Activities can be as simple as watching the night sky, sitting under a large tree, planting some flowers, walking through a garden, listening to ocean waves, or watching or playing with animals.

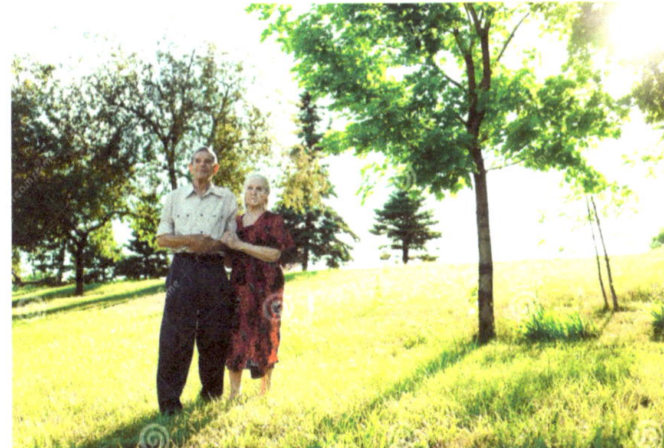

Fig 12.5 Elderly couple spending time with nature

•Meditating: In the Pew Research Center survey referenced earlier, about 53 percent of seniors over 65 said they meditate at least once a week. Among several other benefits, meditation can increase your self-awareness as well as your ability to accept aspects of life that may be out of your control.

•Participating in prayer groups: Praying with other people provides a great opportunity for social engagement. But it can also help you stay encouraged and hopeful since you get to witness and be part of a collective spiritual effort.

•Sharing stories: Talking about good memories with other people can help you feel more grounded and interconnected.

•Playing or listening to music: It's called a universal language for a reason. Music has the power to make almost anybody feel more in tune with the world, especially since it draws people into the present moment. In addition, favorite songs from your past can reawaken positive memories, provide comfort, and renew your spirit.

•Getting a massage: Human touch and physical pleasure can strip away your worries and immerse you deeply in the present moment, which is often a good way to experience a sense of unity with the world.

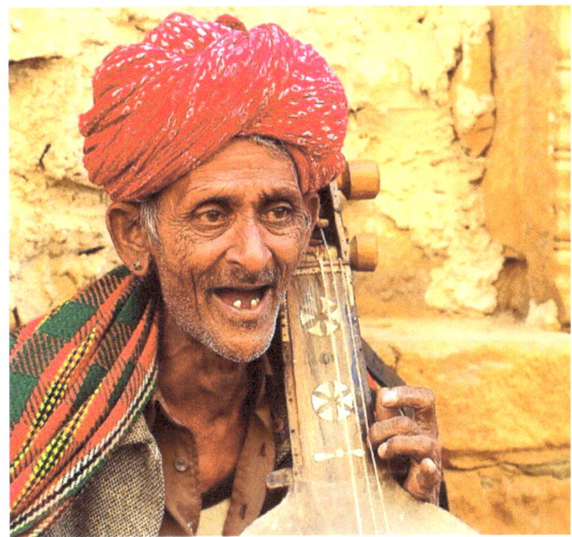

Fig 12.6 Elderly person is enjoying music

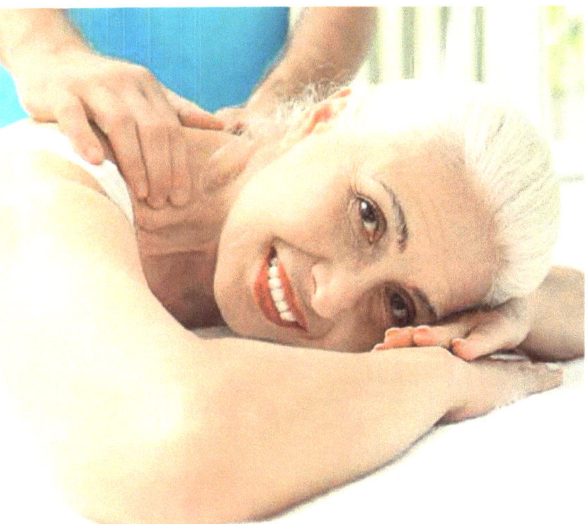

Fig 12.7 Elderly women is enjoying body massage

•**Dancing**: Moving in rhythm to stirring music can make you feel one with the universe. And when you dance with other people, that feeling of unity can become even more intense and expansive.

•**Yoga:** Beyond its many physical benefits, the practice of yoga can help you achieve a higher state of consciousness since it requires strong attention on what's happening in the current moment.

•**Reading or writing:** Words often have a lot of transformative power. Reading the thoughts or stories of good writers can open new pathways for your spiritual core to make itself known. And writing down your own words—as part of your personal reflection or storytelling—can enable you to learn more about yourself, your beliefs, your place in the universe, and what gives you meaning.

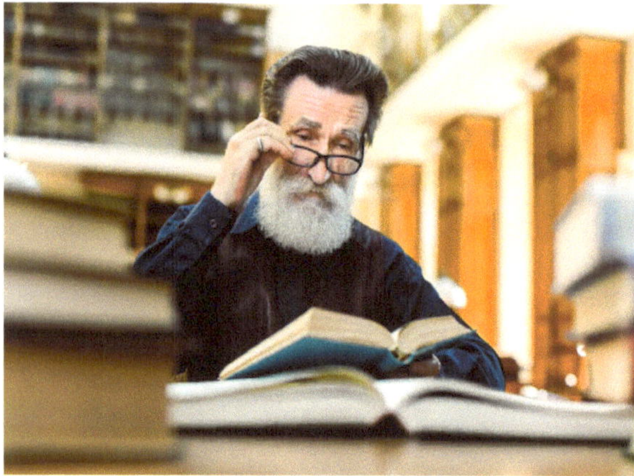

Fig 12.8 Retired prof. is reading a book of a famous author

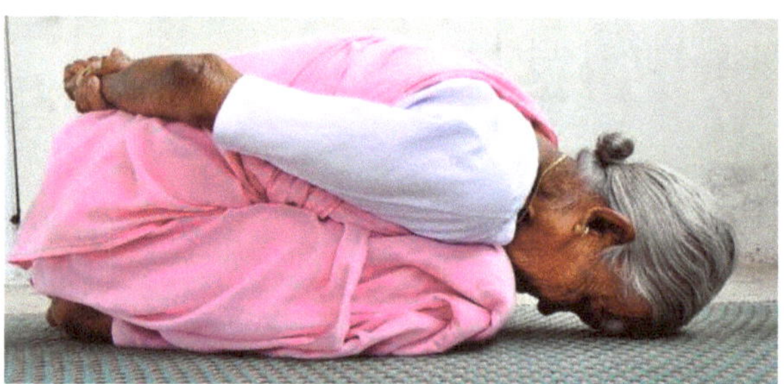

Fig 12.9 Elderly women is practicing Yoga in her daily routine

•Arts and crafts: What could be more spiritual than the act of creation? Making something that has never existed before can generate an energizing sense of harmony and possibility. Drawing, painting, sculpting, and many other kinds of arts and crafts offer the chance to experience meditative and transcendent acts of creation.

•Holding hands or gazing into someone's eyes: Simple yet intimate acts of interpersonal connection offer the chance to feel unified with the spiritual cores of other people.

•**Doing absolutely nothing:** By freeing yourself of distractions and sitting alone, in silence, you can pay closer attention to your thoughts and feelings, which can provide clues to where your spiritual core may be hiding.

Ultimately, no matter what you believe in, the activities that you enjoy most—or that bring you closer to other people or make a positive difference in the world—are the ones that are likely to feel most spiritual to you. So play, laugh, love, create, and remember that almost everyon, regardless of age, shares the same fundamental questions about the deep mysteries of life.

Bibliography and Acknowledgement

- Ali J, Marhemat F, Sara J, Hamid H. The relationship between spiritual well-being and quality of life among elderly people. Holist Nurs Pr. (2015) 29:128–35. 10.1097/
- Andreas S, Schulz H, Volkert J, Dehoust M, Sehner S, Suling A, et al.. Prevalence of mental disorders in elderly people: the European MentDis_ICF65+ study. Br J Psychiatry. (2017) 210:125–31.10.1192
- Bailly N, Martinent G, Ferrand C, Agli O, Giraudeau C, Gana K, et al.. Spirituality, social support, and flexibility among older adults: a five-year longitudinal study. Int Psychogeriatr. (2018) 30:1745–52. 10.1017/S1041610218000029 [PubMed]
- Chen H, Cheal K, McDonel Herr EC, Zubritsky C, Levkoff SE. Religious participation as a predictor of mental health status and treatment outcomes in older persons. Int J Geriatr Psychiatry. (2007) 22:144–53. 10.1002/gps.1704 [
- Dein S. Religion, spirituality and depression: implications for research and treatment. Prim Care Community Psychiatry. (2006) 11:67–72. 10.1185/135525706X121110
- El-Gilany A-H, Elkhawaga GO, Sarraf BB. Depression and its associated factors among elderly: a community-based study in Egypt. Arch Gerontol Geriatr. (2018) 77:103–7. 10.1016/j.archger.2018.04.011
- Foong HF, Hamid TA, Ibrahim R, Haron SA. The association between religious orientation and life satisfaction in older adults living with morbidity and multimorbidity: a gender perspective in Malaysia. Psychogeriatrics. (2020) 20:891–9. 10.1111/psyg.12614
- Glas G. Anxiety, anxiety disorders, religion and spirituality. South Med J. (2007) 100:621–5. 10.1097/SMJ.0b013e31805fe612
- Hafeez A, Rafique R. Spirituality and Religiosity as Predictors of Psychological Well-Being in Residents of Old Homes. (2013). [Google Scholar]
- Idler EL, McLaughlin J, Kasl S. Religion and the quality of life in the last year of life. J Gerontol B Psychol Sci Soc Sci. (2009) 64:528–37. 10.1093/geronb/gbp028 [PMC free article] [PubMed] [CrossRef] [Google Scholar
- King DA, Lyness JM, Duberstein PR, He H, Tu XM, Seaburn DB. Religious involvement and depressive symptoms in primary care elders. Psychol Med. (2007) 37:1807–15. 10.1017/S0033291707000591 [PubMed] [CrossRef] [Google Scholar]
- Lac A, Austin N, Lemke R, Poojary S, Hunter P. Association between religious practice and risk of depression in older people in the subacute setting. Australas J Ageing. (2017) 36:E31–4. 10.1111/ajag.12384
- Mefford L, Thomas SP, Callen B, Groer M. Religiousness/Spirituality and anger management in community-dwelling older persons. Issues Ment Heal Nurs. (2014) 35:283–91. 10.3109/01612840.2014.890472
- Vahia I V, Depp CA, Palmer BW, Fellows I, Golshan S, Thompson W, et al.. Correlates of spirituality in older women. Aging Ment Health. (2011) 15:97–102. 10.1080/13607863.2010.501069
- Zimmer Z, Jagger C, Chiu C-T, Ofstedal MB, Rojo F, Saito Y. Spirituality, religiosity, aging and health in global perspective: a review. SSM Popul Heal. (2016) 2:373–81. 10.1016/j.ssmph.2016.04.009

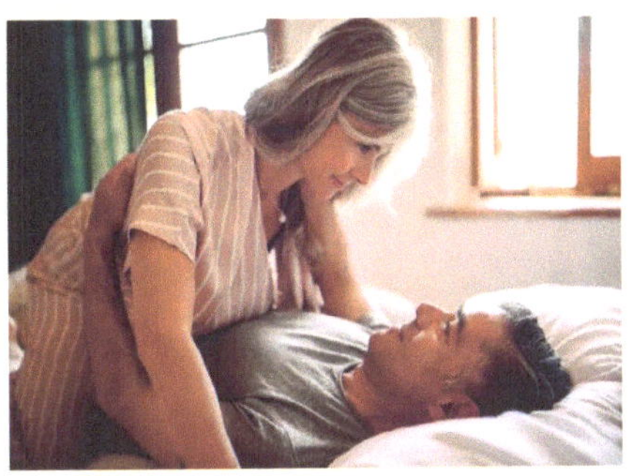

Elderly Sex. Staying Active In The Bedroom

Sex, even well into your senior years, can be a wonderful part of your life. For many older adults, lovemaking is an enjoyable adventure that offers a wide variety of life-enhancing benefits like improved self-esteem, better sleep, and greater overall well-being. Even well into old age, physical intimacy can boost a person's health and happiness. That may be why most older adults between the ages of 65 and 80 see it as a necessity. According to the National Poll on Healthy Aging, 76 percent said that making love—at any age—is an important aspect of romantic relationships. Here's what you should know about having sex after 60, 70, and beyond

1. Physical Changes and Challenges

It's normal and natural to experience physical changes as you get older. And seniors generally tend to have more health problems than younger people. Even so, it's possible to effectively manage (or even overcome) some of the physical issues that could be hindering your intimacy. Single seniors dealing with health issues also have options when it comes to finding partners who understand or share their challenges.

As Men Age:

They naturally produce less testosterone. So, they tend to have a lower sex drive and require more stimulation to achieve and sustain an erection and reach climax.Their orgasms are often shorter and less powerful. And after ejaculating, they tend to need more time before achieving an erection again.

Full or partial erectile dysfunction (ED) can also become a problem. But it can often be effectively treated. In fact, by treating underlying physical or emotional problems, many men can restore some or all of their erectile function.

As Women Age:

Their sexual health may be affected by lower hormone levels.Vaginal dryness can become an issue. (After menopause, many women naturally produce less lubrication during erotic activity. Their bodies simply don't respond to arousal or stimulation in the same way.)Their vaginas may become thinner and less elastic. As a result, vaginal penetration can be painful without enough personal lubrication In addition, some women find it more difficult to become aroused after menopause or surgical procedures such as hysterectomies. It may take them longer to feel excited, and their orgasms may become less intense. Or they may lose interest in sex altogether, at least temporarily. Plus, many women over 60 experience other kinds of physical problems—such as mild urinary incontinence—that cause them extra anxiety during times of intimacy.

Other Health Conditions

Some of the most common medical issues that can affect a person's sexual well-being include:

- Diabetes
- High blood pressure
- Heart disease
- Hormonal imbalances
- Arthritis

That's why it's essential to tell your doctor about any problems you're having with physical intimacy. Even if you aren't experiencing any other symptoms, a decrease in sexual interest or function may be an early sign of a medical problem. (For instance, erectile dysfunction is sometimes an early symptom of heart disease.) Also, if you are recovering from surgery or illness, listen to your doctor's advice about when you can safely start making love again.

Medications

Some antidepressants, antihistamines, acid-blocking meds, and blood pressure drugs can impair a person's libido or sexual function. So it's a good idea to inform your doctor of any issues you may be having in the bedroom. He or she might be able to prescribe something different for you. Of course, you may also be a candidate for certain medications frequently prescribed for intimacy problems. For example, men with erectile dysfunction are often prescribed drugs like Viagra and Cialis. And women with vaginal dryness are sometimes prescribed special gels, creams, or patches as part of hormone replacement therapy. No matter what, you should always talk to your doctorbefore taking any over-the-counter supplements or medications, even if they are marketed as "natural."

Exercise

Regular physical activity can increase your overall energy level, self-confidence, and blood circulation. Plus, it's good for your heart. And anything good for your heart also tends to be good for your sexual health.

Nutrition

A heart-healthy diet is often prescribed for men and women who experience dysfunction during erotic activities. Many dietitians recommend foods low in saturated fat, sodium, and sugar but high in fiber, essential vitamins and minerals, and healthy, unsaturated fats. So eating a wide variety of fruits, vegetables, and nuts can be especially beneficial. In addition, limiting your alcohol consumption to no more than one drink per day is wise.

Sex for Seniors - Frequency

Seeking erotic pleasure more frequently can lead to a stronger libido and better sexual health overall. That's why it can be beneficial to make love even when you aren't in the mood. Every time you engage in intimate activity, you are training your body to respond better to the stimulation. And you don't need to have a partner each time. Solo masturbation can be just as effective.

2. Mental and Emotional Barriers

Sexual problems are often caused or made worse by psychological obstacles. Like many seniors, you may consciously or subconsciously grapple with issues like:

- Self-consciousness
- Performance anxiety
- Relationship problems
- Fear about your health or financial situation
- The death of your partner and the resulting loss of physical intimacy Depression can also be a major barrier. For older adults with this condition, sexual desire, arousal, and pleasure can be very elusive.

Seeking Help

Like other medical conditions, depression can be treated. In addition to medication, talk therapy can sometimes help seniors who have depression that interferes with their ability to be physically intimate.

Seeing a professional mental health counselor or therapist can help you deal with various other obstacles.Mainstream sex therapy is another option. It doesn't involve any physical contact. Sex therapy is aspecialized form of psychotherapy that can help people overcome, cope with, or adapt to challenges or limitations related to erotic intimacy, including functional issues like erectile dysfunction or vaginal pain.

Adults of all ages can benefit from individual or couple's therapy, including seniors and the elderly.

Ask for a referral from your doctor or locate a therapist near you through the American Association of Sexuality Educators, Counselors and Therapists (AASECT) or the Society for Sex Therapy & Research (SSTAR).

For the singles who would enjoy and benefit from companionship but haven't successfully made the leap into the dating world yet, online dating could be a simple, unintimidating place to start. While there are cautions that are important when meeting people from the internet in real life, using a reputable website and service can make a big difference. There are even senior-specific dating sites geared specifically to matching up older singles looking for love, a sexual connection, or both (and a lot more!).

3. Removing Expectations

Making orgasms the driving focus of erotic activity can sometimes backfire. That's why it's often better to focus on exploring all kinds of pleasure rather than trying to achieve one type of outcome. Paradoxically, when people let go of their expectations, they're more likely to experience orgasms and other pleasurable highs.

4. Communicating With Your Partner

Open communication is essential for maintaining good relationships. Lack of honest communication is often one of the biggest causes of a breakup or no-sex marriage. Yet, according to the National Poll on Healthy Aging, only 36 percent of

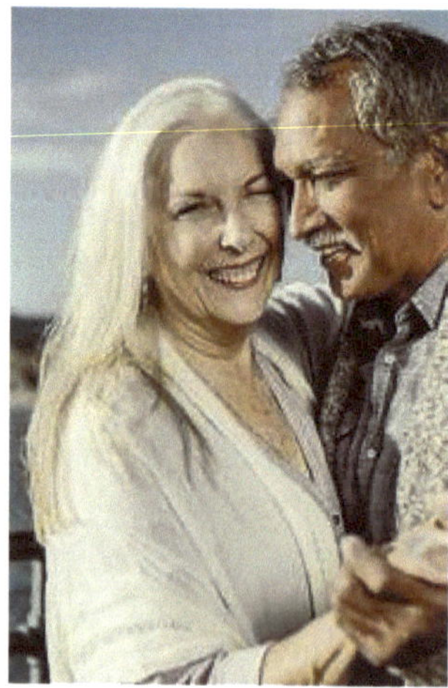

Fig 13.1 Elderly having Open communication in them

seniors between the ages of 65 and 80 would discuss a sexual problem they were having with a spouse or partner.

Before you can experience a satisfying sexual relationship with each other, you and your partner need to share your most intimate feelings. Talk honestly about things like:

- Concerns and anxieties
- Needs and desires
- Boundaries

Make sure your communication is a two-way street by listening to your partner without judgment or interruption. And remember that you can be playful about communicating. A little humor can make the process more comfortable, enjoyable, and reassuring.

5. Changing Your Routine

Particularly for older couples, lovemaking can become boring and predictable. But it doesn't have to stay that way. Purposefully breaking up your routine can help you discover a whole new world of excitement. Even something as simple as choosing a new time of day (for example, you may have more energy for sex in the morning or afternoon vs. the evening). Here are some other things to try:

- New sexual positions
- Different rooms or locations
- Various kinds of outercourse (i.e., physical intimacy without penetration)
- Dates that involve one partner giving pleasure without the other one reciprocating (reversing roles for the next date)
- Fantasy role-playing

Anytime you try something new, be sure to follow up with each other and share your feelings about it. What did you like best? Would you try it again? Did you learn anything about yourself or your partner? What else do you want to try?

6. Setting the Mood

As we get older, many of us experience slower arousal. It may take longer for our desire to ignite during romantic activities. That's why many sexually active seniors make it a habit to do things with their partners that set the mood — like flirting, kissing, or giving each other massages — well in advance of getting naked.

7. Using Protection

Physical intimacy can be risky, regardless of your age. Even for the elderly, it comes with the possibility of sexually transmitted infections (STIs—previously referred to as STDs). In fact, according to athenahealth, among older Americans, infection rates continue to climb for diseases like syphilis, gonorrhea, and chlamydia. Other common STIs include HIV, herpes, HPV, and trichomoniasis. As you age, it becomes harder for your body to fight such infections.

An infected person can pass his or her STI on to you through blood or bodily fluids such as semen or vaginal fluid. And because infected people don't always have symptoms (and may not be aware of their infections), you can't know for sure whether they are healthy or not just based on their word or appearance. So it's crucial to practice safe sex, especially if you are not in a monogamous relationship with someone you completely trust. No method of protection is 100 percent effective. However, you can greatly reduce your risk of contracting an STI by taking steps such as:

- Using a new, unexpired condom for vaginal or anal penetration
- Using a condom or dental dam for oral sex

Before making love with a new partner, always make sure that each of you has been tested for STIs. Be honest with each other. (If you are infected, keeping that information a secret is unethical and dangerous to your partner.) And if either of you has multiple partners, be sure to get tested regularly. Having multiple partners greatly increases the risk of contracting or passing on an infection.

Whenever you see your doctor, be open about your activities so that he or she can appropriately assess your risk and screen you for STIs if necessary. Many infections can be successfully treated.

8. Personal Lubrication

For older women with vaginal dryness, lubrication can be especially vital. Whether having sex with a partner or masturbating solo, lube is a simple way to make the whole experience much more comfortable and pleasurable.

Choosing the right type of personal lubricant for the sexual activity you engage in is crucial. (You may need to buy multiple kinds of lube since they have different uses and limitations.)

9. Sex Toys for Seniors

A good toy can do wonders for your ability to reach maximum pleasure—with or without a partner. Seniors often do best with soft, lightweight, and ergonomic sex toys. Here are a few examples of sex toys that have been recommended as good options for seniors, which are available for purchase through the market

- **Tantus Rumble**
- **PalmPower Massager**
- **Eroscillator**
- **Mimi by Je Joue**
- **Bullet Vibrator with Remote Control**

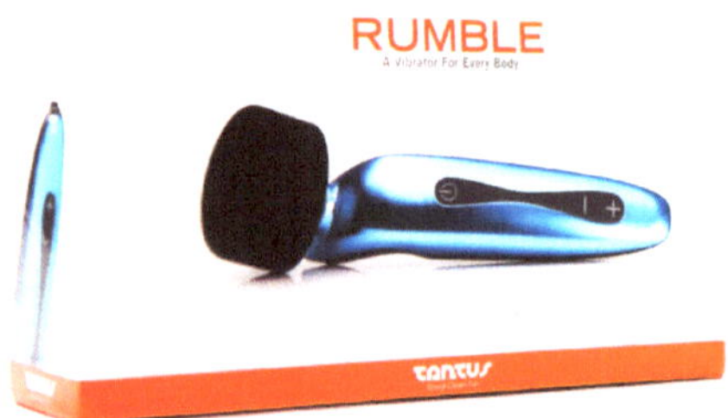

Fig 13.2 For Elderly Rumble is the first-ever featherweight personal massager. Rumble is simple: mid-range power, easily held by most anyone, with controls in a logical place and a contact surface that can be removed and cleaned hygienically. Unlike most other personal massagers, Rumble is accessible to a diverse range of body types as well as abilities.

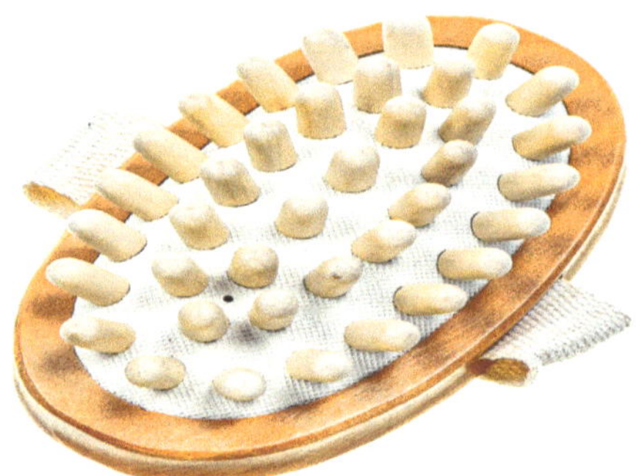

Fig 13.3 For Elderly Palm Held Wood anti-cellulite Massager

10. Going Beyond Intercourse

You don't have to engage in any kind of penetration to have a satisfying erotic life. Outercourse (i.e., sex without penetration) can be incredibly enjoyable. And you can still experience orgasms (maybe even better ones). For a lot of seniors, outercourse eliminates major anxieties. For example, women don't have to worry about vaginal dryness or pain. And men don't have to worry about erectile dysfunction. Even with a flaccid penis, a man can reach climax with the right stimulation.

11. Best Sexual Positions for Seniors

When you want to engage in intercourse but find it hard on your body, it's time to change things up a little. Using new sexual positions often becomes especially important for seniors who want to have sex over 70 years of age. That's because back and knee problems are particularly common among seniors and the elderly. But regardless of age, a new position can make intercourse easier and more comfortable.

Some of the best sex positions for seniors are those in which your weight is evenly distributed over your joints or the strain on your back is alleviated. But every couple is different, so you and your partner may need to try various positions before hitting on one or two that work well for both of you. Here are three of the most commonly recommended positions for older adults:

- **Missionary plank:** With the woman on her back, the man positions himself on top, resting his weight evenly between his forearms on either side of her. He also bends his knees and rests them on either side. This allows his weight to be off his partner and makes it easier to sustain comfortable thrusting. The woman can put her feet on his lower legs for extra traction and comfort. With small tweaks, the missionary plank position can also be reversed to have the woman on top.

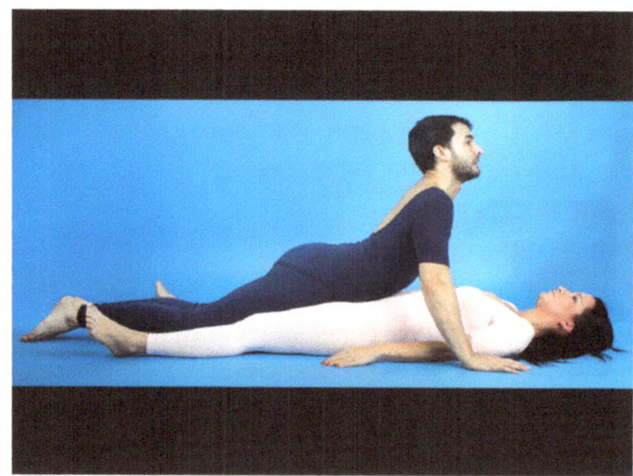

Fig 13.4 showing Arms-Straight Missionary He straightens his arms for more powerful thrusting.

- Spooning: The woman lays on one side of her body while the man cuddles up behind her on the same side of his body. This allows the man to penetrate her vagina comfortably without pressure on his arms or knees. The woman can also lift her top leg over his to make entry easier. From this position, each partner can control the rhythm. For added comfort, the woman can place pillows between her legs, or the man can use pillows or wedge cushions behind his back to help support the weight of their bodies.

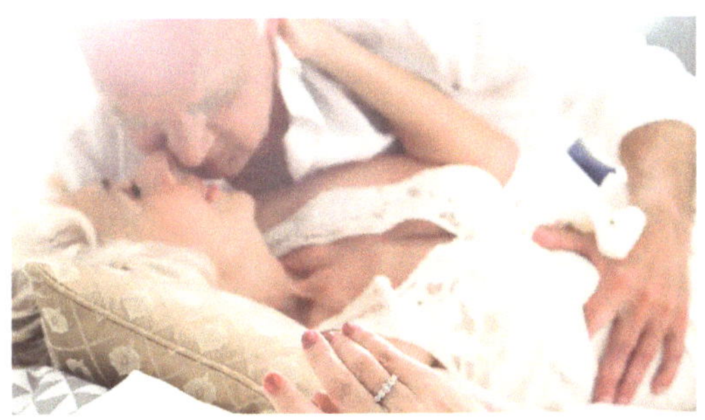

Fig 13.5 Elderly couple having sex in the bed

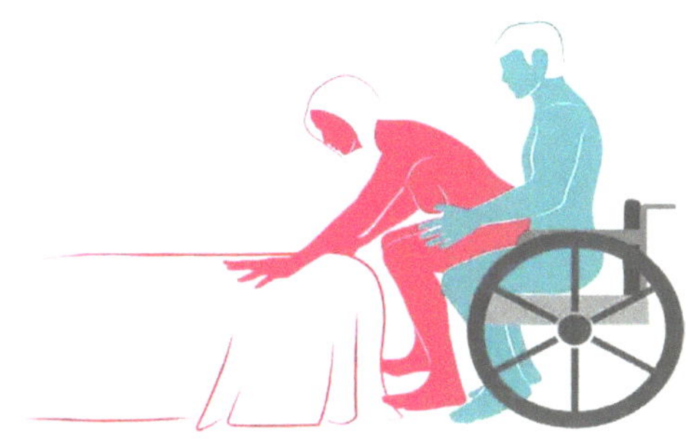

Fig 13.9 Elderly having sex in Modified Sitting Doggy Style

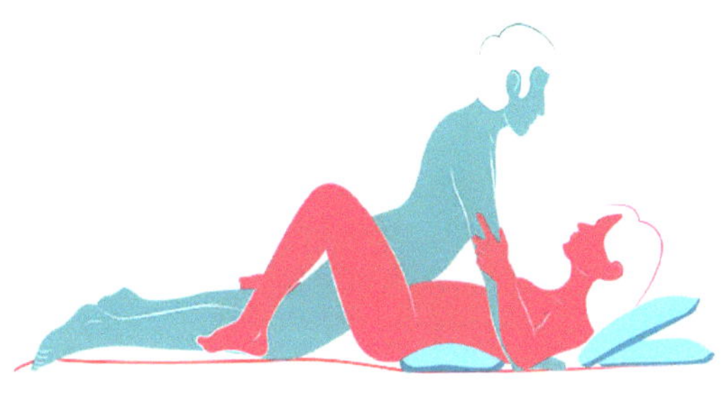

Fig 13.6 Elderly having Missionary sex pose

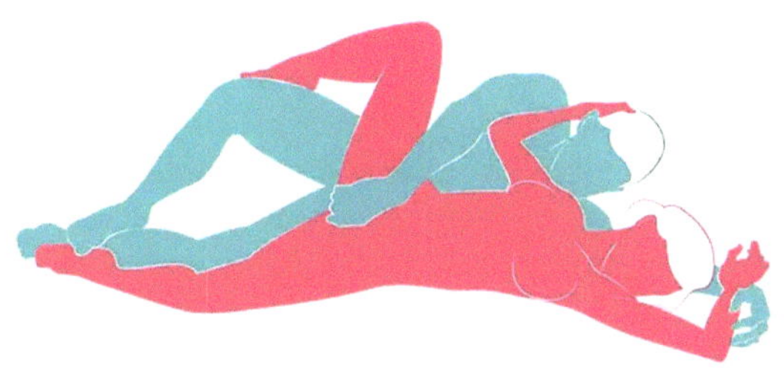

Fig 13.10. Elderly having sex in Spooning Style

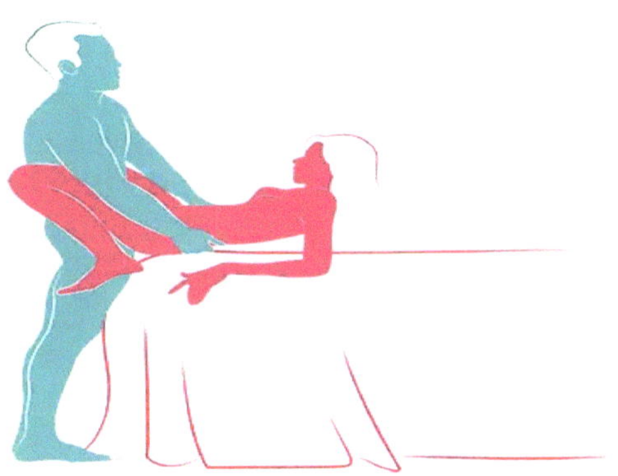

Fig 13.7 Elderly having standing Missionary sex pose

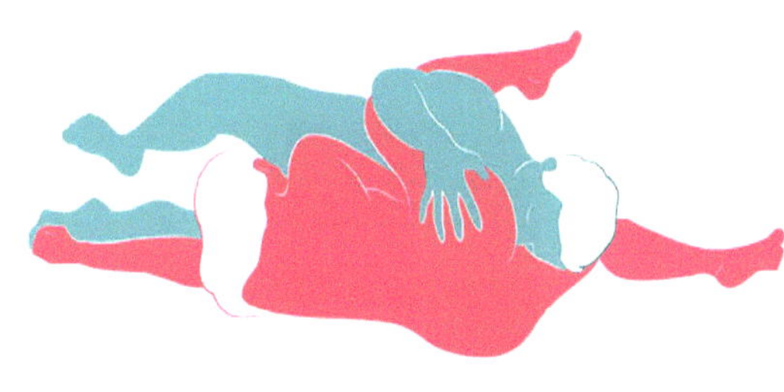

Fig 13.11 Elderly having sex in Sideways 69 style

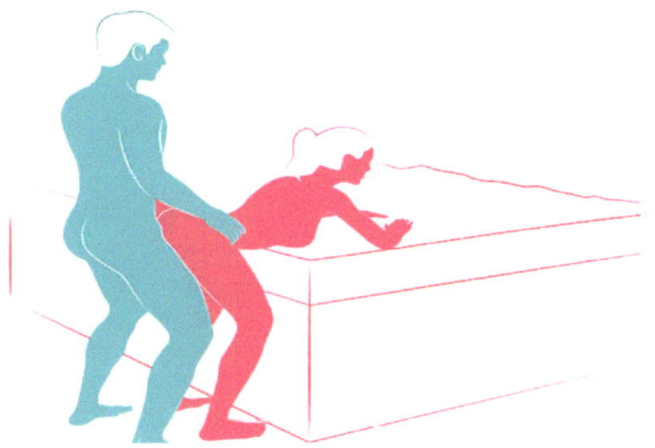

Fig 13.8 Elderly having sex in Standing Doggy Style

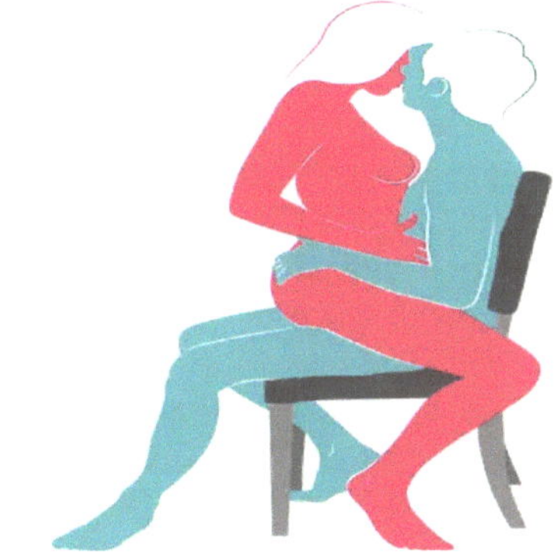

Fig 13.12 Elderly having sex in Sitting Pretzel position

1 – Missionary :- The good ole trusty go-to we all know. While it tops our list of sex positions for seniors, it works well for all ages, but it's especially great if any type of spinal movement causes you pain. The person lying on their back can find an extra boost of support by placing a pillow or two beneath them. Ideally, pillows work well under the lower back or arch of the back. But test it out and see what feels best for you. The person on top has the advantage of using their hands or forearms for support to kneel over their partner.

2. Standing missionary:- If the person doing the penetrating has back or knee pain, another great option is to adapt missionary to a standing position. You'll be perpendicular instead of parallel. The partner lying down comes to the edge of the bed (or other furniture) while the other partner stands upright and thrusts. For the standing partner, this ensures there is no pressure on the back and no weight on the knees.

Standing Doggy style:- Similar to standing missionary, standing doggy style enables one partner to stand in order to do the penetrating. For the partner being penetrated, this takes pressure off the back, but be sure not to arch the back if you have back pain. Adding pillows under the stomach and upper body will add extra support. Bonus: try incorporating the use of a doggy style strap.

Modified Sitting Doggy Style:- This one is great if the penetrating partner is in a wheelchair or has hip pain. Bring a chair or wheelchair to face the edge of the bed. The other partner, with their back facing the seated person, lowers down onto the partner in the chair. The one on top can use their arms and upper body against the bed to thrust up and down on their sitting lover. Again, pillows make for a great prop in any which way you find them to be useful.

Spooning:- Usually thought of as the go-to for after coitus, spooning can be easily enjoyed as a position minimizing any back, wrist, or knee pressure. Lay side by side, parallel, facing the same direction rather than toward each other. The one behind can do the penetrating or the rubbing while the one in front can reach between their legs and rub themselves or their partner. Bonus move: incorporate a fun toy or use those free hands for external clitoral stimulation.

Sideways 69:-Pairs well with a Merlot (like the movie Sideways! Just kidding. Sideways 69 is exactly what it sounds like. You're facing each other's genitals, but instead of being one on top of the other, you're turned sideways. This is great for folks with carpal tunnel or rheumatoid arthritis, as there is no weight burden on each other's hands or wrists. It also enables stimulation with more than just the mouth—spice it up with lube, hands, and toys.

Sitting Pretzel:-Also sometimes referred to as the Time Bomb is another great move if your partner is in a wheelchair or if one partner has limited mobility, lower back, knee, or foot pain, or just feels more comfortable being seated. In in this position, the partner on top faces the partner sitting down. This one makes for extra intimacy as you gaze into each other's eyes. Bonus move: start out slow with a face to face lap dance or make out session to really get things going.

Side-by-Side:-Similar to spooning, except you're facing each other. This is another position where eye gazing can take front and center stage. It's also a good one for people who find sitting for long periods of time to be painful. Any position where partners are lying on their sides tend to be great options for those with back pain. But this one in particular doesn't work for all types of back pain, so don't be afraid to communicate and try something else if it doesn't feel optimal.

What Works Best for You:-You can read expert tips and tricks all day long, but at the end of the day, nobody knows what feels good to your body better than you. Try to look at it as a new fun erotic exploratory journey you get to go on with your body and with your partner. You're discovering new ways of doing things together. Finding the positions that work best for you is all part of the fun!

9 Other Tips for Great Senior Sex

Sex in older age (or any age) is more than just a set of positions, however. The brain is the biggest sex organ and other body parts beyond the genitals also play a part. Here are some tips that go beyond just sex positions for seniors

1.Use Some Toys:- sex toys for seniors

2.Expand the Mind

3.Get Enough Sleep

4.Stretch:- Consider yoga for seniors

5.Relax:-Try take a hot shower together to relax

6.Seek Pain Relief

7.Get Cliterate:- (If your partner owns a clitoris.) Have you heard about the orgasm gap? Do you know that the majority of the clitoris is internal vs. external?1. If your lover is a clitoris owner, remember that most clits need external stimulation in order to reach orgasm. The good ole jackhammer just doesn't do the trick the way mainstream porn has led us to believe.

8.Have an Emotional Quotient

9. Have a Mantra

Bibliography and Acknowledgement

- Arksey H., O'Malley L. Scoping studies: towards a methodological framework. Int J Soc Res Methodol. 2005;8(1):19–32. doi: 10.1080/1364557032000119616. [CrossRef] [Google Scholar]
- Baumle A.K. Springer Netherlands; Dordrecht: 2013. Introduction: the demography of sexuality. International handbook on the demography of sexuality; pp. 3–9. [CrossRef] [Google Scholar]
- Blieszner R. Cambridge University Press; Cambridge: 2006. Close relationships in middle and late adulthood. The cambridge handbook of personal relationships; pp. 211–228. [CrossRef] [Google Scholar]
- Bradford A., Meston C.M. The impact of anxiety on sexual arousal in women. Behav Res Ther. 2006;44(8):1067–1077. doi: 10.1016/j.brat.2005.08.006. [PMC free article] [PubMed] [CrossRef] [Google Scholar]
- Buczak-Stec E., König H.H., Hajek A. The link between sexual satisfaction and subjective well-being: a longitudinal perspective based on the German Ageing Survey. Qual Life Res. 2019;28(11):3025–3035. doi: 10.1007/s11136-019-02235-4. [PubMed] [CrossRef] [Google Scholar]
- Burgess E.O. In: The handbook of sexuality in close relationships. Harvey J.H., Wenzel A., Sprecher S., editors. Psychology Press; Now York: 2004. Sexuality in midlife and later life couples; pp. 447–464. [Google Scholar]
- Cunningham G.R., Stephens-Shields A.J., Rosen R.C., Wang C., Ellenberg S.S., Matsumoto A.M., et al. Association of sex hormones with sexual function, vitality, and physical function of symptomatic older men with low testosterone levels at baseline in the testosterone trials. J Clin Endocrinol Metab. 2015;100(3):1146–1155. doi: 10.1210/jc.2014-3818. [PMC free article] [PubMed] [CrossRef] [Google Scholar]
- DeLamater J. Sexual expression in later life: a review and synthesis. J Sex Res. 2012;49(2–3):125–141. doi: 10.1080/00224499.2011.603168. [PubMed] [CrossRef] [Google Scholar]
- Diamond L.M., Huebner D.M. Is good sex good for you? Rethinking sexuality and health. Soc Pers Psychol Compass. 2012;6(1):54–69. doi: 10.1111/j.1751-9004.2011.00408.x. r
  Dominguez L., Barbagallo M. Ageing and sexuality. Eur Geriatr Med. 2016;7:512–518. doi: 10.1016/J.EURGER.2016.05.013. [CrossRef] [Google Scholar]
- Enzlin P., Mak R., Kittel F., Demyttenaere K. Sexual functioning in a population-based study of men aged 40-69 years: the good news. Int J Impot Res. 2004;16(6):512–520. doi: 10.1038/sj.ijir.3901221. [PubMed] [CrossRef] [Google Scholar]
- Field N., Mercer C.H., Sonnenberg P., Tanton C., Clifton S., Mitchell K.R., et al. Associations between health and sexual lifestyles in britain: findings from the third national survey of sexual attitudes and lifestyles (Natsal-3) Lancet. 2013;382(9907):1830–1844.doi:10.1016/
- Freak-Poli R., Kirkman M., De Castro Lima G., Direk N., Franco O.H., Tiemeier H. Sexual activity and physical tenderness in older adults: cross-sectional prevalence and associated characteristics. J Sex Med. 2017;14(7):918–927.
- Ginsberg T.B., Pomerantz S.C., Kramer-Feeley V. Sexuality in older adults:Behaviours and preferences. Age Ageing. 2005;34(5):475–480. doi: 10.1093/ageing/afi143. [PubMed] [CrossRef] [Google Scholar
- Heidari S. Sexuality and older people: a neglected issue. Reprod Health Matters. 2016;24(48):1–5. doi: 10.1016/j.rhm.2016.11.011. [PubMed] [CrossRef] [Google Scholar]
- Kang J.X., Zeng H. Research progress on sexual health of older adults. Chin Nurs Res. 2010;24(16):1418–1420. https://doi:10.396/j.issn.1009-6493.2010.16.004 [Google Scholar]
- Kang N. The psychology of old age. Modern Science. 2008;1:93–95. [in Chinese] [Google Scholar]
  Kleinstäuber M. Factors associated with sexual health and well being in older adulthood. Curr Opin Psychiatr. 2017;30(5):358–368.doi:10.1097/yco.0000000000000354. [PubMed] [CrossRef] [Google Scholar]
- Lai G. Focus on the social and economic perspective of aging problems. Chinese Journal of Gerontology. 2015;35(2):570–572.
- Laumann E.O., Waite L.J. Sexual dysfunction among older adults: prevalence and risk factors from a nationally representative U.S. probability sample of men and women, 57-85 years of age. J Sex Med. 2008;5(10):2300–2311. [PMC free article] [PubMed] [Google Scholar]
- Papaharitou S., Nakopoulou E., Kirana P., Giaglis G., Moraitou M., Hatzichristou D. Factors associated with sexuality in later life: an exploratory study in a group of Greek married older adults. Arch Gerontol Geriatr. 2008;46(2):191–201. doi: 10.1016/j.archger.2007.03.008. [PubMed] [CrossRef] [Google Scholar
- Ramesh A., Issac T.G., Mukku S.S.R., Sivakumar P.T. Companionship and sexual issues in the aging population. Indian J Psychol Med. 2021;43(5suppl):S71–S77. doi: 10.1177/02537176211045622. [PMC free article] [PubMed] [CrossRef] [Google Scholar
- Sinković M., Towler L. Sexual aging: a systematic review of qualitative research on the sexuality and sexual health of older adults. Qual Health Res. 2019;29(9):1239–1254. doi: 10.1177/1049732318819834. [PubMed] [CrossRef]
- Træen B., Alexandra Carvalheira A., Hald G.M., Lange T., Kvalem I.L. Attitudes towards sexuality in older men and women across Europe: similarities, differences, and associations with their sex lives. Sex Cult. 2019;23(1):1–25. doi: 10.1007/s12119-018-9564-9.
- Wei X., Yang X. Analysis of the related factors of sexual needs in the elderly. Occupational Hygiene and Injury. 2017;32(2):104–105. https://doi:1006-172X(2017)02-104-02 [Google Scholar]
- Yu Z., Yu B. Study on sexual living status and middle-aged and elderly effects on mental health. Chinese Sex Science.2021;30(4):155–157.doi:10.1111/j.1743-6109.2008.00974.x.10.3969/j.issn.1672-1993.2021.04.048.[CrossRef][Google Scholar]
- Zeng Y.L., Yang X. Analysis of the related factors of sexual needs in the elderly. Chongqing Medicine. 2017;46(34):4857–4860.https://doi:10.3969/

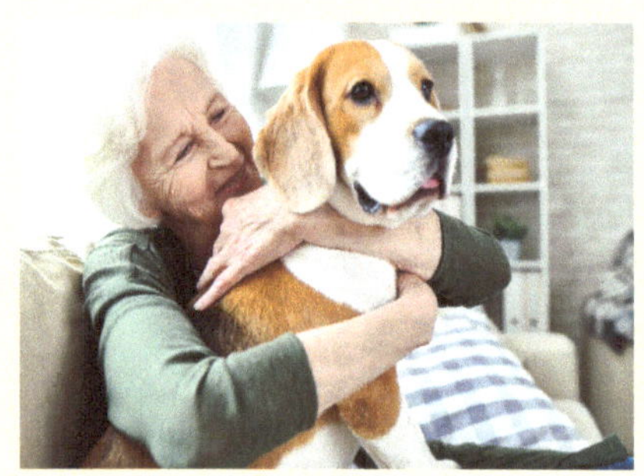

How Pet Therapy Can Benefit Seniors?

Therapy dogs have long been recognized for their ability to provide comfort and promote healing. But did you know that a whole host of other species are beginning to fulfill this important role? These days, the companionship of cats, birds, rabbits, and even robotic animals is being utilized to benefit older adults in numerous therapeutic ways.

Pet therapy for elderly people can boost their well-being and improve their physical, mental, and emotional functioning. Interacting with a kind and affectionate animal can lower people's stress levels, help them become more active, and bring them out of their shells. This can be immensely helpful to seniors who are struggling with loneliness or dealing with health conditions such as heart disease, cancer, chronic pain, or dementia.

The information below will help you understand the various aspects of pet therapy and how it can improve the lives of older adults. You'll learn about the therapeutic role played by dogs, including the unique benefits of robotic dogs for seniors. And the options (both living and robotic) are available in an increasingly wide range of other animal species. You'll gain a better understanding of the unique functions of therapy animals, service animals, and emotional support animals. And you'll get an introduction to the many benefits of robotic pets

What Is Pet Therapy?

Pet therapy is a general term that refers to the use of animals for treatment and companionship. It encompasses both animal-assisted therapy and animal-assisted activities. While these two terms are closely related, they are not technically the same thing.

Animal-assisted therapy (AAT) draws on the aid of animals for therapeutic treatment. It is structured to meet specific therapy goals and is overseen by a health professional who has a keen understanding of the way humans and animals interact. The professional documents each session and tracks patient progress. For instance, a physical therapist might ask an elderly man who is recovering from a stroke to brush a dog's coat or toss a ball to a dog as a way of regaining the mobility in his hands.

Animal-assisted activities (AAA) are more free-form, and they are conducted without any specific treatment goals in mind. Typically, specially trained therapy dogs or cats provide comfort and cheer to elderly people by visiting hospitals, nursing homes, hospices, and assisted living facilities. Facility staff generally provide some guidance and assistance, but they don't keep formal notes.

Essentially, "pet therapy" refers to guided human-animal interactions that are meant to help improve people's quality of life.

What Pet Therapy Can Do for Seniors?

Having animals around can benefit seniors in a whole host of ways. For instance, walking a dog is obviously good exercise. Feeding, brushing, and caring for a pet can also help a senior feel needed and purposeful. Plus, the total acceptance and unconditional love that animals give can go a long way toward lowering people's stress levels and helping shift their focus away from their own problems. Indeed, animal-assisted therapy in nursing homes is becoming increasingly widespread as studies like those in the Journals of Gerontology Series A: Biological Sciences and Medical Sciences and Current Gerontology and Geriatrics Research confirm its effectiveness in combating loneliness and depression in older adults.

Take patients suffering from dementia for example. Research has found that animals can reduce agitation and stress in people with this condition. In a study in the Western Journal of Nursing Research, having a specially trained dog come to live in an Alzheimer's care unit resulted in a significant drop in behavioral issues among the residents. And a separate study in the Western Journal of Nursing Research found that Alzheimer's patients living in nursing homes got more nutrition and gained more weight when fish aquariums were set up in the

facility for residents to look at during meal times.
Animal-assisted therapy benefits for seniors can also include:

- Increased self-esteem
- Reduced feelings of anxiety and isolation
- Decreased blood pressure and heart rate
- Improved motor skills
- Increased social interaction
- Stimulated memory as seniors reminisce about pets they used to have
- Quicker recovery time from injuries
- Higher levels of physical activity

The Role of Therapy Dogs

Research in Learning & Behavior has shown that dogs are attuned to human emotional states and will seek to help people in distress. So it's not surprising that therapy dogs are good for easing anxiety in and providing comfort to older adults. Dogs are used in therapy to offer companionship and affection and enhance people's physical and mental health.

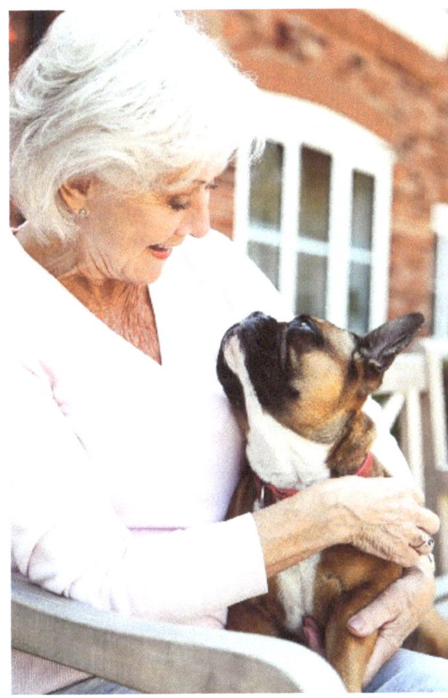

Fig.14.1 Elderly women feeling mentally better after putting the pet dog in her lap.

Commonly, dog therapy programs involve volunteer animals and their handlers coming to spend time with elderly people in hospitals and nursing homes. When a therapy dog visits, the seniors might feed, pet, groom, walk, or play with the animal

These interactions can help speed a senior's recovery from illness or injury or just help lift his or her spirits. Some long-term care facilities have therapy dogs that live on-site and are handled by a trained staff member; in such cases, residents often work together to care for the animals. Other facilities arrange for pet visits from local volunteers or organizations.

Did you know you can also arrange for therapy dog home visits? Organizations like Therapy Dogs International and Alliance of Therapy Dogs offer free services whereby a volunteer handler and therapy dog make periodic visits to seniors who still live in their own homes but are lonely, isolated, or struggling with physical impairments.

To be effective as therapy dogs, the animals must be patient, obedient, calm, friendly, well-socialized, and even-tempered. They must welcome being petted and cuddled by unfamiliar people and take direction well. In addition, a therapy dog trainer must ensure that the dogs become acclimated to equipment like canes, walkers, wheelchairs, and motorized beds. And dogs that work with dementia patients must be comfortable with the mood swings that people with this condition frequently exhibit.

While any breed of dog can be a therapy dog, some breeds are noted for their suitability to serve. Some of the most frequently used dogs for therapy include Labrador retrievers, golden retrievers, St. Bernards, beagles, poodles, pugs, Boston terriers, and greyhounds. (Read more about dog breeds that are well-suited for seniors.)

The law does not mandate that therapy dogs be certified. However, some facilities will only accept dogs that have received formal training and are registered with a therapy dog organization. Here are a few examples of organizations that register or certify therapy dogs:

- Alliance of Therapy Dogs
- Pet Partners (formerly known as Delta Society)
- Bright and Beautiful Therapy Dogs
- Love on a Leash
- Therapy Dogs International

It's important to understand that a certified therapy dog is not the same as a service dog. Learn more about the differences

Other Types of Therapy Animals

While dogs are the most common type of pet used in animal therapy, a growing number of other species are also performing this kind of work. For instance, cats can be good for therapy

They are the only animals that purr, and cuddling with a purring cat can soothe a person's mood. Plus, a study in The Journal of the Acoustical Society of America has demonstrated that when cats purr, they produce a sound frequency that is ideal for promoting bone growth and healing in humans.

Almost any animal can be a therapy animal if it has the right temperament and training. Love on a Leash certifies cats, dogs, and rabbits as therapy pets. Pet Partners provides therapy animal training and registration for nine different species: Dogs, cats, horses, guinea pigs, rabbits, llamas, rats, birds, and miniature pigs can all be used for pet therapy. And Maryland-based non-profit organization Pets on Wheels accepts any breed or species for its therapy teams so long as the animal passes a temperament screening and health check.

There are three types of assistance animals which play separate and distinctive roles.

Therapy animals

A therapy animal is a pet that has been trained to interact with and provide comfort to a wide range of people in different environments. As noted above, therapy animals for seniors are not limited to just dogs; they can be cats, horses, birds, or many other species. Although they provide a valuable service, pets that are involved in therapy work do not have any special rights under the law and can only enter businesses and facilities that they have been invited into, or that allow animals in general.

Service animals

A service animal goes through extensive training so that it can provide specific assistance to a person with a physical or mental disability. Under federal law, only dogs (and in some circumstances, miniature horses) qualify as service animals. Service dogs for seniors can perform tasks such as:

- Guiding a person with low vision
- Alerting a person with diabetes to changing blood sugar levels
- Providing balance and stability help to a person with mobility challenges
- Pulling a wheelchair
- Reminding a person with a mental disorder to take his or her medication
- Helping a person stay safe during an epileptic seizure
- Alerting someone who is deaf or hard of hearing when someone is approaching
- Keeping a person with dementia from walking out of the house unaccompanied

Service dogs are considered working dogs, not pets. They stay with their handlers at all times and are protected by the Americans With Disabilities Act (ADA). Service dogs are legally permitted to accompany their human handlers into public places like stores, restaurants, hotels, hospitals, buses, and airplanes. They also have full access to housing complexes that would not normally allow pets.

While service dogs do not have to wear any special ID tags or vests, doing so can head off unnecessary questions. (A vest or harness can also let people know that the animal is performing an important task and should not be petted.) You should be aware that business owners and employers cannot ask service dog handlers to provide details about the handler's disability. They can only ask if the dog is a service animal required for a disability and what specific service the dog has been trained to render.

In cases where the ADA conflicts with state laws, whichever law offers broader protections will generally apply. For example, Ohio service dog laws stipulate that assistance dogs must be leashed in public places, whereas the ADA allows service dogs to be off leash if being leashed would interfere with the work the dogs are trained to do. (However, the handler must still maintain control of the animal through voice commands or other signals). In such a case, the ADA's more flexible provisions pre-empt the state regulations.

If you're interested in getting a service dog for yourself or someone you love, you can search for non-profit service animal organizations in your area on the website of Assistance Dogs International

Emotional support animals

Emotional support animals (ESAs) are sometimes known as comfort animals. They are pets that provide therapeutic benefits to individuals who have a diagnosed emotional or mental disability. Unlike a therapy animal that is trained to bring comfort to many people, an emotional support animal supports one specific person. And unlike a service animal that is rigorously trained to perform a specific task, an ESA simply provides companionship and comfort, and it requires no specialized training.

To qualify for an ESA, you need a recommendation letter from a licensed mental health professional such as a psychologist, clinical social worker, or psychiatrist. The professional must certify that you suffer from a specific mental health condition that affects your daily activities and that an emotional support animal will help alleviate one or more of the symptoms of your condition. Such letters must be renewed every year.

Table 14.1 Studies on the use of animals on blood pressure

Study	Type of study	*N*	Summary of results
Allen et al.	Randomized, unblinded, prospective, controlled	48	Subjects had lower blood pressure and heart rates in response to an acute mental stressor in the presence of a pet
Friedmann et al.	Controlled, unblinded, prospective	11	Blood pressure lower when animal and acute mental stressor present
Barker et al.	Controlled, unblinded, prospective	10	Pet owners reduced systolic and diastolic blood pressure in the presence of animal when mental stressor present
Anderson et al.	Retrospective chart survey	5741	Pet owners had lower resting blood pressure
Wright et al.	Mail questionnaire	1179	Pet owners had lower systolic, mean arteriolar, pulse pressures, risk of HTN (O.R. = 0.62)

Table 14.2 Studies on the use of animals in cardiovascular disease.

Study	Type of study	*N*	Summary of results
Friedmann and Thomas	Retrospective data analysis	424	Dog owners less likely to die 1 year after MI
Friedmann et al.	In-person interview survey	96	Pet owners had higher 1-year survival after CCU discharge
Ruzic et al.	Prospective, controlled, unblinded, longitudinal study	59	Subjects walking dogs regularly achieved a higher workload on a bicycle exercise test ($P < .06$)
Friedmann et al.	Retrospective data analysis	460	Pet owners implant with deĀbrillator more likely to survive
Cole et al.	Randomized, controlled, unblinded study	76	Subjects exposed to an animal had signiĀcantly better hemodynamic and neurohormonal parameters
Abate et al.	Observational intervention group, historically case-controlled study	69	Subjects with dog-assisted ambulation walked signiĀcantly greater distance
Parker et al.	In-person interview survey	424	Pet owners more likely to have cardiac morbidity and mortality one year after admission for an acute coronary syndrome

Under the ADA, pets that function as emotional support animals are not entitled to any special protection and cannot go into any building or facility where animals are not allowed. However, under the Fair Housing Act, even housing facilities that have a no-pet rule must allow your ESA to live with you. The landlord or housing provider can ask to see your official recommendation letter. Similarly, the Air Carrier Access Act allows your emotional support animal to accompany you into aircraft cabins for free, provided you have a legitimate recommendation letter. (Some airlines require 48 hours' notice as well as verification of your animal's health and obedience training to accommodate it as an ESA, so make sure to check your airline carrier's requirements before your flight.)

Unfortunately, some people claim that their pets are emotional support animals even when they aren't. And plenty of disreputable online sites claim to provide recommendation letters quickly and easily for a fee. To be sure you receive a legitimate letter, talk to the healthcare professional who is treating you

How Robotic Pets for Adults Can Make a Difference

Many older adults enjoy the companionship of animals but can't have any of their own because they have allergies or reside in facilities that don't allow pets. Others simply don't want or can't handle the responsibility of caring for a living creature. In such cases, the ideal solution may be a robotic animal. After all, robots are easily controlled, don't need to be fed or cleaned up after, and don't shed or transmit any diseases. And research studies in the Journal of the American Medical Directors Association and the Journal of Gerontological Nursing have demonstrated that robotic pets have the ability to improve the quality of life for older adults.

For instance, Hasbro's Joy for All Companion Pet line was designed to bring comfort and happiness to older adults through engaging interactions with realistic robotic pets. Soft fur, blinking eyes, and limbs that move are features of both the robotic therapy dog and cat designed by Hasbro.The Joy for All cat, which launched in 2015 and costs $99.99, purrs and meows like a real feline and features built-in sensors in its cheek, back, belly, and head that enable it to respond to human touch. It will nuzzle your hand or even roll over on its back to request a belly rub. It might squirm a bit, but it can't get up and walk around. If left alone for a few minutes, it will drift off to sleep.

The robotic therapy dog version was released in 2016 and costs $129.99. Built to resemble a golden retriever puppy, the dog includes sensors that prompt it to nuzzle your hand when you touch its cheek. If you gently pet the puppy's back, you will even feel a simulated heartbeat. The dog will also turn its head in response to your voice and make realistic barking and puppy sounds. Hasbro has partnered with researchers at Brown University to expand the abilities of the Joy for All pets through artificial intelligence. Armed with a $1-million grant from the National Science Foundation, the group is working toward enabling the robotic pets to perform tasks like locating lost objects and reminding seniors to take their medication. The project has been dubbed Affordable Robotic Intelligence for Elderly Support (ARIES), and researchers say the word "affordable" is key: While no price has yet been set, the hope is to keep it to just a few hundred dollars.

One robotic pet that has long utilized advanced artificial intelligence is PARO the seal. Specifically designed as a therapy animal to comfort people with dementia, PARO resembles a baby harp seal and is remarkably lifelike, with soft white fur, paws that move, and eyes that follow people's movements. It can seek out eye contact, remember faces, respond to touch, and even learn its own name. PARO also gradually learns to repeat behaviors that result in petting.

With a price tag of $5,000 to $6,000, the PARO seal is generally too expensive to be a personal pet. But it is a popular addition to dozens of hospices, long-term care facilities, hospitals, and senior living communities throughout North America. In 2009, it even became certified as a therapeutic medical device by the U.S. Food and Drug Administration. Research, such as a study in the Journal of the American Medical Directors Association as well as one in Frontiers in ICT, has revealed that interacting with the PARO robot makes nursing home residents happier, less lonely, less stressed, more social, and more active. One study by the Front Porch Center for Innovation and Wellbeing even found that the use of PARO reduced the need for psychotropic medications in almost two-thirds of cases where such medications were being considered.

Harness the Healing Power of Animals

As you can see, therapy dogs are far from the only animals that can provide companionship and promote healing. And with the range of available options, from visits with live animals to sessions with robotic creatures, you can enjoy the benefits of pet therapy in any setting.

Table 14.3 Studies on the use of animals on physical activity.

Study	Type of study	N	Summary of results
Temple et al.	Prospective, observational	48	Pet owners more likely to use parks
Reeves et al.	Telephone survey	5902	Dog walkers most likely to perform leisure-time physical activity
Moudon et al.	Telephone survey	608	Dog owners more likely to walk (O.R. = 1.69)
Thorpe et al.	In-person questionnaire survey	3075	Dog owners more likely to engage in physical activity, walking
Feng et al.	Prospective, observational	545	Dog walking associated with physical activity (measured by accelerometer carried by subjects)
Yabroff et al.	Telephone survey	41,514	Dog owners walked longer times
Raina et al.	Telephone survey	1054	Pet owners experienced slower deterioration in activities of daily living
Oka and Shibata	Online survey	5253	Dog walkers had more physical activity
Dembicki and Anderson	Cross-sectional, observational study	127	Dog owners walked longer times
SchoĀeld et al.	Telephone survey	1237	Dog ownership not associated with recommended physical activity large dog owners walked more than small dog owners

Table 14.4 Potential benefits and risks of animals in the elderly.

Potential bene its	Potential harms
Increased physical activity	Cost
Improved survival in cardiovascular disease	Injury to self
Improved circulatory hemodynamic responses	Injury to others
Less behavioral disturbance in demented patients	Damage to property
Improved socialization in demented patients	Damage to environment
Weight maintenance in demented patients	Zoonotic infections
Less anxiety, fear in depressed patients	Adverse psychological event (e.g., grief reaction over loss of pet)
Improved social behavior in schizophrenics	Adverse social event (e.g., friends, neighbors fear pet)
Less loneliness	Greater rehospitalization rate in acute coronary syndrome patients

Bibliography and Acknowledgement

- Anderson W. P., Reid C. M., Jennings G. L. Pet ownership and risk factors for cardiovascular disease. Medical Journal of Australia. 1992;157(5):298–301. [PubMed] [Google Scholar]
- Banks M. R., Banks W. A. The effects of animal-assisted therapy on loneliness in an elderly population in long-term care facilities. Journals of Gerontology—Series A Biological Sciences and Medical Sciences. 2002;57(7):M428–M432. doi: 10.1093/gerona/57.7.M428. [PubMed] [CrossRef] [Google Scholar]
- Cangelosi P. R., Sorrell J. M. Walking for therapy with man's best friend. Journal of Psychosocial Nursing and Mental Health Services. 2010;48(3):19–22. doi: 10.3928/02793695-20100202-05. [PubMed] [CrossRef] [Google Scholar]
- Dembicki D., Anderson J. Pet ownership may be a factor in improved health of the elderly. Journal of Nutrition for the Elderly. 1996;15(3):15–31. [PubMed] [Google Scholar]
- Edwards N. E., Beck A. M. Animal-assisted therapy and nutrition in Alzheimer's disease. Western Journal of Nursing Research. 2002;24(6):697–712. doi: 10.1177/019394502320555430. [PubMed] [CrossRef] [Google Scholar]
- Feng Z., Dibben C., Witham M. D., et al. Dog ownership and physical activity in later life: a cross-sectional observational study. Preventive Medicine. 2014;66C:101–106. [PubMed] [Google Scholar]
- Guay D. R. P. Pet-assisted therapy in the nursing home setting: potential for zoonosis. The American Journal of Infection Control. 2001;29(3):178–186. doi: 10.1067/mic.2001.115873. [PubMed] [CrossRef] [Google Scholar]
- Harris M. D., Rinehart J. M., Gerstman J. Animal-assisted therapy for the homebound elderly. Holistic Nursing Practice. 1993;8(1):27–37. doi: 10.1097/00004650-199310000-00006. [PubMed] [CrossRef] [Google Scholar]
- Johnson R. A., Odendaal J. S. J., Meadows R. L. Animal-assisted interventions research: issues and answers. Western Journal of Nursing Research. 2002;24(4):422–440. doi: 10.1177/01945902024004009. [PubMed] [CrossRef] [Google Scholar]
- Kanamori M., Suzuki M., Tanaka M. Maintenance and improvement of quality of life among elderly patients using a pet-type robot. Japanese Journal of Geriatrics. 2002;39(2):214–218. doi: 10.3143/geriatrics.39.214. [PubMed] [CrossRef] [Google Scholar]
- Kongable L. G., Buckwalter K. C., Stolley J. M. The effects of pet therapy on the social behavior of institutionalized Alzheimer's clients. Archives of Psychiatric Nursing. 1989;3(4):191–198. [PubMed] [Google Scholar]
- Kurrle S. E., Day R., Cameron I. D. The perils of pet ownership: a new fall-injury risk factor. Medical Journal of Australia. 2004;181(11-12):682–683. [PubMed] [Google Scholar]
- Levine G. N., Allen K., Braun L. T., et al. Pet ownership and cardiovascular risk: a scientific statement from the American Heart Association. Circulation. 2013;127(23):2353–2363. doi: 10.1161/CIR.0b013e31829201e1. [PubMed] [CrossRef] [Google Scholar]
- Oka K., Shibata A. Dog ownership and health-related physical activity among japanese adults. Journal of Physical Activity and Health. 2009;6(4):412–418. [PubMed] [Google Scholar]
- Perelle I. B., Granville D. A. Assessment of the effectiveness of a pet facilitated therapy program in a nursing home setting. Society and Animals. 1983;1:91–100. [Google Scholar]
- Reeves M. J., Rafferty A. P., Miller C. E., Lyon-Callo S. K. The impact of dog walking on leisure-time physical activity: results from a population-based survey of Michigan adults. Journal of Physical Activity & Health. 2011;8(3):436–444.
- Miltiades H., Shearer J. Attachment to pet dogs and depression in rural older adults. Anthrozoos. 2011;24(2):147–158.
- Richeson N. E. Effects of animal-assisted therapy on agitated behaviors and social interactions of older adults with dementia. The American Journal of Alzheimer's Disease and other Dementias. 2003;18(6):353–358. doi: 10.1177/153331750301800610. [PMC free article] [PubMed] [CrossRef] [Google Scholar]
- Stasi M. F., Amati D., Costa C., Resta D., Senepa G., Scarafioiti C., Aimonino N., Molaschi M. Pet-therapy: a trial for institutionalized frail elderly patients. Archives of Gerontology and Geriatrics. 2004;38:407–412. doi: 10.1016/j.archger.2004.04.052. [PubMed] [CrossRef] [Google Scholar
- Temple V., Rhodes R., Higgins J. W. Unleashing physical activity: an observational study of park use, dog walking, and physical activity. Journal of Physical Activity and Health. 2011;8(6):766–774. [PubMed] [Google Scholar]
- Thorpe R. J., Jr., Kreisle R. A., Glickman L. T., Simonsick E. M., Newman A. B., Kritchevsky S. Physical activity and pet ownership in year 3 of the Health ABC study. Journal of Aging and Physical Activity. 2006;14(2):154–168. [PubMed] [Google Scholar]
- Villalta-Gil V., Roca M., Gonzalez N., et al. Dog-assisted therapy in the treatment of chronic schizophrenia inpatients. Anthrozoos. 2009;22(2):149–159. doi: 10.2752/175303709X434176. [CrossRef] [Google Scholar]
- Walsh F. Human-animal bonds I: the relational significance of companion animals. Family Process. 2009;48(4):462–480. doi: 10.1111/j.1545-5300.2009.01296.x. [PubMed] [CrossRef] [Google Scholar]
- Wisdom J. P., Saedi G. A., Green C. A. Another breed of "service" animals: STARS study findings about pet ownership and recovery from serious mental illness. American Journal of Orthopsychiatry. 2009;79(3):430–436. doi: 10.1037/a0016812. [PMC free article] [PubMed] [CrossRef] [Google Scholar]
- Wright J. D., Kritz-Silverstein D., Morton D. J., Wingard D. L., Barrett-Connor E. Pet ownership and blood pressure in old age. Epidemiology. 2007;18(5):613–618. doi: 10.1097/EDE.0b013e3181271398. [PubMed] [CrossRef] [Google Scholar]
- Yabroff K. R., Troiano R. P., Berrigan D. Walking the dog: is pet ownership associated with physical activity in California? Journal of Physical Activity and Health. 2008;5(2):216–228. [PubMed] [Google Scholar]
- Zisselman M. H., Rovner B. W., Shmuely Y., Ferrie P. A pet therapy intervention with geriatric psychiatry inpatients. The American Journal of Occupational Therapy. 1996;50(1):47–51. doi: 10.5014/ajot.50.1.47. [PubMed] [CrossRef] [Google Scholar]

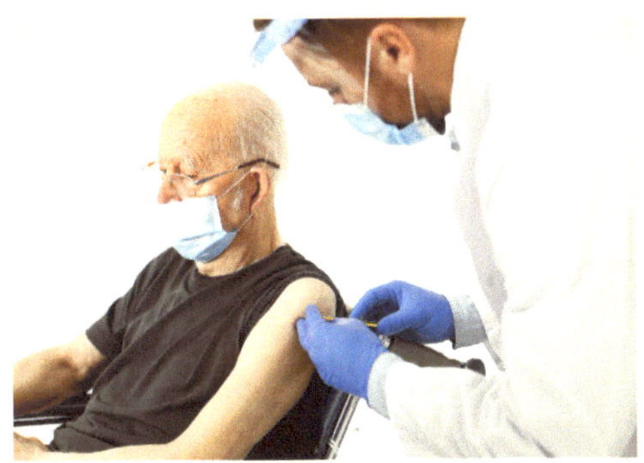

Vaccines For The Elderly.

Current Use and Future Challenges

With increasing life expectancy, the global population ages, and the number of persons older than 60 years of age is expected to double by 2050, reaching 2.1 billion. The number of persons above 80 years is projected to increase even more dramatically from a worldwide total of 125 million in 2015 to 434 million in 2050. The severity of many infections is higher in the elderly compared to younger adults and infectious diseases are frequently associated with long-term sequelae such as impairments in activities of daily living, onset of frailty, or the loss of independence This represents a serious challenge for public health systems, and the prevention of infectious disease is therefore an important measure to ensure healthy aging and improve the quality of life. The tremendous success of childhood vaccination is widely recognized, but the need for life-long vaccination programs and the importance of vaccination for the older population are frequently underestimated. This review summarizes current recommendations for developed countries, gives examples regarding immunogenicity and efficacy data for vaccines currently used for the elderly, and provides an outlook on novel vaccines developed specifically for this age group.

Vaccines specifically recommended for the elderly

Many countries have established vaccination recommendations for adults and most of these also include specific guidelines for older adults. Vaccination against influenza and Streptococcus pneumoniae is usually recommended for persons with underlying diseases and for the elderly with heterogeneous age limits between ≥ 50 years and ≥65 years. Some countries also recommend vaccination against herpes zoster for older adults. Table 1 summarizes current recommendations for Europe and the USA. August is National Immunization Awareness Month. Research tells us that many seniors aren't getting the vaccinations they should and yet, they are one of the age groups where vaccines are most important. As we age, our immune systems tend to become weaker. Vaccines help to fill the gap by

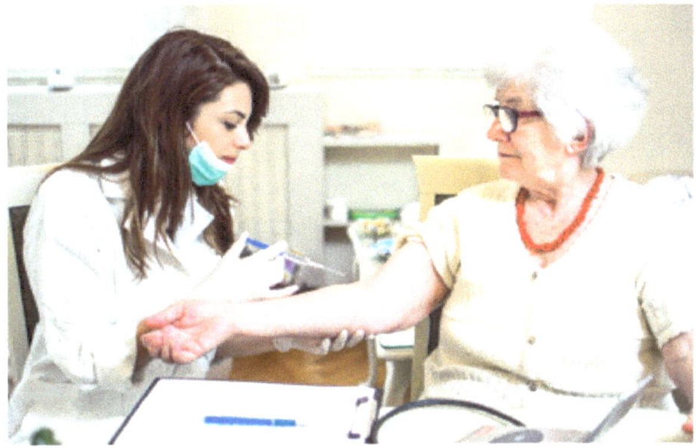

Fig 15.1 Doctor is injecting vaccine in an elderly person

proving added protection against certain diseases. All told, an estimated 45,000 adults die each year from diseases that vaccines can prevent. Many seniors may feel they no longer need vaccinations or they may worry about side effects. Here are the vaccinations the Centers for Disease Control and Prevention (CDC) recommend for adults age 65 and older: Vaccines are an important step in protecting your health and the health of your family. Vaccines are particularly important for older adults. Risks to certain diseases are higher for this age group since it can be more difficult to fight off infections as your immune system naturally weakens as you get older. These infections, such as flu, pneumonia, shingles, tetanus, diphtheria, whooping cough and COVID-19, increase your risk for complications, which can lead to long-term illness and hospitalization.

There are five vaccines adults age 65 and older should consider to prevent certain diseases:

- **Influenza (flu) vaccine**
- **Pneumonia vaccine**
- **Shingles vaccine**
- **Tetanus, diphtheria and pertussis (Tdap) vaccine**
- **COVID-19 vaccine**

The influenza (flu) vaccine is recommended for everyone age 6 months and older every year, starting in the fall. Influenza is a respiratory virus. Getting the vaccine decreases your risk for developing complications from the flu, such as sinus and ear infections, pneumonia, inflammation of the heart, brain or muscle tissues, multi-organ failure or sepsis.

There are two vaccines that are particular for those age 65 and older because they create a stronger immune response: high-dose flu vaccine and an adjuvanted flu vaccine. You can get either of these vaccines in your healthcare provider's office.

Pneumonia

The pneumonia vaccine is recommended as a one-time vaccine for people ages 65 and older.

Pneumonia is caused by a bacteria or virus that infects the lungs. The vaccine is 60 percent to 70 percent effective in preventing invasive disease. You can get this vaccine in your healthcare provider's office.

Shingles

The shingles vaccine is recommended for people age 50 and older even if you had shingles in the past or had the previous shingles vaccine. It is a two-shot series, in which the second shot is given two to six months after the first shot.

Shingles is a viral infection. The chicken pox virus remains inactive in your nerve tissue and can reactivate as shingles, causing a painful, blistery rash on one side of the body. Shingles can also cause postherpetic neuralgia (PHN), which causes severe and debilitating pain where the rash occurred. The vaccine is greater than 90 percent effective in preventing shingles and PHN. Supplies of this vaccine may be limited. Ask your healthcare provider or a pharmacy about vaccine availability.

Tetanus, Diphtheria and Pertussis (Tdap)

The tetanus, diphtheria, and pertussis vaccine combined (Tdap) is recommended if you have not received a tetanus shot in the last 10 years or have only had the tetanus and diphtheria combined (Td) vaccine and not the Tdap in the past.

Tetanus is caused by a bacteria in soil, dirt and manure and can impair the nervous system. Diphtheria is caused by a bacteria that attaches to the lining of the respiratory system, which causes difficulty breathing and swallowing and can get into the bloodstream and damage the heart, kidneys and nerves. Pertussis (whooping cough) can be a very serious disease, especially for vulnerable populations, such as infants, young children and older adults. Pertussis causes coughing fits due to the bacteria attaching to the lining of the upper respiratory system.

The vaccine is greater than 95 percent effective in preventing tetanus and diphtheria and 70 percent effective in preventing pertussis. You can get this vaccine from your healthcare provider.

COVID-19

The COVID-19 vaccine is recommended for ages 12 and older. The risk of severe illness from COVID-19 increases with age, so this is why the Centers for Disease Control recommends the COVID-19 vaccine for older adults too. The COVID-19 vaccine helps prevent severe illness.

It typically takes two weeks after vaccination for the body to build immunity against the coronavirus that causes COVID-19. You are not fully vaccinated until two weeks after the second dose of a two-dose vaccine or two weeks after a one-dose vaccine. The two-dose vaccines are 94 percent to 95 percent effective in preventing COVID-19. The one-dose vaccine is 66 percent effective. You can receive this vaccine from a vaccination clinic set up expressly for this purpose or at a pharmacy

New targets for vaccine development

We still lack vaccines for many pathogens that are of clinical relevance in the elderly.Such as:-

1 Respiratory syncytial virus (RSV)

2.Clostridium difficile,

3.Staphylococcus aureus, which is responsible for infections of prostheses, catheters or surgical wounds

4. S. aureus infection

5.Most vaccine candidates against C. difficile are based on bacterial toxins which are responsible for the clinical symptoms [78]. Vaccines against these and other nosocomial pathogens, such as Klebsiella pneumoniae, Escherichia coli and the fungal pathogen Candida spp. have the potential to substantially reduce healthcare costs and to save many lives

Conclusion

Older adults are at high risk for infectious diseases and vaccination is an important preventive measure to facilitate healthy aging. Childhood vaccination programs are well-accepted and widely used, but unfortunately awareness for adult vaccination is by far less prominent. Several vaccines against influenza, S. pneumoniae and herpes zoster are available for the elderly and vaccines that are used throughout adulthood, such as tetanus, diphtheria and pertussis, are also relevant for the elderly.In addition, vaccines against additional pathogens such as RSV and nosocomial infections could substantially improve health in old age.

Bibliography and Acknowledgement

- Ansaldi F, Bacilieri S, Durando P, Sticchi L, Valle L, Montomoli E, et al. Cross-protection by MF59-adjuvanted influenza vaccine: neutralizing and haemagglutination-inhibiting antibody activity against a(H3N2) drifted influenza viruses. Vaccine. 2008;26:1525–9.
- Bayas JM, Vilella A, Bertran MJ, Vidal J, Batalla J, Asenjo MA, et al. Immunogenicity and reactogenicity of the adult tetanus-diphtheria vaccine. How many doses are necessary? Epidemiol Infect. 2001;127:451–60.
- Chlibek R, Bayas JM, Collins H, de la Pinta ML, Ledent E, Mols JF, et al. Safety and immunogenicity of an AS01-adjuvanted varicella-zoster virus subunit candidate vaccine against herpes zoster in adults >=50 years of age. J Infect Dis. 2013;208:1953–61.
- Cross AS, Chen WH, Levine MM. A case for immunization against nosocomial infections. J Leukoc Biol. 2008;83:483–8.
Cunningham AL, Lal H, Kovac M, Chlibek R, Hwang SJ, Diez-Domingo J, et al. Efficacy of the herpes zoster subunit vaccine in adults 70 years of age or older. N Engl J Med. 2016;375:1019–32.
- Cross AS, Chen WH, Levine MM. A case for immunization against nosocomial infections. J Leukoc Biol. 2008;83:483–8.
De Donato S, Granoff D, Minutello M, Lecchi G, Faccini M, Agnello M, et al. Safety and immunogenicity of MF59-adjuvanted influenza vaccine in the elderly. Vaccine. 1999;17:3094–101
- Esposito S, Principi N. Direct and indirect effects of the 13-valent pneumococcal conjugate vaccine administered to infants and young children. Future Microbiol. 2015;10:1599–607.
Feldman C, Anderson R. Review: current and new generation pneumococcal vaccines. J Inf Secur. 2014;69:309–25.
- Grasse M, Meryk A, Schirmer M, Grubeck-Loebenstein B, Weinberger B. Booster vaccination against tetanus and diphtheria: insufficient protection against diphtheria in young and elderly adults. Immun Ageing. 2016;13:26.
- Halperin SA, Scheifele D, de Serres G, Noya F, Meekison W, Zickler P, et al. Immune responses in adults to revaccination with a tetanus toxoid, reduced diphtheria toxoid, and acellular pertussis vaccine 10 years after a previous dose. Vaccine. 2012;30:974–82.
- Harpaz R, Ortega-Sanchez IR, Seward JF. Prevention of herpes zoster: recommendations of the advisory committee on immunization practices (ACIP). MMWR Recomm Rep. 2008;57:1–30.
- Haynes L, Eaton SM, Burns EM, Randall TD, Swain SL. CD4 T cell memory derived from young naive cells functions well into old age, but memory generated from aged naive cells functions poorly. Proc Natl Acad Sci U S A. 2003;100:15053–8.
- Haynes L. The effect of aging on cognate function and development of immune memory. Curr Opin Immunol. 2005;17:476–9.
- Hennessy S, Liu Z, Tsai TF, Strom BL, Wan CM, Liu HL, et al. Effectiveness of live-attenuated Japanese encephalitis vaccine (SA14-14-2): a case-control study. Lancet. 1996;347:1583–6.
- Iob A, Brianti G, Zamparo E, Gallo T. Evidence of increased clinical protection of an MF59-adjuvant influenza vaccine compared to a non-adjuvant vaccine among elderly residents of long-term care facilities in Italy. Epidemiol Infect. 2005;133:687–93.
- Kaml M, Weiskirchner I, Keller M, Luft T, Hoster E, Hasford J, et al. Booster vaccination in the elderly: their success depends on the vaccine type applied earlier in life as well as on pre-vaccination antibody titers. Vaccine. 2006;24:6808–11.
- Kanitz EE, Wu LA, Giambi C, Strikas RA, Levy-Bruhl D, Stefanoff P, et al. Variation in adult vaccination policies across Europe: an overview from VENICE network on vaccine recommendations, funding and coverage. Vaccine. 2012;30:5222–8.
- Levin MJ, Schmader KE, Pang L, Williams-Diaz A, Zerbe G, Canniff J, et al. Cellular and Humoral responses to a second dose of herpes zoster vaccine administered 10 years after the first dose among older adults. J Infect Dis. 2016;213:14–22.
- Osterholm MT, Kelley NS, Sommer A, Belongia EA. Efficacy and effectiveness of influenza vaccines: a systematic review and meta-analysis. Lancet Infect Dis. 2012;12:36–44.
- Pinchinat S, Cebrian-Cuenca AM, Bricout H, Johnson RW. Similar herpes zoster incidence across Europe: results from a systematic literature review. BMC Infect Dis. 13:2013, 170.
- Rafferty E, Duclos P, Yactayo S, Schuster M. Risk of yellow fever vaccine-associated viscerotropic disease among the elderly: a systematic review. Vaccine. 2013;31:5798–805.
- Schmader K, Gnann JW Jr, Watson CP. The epidemiological, clinical, and pathological rationale for the herpes zoster vaccine. J Infect Dis. 2008;197(Suppl 2):S207–15. S207-S215
- Trucchi C, Alicino C, Orsi A, Paganino C, Barberis I, Grammatico F, et al. Fifteen years of epidemiologic, virologic and syndromic influenza surveillance: a focus on type B virus and the effects of vaccine mismatch in Liguria region, Italy. Hum Vaccin Immunother. 2017;13:456–63.
- Van Damme P, Burgess M. Immunogenicity of a combined diphtheria-tetanus-acellular pertussis vaccine in adults. Vaccine. 2004;22:305–8.
- Waight PA, Andrews NJ, Ladhani SN, Sheppard CL, Slack MP, Miller E. Effect of the 13-valent pneumococcal conjugate vaccine on invasive pneumococcal disease in England and Wales 4 years after its introduction: an observational cohort study. Lancet Infect Dis. 2015;15:535–43.
- Weinberger B, Keller M, Fischer KH, Stiasny K, Neuner C, Heinz FX, et al. Decreased antibody titers and booster responses in tick-borne encephalitis vaccinees aged 50-90 years. Vaccine. 2010;28:3511–5.
- Weinberger B, Schirmer M, Matteucci GR, Siebert U, Fuchs D, Grubeck-Loebenstein B. Recall responses to tetanus and diphtheria vaccination are frequently insufficient in elderly persons. PLoS One. 2013;8:e82967.
- Weinberger B. Adult vaccination against tetanus and diphtheria: the European perspective. Clin Exp Immunol. 2017;187:93–9.
- Wiersma LC, Rimmelzwaan GF, de Vries RD. Developing universal influenza vaccines: hitting the nail, not just on the head. Vaccines (Basel). 2015;3:239–62.
- Wolters B, Junge U, Dziuba S, Roggendorf M. Immunogenicity of combined hepatitis a and B vaccine in elderly persons. Vaccine. 2003;21:3623–8.
- Yao X, Hamilton RG, Weng NP, Xue QL, Bream JH, Li H, et al. Frailty is associated with impairment of vaccine-induced antibody response and increase in post-vaccination influenza infection in community-dwelling older adults. Vaccine. 2011;29:5015–21.

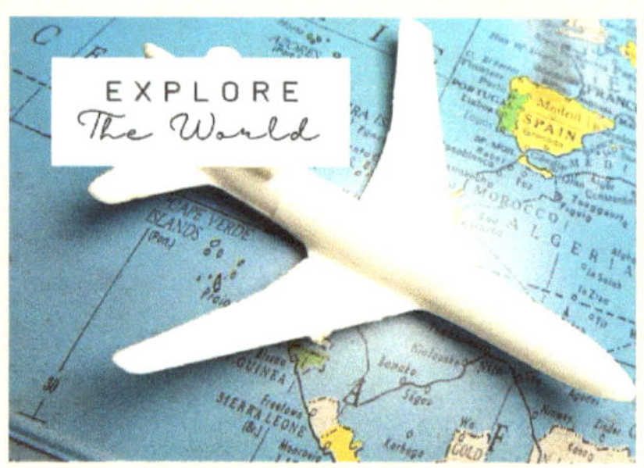

Guidelines of Travelling by Seniors

Travel can be an incredibly rewarding experience, especially for seniors. Exploring different countries and cultures can create lifelong memories and introduce us to new ideas and perspectives. However, seniors must take the necessary precautions to ensure a safe and enjoyable trip. From researching the destination to staying healthy while traveling, senior travelers should always have a plan in place before heading off on their journey.

How To Travel As A Senior: Here are our top travel tips for seniors to make the most of their travels:

1.Start planning early.

Book flights and accommodations as far in advance as possible, so that you have plenty of time to research and compare your options. Also be sure to familiarize yourself with the destination you're traveling to, so you know what to expect. Do some research on your destination, including climate information, any required vaccinations, and any other characteristics or requirements of the area. Also, take some time to investigate the different transportation options available, both for getting to your destination and while you're there.If you'll be traveling by public transit, ask about any senior discounts you may qualify for.You should also plan ahead if you'll need assistance getting around at your destination.

2. Make sure you have a valid passport/ ID card:-

if you'll be traveling outside of the country. Many countries require at least six months of validity left on your passport beyond when you'll be leaving their country after your trip.Check early to be sure you'll have that much time left on your passport so you can start the renewal process if you won't.Right now, passport renewals are taking several months to complete. You can expedite the process, but it will cost you to do so. Make at least two photocopies of your passport and keep one copy in your possession when you're out walking or on a tour at your destination. Lock your original passport in the hotel safe and never carry it with you!If you are pickpocketed, it will be a huge hassle and trip interruption if you have to go to the embassy in the country you're visiting to replace it.A friend of mine just went through that daunting experience on her birthday trip to Italy and she had to alter her travel plans to get her passport replaced. Don't be that person!

What other important documents are needed?

Bring a valid form of identification, such as your driver's license and current insurance cards.Keep them with you at all times during the trip, in case you need them for security reasons or other reasons.It's always a good idea to leave copies of them in your suitcase or in the safe at the hotel, and also with family or friends at home for added protection.

3. Pack light!

It's no fun trying to lug heavy bags around airports or through narrow train or bus aisles, so limit yourself to one checked bag and one piece of carry-on luggage, if possible.When my husband and I travel – even to Europe – we take one carry on suitcase apiece. We've both spent enough time dragging our suitcases around from airport to hotel that we do not want to have to manage anything bigger than this. In fact, this was just reinforced to us when we recently visited Iceland and took a family-sized suitcase instead (because of all that bulky winter clothing!).Neither of us wore half of what we packed and hubby's shoulder strain wasn't worth it.That said, if you're traveling by air, be familiar with the airline's baggage restrictions before packing. They have a weight limit and you'll be charged if you're over that weight.Also, don't forget all the essential items like prescription medication and copies of health records. Organize this paperwork and consider how you'll store them during the trip. **TIP:** it's best to pack enough medication in a carry-on bag so you have them in hand if you go to London and your baggage ends up in Bangkok!

4. Check with your doctor before you go.

Make sure you're healthy enough to travel and that you have had the necessary vaccines and medications. In the post-covid era, some tour groups and countries are still requiring copies of covid vaccination cards for entry.Also, there are certain air travel risks that the elderly face, so you'll want to be sure it's safe for you to fly. Your doctor may be able to suggest additional tips to help you stay healthy in your particular situation while traveling.

5. Check in advance whether your hotel room will have special services available like accessible bathrooms, ramps, elevators, etc, that may be needed due to mobility challenges Also, confirm what type of transportation service the hotel offers and if they have any discounts or special promotions for seniors.

6. Make sure your mobile phone is unlocked if you'll be using it abroad. Purchasing a local SIM card at each of your travel destinations is a great way to avoid expensive roaming charges. Also, make sure to inform your cellphone provider and your family back home of your travel dates and contact information in case of an emergency. And, turn your phone off when it's not in use to save battery life.

7. **Stay flexible.** Don't plan too many activities or sightseeing trips in advance, as this can make it difficult to adjust if something unexpected comes up. Leave time for spontaneous adventures!

8. **Invest in travel insurance that covers out-of-country** medical expenses in case of an emergency.This is especially important for seniors, who are more likely to face medical emergencies on their trips due to age-related conditions.A comprehensive travel insurance policy can help protect you from costly fees and help ensure your safety while abroad.

TIP: Be sure it has emergency evacuation coverage in case you get sick in another country and must get home.My 89-year old uncle recently had chest pains while on a cruise. The ship took him to a hospital when they docked in Panama City, Panama, where it was decided that he needed a heart bypass. He didn't want to do the surgery while overseas, but they did NOT have a travel insurance policy that covered evacuation, so they had to foot the (very, very expensive) bill for an air-ambulance flight back to the USA!But travel insurance isn't just about medical coverage. What if that Mediterranean cruise you were so excited about gets cancelled due to bad weather? Or your luggage gets lost in transit? A comprehensive travel insurance policy can cover trip cancellations, lost or delayed luggage, and even services like that emergency evacuation my uncle needed. It's like a safety net, ready to catch you when unexpected events try to knock you off your travel plans.

9. **Be aware of your surroundings,** just like you should do when you're home. Stay alert while in crowded or unfamiliar areas and stay safe by avoiding late-night activities or walking alone at night.

10. **In the event of an emergency,** it's important to know how to contact local help. Make sure you learn (or have at least written down and bought with you) the local emergency services number before traveling (hint: 911 is only the emergency number in the United States. Each country has its own emergency number). Store it in a secure place where you can access it easily if needed. This way, you can quickly get in touch with local authorities if needed.

11. **Let a family member and/or a friend know your travel details** and when you'll be back home. This way, someone knows where you are at all times if there is an emergency back home. And, they can check in with you if needed. It's also a good idea to keep in touch with them regularly so that they know you're safe and having a great time.

12. **Avoid carrying large amounts of cash or valuable items with you.** Use a money belt or pickpocket-proof purse or wallet for your money and valuables.

13.**Only exchange money at legitimate businesses**, like banks or currency exchanges. If you plan in advance, you can typically order foreign currency from your bank. In addition, there are usually currency exchanges at the airport when you land in a foreign country (expensive) or you can exchange currency at a local bank in the city you are visiting (cheaper, but still pricey).

Air Travel Risks For Elderly

As a senior, you have plenty of reasons to fly. Maybe you're heading out on that dream vacation or traveling to see a loved one.Air travel isn't the same for you as it was when you were younger, though. Now your body will react differently to the stresses of flying than it did years ago.

Elderly fliers have the following air travel risks:

- **Severe jet lag**
- **Bodily pain and discomfort**
- **Higher illness risk**
- **Dehydration**
- **Temporary hearing loss**
- **Hypoxia**
- **Cardiac stress**
- **Deep vein thrombosis**

Age changes one's body in so many ways, and that includes a person's flight tolerance. According to a Frontiers in Physiology study from 2019 on the subject, the air pressurization changes that occur at a high altitude of even 7,000 to 8,000 feet can affect older adults in a multitude of ways.

If not that, then long flights and exposure to other people put senior travelers at a higher risk of medical issues.

Severe Jet Lag

A Washington Post article from 2019 reported data from MIT that correlates age with the severity of jet lag.In other words, the older an individual, the higher the risk for severe jet lag when changing time zones.Jet lag can cause memory and concentration issues (which can be scary for adult children if you're concerned about your senior developing dementia), reduced sleep quality, difficulty keeping awake during the day, and exhaustion.

Bodily Pain And Discomfort

Airline seats are designed for user comfort, but even still, senior citizens might find themselves with aches and pains from sitting, especially particularly after long-haul flights. The discomfort can persist even after exiting the plane, which will make getting around the airport particularly difficult.

Higher Illness Risk

According to travel resource FLIGHTFUD, the average person is at an elevated 10x risk of developing an illness from flying on a plane. Colds are the most common illness one can pick up, but plenty of people can develop COVID-19. Trust me, I know this firsthand, because I got it on the flight home after our trip to Iceland.I was seated next to teens who were complaining to their parents about how yucky they were feeling. Two days later, I came down with it.The reason illnesses follow frequent travelers around? You're stuck in a confined space with hundreds of other strangers for hours. That doesn't exactly give you much reprieve from illness-causing germs While an illness is a minor inconvenience for most adults, it could be more serious for elderly passengers.

Dehydration

The elderly are at greater risk of becoming dehydrated more easily compared to younger adults. A senior might not have access to fluids for hours at a time when flying, or they do, but not in a significant enough quantity to ward off dehydration. Or, if you're like me, you don't drink much because you don't want to use the plane's restroom a dozen times before you land. If you have developed papery skin, sunken eyes, and dry lips and tongue while traveling, you're dehydrated.

Temporary Hearing Loss

The National Institutes of Health found that one-third of seniors already have hearing loss. Flying on an airplane can only have more impact hearing issues for the elderly.Some flyers experience airplane ear, which can cause a degree of hearing loss and ear pain and pressure. The hearing loss is only temporary and it's caused by air pressure changes in the airplane cabin, but considering seniors are already at risk for hearing issues, any type of hearing loss can be scary.

Hypoxia

A much more severe air travel risk for the elderly is hypoxia, which occurs when the body doesn't have enough oxygen to maintain homeostasis in the tissue. The same team that did the Frontiers in Physiology study found that flying can cause mild hypoxia. An elderly traveler who already has breathing issues, whether from age or a medical condition, could experience more severe breathing issues on a plane.

Cardiac Stress

In the same study, the researchers found that an altitude of at least 7,000 feet increased one's cardiovascular risk. Seniors involved in the study had a decreased heart-rate variability and a higher heart rate. These are indicative of cardiac stress. Since planes often fly at elevations of at least 35,000 feet over sea level, a senior risk of cardiac stress goes up exponentially, especially if they already have a heart condition.

Deep Vein Thrombosis

It's not only that sitting for long periods on a plane can cause bodily pain and discomfort in older people. They also run the potential risk of deep vein thrombosis (DVT). DVT causes blood clots in deep veins such as the arm, pelvis, thigh, or lower leg. The symptoms include swelling and pain in the affected site, although some patients are asymptomatic. Per the CDC, to help prevent the risk of blood clots and DVT if you're flying long distances, it's a good idea to get up and walk around the aircraft cabin every 2 to 3 hours (the same applies to driving – stop and walk around for a few minutes every couple of hours).

You might also consider wearing compression socks. The mild squeezing action promotes blood flow and prevent or reduce swelling and fatigue in your legs and feet.

What Seat On The Plane Is Best For The Elderly?

If you are traveling with an elderly parent and will be flying, you'll want to be sure you're as comfortable as you can be – especially on a cross country flight or for international travel. On that note, what is the best seat in the house for older people?

The closer to the front that a senior can be when flying on a plane, the better. Why is that? For several reasons. For one, you won't have to go as far to get to the bathroom. Also, seats nearer the front of the plane usually have a little more legroom. You will have the space to stretch out you legs and sit more comfortably. Of course, it's not only seniors who enjoy these benefits but any traveler. Therefore, you can expect that seats near the front of the plane will usually be reserved quicker. Therefore, if you want to book yourself or a senior family member a seat near the front of the plane, don't delay.

What Medical Conditions Would Prevent You From Flying?

TIP: Because seniors are more likely to suffer from health conditions of any kind, we highly recommend purchasing travel insurance whenever you travel.Earlier, we talked about how a senior can fly on a plane at any age. Well, almost any age. Certain medical conditions can preclude the elderly from flying, regardless of age. Let's go over these health concerns now.

Heart Conditions

If a senior has a history of cardiovascular disease, including arterial hypertension, heart rhythm or heart rate disorders, chest pain or angina at rest, stroke, recent heart attack, or heart failure, they likely should not go on an airplane. We recommend speaking to your senior's healthcare provider and asking for their medical opinion before booking a flight.

Recent Surgeries

If the senior in your life just received surgery, even if it was minor, they shouldn't be eager to jump on a plane right away. That's especially true for more serious procedures. In that case, older travelers should wait up to three months before they fly on any commercial flights.

Infectious Diseases

For the safety of everyone on board, an elderly person who has or very recently had an infectious disease should reconsider flying. If the senior is serious about flying, even with their infectious disease history, they should wear a face mask. Be aware that they may also need a Fit-to-Fly Certificate. We'll talk more about these certificates in the next section.

Deep Vein Thrombosis

Before making up your mind about whether someone with DVT should fly, schedule an appointment with their primary care physician and ask for their thoughts. A doctor can review the senior's current health and circumstances to decide. If they have travel plans that involve a long flight, their health care provider might disapprove of the flight.

Respiratory Diseases

The high rate of air pressurization and being stuck sharing the same air with other people on a plane for hours means flying may not be safe if a senior has or recently had a respiratory disease. If they have shortness of breath and are using supplemental oxygen, especially, it can make flying dangerous.

Stroke

If your senior parent or loved one recently had a mini-stroke or a full stroke, they're at an elevated risk of developing blood clots and DVT. Getting on a plane isn't the safest or smartest idea right after a stroke, but let the senior's doctor make the final call.

Chronic Obstructive Pulmonary Disease

Pressurized air can worsen COPD, especially at certain elevations and plane sizes. An elderly person may find themselves unable to breathe in the less oxygenated air. Your senior's doctor will likely recommend skipping long flights if they have COPD.

Fit-To-Fly Certificate For The Elderly: Who Needs One?

As promised, let's take a deeper look at the Fit-to-Fly Certificate. What exactly is this medical certificate, and who needs it? A Fit-to-Fly Certificate allows certain flyers entry into various parts of the world, including the United States. The certificate became a requirement after the COVID-19 pandemic began in 2020. It proves that the holder does not have COVID and that they have tested negative for the condition. If required to have this certificate, the traveler must have had a negative test in at least the last 72 hours before their flight, but possibly more recently than that. In some parts of the world, in addition to showing a negative COVID test and a Fit-to-Fly certificate, a person may also have to be subject to a physical.It's up to the airlines to require Fit-to-Fly Certificates and they're not exclusive to the elderly.

How To Stay Healthy While Traveling

Staying healthy on the road is just as important as staying safe. It can be a bit of a challenge, though.

Here are some tips for senior citizens to keep in mind when preparing for their next trip:

1. Stay hydrated – Dehydration is one of the most common causes of health issues on the road, especially during long flights or days spent sightseeing. Make sure to bring along a reusable water bottle and refill it often throughout your travels. Consider bringing a filtering water bottle along like this one. Many countries have water that isn't filtered the same as it is at home. This means you can end up with diarrhea and stomach problems if you drink the water, eat a salad or other food that was washed in local water, brush your teeth, or have a drink containing ice cubes. A self-filtering water can eliminate a lot of problems.

2. Get plenty of rest – Traveling can take its toll on our bodies and minds, so factor in some rest periods during your trip. Wherever possible, try to book accommodations in quieter areas and don't be afraid to take a nap during the day.

3. Eat healthily – When possible, opt for fresh produce instead of processed snacks and drinks during your trip, but stick to fruits and vegetables that you can peel (see the TIP under "stay hydrated" above).

4. Be prepared – Make sure to pack any essential medications in your carry on that you might need during your travels. Also, check with your doctor before traveling to make sure you're up-to-date on vaccinations for the countries you are visiting.

5. Bring an emergency contact list with you in case of any medical issues that come up while you're traveling. This should include the numbers for your doctor, your health insurance provider, and family and/or close friends you might need to contact.

6. You also should always carry a list of your current medication names and dosages, no matter if you're at home or on a trip. This way first responders won't give you anything that will interact with a medication you're taking should you have a medical emergency. Having this information accessible could prove invaluable in the event of a medical emergency while abroad.

7. Now, let's talk about medication and time zones. If you're traveling across several time zones, your medication schedule could get a bit tricky. But here's a tip: set reminders on your phone based on your home time zone. So, if you usually take a pill at 8 AM in New York and you're now in London, your alarm should ring at 1 PM local time. And remember, it's always a good idea to bring a little extra medication than you think you'll need, just in case of delays or unexpected events.

Long Flights

Long flights can be especially exhausting, so it's important to take steps to stay healthy and safe.

One of the most serious risks associated with long flights is deep vein thrombosis (DVT), which is when a blood clot forms in one of the body's veins. This can cause pain, swelling, and even death if not treated quickly.

To prevent DVT while flying:

- Stay hydrated and avoid alcohol
- Wear comfortable clothing that allows you to move around easily while seated
- During the flight, stand up and stretch your legs every hour or two – this helps get your circulation going again.
- Pumping your legs and moving your feet up and down and back and forth while seated can also help to keep blood moving.
- Consider wearing compression socks or stockings during longer flights to help reduce the risk of DVT.

If you experience any symptoms such as pain, tenderness, or swelling in your legs during or after a long flight, make sure to consult with a doctor immediately. These can be signs of DVT and should not be ignored! In addition to the tips above, seniors should also avoid sitting in one position for too long throughout their trip. Try to shift positions and move around 20 minutes or so. It's also important stay away from caffeine and sugary snacks, which can cause dehydration, headaches, and other issues. If possible you may want to consider bringing a pillow along on your flight – this can help keep your neck in a comfortable position during take-off and landing as well as during naps.

Senior Travel With Mobility Issues

If you have mobility concerns, you don't have to give up traveling. You can opt for taking vacations with little walking (read our suggestions for USA trips) or relax at an all-inclusive resort. Did you know you can even take European tours with limited mobility?

Mobility Aids

If you have mobility concerns when traveling, it might be helpful to bring a wheelchair or walker along during your travels – even if you don't generally use one at home. They can help make navigating public spaces, airports, and other areas much easier. If you plan on bringing a wheelchair or walker with you, make sure to check with your airline in advance to find out their policies and procedures for traveling with such items. Some airlines may require that the mobility aid be folded down and stored as checked luggage, while others may allow it to be brought on board as carry-on luggage.Also, it's worth the time to research any public transportation options that may be available in your destination city

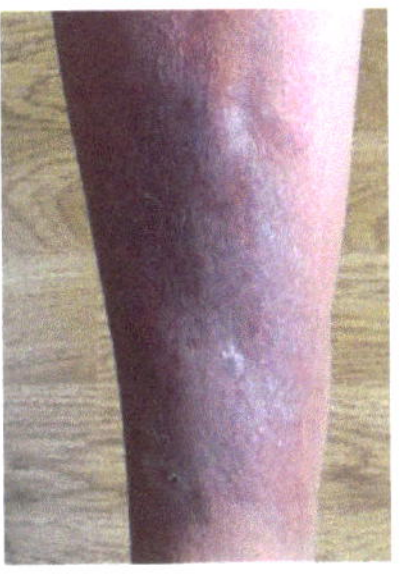

Fig 16.1 Development of deep vein thrombosis during Air travel

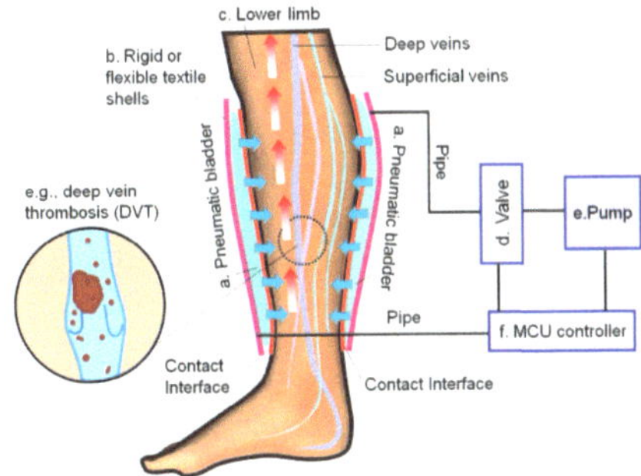

Fig 16.2 Intermittent pneumatic compression in reduction of risk of deep vein thrombosis

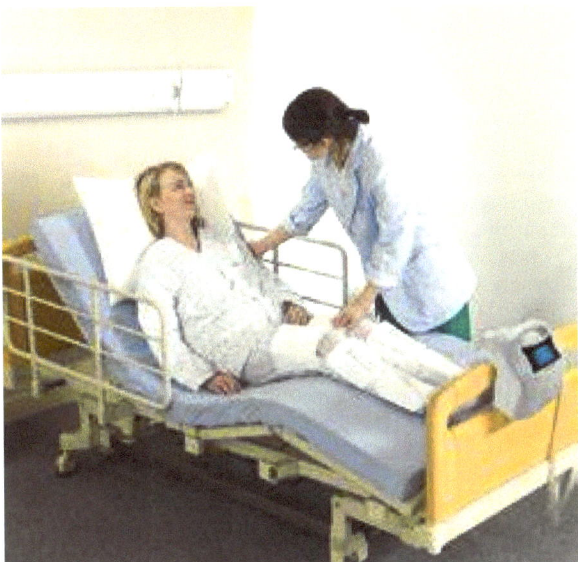

Fig 16.3 Intermittent pneumatic compression DVT

many of these have access ramps and other features designed specifically for those with mobility issues. Finally, if you need assistance getting around during your stay, consider hiring a local service like Uber Assist or Lyft Access – they provide rides from certified drivers who specialize in helping passengers with disabilities.

Tips For Traveling With Limited Mobility

1.When traveling with mobility concerns, look out for uneven surfaces and raised thresholds that can be difficult to navigate.

2.Watch out for narrow pathways and doorways as these can also pose a challenge if you are using a wheelchair or walker.

3.Be aware of any stairs or large bumps in the ground that may require assistance when navigating them.

4.Be sure there is enough space to turn around when using a wheelchair or walker so that you don't get stuck in tight spaces.

5.Ensure your hotel room has adequate accessibility features such as grab bars in the bathroom, ramps up to the entrance if necessary, and wide door openings for easy access with mobility devices.

Hotel Room Safety For Elderly

Seniors should always be mindful of their personal safety when checking into a hotel or motel.

Here are some tips for staying safe in a hotel room:

1. Avoid staying on the ground floor as it makes your room more vulnerable to break-ins.
2. Make sure the door has a deadbolt lock and is properly secured after entering the room.
3. Consider using the hotel's in-room safe (if there is one) to store valuables like credit cards, money, jewelry, phones and other items that you won't be carrying with you in public spaces. And try to minimize how many of these things you carry with you when you're out in public.
4. Always check around the room for potential hazards, such as exposed wires or cords, slippery floors, broken furnishings, and any signs of water damage. If anything doesn't feel right, contact the front desk immediately.
5. Do your research before booking a room – be sure to check reviews and ratings of the hotel/motel you plan on staying at. This will help ensure you are staying at a place in a safe area.
6. When out and about in the city, make sure to stay in well-lit areas with other people around. Avoid walking alone late at night or in any sketchy locations.
7. Be aware of your surroundings when returning to your hotel room and always use the peephole before opening the door.
8. Night lights can help make it easier for seniors with impaired vision to navigate throughout the room at night. Personally, I always bring either a battery powered or plug-in LED night lightalong in my suitcase. Most hotel rooms will have a night light in the bathroom, but bringing your own means you have one if they don't provide one.
9. Keep personal items, such as IDs and passports or wallets and money belts, out of view of the hotel cleaning staff by using the in-room safe if there is one. You might also consider bringing your own portable safe that attaches to the bed frame.

Bibliography and Acknowledgement

- Aalen O., Borgan O., Gjessing H. Survival and Event History Analysis: A Process Point of View. Springer Science & Business Media; New York, NY, USA: 2008.
- Antonovsky A. The salutogenic model as a theory to guide health promotion. Health Promot. Int. 1996;11:11–18. doi: 10.1093/heapro/11.1.11. [CrossRef] [Google Scholar]
- Ashrafi T.A., Myrland Ø. Determinants of trip duration for international tourists in Norway; a parametric survival analysis. Eur. J. Tour. Hosp. Recreat. 2017;8:75–86. doi: 10.1515/ejthr-2017-0008. [CrossRef] [Google Scholar]
- Barros C.P., Butler R., Correia A. The length of stay of golf tourism: A survival analysis. Tour. Manag. 2010;31:13–21. doi: 10.1016/j.tourman.2009.02.010. [CrossRef]
- Barros C.P., Correia A., Crouch G. Determinants of the length of stay in Latin American tourism destinations. Tour. Anal. 2008;13:329–340. [Google Scholar]
- Canham S.L., Fang M.L., Battersby L., Woolrych R., Sixsmith J., Ren T.H., Sixsmith A. Contextual Factors for Aging Well: Creating Socially Engaging Spaces through the Use of Deliberative Dialogues. Gerontologist. 2018;58:140–148. doi: 10.1093/geront/gnx121. [PubMed] [CrossRef] [Google Scholar]
- Chen N., Qaio G., Zhang Y. Research on the relationship between tourism barriers and tourism participation intention of disabled people based on helplessness theory—Application of structural equation model. Tour. Trib. 2009;24:47–52. [Google Scholar]
- Chen S.C., Shoemaker S. Age and cohort effects: The American senior tourism market. Ann. Tour. Res. 2014;48:58–75. doi: 10.1016/j.annals.2014.05.007.
- Cleves M., Gould W., Gutierrez R.G., Marchenko Y.V. An Introduction to Survival Analysis Using Stata. Stata Press; Lakeway Drive College Station, TX, USA: 2010.
- Du M., Tao L., Liu M., Liu J. Tourism experiences and the lower risk of mortality in the Chinese elderly: A national cohort study. BMC Public Health. 2021;21:996. doi: 10.1186/s12889-021-11099-8. [PMC free article] [PubMed] [CrossRef]
- Escuder M.P. Modelling the impact of lifelong learning on senior citizens' quality of life. Soc. Behav. Sci. 2012;46:2339–2346. doi: 10.1016/j.sbspro.2012.05.481.
- Fernández-Ballesteros R., Sánchez-Izquierdo M. Health, Psycho-Social Factors, and Ageism in Older Adults in Spain during the COVID-19 Pandemic. Healthcare. 2021;9:256. doi: 10.3390/healthcare9030256. [PMC free article] [PubMed]
- Fleischer A., Pizam A. Tourism constraints among Israeli seniors. Ann. Tour. Res. 2002;29:106–123. doi: 10.1016/S0160-7383(01)00026-3. [CrossRef] [Google Scholar]
- Foster L., Walker A. Gender and active ageing in Europe. Eur. J. Ageing. 2013;10:3–10. doi: 10.1007/s10433-013-0261-0. [PMC free article] [PubMed] [CrossRef] [Google Scholar]
- Hsu C.H.C., Cai L.A., Wong K.K.F. A model of senior tourism motivations—Anecdotes from Beijing and Shanghai. Tour. Manag. 2007;28:1262–1273. doi: 10.1016/j.tourman.2006.09.015. [CrossRef] [Google Scholar]
- Huber D., Milne S., Hyde K.F. Constraints and facilitators for senior tourism. Tour. Manag. Perspect. 2018;27:55–67. doi: 10.1016/j.tmp.2018.04.003. [CrossRef] [Google Scholar]
- Hunter-Jones P., Blackburn A. Understanding the relationship between holiday taking and self-assessed health: An exploratory study of senior tourism. Int. J. Consum. Stud. 2010;31:509–516. doi: 10.1111/j.1470-6431.2007.00607.x. [CrossRef] [Google Scholar]
- Jang S., Bai B., Hu C., Wu C.M.E. Affect, travel motivation, and travel intention: A senior market. J. Hosp. Tour. Res. 2009;33:51–73. doi: 10.1177/1096348008329666.
- Kim H., Woo E., Uysal M. Tourism experience and quality of life among elderly tourists. Tour. Manag. 2015;46:465–476. doi: 10.1016/j.tourman.2014.08.002.
- Lee S.H., Tideswell C. Understanding attitudes towards leisure travel and the constraints faced by senior Koreans. J. Vacat. Mark. 2005;11:249–263.
- Nimrod G. Retirement and tourism Themes in retirees' narratives. Ann. Tour. Res. 2008;35:859–878. doi: 10.1016/j.annals.2008.06.001. [CrossRef] [Google Scholar]
- Peterson M., Lambert S.L. A demographic perspective on U.S. consumers' out-of-town vacationing and commercial lodging usage while on vacation. J. Travel Res. 2003;42:116–124. doi: 10.1177/0047287503254957.
- Qiao G., Li F., Xiao X., Prideaux B. What does tourism mean for Chinese rural migrant workers? Perspectives of perceived value. Int. J. Tour. Res. 2021 doi: 10.1002/jtr.2496. [CrossRef] [Google Scholar]
- Ryu E., Hyun S.S., Shim C. Creating New Relationships Through Tourism: A Qualitative Analysis of Tourist Motivations of Older Individuals in Japan. J. Travel Tour. Mark.2015;32:325–338.
- Sie L., Patterson I., Pegg S. Towards an understanding of older adult educational tourism through the development of a three-phase integrated framework. Curr. Issues Tour. 2015;19:1–37. doi: 10.1080/13683500.2015.1021303. [CrossRef] [Google Scholar]
- Tung V.W.S., Ritchie J.R.B. Investigating the memorable experiences of the senior travel market: An examination of the reminiscence bump. J. Travel Tour. Mark. 2011;28:331–343. doi: 10.1080/10548408.2011.563168. [CrossRef] [Google Scholar]
- World Health Organization Ageing: Healthy Ageing and Functional Ability. [(accessed on 30 September 2015)]. Available online: https://www.who.int/zh/news/item/30-09-2015-who-number-of-people-over-60-years-set-to-double-by-2050-major-societal-changes-required
- Xu C., Liu D., Mei X. Exploring an Efficient POI Recommendation Model Based on User Characteristics and Spatial-Temporal Factors. Mathematics. 2021;9:2673. doi: 10.3390/math9212673. [CrossRef] [Google Scholar]
- Yoon H., Huber L., Kim C. Sustainable aging and leisure behaviors: Do leisure activities matter in aging well? Sustainability. 2021;13:2348. doi: 10.3390/su13042348.
- Zeng Y., Poston D.L., Jr., Vlosky D.A., Gu D. Healthy Longevity in China: Demographic, Socioeconomic, and Psychological Dimensions. Springer; Dordrecht, The Netherlands: 2008. [Google Scholar]
- Zhang Q., Zhang H., Xu H. Health tourism destinations as therapeutic landscapes: Understanding the health perceptions of senior seasonal migrants. Soc. Sci. Med. 2021;279:113951. doi: 10.1016/j.socscimed.2021.113951. [PubMed] [CrossRef] [Google Scholar]

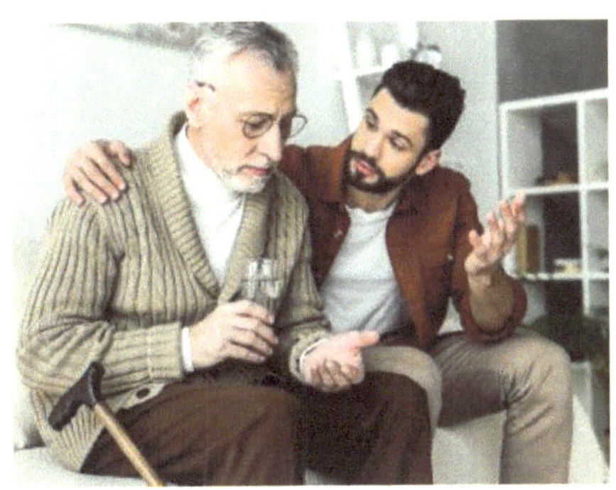

Grown Children Who Ignore Their Parents And Seniors

Grown children who ignore their parents can provoke a great deal of emotional distress and even physical health problems in elder loved ones. And adult children whose older or elderly parents don't communicate with them can undergo similar feelings of loss and bewilderment. Although some seniors struggle with feeling abandoned, others face the opposite problem—realizing that cutting off contact with a family member is the best course of action to protect their own well-being.

These topics can be hard to talk about. Whether you're feeling ignored or dealing with family estrangement, the emotions can take a toll. And many people feel too ashamed to seek help. If you're experiencing an estranged relationship with a parent or child, the following information can help you explore why there is a division, and how to handle it.

When You Feel Ignored

Many seniors experience feelings of chronic loneliness. And one common complaint among lonely seniors is that their adult children ignore them. Of course, everyone has different criteria for what being ignored actually means. Consider the results of a study that asked Americans how often grown children should call their parents. Almost one quarter of those surveyed said that grown children should call their parents at least once a day, while 12 percent thought once a month or less was adequateSimply put, your perception may not match the reality of your loved one's feelings and intentions. So if you feel like you want more contact with certain family members, talk to them about it. They likely won't know that you want to talk or visit more often unless you tell them.

After all, in today's busy world, it's easy for people to get caught up in their own lives and as a result, spend less time with other friends and family. That fact can be hard to accept for a parent especially. In fact, psychologists say that the parent-child relationship is typically more important to the parent —and that's a perfectly normal part of human psychological development. But it also means that absence is often felt more strongly by the parents than by the adult children.So, you might have to be proactive when it comes to having more contact with your children. Some families find that it helps to have a set schedule for calls or visits. That way, staying in touch becomes part of everyone's routine. So if your child is not always there when you call, ask about a good time to call and try to stick to that time.Of course, adult children should also listen carefully to parents who express concerns about feeling ignored. After all, loneliness can lead to many physical and mental health problems in seniors. Taking some time to reach out to older parents can help your family avoid more serious issues later on.

Family Estrangement

Family estrangement goes well beyond one person feeling ignored. When a family member is estranged, those bad feelings are magnified, often to a degree that can seem almost unbearable.

What does "estranged" mean? Here's a short explanation: You are estranged from a family member when one person in the relationship feels that something about the other person justifies cutting off all contact. In other words, you don't communicate with each other, and any communication that does happen is tense, without any trust or intimacy.

Estrangement is usually a conscious decision. If you're simply too busy to keep in touch, that's not necessarily estrangement. A person initiating an estrangement could contact the other person but chooses not to.

A study in the Journal of Marriage and Family used the **following criteria to determine if a mother was estranged from an adult child:**

- The pair hadn't had any contact (in person or by phone) for at least a year;
- Or the pair was in contact less than once a month, and the mother rated the quality of the relationship as less than a four on a scale of one to seven.

Additionally, many people feel that family bonds are becoming more fragile than they used to be. Check out these facts:

- A Journal of Psychology and Behavioral Science study found that more than 40 percent of surveyed college students (ranging in age from 18 to 56) had experienced some kind of family estrangement during their lives.
- Around 10 percent of participating mothers were estranged from at least one of their children at the time of the Journal of Marriage and Family study.

Why Do Family Members Become Estranged From Each Other?

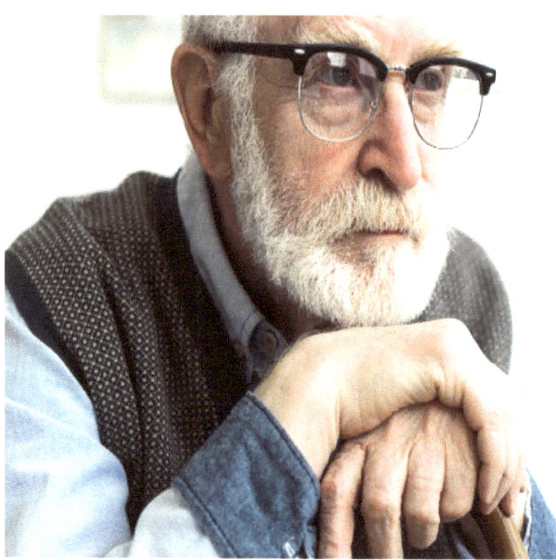

Fig.17.1 Showing a old man feeling depressed after becoming estranged from the family on differences of opinion.

Why do children abandon their parents? And why do parents stop talking to their grown children? Ask a dozen families these questions and you'll likely get a dozen different answers. After all, each family is unique, and relationships can break down in countless different ways. But you may be surprised to learn that many people don't know why a family member has stopped talking to them. They have no idea what has caused the child or parental estrangement. So it can be particularly heartbreaking for anyone who has felt secure in a family relationship to suddenly have to ask, "Why does my family hate me?"

But here's an interesting fact: In a University of Cambridge survey, a significant percentage of estranged parents and children weren't even sure who had initiated the estrangement. In other words, the path to an estranged relationship isn't always clear.The same survey found that emotional abuse is the most common reason given by people who are estranged from their parents. The other reasons named were:

- Conflicting expectations regarding family roles
- Differences in values
- Neglect
- Problems related to mental health issues
- A traumatic family event

Parents who said they had estranged relationships with their children named divorce as the top reason. (For example, a child may not have approved of a parent's decision to get divorced.) Other reasons include:

- Mismatched expectations about family roles
- Traumatic events
- Mental health issues
- Emotional abuse
- Issues related to in-laws
- Issues related to marriage

Many other factors can lead to estrangement within families, including:

- Political disagreements
- Disapproval of sexuality or religion
- Judgments about career and relationship
- Substance abuse
- Financial stress

As well, many people blame general societal changes for the increase in the number of families experiencing estrangement. In a lot of cases, we simply don't need to rely on family members the way we used to. That's partly because, in general, we're a lot more mobile than we once were. (For example, it's a lot easier to ignore a family member who lives across the country than to ignore a relative who works and lives on the same farm.)

In addition, some seniors feel that recent years have seen an increase in entitled adult children who stop talking to their parents for selfish reasons. But many adult children disagree with this sentiment and present a counterargument: Older parents don't recognize that their adult children have their own busy lives and that life has changed since those parents were their children's age.

When Grown Children Stop Talking to Their Parents

If you've devoted years to raising a family, feeling like you have ungrateful adult children who won't talk to you can seem strikingly unfair.

Consequences

Family tensions can take a toll on older or elderly parents. Consider these facts on the impact of estrangement:

- Almost one-third of parents who are estranged from their offspring have considered suicide.
- According to the University of Cambridge survey noted earlier, 90 percent of people with estranged family members find the holidays difficult.
- The same survey found that 68 percent of people with estranged family members feel judged by others.

According to a study in the Journal of the American Geriatrics Society, social contact with family members helps seniors who are over 70 years old avoid depression. (Prior to the age of 70, social contact with friends may help prevent depression, but family ties become more important with age.)

Many people who've experienced estrangement say that the feelings are similar to experiencing a death in the family. After all, you're mourning what feels like the end of a relationship. But the stress of estrangement often lacks resolution because the relationship remains uncertain. That can make the healing process difficult. (Grief counselors call this type of loss an "ambiguous loss.")

And one complicating factor for abandoned parents is that many seniors rely on family members for at least some elements of their caregiving. When family relationships break down, seniors can experience difficulties in arranging the care they need.

Coping with estrangement

Parents whose children stop talking to them are often left wondering what they did wrong, or if their children hate them. Most people truly just want a normal parent/adult-child relationship. However, one of the biggest steps you can take toward a more functional relationship is to accept that you can't control the situation.

So, what can you do? In simple terms, you deal with rejection from a child by keeping the lines of communication open and respecting his or her autonomy.

Here are some additional tips that might apply to your situation.

1. Don't push too much.

You should respect your estranged child's boundaries, even if you may not think that those boundaries are very fair. Don't keep reaching out if he or she has told you not to. (Being repeatedly rejected can be harmful to your own mental well-being.)

2. Try not to be defensive.

Wanting to defend yourself a perfectly normal reaction. However, if your child tells you why they no longer want to be in contact, don't deny how they are feeling—listen carefully.

3. Apologize when needed.

Saying you're sorry isn't necessarily an admission of guilt. Rather, it can be the first step toward reconciliation. Sometimes, it helps just to acknowledge that your child is hurting and that you're sorry if you played a role in that pain—even if you never intended to hurt anyone.

Also, remind yourself that societal expectations around parenting have changed. Your child may view the world through a different lens than you did when you were raising them.

4. Ease back on any guilt trips.

Guilt can make adult children less likely to want to engage with their parents.

5. Look after yourself.

You're a valuable person in your own right, and in your senior years it's important to have a fulfilling life that doesn't center around your children. So try to develop interests of your own.

Talk to your healthcare provider about what you're going through and be alert to symptoms of mental health issues, such as trouble sleeping or unexplained fatigue.

6. Watch your judgment.

Unless you're specifically asked, there is no need to comment on things like your child's sexual orientation, appearance, parenting, finances, or any of the countless other areas which your child is now responsible for.

Parents who don't respect boundaries can add more stress to their adult children's day-to-day experiences.

7. Don't try to buy your child's attention.

About two-thirds of Americans over the age of 50 provide at least some financial support to a child who is older than 21. But this type of financial support should not be connected to the amount of contact that your children have with you.

8. Stay positive and seek help when needed.

Admittedly, this can be difficult. But the stress of family estrangement can affect your physical health. Talking to a counselor or to your doctor can help relieve any negative feelings. Seeking professional support can also help you gain a new perspective on the relationship, which might make reconciliation more likely.

When Parents Ignore Their Grown Children

We're often raised to think that it's our parents' job to look after us, even as we grow older. So parents walking away from adult children can feel like a a violation of the natural order of things.

Parents who ignore their child or choose not to make contact can provoke a lot of difficult feelings. If you're an adult child in this type of situation, your emotions may be all over place. Estranged children can feel:

- Hurt
- Isolated
- Guilty
- Insecure
- Sad
- Worried
- Angry
- Anxious
- Forgotten

Here are some tips that can help.

1. Don't be ashamed.

Remember, family estrangement is surprisingly common. It doesn't mean that you're not worth loving or that you're not capable of having loving relationships. So try not to take it personally. Your parents may have experienced trauma in their own lives that affects the way they treat you.

2. Talk to others.

If a parent suddenly stops communicating with you without giving an explanation, consider talking to other people, such as relatives or caregivers, to determine a reason. (For example, it's possible that your parent is experiencing early signs of dementia.)

3. Get support.

Even when you're an adult, strained relationships with your parents can hurt. So don't hesitate to seek counseling if you feel overwhelmed. Also, tell other people close to you how you feel. (Up to 73 percent of married people experiencing estrangement find that talking to a spouse is helpful, according to the University of Cambridge survey referenced earlier.)

Deciding to Cut Off Contact With a Family Member

As an adult, particularly as a senior, you have earned the right to control your own relationships. Sometimes that means taking steps toward protecting your own physical and mental health by cutting off contact with family members who harm your well-being.People choose to stop talking to family members for many different reasons, including:

- Substance abuse
- Physical abuse or threats

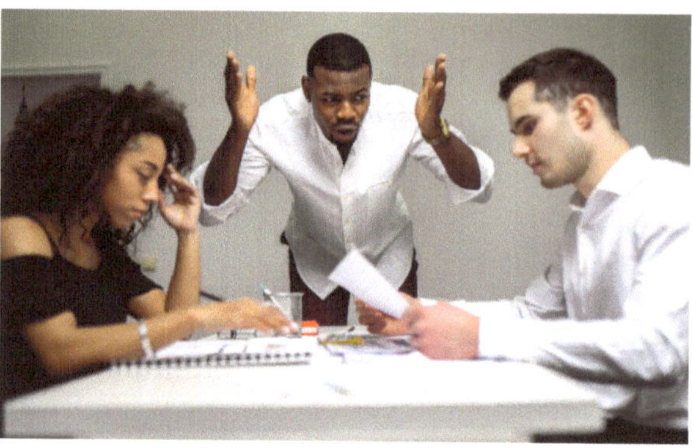

Fig.17.2 Imagine noticing an unsettling silence at family gatherings where laughter and conversation once flourished

- Feeling unsafe
- Being used financially
- Mental health conditions
- Wanting to avoid unnecessary drama that some people create

Even so, this is usually not an easy decision. After all, we're supposed to love our family members unconditionally. But choosing not to have contact with someone doesn't necessarily mean that you don't love that person. Sometimes, it's the best course of action for everyone involved. (In fact, the University of Cambridge study found that 80 percent of people who are estranged from at least one family member said it had some positive aspects.)

Making the decision to cut off contact is best done with the help of a mental health professional. Also, keep in mind that it doesn't have to be a sudden or dramatic split. If you're not sure whether you want a family member in your life, it's OK to just cut back on the amount of contact you have. Here's the most important word when it comes to learning how to deal with a disrespectful grown child or disrespectful parents: Boundaries. It means not putting up with being treated poorly or without consideration. Feeling as if you don't love your child anymore is also a signal that it's time to talk with a counselor. And always remember this: If someone is hurting you physically or emotionally, you should not be alone with them.And if you're an older parent, disowning a child is sometimes the best decision if your own health or financial welfare is being harmed.How can you disown a father, mother, son, or daughter? Here are some actions that might work for you:

- Tell the person in writing (such as through a letter sent by certified mail) that you wish to sever your connection and will no longer accept any contact with them.

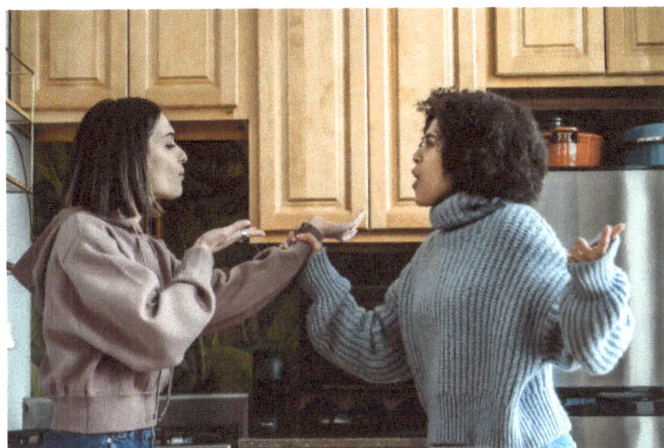

Fig.17.3 A significant factor in why you might find children ignoring their parents is a breakdown in communication.

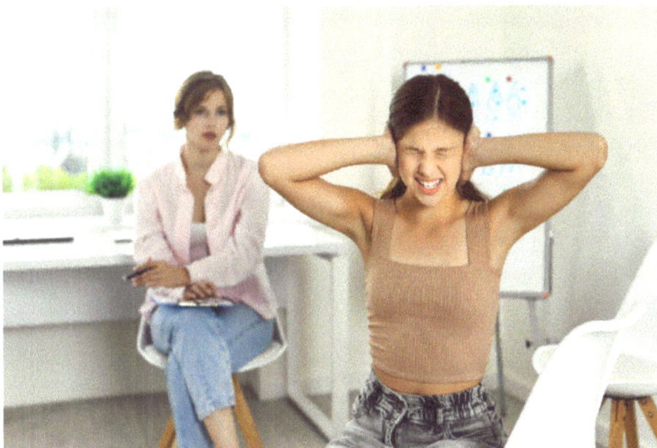

Fig.17.4 Signs of Disconnection When your child starts to drift away, it might not be immediately noticeable. However, certain behaviors can signal a growing disconnection between you and your child.

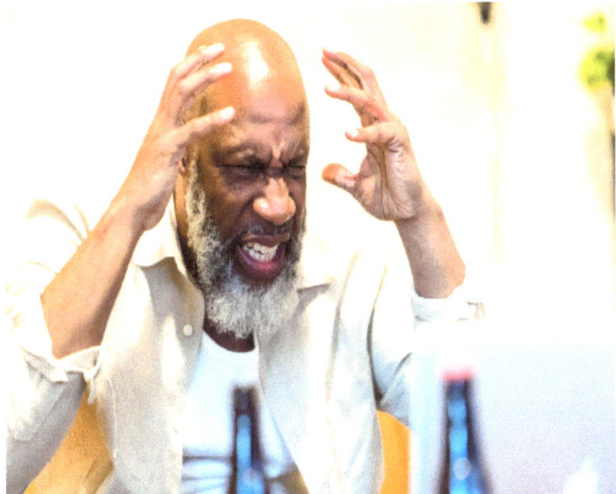

Fig.17.5 Consequences of Parent- Child Estrangement The estrangement between you and your children can lead to profound emotional repercussions and alter family dynamics significantly.

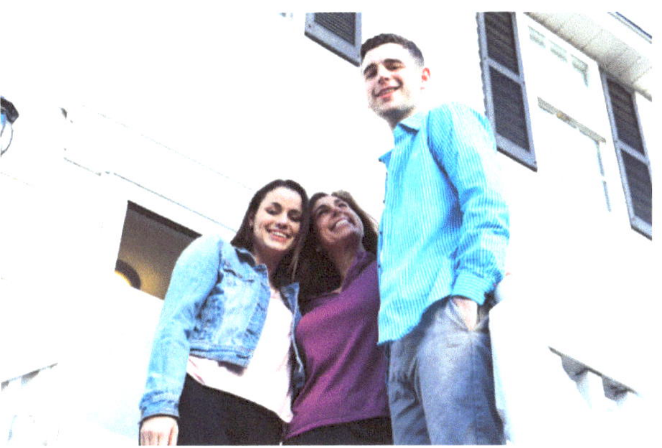

Fig.17.6 Adopting Adult-to-Adult Relationships.Redefining your relationship involves transitioning from a parent-child dynamic to an adult-to-adult one. This shift entails respecting boundaries and engaging in conversations that recognize your grown child's autonomy.

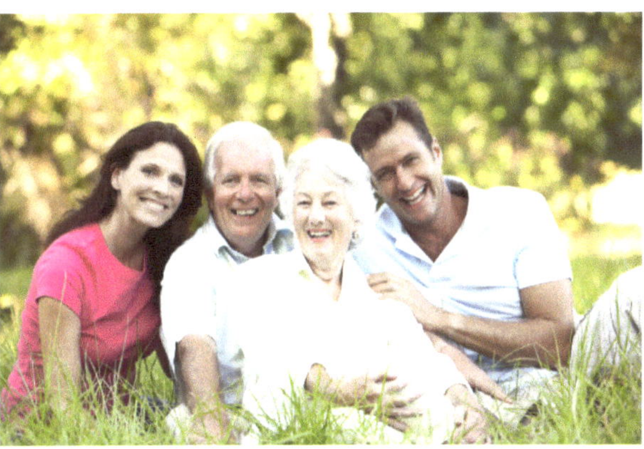

Fig.17.7 Strategies to Reconnect .When your grown children have become distant, the pathway to a restored relationship often starts with careful and considered approaches to re-establishing communication and setting healthy boundaries.

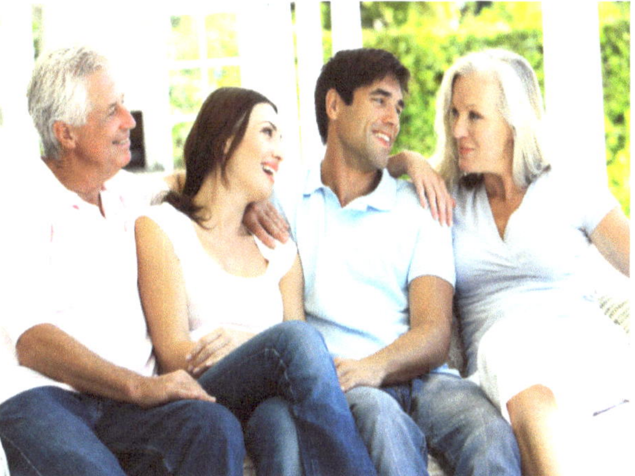

Fig.17.8 Moving ForwardIn the journey to move forward when your grown children refuse communication, it's crucial to focus on personal healing and reshaping your life toward fulfillment.

• Stop contact by refusing to accept calls, mail, or emails from the person.
• Obtain a restraining order or peace bond if you are being harassed or stalked or experiencing abuse.
• Change your will to ensure that the person doesn't receive any inheritance from you. (If you have young children and want to disown your older parents, ensure that your will makes it clear that someone else will be your children's guardian if you die.)• Block the person on all social media.
• Stay active socially. Holidays, in particular, can be difficult when you're estranged from a family member, even if you're the one who initiated it. Creating a "family of choice" composed of friends and other relatives can give you opportunities to feel the close connections you need.
• Be open and honest with other family members. It's common to want to cut ties with one family member while staying in contact with others. But that can sometimes feel awkward for the rest of the family, so keep the lines of communication open.

Helpful Resources

You don't have to experience family relationship problems alone. Plenty of assistance is available.
If you're over 60 and need someone to talk to right away, the Institute on Aging offers a Friendship Line for seniors in crisis.
Family estrangement support groups exist online and in-person. However, keep in mind that feelings about family breakdowns can be very intense, so consider observing a group for a while before sharing your own experiences. As well, here are some books that have helped others:

1. Done With the Crying: Help and Healing for Mothers of Estranged Adult Children by Sheri McGregor
2. Healing from Family Rifts: Ten Steps to Finding Peace After Being Cut Off from a Family Member by Mark Sichel
3. When Parents Hurt: Compassionate Strategies When You and Your Grown Child Don't Get Along by Joshua Coleman
4. But It's Your Family...: Cutting Ties with Toxic Family Members and Loving Yourself in the Aftermath by Dr. Sherrie Campbell
5. When Our Grown Kids Disappoint Us: Letting Go of Their Problems, Loving Them Anyway, and Getting on with Our Lives by Jane Adams

Bibliography and Acknowledgement

- Anetzberger, Georgia J. The Etiology of Elder Abuse by Adult Offspring. Springfield, IL: Charles C. Thomas Publishing, 1987.
- Austin MA, Riniolo TC, Porges SW. Borderline personality disorder and emotion regulation: Insights from the Polyvagal Theory. Brain and Cognition. Published online October 2007:69-76. doi:10.1016/j.bandc.2006.05.007
- Brandl, Bonnie, and Loree Cook-Daniels. Domestic Abuse in Later Life: Who Are the Abusers? Washington DC: National Center on Elder Abuse, 2003.
- Bunford N, Evans SW, Langberg JM. Emotion Dysregulation Is Associated With Social Impairment Among Young Adolescents With ADHD. J Atten Disord. Published online March 29, 2014:66-82. doi:10.1177/1087054714527793
- Burns EE, Jackson JL, Harding HG. Child Maltreatment, Emotion Regulation, and Posttraumatic Stress: The Impact of Emotional Abuse. Journal of Aggression, Maltreatment & Trauma. Published online November 18, 2010:801-819. doi:10.1080/10926771.2010.522947
- Fingerman, Karen. "Millennials and Their Parents: Implications of the New Young Adulthood for Midlife Adults." Innovation in Aging. 2017, vol. 1(3), 1-16.
- Fletcher K, Parker G, Bayes A, Paterson A, McClure G. Emotion regulation strategies in bipolar II disorder and borderline personality disorder: Differences and relationships with perceived parental style. Journal of Affective Disorders. Published online March 2014:52-59. doi:10.1016/j.jad.2014.01.001
- Gibson LC. Adult Children of Emotionally Immature Parents: How to Heal from Distant, Rejecting, or Self-Involved Parents. New Harbinger Publications; 2015.
- Gottman, John. Why Marriages Succeed or Fail. New York: Fireside Books, 1994.
- Joormann J, Stanton CH. Examining emotion regulation in depression: A review and future directions. Behaviour Research and Therapy. Published online November 2016:35-49. doi:10.1016/j.brat.2016.07.007
- Kober H. Emotion regulation in substance use disorders. In: Handbook of Emotion Regulation. The Guilford Press; 2014:428–446.
- Li D, Li D, Wu N, Wang Z. Intergenerational transmission of emotion regulation through parents' reactions to children's negative emotions: Tests of unique, actor, partner, and mediating effects. Children and Youth Services Review. Published online June 2019:113-122.
- Marcell, Jacqueline. Elder Rage, or Take My Father . . . Please: How to Survive Caring for Aging Parents. Irvine, CA: Impressive Press, 2001.
- Payne, Brian K. Crime and Elder Abuse: An Integrated Perspective. Springfield, IL: Charles C. Thomas Publishing, 2000.
- Quinn, Mary Joy, and Susan K. Tomita. Elder Abuse and Neglect: Causes, Diagnosis, and Intervention Strategies. New York: Springer Publishing Company, 1986.
- Rancew-Sikora D, et al. (2022). Adult children move out: Family meals and reflections on parental self-sacrifice at the moment of transition.https://journals.sagepub.com/doi/abs/10.1177/13607804211065050

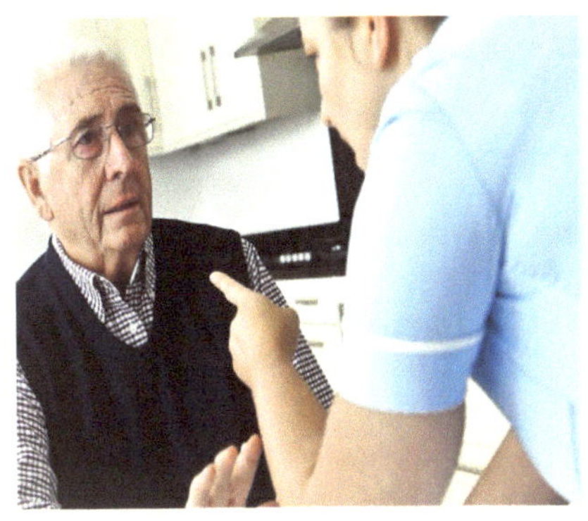

Elder Abuse: Types, Warning Signs, and How to Report It

Have any types of elder abuse ever affected you or anyone you know? Have you ever suspected that you or a vulnerable senior in your life might be suffering from neglect or mistreatment? Do you feel conflicted, afraid, embarrassed, or unsure of what to do about it? Each day, millions of older people in America and around the world are negatively impacted by elder abuse. It's an ugly problem that needs to be better understood and taken more seriously by everyone, in every community. Nobody deserves to be neglected, exploited, or abused.

Unfortunately, the warning signs of abuse are often missed, ignored, or rationalized away—even by well-meaning people. In fact, it's likely that most cases of elder mistreatment go unreported, which means that Adult Protective Services, law enforcement agencies, and other relevant authorities often don't get the chance to intervene on behalf of seniors who need help. As a result, countless older adults experience a poorer quality of life and worse health outcomes than they otherwise would. (For victims of elder abuse, the risk of premature death is estimated to be three times higher than for seniors who haven't been abused, according to the U.S. Department of Justice.)

By learning more about this subject, you can better protect yourself or those you care about. Plus, our communities need more advocates for the elderly. People like you can be lights who shine hope in the darkness and help create positive change. This article will teach you what constitutes abuse and neglect, who and what to pay attention to, how to report elder abuse, and how to potentially prevent it from happening.

What Is Elder Abuse? How Prevalent Is It?

Currently, there isn't one universally accepted definition of elder abuse. Legal definitions vary from state to state, and different researchers, government agencies, and non-profit organizations often have their own sets of criteria for defining elderly abuse. However, many basic definitions are similar to this one:

Elder abuse is any action or inaction that harms, endangers, or causes distress to a person over the age of 60 or 65 and is done intentionally by someone who is known to the victim and in a position of trust.

Crimes like burglary, street robbery, and assault by strangers are generally not considered elder abuse. But physical assault by a family member, neighbor, or caregiver definitely is considered elder abuse if it happens to a senior. Neglect is also frequently considered a form of elder abuse, as is sexual assault, psychological mistreatment, and financial exploitation when there is an expectation of trust between the victim and perpetrator.

How many seniors experience elder abuse? Nobody really knows. Estimates vary substantially since certain actions may be considered elder abuse according to some definitions but not according to others. Plus, the defined age for elder abuse victims varies: Some agencies and researchers say that anyone 55 or older can experience elder abuse, whereas others peg the age at 60, 65, or 70 and older. In addition, it's believed that for every case of elder abuse that gets reported, several more are never brought to light.

Even so, an article in The Lancet Global Health estimates that about 1 in every 10 older Americans experience elder abuse. Worldwide, the rate is estimated to be about 1 in every 6 older people. Among seniors who are ill or disabled, the rate is even higher. For example, the National Center on Elder Abuse (NCEA) says that depending on the particular study, between 27.5 percent and 55 percent of seniors who have dementia are estimated to suffer from elder neglect or abuse.

The consequences of elder abuse can be costly and far-reaching. In America alone, elder abuse causes so many injuries that it may be directly responsible for more than $5 billion in medical costs each year.

How Many Types of Elder Abuse Are There?

Elder abuse can take several different forms, and some seniors experience multiple kinds of abuse at the same time. Here are 7 types of elder abuse that are among the most commonly reported:

1.Financial exploitation: Also known as financial abuse, this type of mistreatment can involve scams, fraud, coercion, theft, or improper use of a senior's money, property, or other valuable resources. It affects about 1 in 18 cognitively healthy, non-institutionalized seniors every year. However, the prevalence rate among all seniors may be much higher than that. Essentially, financial exploitation of an elderly person is any intentional act in which a perpetrator improperly reaps financial benefits at the expense of a victim's livelihood or well-being. Perpetrators often get their victims to trust them by using deception or providing offers of help that are based on false pretenses. They also may use scare tactics or make wildly overstated claims in order to get seniors to give them money or hand over control of their assets. Many scams involve telemarketing, but most financial abuse is carried out by people that seniors already know and trust, such as family members and service professionals.

2.Neglect: This type of abuse happens when a vulnerable senior is deprived of essential necessities like food, water, medical treatment, proper clothing, or a safe, clean, and comfortable living environment. Neglect in the elderly is often intentional, perpetrated as a way to exert power, push a senior toward an earlier death, or coerce a senior into signing away his or her financial assets. But neglect can also happen unintentionally as a result of caregiving failures caused by factors like improper training, a lack of resources, or mental or physical problems that impact a caregiver's ability to do his or her job.

3.Emotional abuse: Also known as psychological abuse, this kind of mistreatment harms a senior's mental health. Perpetrators may ridicule, humiliate, blame, yell at, or threaten their victims. Or they may employ more passive-aggressive tactics like shunning their victims, holding back affection, or remaining silent and disinterested in the face of pleas for help or attempts at reconciliation. Emotional abuse is sometimes used as a way to bully and pressure a senior into doing something that is against his or her wishes or best interests.

4.Physical abuse: Willful infliction of bodily pain or injury can happen to almost any senior, especially a vulnerable elder. Physical abuse can take many forms: Pushing, slapping, punching, choking, kicking, pulling hair, and burning are just a few examples. It can also take the form of a perpetrator inappropriately restraining or imprisoning a victim. And some perpetrators of physical abuse give their victims incorrect or improper doses of medications, which can lead to harmful (and sometimes fatal) side effects.

5.Sexual abuse: Some seniors are raped, molested, or forced to participate in activities of a sexual nature without their consent. Even a conversation about sex can be considered abusive if a senior is uncomfortable or unwilling to engage in the discussion and can't get out of the situation. Sexual abuse also happens to seniors who aren't capable of giving consent, such as those who have dementia or other conditions that make them mentally or physically incapacitated.

6.Abandonment: Many people consider abandonment to be a form of neglect. Indeed, it could probably be classified as extreme elderly neglect. It goes beyond family estrangement. Perpetrators will intentionally desert vulnerable seniors who depend on their care, leaving them with little or no assistance—often for long stretches of time. Abandonment can greatly erode a senior's health and well-being; it can even lead to premature death. Some perpetrators have taken their victims to entirely different states and abandoned them in completely unfamiliar places where they have no support.

7.Rights abuse: Some seniors are denied their basic legal rights. For example, in an institution like a nursing home, abuse of this nature can involve ignoring a vulnerable senior's requests for information or blocking his or her attempts at making official complaints. It can also involve denying proper health care, social activities, privacy, or access to one's money or possessions.

Self-neglect is also a form of elder mistreatment. However, in the case of self-neglect, there is no outside perpetrator; affected seniors cause harm to themselves. They may ignore their own basic needs or even refuse essential care, which can lead to new or worsening illnesses or injuries. In some cases, self-neglect is ultimately fatal. But it isn't always caused by mental or physical decline. Many seniors are poor or socially isolated, don't have the resources to meet all of their basic needs, and don't know where to find help, which means they have to make tough choices. For instance, they may go without heat in order to pay for food and medication. Or they may deny themselves essential medications in order to stay warm.Some people also categorize healthcare fraud as a type of elder abuse or financial exploitation. Like other types of mistreatment, healthcare fraud can take many forms. For example, dishonest medical professionals may take advantage of elderly patients by providing insufficient care yet billing Medicare or Medicaid as if those patients were given full and proper care. Or unscrupulous pharmacists may under-fill prescriptions while charging full price for them.

What Are the Signs of Elder Abuse or Neglect?

Sometimes it's obvious that elder abuse is taking place. However, in many cases, it isn't so easy to recognize abuse or neglect by others. Signs and symptoms can often mirror or get obscured by existing medical conditions, or they can be hidden by the efforts of devious perpetrators.

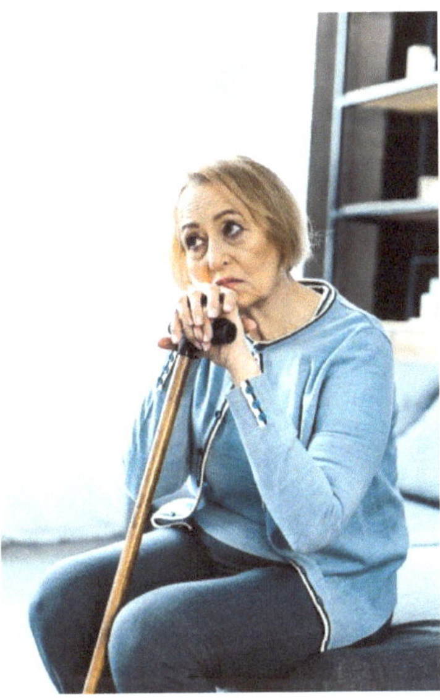

Fig.18.1 Elderly women feeling depressed and lonely after being neglected by family members

But it's important to follow your intuition, take clues seriously, and make note of any troubling patterns you observe. Generally speaking, the signs of abuse or neglect in the elderly are associated with particular types of mistreatment. For example, consider the following warning signs.

When it comes to financial exploitation of the elderly, you may observe signs such as:

•Unusual spending habits, especially for unnecessary products or services
•Confusing bank transactions, including unexplainable transfers or withdrawals
•Missing bank statements or other financial documents
•A large amount of unopened mail or sweepstakes offers
•Unpaid bills or warning letters from creditors or utility companies
•A new "friend" who offers to provide low- or no-cost care
•Missing property or personal possessions
•Suspicious legal documents related to asset control or powers of attorney
•Signatures on documents that look like they were forged or made under duress
•Confusion about recent financial arrangements
•A reduced level of care despite the ability to pay for better service

Signs of neglect in adults over the age of 60 can include things like:

•Rapid or unexpected weight loss
•A sudden decrease in appetite
•Dehydration
•Unexpected breathing problems
•Dirty or inappropriate clothing
•Lack of personal hygiene
•Frequent skin rashes
•Untreated injuries or infections
•Bedsores
•Expired prescriptions
•Faster-than-expected health decline
•Lack of assistive devices
•Missing or broken eyeglasses, dentures, or hearing aids
•Filthy or unsafe living conditions
•Pest infestations
•Lack of attention to needed repairs
•Uncharacteristic confusion, despair, social withdrawal, or sleeping problems

Emotional abuse can be one of the most challenging types of mistreatment to detect. However, it often occurs alongside other forms of abuse that are easier to spot. Signs of emotional neglect in adults aged 60 or above may include:

•Heightened fear or agitation when around a particular person
•Greater-than-expected weight gain or loss
•New or worsening depression or social anxiety
•Significant personality changes
•Uncharacteristic disorientation or confusion
•Strange behaviors like rocking back and forth, sucking a thumb, or biting oneself
•Blood pressure that's consistently higher than what would be expected
•New or worsening sleep problems

When it comes to physical abuse, the signs can sometimes be mistaken for the results of accidents or unintentional injuries. That's why it's important to look for patterns, unusual behaviors, or injuries that are unlikely to be the result of accidents. You may see signs like:
•Bruises or abrasions that wrap around the person's wrists, arms, ankles, legs, or torso
•Bruises that are in the same places on both sides of the body
•Bruises that are multicolored
•Cigarette burns
•Other unexplainable burns, bruises, abrasions, or scars
•Frequent sprains or bone fractures
•Unusual bleeding
•Broken dentures or eyeglasses
•Unexpected tooth loss
•Strange hair loss in just one small part of the head
•Frequent hospitalizations for the same types of injury
•Injuries that haven't been treated right away
•Changing stories or excuses that don't make sense
•Suspicious patterns of medical treatment (such as getting treated at a variety of different facilities for no clear or credible reason)

Sexual abuse in adults is a type of mistreatment that can remain hidden for a long time, often because of embarrassment, fear of further humiliation, or memory problems caused by dementia. Plus, the most tell-tale signs are usually out of view unless you're a trusted caregiver, medical professional, or intimate partner. Indications of sexual abuse may include:
•Groin or inner-thigh bruises
•Pain, irritation, or unusual bleeding in the buttocks or genital area
•Bruises or cuts around the breasts
•Unexplained infections such as sexually transmitted diseases (STDs)
•Bloodied, stained, or ripped clothing, especially underwear
•Uncharacteristic behavior of a sexual nature

It's also important to know what to look for in the behavior of potential abusers. People who abuse or neglect seniors may:
•Refuse or try to delay visitations or social activities
•Unfairly criticize or express frequent frustration with family members or care providers
•Resist outside assistance
•Display little or no kindness, compassion, or affection
•Act excessively or inappropriately affectionate
•Show poor caregiving abilities
•Claim that care is adequate when it clearly needs to improve
•Complain of exhaustion
•Get angry easily
•Change the stories they tell about the same incidents
•Make seemingly out-of-context excuses
•Abuse drugs or alcohol

Who Are the Most Common Abusers?

Chances are good that you already know someone who has the motive and opportunity to mistreat or take advantage of a vulnerable senior. Abuse can be inflicted by almost anybody who benefits from having power, authority, or an expectation of trust. For example, potential elder abusers can include:
•Spouses or romantic partners
•Sons or daughters
•Brothers or sisters
•Nieces, nephews, or other blood relatives
•In-law relatives
•Paid or volunteer caregivers
•Friends
•Legal guardians
•Neighbors or other acquaintances
•Financial advisors
•Salespeople
•Healthcare practitioners
•Religious leaders

In most cases of elder abuse, the victims know the perpetrators very well. That's even true when it comes to financial abuse. In fact, according to the NCEA, family members account for close to 60 percent of those who financially exploit seniors. And friends, neighbors, and home care aides collectively account for nearly 32 percent of financial abusers who target the elderly. Financial abusers are often motivated by a sense of entitlement, the opportunity for a sizeable inheritance, a lack of money caused by unemployment, or the need to pay off debts or fuel an addiction to drugs, shopping, or gambling.Many elderly people experience domestic violence. Couples who retire together often deal with new financial challenges, disabilities, or changes to their roles that strain their relationships. Physical or emotional abuse can become a problem as tensions escalate and frustration sets in. Adult children who live with their elderly parents can also become violent and frustrated when faced with the costs and demands of caregiving, especially if they depend on their parents' financial resources. In some cases, the elder abuse is merely a continuation of past domestic violence.Some residents of long-term care facilities experience violent assaults or verbal aggression by other residents. Whether or not resident-on-resident violence should be considered elder abuse is still open for debate among many researchers. Such violence is often caused by dementia or other types of mental illness or cognitive decline.

Why Are Some Seniors More Vulnerable to Abuse Than Others?

Most of us like to imagine growing old peacefully, with few worries and lots of freedom to enjoy our most cherished personal interests. But the reality is that, for many of us, our senior years will be different than what we envisioned. We may face new challenges that we didn't expect. And we may increasingly need to rely on the help of other people. As a result, we may become targets for abuse, neglect, or exploitation. Here are some of the risk factors:

•Chronic illness or disability
•Dementia
•Depression or other mental health issues
•Recent losses of friends or loved ones
•Loneliness or social isolation
•Poor relationships with family members
•Lack of cultural or community support
•Substance abuse
•Anything that's extra challenging for caregivers (such as incontinence or sundowners syndrome)
•Poor financial or technological literacy
•Predictable financial deposits
•Low income
•Valuable assets
•Sharing a living space
•Having caregivers who lack the necessary skills, feel tired and overwhelmed, abuse drugs or alcohol, or have financial or mental health problems

Remember: Nobody who is abused or neglected is ever to blame. No matter how vulnerable you may be due to your circumstances, you never deserve to be mistreated. If you're a victim, it's not your fault. There is never a good excuse for anyone to abuse or neglect someone else.

What Should I Do If I See, Suspect, or Experience Elder Mistreatment?

Trust what you're seeing or feeling. Elder abuse can sometimes be subjective, but it's usually better to err on the side of caution. That's even true for potential elderly neglect by family members. Your emotions may be conflicted, but choose to do what's necessary in order to protect yourself or the senior in your life who you suspect is being mistreated. Don't stay silent.

If there is an immediate danger to life, limb, or property, ***call local help number.***

Otherwise, call Adult Protective Services (APS) in your state. APS exists to protect vulnerable seniors and investigate reports of alleged abuse or neglect. The APS agency in your region may have its own elder abuse hotline, allowing you to maintain confidentiality while reporting mistreatment. In many states, APS workers will:

•Evaluate the level of danger
•Take steps to ensure the safety of you or the alleged victim
•Help relieve the immediate effects of emotional trauma
•Gather evidence and assess the nature and scope of the alleged abuse
•Determine what social services may be needed
•Make arrangements for any necessary services, whether legal, financial, social, or medical in nature
•Work as advocates to help protect you or the alleged victim from future harm

Table 18.1 Definition and type of abuse faced by elders.

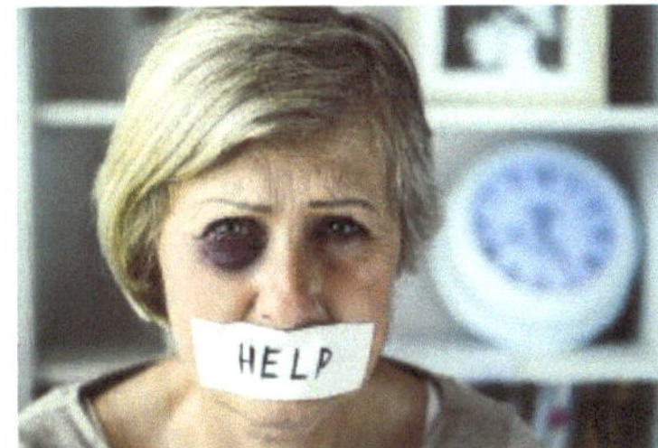

Type of abuse	Definition of abuse
Physical abuse	Intentional bodily injury
Sexual abuse	Nonconsensual sexual contact (any unwanted sexual contact).
Emotional abuse	Infliction of mental anguish or pain
Financial abuse / exploitation	Illegal or improper use of funds or other resources
Neglect	Through action or inaction, depriving care necessary to maintain the person's physical or mental health
Self-neglect	Behavior that threatens one's own health or safety
Abandonment	Action or inaction that leaves the vulnerable person without the ability to obtain food, clothing, shelter or care

When it comes to nursing home abuse, reporting can also be done through your state's Long-Term Care Ombudsman Program (LTCOP). Residents of nursing homes, assisted living communities, and other long-term care facilities can contact their region's LTCOP to make complaints and get independent advocates working on their behalf. The LTCOP in your region may even operate a confidential nursing home abuse hotline.

It's also a good idea to know your state's laws as they pertain to elder abuse. Explore the resources in your state so that you can learn your rights and know where to turn for help.

How Can Elder Abuse Be Prevented?

Increased awareness of this problem is essential. So don't be afraid to share what you know. Reach out to other seniors or younger adults. Even many politicians and professionals in the fields of healthcare, criminal justice, and financial services need reminders about the problem of elder abuse and neglect. They also need to be encouraged to report it when they suspect it.

Some of the ways to lower your risk of being abused or neglected as a senior include:

•Taking care of your physical health by going for regular check-ups, exercising, and eating a nutritious diet

•Maintaining close friendships, having fun, and interacting with your community

•Keeping a senior-friendly cell phone to ensure a connection to the outside world if you need to reach out for help or even get perspective on a potentially abusive situation

•Getting legal assistance to create a living will and other documents that clearly outline what should happen to you and your assets if you ever become incapacitated

•Seeking counseling or therapy for relationship troubles, substance abuse problems, or mental health issues

•Registering your phone number with the National registry

•Empower yourself by staying connected and informed on the latest news by joining e-newsletters such as the Elder Justice Coalition

When all is said and done, you may not be able to fully prevent mistreatment. But seniors who stay active and involved in their communities often make poor targets for abusers. Help look after other people so that they'll help look after you.

Bibliography and Acknowledgement

- Baker PR, Francis DP, Hairi NN, Othman S, Choo WY. Interventions for preventing abuse in the elderly. Cochrane Database Syst Rev. 2016 Aug 16;2016(8):CD010321. [PMC free article] [PubMed]
- Bows H. The other side of late-life intimacy? Sexual violence in later life. Australas J Ageing. 2020 Jun;39 Suppl 1:65-70. [PubMed]
- Chen AL, Koval KJ. Elder abuse: the role of the orthopaedic surgeon in diagnosis and management. J Am Acad Orthop Surg. 2002 Jan-Feb;10(1):25-31. [PubMed]
- Dong X, Simon MA. Vulnerability risk index profile for elder abuse in a community-dwelling. J Am Geriatr Soc. 2014 Jan;62(1):10-5. [PMC free article] [PubMed]
- Dong XQ. Elder Abuse: Systematic Review and Implications for Practice. J Am Geriatr Soc. 2015 Jun;63(6):1214-38. [PMC free article] [PubMed]
- Janofsky JS, McCarthy RJ, Folstein MF. The Hopkins Competency Assessment Test: a brief method for evaluating patients' capacity to give informed consent. Hosp Community Psychiatry. 1992 Feb;43(2):132-6. [PubMed]
- Lee M, Rosen T, Murphy K, Sagar P. A new role for imaging in the diagnosis of physical elder abuse: results of a qualitative study with radiologists and frontline providers. J Elder Abuse Negl. 2019 Mar-May;31(2):163-180. [PMC free article] [PubMed]
- Met Life. Broken Trust: Edlers, Family, and Finances. March 2009. Found on the internet at https://www.giaging.org/documents/mmi-study-broken-trust-elders-family-finances.pdf
- Mileski M, Lee K, Bourquard C, Cavazos B, Dusek K, Kimbrough K, Sweeney L, McClay R. Preventing The Abuse Of Residents With Dementia Or Alzheimer's Disease In The Long-Term Care Setting: A Systematic Review. Clin Interv Aging. 2019;14:1797-1815. [PMC free article] [PubMed]
  Mion LC, Momeyer MA. Elder abuse. Geriatr Nurs. 2019 Nov-Dec;40(6):640-644. [PubMed]
- Rodríguez MA, Wallace SP, Woolf NH, Mangione CM. Mandatory reporting of elder abuse: between a rock and a hard place. Ann Fam Med. 2006 Sep-Oct;4(5):403-9. [PMC free article] [PubMed]
- Storey, J. E. Risk factors for elder abuse and neglect: A review of the literature. Aggression and Violent Behavior. January-February 2020. Found on the internet at https://www.sciencedirect.com/science/article/abs/pii/S1359178918303471?via%3Dihub
- True Link. True Link Releases Elder Abuse Findings. Jan. 28, 2015.Foundontheinternetathttps://www.truelinkfinancial.com/blog/true-link-releases-latest-elder-financial-abuse-findings-losses-discovered-to-be-much-worse-than-originally-thought
- Wysokiński A, Sobów T, Kłoszewska I, Kostka T. Mechanisms of the anorexia of aging-a review. Age (Dordr). 2015 Aug;37(4):9821. [PMC free article] [PubMed]
- XinQi Dong, MD, et. al. Elder Self-neglect and Abuse and Mortality Risk in a Community-Dwelling Population. JAMA. Aug. 5, 2009. Found on the internet at https://www.ncbi.nlm.nih.gov/pmc/articles/PMC2965589/

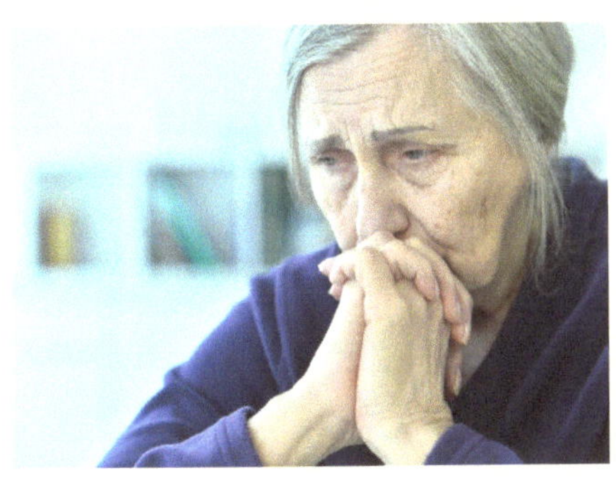

Elderly Suicide vs. Death With Dignity

Elderly suicide has an enormous impact on the families and friends of seniors who take their own lives prematurely. That's why it deserves our attention. How many heartbreaking tragedies might we prevent if we simply knew what to look for and how to take action?

Yet, our feelings about this complex and sensitive issue are often influenced by cultural biases, misconceptions, and the language we use when talking about it. As a result, many of us have conflicted feelings about the controversial issues of euthanasia and death with dignity, sometimes overlooking the factors that make them different than traditional notions of suicide. In fact, Gallup surveys have shown that our opinions about such matters can depend a lot on how those topics are framed.

This chapter will help you better understand the issues surrounding suicide and physician-assisted dying among older adults. That way, you can better support your elderly friends and loved ones—or find the help you may desperately need to obtain your own peace of mind.

Suicide vs. Euthanasia vs. Death With Dignity:

How They Differ

The words we use matter—often more than we realize. In relation to this topic, they are especially important. That's because they evoke strong feelings, and they are associated with entirely different contexts and situations.The distinctions may seem subtle, but they have a large significance in the personal lives of those they impact. So although it's easy to find examples of the following terms being used loosely or interchangeably, many people believe that it behooves all of us to use them within their appropriate contexts.

Here's what you should understand:

Suicide, according to the simplest definition, is the act of intentionally killing yourself. Although many different factors can converge to motivate people to commit suicide, mood disorders such as depression are usually the biggest driving forces in that outcome, according to an article in Psychiatric Clinics of North America.Unable to effectively cope with their despair, people eventually lose all hope and view suicide as their last remaining option. But although suicide seems like a logical choice to them, studies noted by an article in Clinical Interventions in Aging have shown that people with depression who have recently attempted suicide tend to exhibit cognitive impairments related to their memory, attention, and quality of decision-making.That's why suicide is generally considered a tragic result of untreated or poorly treated mental illness. Lacking appropriate support, those attempting suicide often feel powerless to choose any other course of action. Suicide can also have lasting and traumatic effects on the friends and loved ones left behind.

Euthanasia (also known as mercy killing) is the intentional act of painlessly causing the death of someone who is in an irreversible coma or suffering unbearably from a painful and incurable medical condition. The action, where legally carried out, is usually performed by a physician or other health care professional when reasonable alternatives or expectations for improvement are absent. But there are different types of euthanasia: active and passive, which can each be either voluntary or non-voluntary.

- **Active euthanasia:** This is when someone (generally a medical professional) directly and intentionally causes the death of a patient, such as by administering a lethal dose of medication.
- **Passive (or non-active) euthanasia:** Under the most common definitions, this is when a patient's death is caused through the deliberate withholding of treatments that may otherwise sustain his or her life, even if just for a little while. So the difference between active euthanasia and passive euthanasia is that the former type requires a new and tangible lethal action, whereas the latter type involves stopping one or more life-sustaining measures that are already in use.
- **Voluntary euthanasia:** This occurs when a patient's death is hastened with his or her informed

consent (i.e., approval).

•Non-voluntary euthanasia: This happens when a patient's medical condition makes it impossible for him or her to provide consent, so someone else makes the decision on his or her behalf in light of factors such as poor quality of life that is unlikely to get better.Some people also use the term "involuntary euthanasia" to describe an action that is, essentially, murder. Under this scenario, the patient may have been capable of providing consent, but he or she wasn't given the opportunity. Or the patient may have stated a desire to live, but he or she was killed anyway. Either way, the patient's best interests were not put first—taking the action out of the domain of euthanasia and into the realm of something much more sinister.

Death with dignity gives some terminally ill people the option of legally hastening their own death with the assistance of a licensed physician. But death with dignity laws vary between the relatively few regions where they've been enacted. In Canada, for instance, the law makes it possible for a medical provider to perform voluntary euthanasia for certain kinds of patients, although the preferred term for it is medical aid in dying.

In the states where it is legal in the U.S., the typical death with dignity definition excludes any form of euthanasia. So, in those regions, the difference between euthanasia and death with dignity is that, with the latter form of dying, patients themselves must administer the lethal medication. Licensed physicians prescribe the lethal substances for their patients to self-administer once all the steps in a mandatory process have been followed.

In addition to medical aid in dying, death with dignity is also known as:

- Physician aid in dying
- Medical assistance in dying
- Physician-assisted dying
- Physician-assisted death

Of course, you are also likely to run across terms such as "assisted suicide," "doctor-assisted suicide," or "suicide with dignity" when reading about this issue. But to many of the terminally ill seniors who choose the path of dying with dignity, terms that include "suicide" are inaccurate and disrespectful. Their friends and family members also frequently find such terms to be offensive.After all, "suicide" tends to carry negative connotations of emotional despair, impaired judgment, and immorality. But those who choose to die with dignity are required to be of sound mind. And they get the comfort of knowing that they do not have to experience unbearable agony, an unacceptable quality of life, or an unpeaceful death. In a sense, they do not see themselves as the ones causing their death; that blame falls on their terminal illness. Rather, they are merely decreasing the amount of time that they must suffer. They will die soon anyway. That's the meaning of death with dignity: being able to exercise your right to die a peaceful death when your fatal illness cannot be cured and you still have the freedom and capability to make such a decision. It's a personal choice that's exercised by rational people of legal age, from young adults to the elderly. "Assisted suicide," in their view, doesn't accurately describe the legal, medical, and conceptual choice they're making.

Still, whether you're talking about death with dignity or euthanasia, debate swirls around this topic. So it's only by understanding the arguments for and against dying with dignity that you can truly appreciate what it all means for the patients, loved ones, physicians, and caregivers impacted by it.

Elderly Suicide Facts and Statistics

As a culture, we tend to think of suicide as primarily occurring among young individuals. Many people also view suicide in the elderly population as somehow being less tragic than youth suicide. Some people even believe, mistakenly, that depression is a normal part of aging or, on the flip side, that seniors are able to cope much better with life's stressors than younger adults. Unfortunately, those beliefs cause too many of us to overlook the very real and widespread problem of suicide among older adults.In fact, according to the most recent data on suicide rates from the Centers for Disease Control and Prevention , elderly men over 75 kill themselves at the highest rate of any age group in the U.S. (39.7 deaths per 100,000 people).

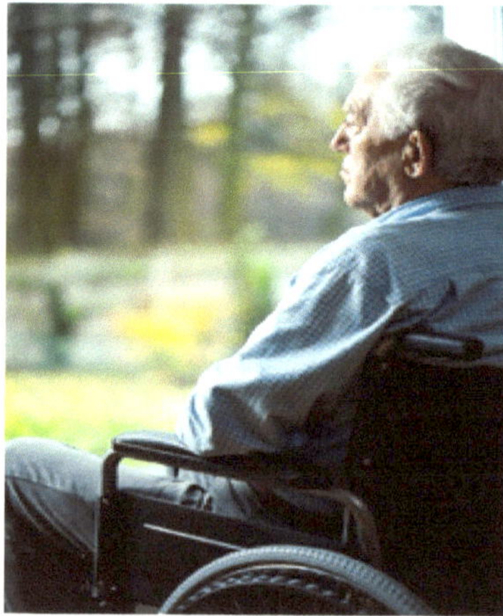

Fig.19.1 Sitting alone on the chair ,having mental depression and is more prone to suicide

And although older women have much lower rates of suicide than men, the rate of suicide among females peaks between the ages of 45 and 64 at 9.7 deaths per 100,000 people.

In many other countries around the world, elderly suicide rates are even higher. Worldwide, the senior citizen suicide rate (for those 70 and older) is about 27.5 deaths per 100,000 people, according to Our World in Data. Yet, in some nations, the rate is even more staggering. So, around the globe, which country has the highest rate of elderly suicide? That would be South Korea, with about 86 deaths per 100,000 people.

Here's another important stat: The article in Psychiatric Clinics of North America says that when it comes to completing suicide, elderly people die from their attempts at a much higher rate than young adults (25 percent vs. 0.5 percent).

Keep in mind that none of these statistics include physician-assisted death (i.e., so-called "assisted suicide"). For elderly people and younger adults with painful or debilitating terminal illnesses, the decision to seek medical aid in dying is an altogether different situation than contemplating suicide when comparatively healthy.

That's why it's essential that we all do a better job of understanding and recognizing the risk factors and warning signs that can affect or be displayed by a troubled senior. Suicide is not an inevitable consequence of mental health problems. Often, it can be prevented.

Why Suicide in the Elderly Happens

Despite progress in many other areas, our modern society still has shortcomings when it comes to how we think about aging, mental illness, and death. For example, many people stigmatize depression and mistakenly believe that suffering is always part of the aging process, which can make older adults reluctant to seek the right kind of help.

According to the article in Clinical Interventions in Aging, when it comes to suicide, senior citizens who've taken their own lives were much less likely to have visited a mental health professional in the month before their death than to have seen a primary care physician.

Some people also have romanticized notions about suicide, which may be holdovers from the past. For instance, in ancient Rome, suicide was often seen as a way to die with honor—as long as you didn't have any mental problems. A traditional Roman suicide ritual may have involved appeasing the gods for shameful actions and being surrounded by your loved ones, ensuring that one of them heard your final words. Today, the reasons for late-life suicide are as diverse as the individual seniors who attempt it. But the risk of suicide is cumulative, meaning that multiple factors are usually involved. The Psychiatric Clinics of North America article says that each new risk factor affecting a senior increases the probability that he or she will attempt suicide. Adding to the overall risk is this fact according to an investigation by Kaiser Health News and PBS NewsHour (KHN): Baby boomers have committed suicide at higher rates than those in other generations, which may continue into their senior years.The KHN/PBS NewsHour investigation reveals that among older adults, suicidal behavior is mainly associated with:

- **Depression:** This mental health condition is often the biggest risk factor for suicide. Affected seniors come to feel a sustained sense of hopelessness or a lack of meaning and purpose in their lives. They may not see any kind of path to a satisfying future or any new goals to pursue. They feel powerless to solve their problems, and they may even feel angry with themselves for not being stronger. But depression isn't the only mental health issue that can play a major role in suicidal behavior. Other psychiatric conditions that cause sustained psychological pain or discomfort (such as generalized anxiety disorder) can lead to suicidal ideation.
- **Frailty:** Feeling weak or consistently fatigued makes life harder and less enjoyable. Many physical illnesses can cause persistent debility in seniors, contributing to a sense of despair.
- **Detachment:** Some seniors feel secluded or disconnected from life, particularly in a social sense. They may suffer from chronic loneliness or feel ignored by their grown children or other loved ones. According to the Clinical Interventions in Aging article, one study found that seniors who attempt suicide are less likely to have children, be married, or participate in religion.
- **Access to lethal means:** When a senior has suicidal thoughts, he or she is more likely to attempt suicide if the means to do so are readily available. That's why guns are involved in 46 percent of all suicides in America, according to Our World in Data. But several other means are often available to older adults who seek to take their own lives. The article in Clinical Interventions in Aging says that seniors who've lost a close family member within the previous six months have the highest risk of suicide. Other factors that can

increase an older adult's risk of suicide include:

- Alcohol abuse
- Chronic pain
- Cognitive impairment
- Divorce
- Elder abuse
- Employment changes
- Family conflict
- Fear of being a burden on others
- Lack of access to mental health care
- Loss of independence
- Loss of friends or pets
- Being male
- Money problems
- Physical disability
- Regret
- Shame
- Stress
- Stubbornness
- Trouble adapting to change

Warning Signs of Potential Elder Suicide

When it comes to the potential for suicide in older adults, the danger signs can sometimes be easy to miss. After all, many seniors have fewer social interactions than younger people, and they may have extra determination to take their own lives. They may even work harder at hiding their intentions so as not to ruin their plans. Plus, seniors who live independently or semi-independently often have more ability to keep their suicidal thoughts and preparations to themselves.

Even so, it is possible to assess the risk of suicide. In elderly people, the potential for suicide can reveal itself in many different ways. Some of the things to watch out for include:

•Communication of suicidal thoughts or intentions: This is usually the clearest indication that someone may be seriously considering suicide. For example, you may hear a senior say things like, "Maybe you won't see me after this" or "I wish I wasn't alive" or "You'll be happier when I'm gone." Such statements aren't always related to suicidal contemplation, but they are definitely red flags that warrant the attention of a mental health professional right away.

•Problematic changes to the usual routine: Seniors who are contemplating suicide sometimes quit performing normal daily habits related to their self-care. For example, they may not pay as much attention to their appearance or personal hygiene. They may adopt poor eating habits. They might stop taking essential prescription medications. Or they may have trouble sleeping or adopt an unhealthy sleep schedule.

•Unusual behavior or changes in mood or personality: Some older adults with suicidal thoughts or intentions begin to take risks that are out of the ordinary for them. Or they display other patterns of thought or behavior that their friends and loved ones perceive as inconsistent with their typical personalities. For example, a troubled senior might hoard medications, start abusing drugs or alcohol, give away cherished belongings, drive recklessly, display a sudden fascination with dark topics, or act in a high-strung manner.

•Loss of interest in current or future activities: This can be a symptom of depression, which is a big red flag. But a senior who is seriously contemplating suicide due to a combination of other factors may also display a lack of desire in doing things that he or she would ordinarily pursue.

•Grief over family-related issues: The recent loss of a spouse or other close family member can cause intense sorrow and/or loneliness for a surviving senior, which may contribute to suicidal ideation. But conflicts among living family members can also lead to deep feelings of distress, social isolation, and thoughts of escape.

•Despair over recent changes in health or independence: Anything that significantly diminishes the quality of life that a senior previously enjoyed can cause deep grieving. For example, having a chronic or terminal illness can trigger a large range of troubling emotions, as can an unwanted change in lifestyle or living arrangements (especially if it involves losing personal autonomy).

Seniors who have previously attempted suicide may also be at higher risk of making future attempts.

Elderly Suicide Prevention

If you suspect that a senior is seriously thinking about taking his or her own life, it's essential to respond to the issue as quickly as possible. Preventing suicide in the elderly often requires action on multiple fronts. According to Mayo Clinic, intervening is always the most appropriate option—even if you have doubts about what to do. You're unlikely to make things worse; on the contrary, you may help reduce the person's suicidal impulses.

Get immediate help if you believe that a suicide attempt is imminent. Otherwise, here are some actions you may be able to take:

•Have a compassionate conversation: Gently asking relevant questions and listening attentively to the answers is a great way to show the person that you care. Just make sure you do so without interrupting or

passing judgment. Allow the person to freely express his or her thoughts
and emotions, but listen for clues that may indicate the seriousness of his or her intentions. Ask how the person is coping, what's going on to trigger the distressing feelings, whether death or suicide are explicitly being thought about, what kind of harmful or lethal means may be readily available, and so on.

•Refer the senior to the Institute on Aging's toll-free Friendship Line (1-800-971-0016): This 24-hour service is one of the best resources for suicide prevention. Elderly people and seniors who are 60 or older can call at any time for friendly emotional support or crisis intervention. For many seniors, ongoing outreach can also be set up so that they regularly receive calls from volunteers who check in on their well-being.

•Make it harder for the person to access lethal means: The longer it takes for someone to act on a suicidal impulse, the less likely it is that he or she will die from an attempt. That's why, whenever possible, it makes sense to remove weapons and other potentially lethal items from a troubled senior's home environment. If that isn't possible, you still may be able to make the items harder to use. For example, guns can be stored in a locked cabinet or closet with trigger locks on each gun (and the ammo and keys can be stored in separate places). Prescription medications can be left with a caregiver who only provides them as needed. In some situations, access to alcohol or illicit drugs might also need to be managed since the person may be more likely to attempt suicide while under the influence.

• Encourage participation in a support group: A sense of belonging can help prevent suicidal ideation in an older adult, according to the Clinical Interventions in Aging article. So it may be useful to find a local support group where the senior you care about can meet and talk with people who share similar experiences. Look for support groups related to the specific problems that are contributing to the person's distress (such as grief or a particular illness). Many people who are at risk of suicide also benefit from attending groups for survivors of attempted suicide, even if they haven't made an attempt themselves.

•Invite the senior to attend physically and mentally stimulating activities with you: Whether it's a yoga or exercise class or a workshop related to a new or existing hobby, getting the person out and engaged in fresh pursuits can help revive his or her appreciation for life, at least temporarily.

•Help the person find a mental health professional: Regardless of what else you do, always help connect a troubled senior with professional counseling or therapy. One place to start is the Institute on Aging, which offers both in-home and outpatient therapy services for seniors.

Getting Immediate Help

First, take a slow, deep breath and tell yourself that you can get through this—no matter how upsetting the situation may be.

If the person intends to commit suicide but hasn't yet made an attempt:

•Encourage the senior to call the Friendship Line.

•Call Call emergency no. on a separate phone, if possible.

•Stay close by. Do not leave him or her alone until help arrives.

If the person has already attempted suicide:

•Call emergency no. and stay with the senior, following the instructions you're given.

•Alternatively, drive the senior to the emergency department of a nearby hospital (but only if you can do so safely).

•Take notice of any medications, alcohol, or other substances the senior may have used. In the event that someone you care about doesn't survive a suicide attempt, seek grief counseling as soon as possible. Also, you may benefit from attending a local support group for survivors of suicide loss. If you have the impulse to attempt suicide:

•Go to a place where other people are nearby. Do not isolate yourself.

•Call your counselor or therapist if you have one.

•Alternatively, call the Friendship Line

Death With Dignity Facts and Laws

Death with dignity (i.e., physician-assisted dying) takes place in a completely different context than suicide. It empowers eligible terminally ill adults to plan peaceful deaths at the times and locations they choose.

In the U.S., Oregon's Death with Dignity Act was the first law of its kind. It came into effect in 1997. Washington state followed with its own law roughly a decade later.

At the time of this writing – September 2023 – death with dignity was legal in the following states and jurisdictions:

- California
- Colorado
- Hawaii
- Maine
- Montana

- New Jersey
- New Mexico
- Oregon
- Vermont
- Washington
- Washington, D.C.

In addition, death with dignity is legal in Canada, where it's known as medical assistance in dying (MAID). According to an article from The Conversation, it is also legal in Columbia, the state of Victoria in Australia, and a few European countries, including Belgium, the Netherlands, and Luxembourg. In Switzerland, the practice isn't explicitly authorized by law, but it also isn't forbidden as long as it is carried out for so-called "non-selfish" reasons.

Basic Eligibility

According to the Death with Dignity National Center, in the places where it is legal in the United States, the requirements for death with dignity are generally that you must be:

•At least 18 years old

•A resident of a state (or DC) that has a death with dignity law

•Terminally ill with a medical prognosis of six months or less to live

•Mentally capable of making and communicating your own medical decisions

•Physically capable of self-administering and ingesting the lethal medication prescribed for you

In terms of the residency requirements, you simply need to prove that you currently live in the region where you intend to die with physician assistance. It isn't necessary to show that you've been a resident for any minimum length of time. But you do need to provide documentation of your current residence.For example, if you want physician-assisted death in Oregon, your proof of residency could be an Oregon driver's license or ID card, a copy of your recent state tax return, proof of voter registration in the state, or papers that show that you currently own or rent a home in the state. But to qualify for death with dignity, you do not have to live in Oregon for any specific amount of time.

California, Colorado, Hawaii, and Washington have the same residency requirements as Oregon. In the other regions where death with dignity is legal, the documentation requirements are similar but a little more varied. In addition to the above requirements, you must follow all of the required steps in the process, which include getting approval from two physicians and adhering to two waiting periods.

In Canada, the law is more flexible. For example, it allows for voluntary euthanasia, meaning that a doctor or nurse practitioner can administer the lethal medication if you prefer not to self-administer it. Also, you do not have to be terminally ill for euthanasia or medical assistance in dying in Canada, but you do have to meet certain requirements, including:

•Being at least 18 years old

•Qualifying for publicly funded health care in Canada

•Having a serious illness or disability that has progressed to a state of irreversible functional deterioration, causes intolerable physical and mental suffering, and makes your natural death "reasonably foreseeable"

•Making a voluntary, uncoerced request for medical assistance in dying

•Providing informed consent after being told that other options like palliative care are available to help ease your suffering

•Having the ability to provide informed consent at the moment when medical assistance in dying is to be carried out

Some Canadian courts have ruled that the "reasonably foreseeable" clause is invalid if interpreted to mean that someone has to be at or near the end of life. So going forward, that clause may not be an obstacle to eligibility for certain patients who are experiencing intolerable suffering but are not expected to die from their conditions in the near future.

Simply put, a wide variety of suffering patients qualify for voluntary euthanasia in Canada if they don't want (or are physically unable) to self-administer lethal medications. But they must be evaluated by at least two independent health care practitioners in order to qualify for medical assistance in dying. Canadian law also has other requirements that must be followed, such as a waiting period and independent witnesses to your request.

Additional Facts

Under state laws for death with dignity, it is incorrect to label the practice as physician-assisted "suicide." Statistics, moreover, show no indication of these laws being widely abused, according to an article in JAMA: The Journal of the American Medical Association. In fact, you may be surprised to learn that:

•In the places where euthanasia and/or physician-assisted dying are legal, they account for only 0.3 to 4.6 percent of all deaths, according to the JAMA article.

•The Death with Dignity National Center says that about 90 percent of people who choose death with dignity are receiving hospice care at the time of their passing. And the article in JAMA says that over 70 percent of them have cancer.
•The JAMA article notes that fewer than one in five physicians have received a request for medical aid in dying or euthanasia. And only five percent or less of physicians have ever complied with such a request.
•Only patients themselves can request death with dignity; no proxies are allowed, according to the Death with Dignity National Center. (Even if a person has medical power of attorney, he or she cannot make such a request on behalf of someone else.)
•As long as death with dignity is carried out in a state where it is legal (and where you requested it), it doesn't have any effect on life insurance or similar policies. That's because, legally, your death will not be considered suicide, according to the Death with Dignity National Center.

As previously mentioned, among other places, death with dignity is legal in California, Colorado, Oregon, Vermont, and Washington. ProCon.org says doctors have written thousands of prescriptions for self-administered lethal medications under laws for physician-assisted dying. However, only about 66 percent of people who receive such prescriptions have used them to end their life. (Many people request death with dignity but ultimately choose not to go through with it.)

Why Death With Dignity Is Different Than Archaic Cultural Customs

It's important to distinguish today's medical aid in dying laws from past cultural customs and practices that many people associate with elderly euthanasia. History, after all, includes unsettling stories from various cultures around the world about the killing of old people.Also known as senicide or geronticide, the practice of killing elderly people through abandonment or other means (sometimes at their request) has shown up in many historical narratives. According to an article from Nowhere, although reliable information about such practices is relatively sparse, some cultures from the past have been said to engage in traditions like:

•Leaving elderly people alone on the top of mountains
•Sacrificing and eating old men
•Ritualistically killing older adults with certain weapons
•Having children slay their elderly parents with swords
•Throwing elderly people to dogs that have been trained to kill them

Most of us who are alive today would probably view such practices as grisly and barbaric. But those customs didn't always constitute murder; sometimes they were a form of voluntary euthanasia. Elderly people, in certain cultures, wished to die in accordance with traditions that would be outrageous and illegal by today's standards.

One of the most widely circulated stories concerns the Inuit (often referred to by terms that many people find derogatory, such as "Eskimo"). The Nowhere article notes that elderly Inuit people are said to have been put on ice floes and left to die from freezing and starvation—a rare, abandoned practice that some Inuit people and anthropologists have verified but that some scholars have disputed. For those who believe the practice took place, it's thought that some Inuit elders viewed that form of death as an appropriate way to end a life that had become "too much." Other Inuit death rituals involved placing a deceased person's body within a ring of rocks so that the wind wouldn't blow away his or her disintegrating bones.

Today, when debating whether to make physician-assisted death or voluntary euthanasia legal, some opponents of the idea like to equate it with archaic cultural customs (such as those just mentioned). But proponents of dying with dignity believe that such characterizations are unfair and intellectually dishonest. They argue that death with dignity laws allow for humane, non-violent deaths—without cultural coercion—for those who will die soon anyway and don't wish to prolong their suffering (not for those who feel they've gotten "too old").

Arguments For and Against Death With Dignity

Although it's legal in multiple states, physician-assisted dying remains highly controversial. Still, most Americans support the idea of allowing physicians to help terminally ill patients end their lives. In fact, when the phrase "commit suicide" isn't part of Gallup's survey questions about this issue, more than 70 percent of Americans express support for death with dignity. Even when that phrase is included, about 65 percent of Americans still support the concept.Death with dignity is a particularly divisive issue among physicians. The American Medical Association is against the practicehowever, many other medical associations in the U.S. and elsewhere have endorsed the idea.A lot of physicians believe that medical aid in dying goes against the Hippocratic Oath, which, in some modern variations, says:

If it is given to me to save a life, all thanks. But it may also be within my power to take a life; this awesome responsibility must be faced with great humbleness and awareness of my own frailty. Above all, I must not play at God.

Yet, opinions vary as to whether the oath is adequate or even still relevant. That's partly why, according to one poll by Medscape Medical News, about 56 percent of physicians have a positive opinion of death with dignity laws. And among physicians in states that don't have such laws, more than 60 percent say that they've had cases in which they would have liked their patients to have the option of physician-assisted death. But the many arguments for and against making death with dignity legal can be incredibly varied.

Arguments in Support of Physician-Assisted Dying

•Peaceful death should be a human right. Proponents believe that terminally ill people who don't want to endure needless suffering deserve the freedom to choose to die with dignity, on their own terms. If a person is still mentally competent and physically capable of making that decision, why should anyone else have the right to say no?

•Patients already have the right to refuse treatment. As long as medical patients are deemed mentally competent and have been adequately informed of their rights and options for care and treatment, they can decline any further medical interventions that might prolong their lives. That's why some people argue that a physician withholding treatment isn't that much different than a physician providing medical aid in dying. Whether the deed is passive or active, the final outcome is the same. But the active deed often involves less suffering.

Some patients request physician-assisted death because it means that they won't have to go through treatments (or any withholding of treatments) that might prolong or add to their pain or distress. They don't want to experience a lower quality of life that they find unacceptable. Besides, death with dignity laws provide safeguards to confirm patients' prognoses as well as their mental fitness for decision-making.

•It's humane. Most people would never want their friends or loved ones to suffer unbearably for any amount of time. Yet, sometimes patients' expressions of pain or distress aren't taken as seriously as they should be, especially when their loved ones can't bear the thought of losing them. Proponents argue that offering dignity in dying is a greater act of compassion than forcing someone to endure an intolerable quality of life when healing is no longer possible. Plus, physician-assisted deaths tend to be peaceful and relatively easy (in comparison to a lot of deaths in which intensive medical care is involved).

•We provide it for our pets. When it comes to our animal companions, we tend to be far more willing to act with compassion in order to prevent additional suffering and poor quality of life. Shouldn't we extend that kindness and compassion to human beings? Why do we find it easier to recognize that an animal's life doesn't need to continue at any cost? Like us, animals suffer. According to an article in Animal Sentience, there is even evidence for the possibility that some animals choose to take their own lives.

•Intolerable suffering is painful for everyone involved. Needless pain and distress is hard for terminally ill patients, of course. But it also causes significant distress for their friends and loved ones. That's one reason why some people who've witnessed the prolonged deaths of those they care about are proponents of dying with dignity. They recognize that, when chosen by a patient and supported by loved ones, it can reduce the amount of time that everyone spends grieving.

•It can improve other end-of-life care options. Many proponents like to point out that, in the places where death with dignity is legal, other options like pain management, palliative care, and hospice services get better. After all, it provides extra motivation for physicians and patients to talk about the full range of end-of-life care options—openly and honestly. Plus, even though most patients won't ever choose physician-assisted death, having it as an option can greatly improve their peace of mind.

Arguments Against Physician-Assisted Death

•It might make us undervalue human life. Many opponents of death with dignity laws believe that it is immoral for people to take their own lives or for anyone to assist someone else in doing so—regardless of the circumstances. In a lot of cases, their opposition is based on religious teachings about the sanctity of human life. They find the ideas of physician-assisted dying to be a sort of "phony compassion" that actually dehumanizes those who are suffering. And they worry that such laws may initiate a "slippery slope" in which assisted dying is eventually encouraged as an option for a much wider range of people.

•Physicians are meant to heal, not take lives. Many medical practitioners wonder why "doctor-assisted suicide" should be legal since it seems to go against the practice of doing no harm. They refuse to violate the Hippocratic Oath or undermine their professional values by actively causing a patient's death. In their view, suffering can be alleviated by proper palliative care, and they don't want assisted death to become an appealing default option.

Similar arguments are made with regard to the death penalty. In some states, doctors can perform executions (or assist with them), primarily through lethal injection. In fact, physician involvement is required by law for executions in some states. However, participating doctors usually keep their involvement confidential since it violates the American Medical Association's code of ethics and goes against the views of many in the general public.

•It may demean people with disabilities or chronic illnesses. Some opponents worry that assisted-death laws will expand or intensify incorrect assumptions that those with disabilities or long-term medical issues always have a poor quality of life and would rather be dead. They're concerned that the lives of people with disabilities will be less valued, resulting in more discrimination.

•The practice may become overused as a way to lower health care costs and reduce caregiving burdens. Opponents sometimes equate all assisted-death laws with euthanasia and wonder why euthanasia should be legal when financial and caregiving obligations may provide incentives for families to coerce their sick loved ones into that option.

•It can be difficult to judge someone's mental competence. This is especially true if a patient has an undiagnosed illness like dementia or depression that affects his or her abilities to understand all care options and make rational decisions. In some cases, it also may be hard to tell whether a person has been coerced into pursuing physician-assisted death.

•Medical diagnoses are sometimes wrong. Some opponents of physician-assisted death point out that doctors, albeit relatively rarely, sometimes incorrectly diagnose certain patients as being terminally ill. So there is a risk that some patients may choose assisted dying based on false information.

Dying With Dignity: The Typical Process

Before going down this path, it's important for terminally ill seniors to carefully consider all available options for their end-of-life care. This is especially critical if you have a progressive illness that might make you unable to provide informed consent, make decisions, or ingest the lethal medication prescribed for you when the time comes to do so. Under state death with dignity laws, you must be mentally competent and physically capable of ingesting the necessary medications at the time of your planned death.

So make sure you explore your options for palliative and/or hospice care. Besides, even if you choose physician-assisted dying, you can still benefit greatly from such care in the weeks or months leading up to your death—especially if your illness causes pain or other distressing symptoms. On average, palliative care costs about $95 per day. But that cost is frequently covered by Medicaid, Medicare, or private insurance.

In the states where death with dignity is legal, the entire process often takes at least a few weeks. Here's what you typically need to do:

1. Speak with your physician, make your first verbal request, and get authorization.

A good time to bring up death with dignity is when you and your doctor are talking face-to-face about other end-of-life options like palliative and hospice care. Just remember that a lot of physicians aren't receptive to this idea, at least initially. You'll need to share your reasons for wanting physician-assisted death, making it clear that you understand your prognosis, have been considering the alternatives, and don't wish to suffer needlessly. Verbally ask your physician whether he or she would be willing to support your decision to die with dignity by writing you a prescription for lethal medication in accordance with the applicable state law. Request a simple answer: yes or no. If your physician says no, accept his or her decision. But make sure that your request gets documented as part of your medical record.

It's possible that your doctor will not be willing to prescribe the lethal medication for you but would still be willing to act as a consulting physician—confirming your mental competence, diagnosis, and prognosis. Regardless, you will need the participation of two physicians. Both will need to evaluate your medical condition and mental judgment. But only one (the attending physician) will need to be willing to prescribe lethal medicationSince you need two participating doctors, ask for a referral to another physician, no matter how he or she answers. And keep in mind that any type of licensed physician can participate, regardless of specialty. You won't be able to proceed until you receive physician authorization.

2. Tell your friends and family.

Although it isn't legally required, talking to your loved ones about your plans for a physician-assisted death is highly recommended. After all, they'll need time to digest the information and process their feelings, regardless of whether they support the idea. In the best-case scenario, your loved ones will come to understand your decision, stand by you, and provide aid in planning the peaceful death that you want and deserve.

3. Comply with the first waiting period.

After receiving physician authorization, you typically need to wait at least 15 to 20 days before proceeding to the next step. The exact waiting period depends on your state's death with dignity law.

4. Make your second verbal request.

Speak to your attending physician, again requesting assistance to die with dignity in accordance with the relevant law in your state.

5. Submit a request in writing.

Each state with a physician-assisted dying law has its own forms to use for this purpose. So the requirements vary a little, depending on where you're going through this process. Generally, you must wait to submit your written request until any time after you've made your first verbal request. However, in the District of Columbia, you must also make this written request before your second verbal request. In addition, you may need to have your signature witnessed by two people who meet specific requirements.

6. Observe the second waiting period.

This doesn't apply in Colorado or California. For other regions where death with dignity is legal, your attending physician can only write the prescription for your lethal medication after waiting at least two full days from the time of receiving your written request.

7. Pick up your prescribed medication.

Under state laws for death with dignity, medication prescriptions must be delivered directly by your attending physician to a pharmacy. Once your pharmacy has the prescription, you can choose when to have it filled. And you can designate someone else to pick up the medication when it is ready. But remember: You do not have to fill the prescription if you end up having a change of heart.

Physicians aren't required to prescribe any specific medications. So prescriptions can vary from patient to patient and region to region. And the preferred medications for physician-assisted dying have changed over the years Today, a commonly recommended combination of diazepam, morphine, digoxin, and amitriptyline is given for death with dignity in the U.S., according to a MarketWatch article. (Another common protocol uses propranolol instead of amitriptyline.)

The MarketWatch article notes this fact: Using that four-drug cocktail means that it costs roughly $700 to $750 to die with dignity, unless you can afford and access the medications commonly used in Europe. According to the Death with Dignity National Center, Seconal is frequently unavailable in the U.S., and even if you can access it, it tends to cost between $3,000 and $5,000. Pentobarbital is also notoriously hard to access in America because the European Union has banned its export. Both of those medications are known to be fast-acting and provide for painless deaths. That's why a non-profit organization in Switzerland called Dignitas often uses pentobarbital to kill patients who seek their help in dying with dignity. But it can cost thousands of dollars for assisted dying if you're an American who wants to die overseas by using that medication. (Most of your expenses would be travel-related.) By staying back in the U.S., you'll be able to die with dignity at home, a lot more affordably. At this point in the process, you just have to decide when the time is right to commence your final act.

8. Plan a time and location, then ingest your medication.

Remember that in order to retain your legal protections, you can only take the lethal medication in the state where you received it. Otherwise, you are free to choose when and where you wish to die—if you still want to. (A significant number of patients ultimately choose not to end their lives this way. You're under no obligation to ingest the medication, even if you've come this far in the process.)Many patients choose to be surrounded by close family and friends during their final moments. Others prefer to have privacy for this part of their journey. Whatever you decide is OK. Either way, you will need to administer the medication yourself. You can, however, have someone help you prepare it. You may need to ingest multiple medications in a particular sequence, including meds to prevent nausea, to put you to sleep (and keep you asleep), and to ensure that you don't feel pain. The time it takes to fall asleep and pass away varies depending on the patient. Regardless of how long it takes for you to pass away, the medications should keep you in a comfortable state of painless, unconscious sleep until your peaceful end finally comes.

Bibliography and Acknowledgement

- ÁRamis.https://www.biobiochile.cl/noticias/opinion/tu voz/2021/01/19/libertad-y-muerte-digna-en-chile-estar-a-favor-de-la-vida-o-de-la-conciencia.shtml Libertad y muerte digna en Chile [Internet]. BioBioChile. 2021 [Cited 28 Dec 2021].
- Agencia estatal Boletín Oficial del Estado Ley Orgánica 3/2021. https://www.boe.es/eli/es/lo/2021/03/24/3 de 24 de marzo, de regulación de la eutanasia [Internet]. 2021 [Cited 28 Dec 2021].
- Barrio Cantalejo I.M., Simón Lorda P. Ethical criteria for substitute decision-making in people without capacity. Rev. Esp. Salud Publica. 2006;80(4):303–315. [PubMed] [Google Scholar] Bergdolt K. Current and historical aspects of euthanasia. Ars. Med. 2016;32(2):199. [Google Scholar]
- Bont M., Dorta K., Ceballos J., Randazzo A., Urdaneta-Carruyo E. Euthanasia: a historic Hermeneutical. Salud comunidad. 2007;5(2):36–45. [Google Scholar]
- Brandalise V.B., Remor A.P., Carvalho D de, Bonamigo E.L. Suicídio assistido e eutanásia na perspectiva de profissionais e acadêmicos de um hospital universitário. Rev Bioét. 2018;26(2):217–227. [Google Scholar]
- Brinkman-Stoppelenburg A., Evenblij K., Pasman H.R.W., van Delden Jjm, Onwuteaka-Philipsen B.D., van der Heide A. Physicians' and public attitudes toward euthanasia in people with advanced dementia. J. Am. Geriatr. Soc. 2020;68(10):2319–2328. [PMC free article] [PubMed] [Google Scholar]
- Calati R., Olié E., Dassa D., Gramaglia C., Guillaume S., Madeddu F., et al. Euthanasia and assisted suicide in psychiatric patients: a systematic review of the literature. J. Psychiatr. Res. 2021;135:153–173. [PubMed] [Google Scholar]
- Campos-Pérez M. Universidad Pública de Navarra; 2014. Eutanasia Y Nazismo.https://academica-e.unavarra.es/xmlui/handle/2454/11239 [Internet] [Cited 28 Dec 2021]. Available in: [Google Scholar]
- Carrasco M.V.H., Crispi F. Euthanasia in Chile. Rev. Med. Chile. 2016;144(12):1598–1604. [PubMed] [Google Scholar] Castellón V.M. Analysis of euthanasia. Anál econ. 2020;1(41):121–132. [Google Scholar]
- Dalfin W., Guymard M., Kieffer P., Kahn J.P. Droit à mourir et suicide assisté : état des lieux et analyse critique [The right to die and assisted suicide: review and critical analysis] Encephale. 2021;S0013(21) 7006. 00167. [PubMed] [Google Scholar]
- Di Paolo M., Gori F., Papi L., Turillazzi E. A review and analysis of new Italian law 219/2017: 'provisions for informed consent and advance directives treatment. BMC Med. Ethics. 2019;20(1):17. [PMC free article] [PubMed] [Google Scholar]
- Emanuel E.J., Onwuteaka-Philipsen B.D., Urwin J.W., Cohen J. Attitudes and practices of euthanasia and physician-assisted suicide in the United States, Canada, and Europe. JAMA. 2016;316(1):79–90. [PubMed] [Google Scholar]
- Fontalis A., Prousali E., Kulkarni K. Euthanasia and assisted dying: what is the current position and what are the key arguments informing the debate? J. R. Soc. Med. 2018;111(11):407–413. [PMC free article] [PubMed] [Google Scholar
- García Farrero J., Lafuente Nafría B., Vilanou Torrano C. Catholic universities in Europe: Louvain, Freiburg and Milan. Its repercussions in Spain at the beginning of the 20th century. Foro educ. 2018;16(25):141. [Google Scholar
- García Pereáñez J.A. Considerations of bio-law on euthanasia in Colombia. Rev Latinoam Bioet. 2016;17(32–1):200–221. [Google Scholar]
- Grosse C., Grosse A. Assisted suicide: Models of legal regulation in selected European countries and the case law of the European Court of Human Rights. Med. Sci. Law. 2015;55(4):246–258. [PubMed] [Google Scholar]
- Lavery J.V., Dickens B.M., Boyle J.M., Singer P.A. Bioethics for clinicians: 11. Euthanasia and assisted suicide. CMAJ (Can. Med. Assoc. J.) 1997;156(10):1405–1408. [PMC free article] [PubMed] [Google Scholar]
- Letter "Samaritanus bonus" of the Congregation for the Doctrine of the Faith on the care of persons in the critical and terminal phases of life. https://press.vatican.va/content/salastampa/es/bollettino/pubblico/2020/09/22/carta.html [Internet]. [Cited 28 Dec 2021]. Available in:
- Licata M., Nicoli F., Armocida G. Forgotten episodes of euthanasia in the 19th century. Lancet. 2017;390(10096):736. [PubMed] [Google Scholar]
- Merino S., Aruanno M.E., Gelpi R.J., Rancich A.M. The prohibition of euthanasia" and medical oaths of Hippocratic Stemma. Acta Bioeth. 2017;23(1):171–178.
- Oduncu F.S., Sahm S. Doctor-cared dying instead of physician-assisted suicide: a perspective from Germany. Med. Health Care Philos. 2010;13(4):371–381. [PubMed] [Google Scholar]
- Parreiras M., Antunes G.C., Marcon L.M.P., Andrade L.S., Rückl S., Andrade V.L.Â. Eutanásia e suicídio assistido em países ocidentais: revisão sistemática. Rev Bioét. 2016;24(2):355–367. [Google Scholar]
- Picón Jaimes Y., Orozco Chinome J., Lozada Martínez I., Moscote Salazar L. Disease, euthanasia and abortion: a reflection from bioethics. Revista Médica De Risaralda. 2021;27(1):4–9. [Google Scholar]
- Sabriseilabi S., Williams J. Dimensions of religion and attitudes toward euthanasia. Death Stud. 2020:1–8. Sabriseilabi S., Williams J. Dimensions of religion and attitudes toward euthanasia. Death Stud. 2020:1–8.
- Solorzano Navarro H., Manuel Vivanco Crítica a la moral conservadora. Aborto, eutanasia, drogas, matrimonio igualitario. Rev. Cien. Soc. 2017;38:138. [Google Scholar]
- Turillazzi E., Maiese A., Frati P., Scopetti M., Di Paolo M. Physician-patient relationship, assisted suicide and the Italian constitutional court. J. bioeth. Inq. 2021 Oct 21.
- Velasco Bernal C., Trejo-Gabriel-Galan J.M. Leyes de eutanasia en España y en el mundo: aspectos médicos [Euthanasia laws in Spain and in the world: medical aspects] Atención Primaria. 2022;54(1):102170. [PMC free article] [PubMed] [Google Scholar]
- Von-Engelhardt D. Euthanasia in between shortening life and aiding death: past experiences, present challenges. Acta Bioeth. 2002;8(1) [Google Scholar]
- Yildirim J.G. Knowledge, opinions and behaviors of senior nursing students in Turkey regarding euthanasia and factors in Islam affecting these. J. Relig. Health. 2020;59(1):399–415. [PubMed] [Google Scholar]

Management Of Terminal End-Stage Medical Conditions In Elderly

Having a terminal illness is definitely life-altering. Whether you're a terminally ill senior or a close friend or family member of one, the impact is significant. It's normal to experience a huge range of emotions and have trouble knowing what to do. After all, dealing with a terminal illness often means coping with a lot of change and uncertainty. Yet, it's also possible to get through the experience with some dignity and greater peace of mind.

Reliable information and good communication are essential. Seniors with terminal cancer, Alzheimer's disease, advanced heart and lung conditions, or other terminal diseases often need the support and broader perspective fostered through open dialogue with their doctors, caregivers, and loved ones. Families of terminally ill seniors also benefit from having honest conversations and learning more about their loved ones' conditions.

That's why this article covers a variety of topics to help you and your loved ones navigate the challenges and make the best of your remaining time. You'll learn more about what to expect, what to ask, and what to consider when making hard decisions (such as whether to fight for as much time as possible or place a higher priority on quality of life).

What Is a Terminal Illness?

Persistent, irreversible medical conditions come in two varieties: chronic and terminal. The main difference is that a chronic illness, in and of itself, isn't considered to be fatal. With treatment, many people who have chronic diseases live their full lives. In contrast, terminal conditions directly cut many people's lives short.

So, what is terminal disease? Here's a common terminal illness definition: a progressive, incurable medical condition that typically leads to death within a relatively short amount of time. Depending on the particular factors involved, terminal illnesses (also called end-stage or life-limiting diseases) can bring about the end of patients' lives days, weeks, months, or, in some cases, years after diagnosis.

Some of the most common terminal illnesses are:

- Late-stage cancers
- Advanced heart and circulatory conditions
- Dementia
- Advanced respiratory diseases
- Irreversible damage from stroke
- Advanced kidney disease
- Advanced liver disease

Additional medical conditions that merit inclusion on a terminal illness list are amyotrophic lateral sclerosis (also known as ALS or Lou Gehrig's disease), certain other neurodegenerative disorders, and some kinds of drug-resistant bacterial infections. Some viruses, such as Ebola, can also cause terminal illness.

Complications That Become Terminal

Having a combination of multiple medical conditions and/or complications that will likely lead to death in a short amount of time also qualifies as "terminally ill." In fact, someone with a progressive chronic illness may eventually experience complications that endanger his or her life. So even though a chronic illness itself is not a terminal disease, complications arising from it (such as infections) may lead to a terminal condition.

That's why Alzheimer's is a terminal illness, but Parkinson's disease is not. Alzheimer's always leads to death as a result of the disease itself, often at an earlier age than would otherwise be expected. In contrast, Parkinson's progresses in a way that, slowly, over time, reduces a person's movements until he or she can eventually no longer stand or walk. With late-stage Parkinson's, a patient becomes more vulnerable to potentially fatal complications like infection, blood clots, and falls. But Parkinson's is considered a chronic illness because the disease itself doesn't directly lead to death, and advances in treatment have greatly extended patients' life expectancies.

Similarly, Crohn's disease is not terminal, but some people eventually develop life-threatening complications from it. Diabetes is not a terminal illness, but it can cause fatal secondary conditions if it isn't managed well. And multiple sclerosis (MS) is not a terminal illness, but some patients at the advanced stage of the disease can pass away from infections or other complications.

What It All Means

Basically, a terminal medical condition is a single illness or combination of medical problems that will directly lead to death in a relatively short period of time. There are no cures for conditions like dementia or terminal cancer, meaning that people who are diagnosed with them will generally pass away a lot sooner than they would if they were healthy.

Of course, not all cancers are fatal. Many early-stage cancers can be successfully treated and put into remission. But many stage 4 (IV) cancers are terminal because they have metastasized (i.e., spread) to other regions of the body, making treatment much more difficult, ineffective, or even impossible. Any type of cancer can progress to a late stage and become fatal.

By the same token, heart disease is fatal for many older adults when it advances to a point at which effective treatment options no longer exist. That's also true for a lot of patients with other advanced organ diseases. For them, being terminally ill means not having options like organ transplants or other potentially life-saving treatments or procedures.

How Long Can a Terminally Ill Senior Live?

This can be hard to predict—even for doctors. It depends on all kinds of different factors, including the person's age, his or her particular diagnosis and treatments, the stage of the illness, and his or her other physical and/or mental conditions. In the elderly, terminal illness often leads to death in six months or less. In younger seniors, terminal diseases sometimes last longer than expected—sometimes for years. But no two terminally ill patients are exactly the same. Survival times vary for everyone.

The Trouble With Predictions

Physicians often make inaccurate predictions about their patients' survival time. In fact, numerous studies have shown that physicians tend to be too optimistic when estimating how long their terminally ill patients have to live. They frequently overestimate, which can make their prognoses unreliable.

On the other hand, some doctors are accurate in their estimates, and some are even too pessimistic. So any prognosis you receive is only an educated guess, not a precise determination of your actual longevity. Doctors try to know how much time you have to live by:

- •Looking at the median survival time of people your age, with your illness
- •Judging the progression and stage of your illness
- •Evaluating the potential impacts of other conditions you may have
- •Weighing your family history
- •Determining whether you can handle proposed treatments
- •Analyzing whether treatments may extend your survival time
- •Using intuition based on clinical experiences with similar patients

A study in the Journal of Palliative Medicine found that about 13.4 percent of terminally ill patients survive more than six months after beginning hospice care. But, like physicians, hospice teams are often inaccurate at predicting death within a specified period of time, especially when it comes to stroke and dementia patients.

According to the National Hospice and Palliative Care Organization, the median length of hospice care in the U.S. is 18 days. That means half of all hospice patients survive longer than that and half survive for less time. The median length of hospice care also varies by the type of terminal illness, as highlighted in the following examples:

- •Kidney disease: 8 days
- •Cancer: 18 days
- •Respiratory illness: 21 days
- •Stroke: 26 days
- •Heart or circulatory disease: 31 days
- •Alzheimer's, Dementia, and Parkinson's: 55 days

Survival

It's true that many terminally ill patients are able to live for a while before requiring hospice or end-of-life care. With some illnesses, it can take several months or even years to reach that point. But regardless of how long it lasts, you cannot survive a terminal illness if it was accurately diagnosed.By definition, terminal cancer is incurable (as are other terminal medical conditions). Depending on the particular circumstances, a person can survive stage 4 cancer for five years or longer. However, you cannot recover from terminal cancer if it is truly incurable and/or untreatable.After age 65, the life expectancy of a person with stage 4 cancer is often two years or less at the time of diagnosis, according to survival statistics from the National Cancer Institute n fact, only 43.8 percent of all American seniors with late-stage cancer would be expected to survive at least one year. And only about 20 percent would be expected to live at least five years. However, those numbers are for all cancers in general. Certain cancers come with significantly better or worse expectations.

For example, data from the National Cancer Institute shows that the one-year survival rate for seniors with metastatic lung cancer is 24.6 percent. And only about 4.3 percent would be expected to live five years. For late-stage pancreatic cancer (one of the deadliest types), the numbers are even worse: Only 13.6 percent of seniors would be expected to live one year, and only 1.8 percent would be expected to live five years.

So-called "medical miracles" have certainly been reported. These are cases in which patients diagnosed with terminal illnesses seem to have recovered without any logical explanation. But those types of cases are rare; they are extreme outliers. And many of them may just be the result of mistaken diagnoses, meaning that the physicians involved were wrong in their assessments. (Their patients may not have been terminally ill to begin with.)

What Are the Main Stages of Terminal Illness?

Most terminal diseases are experienced as a progression of various emotions and physical changes. But terminal illness stages can look very different from one patient to another. Each disease progresses in its own way, and not all patients experience exactly the same symptoms and changes.

For example, certain terminal illnesses are painful for some patients but not for others. And each terminal patient experiences a unique range and intensity of emotions, which can change quickly and fluctuate over time.

Mental and Emotional Stages

People respond in different ways after learning they are terminally ill. But nearly every feeling is normal. So there isn't one universal set of mental and emotional phases; they can come and go without any apparent rhyme or reason. However, most terminally ill patients do experience at least some of the following mental or emotional states, though not necessarily in this order:

•**Shock:** After being diagnosed with a terminal illness, it's common to feel surprised and disturbed. Getting that kind of news is upsetting, and it can feel very sudden, even if you thought it was a possibility beforehand.

•**Confusion:** Knowing that you're terminally ill can make you feel disoriented, kind of like being lost in time and space. You might have trouble concentrating. And some seniors experience temporary hallucinations or say or do things that are confusing to other people.

•**Denial:** You may not be able to acknowledge the uncomfortable truth of your terminal illness, at least for a little while. Denial is a natural defense mechanism when we're faced with what we deem to be an unacceptable reality.

•**Fear:** The change and uncertainty that comes with having a terminal medical condition can definitely be scary. After all, you might be afraid of what will happen to you physically, whether you'll be in pain, how your illness will affect your family, what death will be like, and more. Your fear may trigger feelings of anxiety, distress, restlessness, and agitation as you ponder your future.

•**Anger:** Some terminally ill patients look for people or things to blame for their conditions. They may even resent the healthy people around them or feel irritated by having to disrupt their plans, hobbies, lifestyles, or relationships in order to deal with their illnesses.

•**Hope:** Many seniors with terminal illnesses eventually feel a sense of optimism about their future, which can certainly be a positive way of coping. But for some patients, hope can manifest as bargaining; that is, they would give or do anything in exchange for a cure or extra time, even when all of the evidence points to that not being a realistic possibility.

•**Frustration:** Knowing that you can't change the reality of your terminal medical condition can create a significant amount of inner tension, making you feel annoyed. That can be especially true when you have to cancel plans or do things in a different way than you ordinarily would.

•**Guilt:** Terminally ill seniors often feel like they are a burden on their families and caregivers, blaming themselves for the adversity experienced by others due to their conditions.

•**Helplessness:** You might have days when you feel powerless or extra vulnerable, without a sense of control over your life.

•**Sadness or depression:** It's common to feel down in the dumps when you have a terminal disease.

But some patients feel sad or disinterested in their daily activities for more than two weeks at a time, which can mean they have clinical depression.

•**Detachment:** Feeling a general sense of indifference, some terminally ill seniors stop pursuing social engagements or try to avoid even simple interpersonal interactions.

•**Loneliness:** Some patients think that nobody could truly understand what they are experiencing, so they avoid socializing or sharing their feelings with others. Or they may feel isolated, even if they have the support of people who care about them.

•**Reflectiveness:** Confronted with your mortality, you may ponder the meaning and purpose of your life. That might involve thinking about cherished memories and all of the people, events, and achievements that have mattered most to you. You might also begin to question your personal philosophies or spiritual beliefs.

•**Regret:** Reflection can lead to many positive feelings, but it can also lead to feelings of remorse, disappointment, or dissatisfaction. For example, you might regret personal conflicts that haven't been resolved or major goals that you haven't fulfilled.

•**Acceptance:** Eventually, some terminally ill seniors are able to fully acknowledge their mortality and embrace their approaching deaths. Once they do, they often feel more positive, at peace, and in greater control of their circumstances.

Combined with a terminally ill senior's spiritual convictions, intense emotions can sometimes play a role in bringing about dreams or visions that seem to have deep meaning. Often, such experiences are comforting. But having confusing or upsetting dreams or visions is sometimes a side effect of medication or a sign of a new, underlying medical complication that needs attention.

Physical Changes

The physical experiences of terminally ill patients vary widely. Each circumstance is different. Some people have a relatively smooth transition to the end of life; others have challenging complications. But with proper care, most challenges can be managed in a way that greatly improves a patient's level of comfort.

Still, it's helpful to know what you might experience. That way, you aren't caught off guard by physical changes that you weren't expecting.For example, terminal cancer symptoms are often wide-ranging, but many patients experience worsening pain and fatigue as their conditions progress. They also may experience fatal complications. That's because cancer can cause death in a variety of ways. Depending on where it has spread in your body, terminal cancer kills you by triggering irreversible complications like:

•Anemia
•Infections
•Brain impairment
•Severe dehydration
•Uncontrolled bleeding
•Severe malnutrition
•Organ failure (such as of the heart, lungs, or liver)
•Blood clots that cause stroke or obstruction of an artery

Other terminal diseases can cause the same or similar complications, especially as patients get closer to passing away. But most of the physical changes caused by terminal conditions aren't directly fatal; they may just be indications that the body is compensating as best as it can. For example, in the final months, weeks, or days of life, a terminally ill senior might experience or display symptoms such as:

•Pain
•Nausea
•Constipation
•Fatigue
•Dry mouth
•Loss of bladder control
•Difficulty swallowing
•Weight loss
•Swelling and puffiness
•Noisy breathing
•Weakness
•Shortness of breath
•Loss of appetite
•Feeling too hot or cold

Pain isn't experienced by all terminally ill patients. But it can come about in a lot of different ways. For instance, it may come on suddenly and dissipate in a matter of weeks, days, or hours. Or it may come on gradually or intermittently and last for the length of a patient's remaining life.

Pain can be caused by inflammation or damage to nerves, bones, or organs. It can also "break through" when a patient is on painkillers. And pain can be felt in one area of the body even though the root cause is in a different area. But regardless of a person's condition, pain and other symptoms can often be managed through proper treatment and care.

When it comes to a terminally ill senior's last hours or minutes of life, loved ones and caregivers may notice changes such as:

- Cold hands and feet
- Blotchy or pale-blue skin
- Loud, "rattly" breathing

- Unconsciousness
- Slow, shallow, inconsistent breathing
- Delirium or out-of-character behavior

What Should I Do After Being Diagnosed With a **Terminal Illness?**

It's normal to wonder how to move forward when presented with the unpleasant revelation of your terminal condition. You might feel stuck in time, unsure of the actions to take next. But take heart; you can reclaim a sense of control. Your goal should be to eliminate as much uncertainty as possible while drawing upon the strength of others. That way, you can make room for greater comfort and peace of mind for you and your loved ones. Here's how to achieve that:

1. Get a second opinion.

Doctors and other medical professionals aren't perfect. Sometimes they get things wrong. And this is your life we're talking about. So you shouldn't have to wonder about your diagnosis.

By getting a second opinion from a doctor at a different institution, you'll either get your diagnosis confirmed or learn that your medical condition might be something else. If your terminal illness is confirmed, you'll know for sure—eliminating some of your doubts. And if the second opinion includes roughly the same prognosis, you'll probably have a better idea of how much time you have left.

2. Ask for honesty.

The truth isn't always easy to hear. Even so, the vast majority of patients with advanced cancer want accurate and honest communication about their prognosis, according to an article in the Annals of Palliative Medicine. (The same is probably true of other terminally ill patients.)

Yet, according to a study in the Journal of Clinical Oncology, very few patients fully understand their prognosis unless it is discussed with the appropriate physicians on an ongoing basis. In part, that's because many doctors lean too heavily in the direction of optimism (at least initially), sometimes sugarcoating what a prognosis actually means. They're afraid to crush their patients' hopes.

When discussing terminal diagnoses, doctors do tell patients they are dying. But they don't always say it so bluntly or directly. For instance, instead of telling a patient that he or she will likely pass away in under a year, a doctor might say that the illness probably isn't curable. Unfortunately, that can provide a patient with just enough hope to move him or her in a direction that is more destructive than beneficial.

For example, without a candid prognosis, a patient may decide to pursue costly or risky treatments that aren't supported with scientific evidence or that greatly reduce his or her remaining quality of life. Or a patient might not take the time to consider or plan for the kind of end-of-life care that he or she would really want—and deserve.

According to the Stanford ML Group, about 80 percent of Americans want to live their last days at home, yet as many as 60 percent of all deaths occur in acute-care hospitals. And most of those hospital patients receive aggressive treatments in their last days. Such treatments often do little to extend patients' lives by any significant margin. Instead, they frequently prolong the suffering in an environment that is anything but peaceful.

So as a terminally ill patient, it may be in your best interests to insist on honesty from your physicians. Get them to tell it to you straight, no matter how difficult the news will be to hear. Ask about the full range of potential outcomes. Or at least specify how much knowledge you want your doctors to share with you.

That way, you'll be more grounded when considering your next steps. And you'll likely have more of an opportunity to make arrangements, such as for palliative care, that can maximize your quality of life going forward.

(Many terminally ill patients and families that are driven by unjustified hope and the potential of alternative, experimental, or aggressive treatments try to schedule palliative care when it's too late. That can result in medical crises, distressing visits to the hospital, and unpeaceful death.)

Discuss your care and treatment options.

After the initial shock of your diagnosis wears off, schedule appointments with your doctors in order to have conversations about the courses of action that are available and realistic for you. Depending on your condition, you may have the option of pursuing treatments to extend your life or shifting your focus entirely to the management of your symptoms. (You also may have the option of pursuing both symptom management and ongoing treatment concurrently.)

But in order to make that kind of decision, you should learn all you can about what to expect from your particular illness as it progresses. Your doctors can talk to you about subjects like:

- Continuing treatment: Being terminally ill means not having access to curative treatments. At best, certain treatments might extend your life a little, potentially giving you some extra weeks, months, or years. But there is often a tradeoff for that extra time: lower quality of life. That's because many treatments come with negative side effects that can make it difficult or impossible to carry out normal daily activities or have any fun. For some patients, clinical trials for experimental treatments are an option. But a lot of clinical trials come with low odds of success. Some clinical trial patients die even sooner than they would without the experimental treatment.

•**Potential care environments:** Your residential and caregiving options may be limited by the type of illness and symptoms you have. For example, certain kinds of pain can only be managed effectively in hospitals, nursing homes, or other settings with skilled nurses on hand. But if you have the option, you might prefer to receive care at home or in an assisted living facility that feels more comfortable and familiar to you. As your illness progresses, however, your options may change.

•**Palliative care:** This type of care is all about soothing, managing, or alleviating the symptoms of terminally ill patients so that they can have the best quality of life possible during their remaining time. Palliative care professionals can also help connect terminally ill seniors and their families with spiritual, psychological, and social assistance. Patients can schedule palliative care right after they're diagnosed if they want, and they can receive it while also undergoing treatments. Plus, receiving palliative care makes it less likely that you'll need to be hospitalized or visit the emergency room.

•**Hospice care:** With this type of care, the emphasis is also on palliative support and quality of life. But patients don't receive it until they have stopped treatments and are expected to pass away in a matter of months, weeks, or days. The focus is solely on providing compassion, peace, and comfort, rather than pursuing any potential cures or life extensions. Depending on a patient's needs and wishes, hospice care can take place in a special hospice facility, in a skilled-nursing environment, or even at home. A hospice team often includes a variety of health and support professionals, such as doctors, nurses, counselors, social workers, aides, and volunteers.

•Physician-assisted dying: Currently, this option is only available in a few states. Also known as "death with dignity," it stirs a lot of controversy, even in the states where it is legal. In fact, many doctors are totally against this option. But some terminally ill seniors view physician-assisted dying as a compassionate and desirable choice, enabling them to pass away where and when they want—before their symptoms make it impossible to decide things for themselves or to have the minimum quality of life that they find acceptable.

Figure out what matters most to you going forward.

Some people are fighters all the way to the end, doing anything possible to extend their lives. Others seek to maximize the quality of their remaining time, even if it means they might die a little sooner. And a lot of people choose a path somewhere in the middle—pursuing reasonable treatments up until a certain point, then shifting their focus toward having a "good death."

Remember: You probably can't predict how much time you really have left. And not all "life-extending" treatments work. Sometimes, they do the opposite of what they're meant to do and make patients feel worse on a day-to-day basis. On the other hand, some terminally ill seniors live much longer than anyone expects without pursuing any extra treatments. A focus on quality of life can sometimes have positive, life-extending impacts on people's minds and bodies.

So, after talking about the various options with your doctors, it's really important to prioritize what you want. How do the potential benefits and downsides of each possible course of action align with what you envision for your remaining time? Will they aid or obstruct your deepest wishes? Your priorities may differ from other terminally ill adults you've known. And that's OK. For example, different patients have top priorities as diverse as:

•Proving that they're fighters
•Staying alive long enough for particular events or milestones
•Nurturing their relationships
•Being mentally present for and with the people they love
•Resolving conflicts
•Having fun
•Finishing major creative projects
•Traveling to places they've always wanted to see
•Crossing off items on their bucket lists
•Achieving other long-held goals
•Enjoying an ordinary day-to-day routine
•Helping others do what they love
•Living as comfortably and privately as possible

Many terminally ill seniors find that it helps to talk about all of this with a mental health professional. A licensed counselor or therapist can help you sort out your feelings and imagine a path forward.

Make a care plan.

With your top priorities figured out, you can start supporting them. Whether that means getting treatment, scheduling palliative care, or doing a combination of both, taking action to cope with your terminal illness will help ground you. Plus, the plans you make now don't have to be set in stone. As you move forward, you might change your mind or discover that you need types of support that you hadn't considered before.

When making your plan, think about where and how you want to be cared for, especially as your illness progresses and makes you less independent. Be realistic about your options, reflecting on your discussions with your doctors. And consider who you want to be around, what kind of spiritual support you'll need (if any), and who might be able to carry some of the burden on your behalf.

Also, remember that there may come a point at which you no longer have the physical and/or mental ability to inform people of your wishes or to handle your own affairs. That's why it's a good idea to explore giving someone you trust power of attorney (POA). It's also smart to prepare advance directives so that there are no questions about your wishes when it comes to end-of-life medical decisions.

Planning all of this stuff now will help you and your family; things will just feel a little easier for everyone. And if you have the financial resources to afford it, you can even hire a care manager to help arrange and coordinate all aspects of your care going forward. A care manager can act as your advocate, interacting with you, your loved ones, your doctors, and other people who are part of your support team.

6. Decide who to tell.

Mortality isn't an easy subject to discuss. In fact, according to a survey by The Conversation Project, even though more than 90 percent of people believe it's important to discuss end-of-life care with loved ones, only about a third of people actually ever have. But, of course, being diagnosed with a terminal illness kind of forces the issue.

So it's normal to feel apprehensive about sharing your news with others. But even though telling people that you're terminally ill can be hard, it can also provide some comfort. After all, it can relieve you of some of the mental burden you've been carrying around, and it can deepen your connections with the people who care about you.

Keep in mind that you don't necessarily have to tell everybody all at once. You may decide that, at least ber that it's OK to show your feelings. Don't worry if you're unable to answer all the questions you receive. Some terminally ill seniors find it beneficial to have a counselor or care manager present when telling friends and loved ones about their conditions and the plans they've started making. It can also help to discuss your end-of-life options with people you love and trust before finalizing any plans. The Conversation Project offers a conversation starter guide that provides a useful framework for preparing to have this kind of discussion.

7. Prepare advance directives.

Also known as a living will, an advance directive is a legal document that expresses what you want to happen in the event that end-of-life decisions need to be made when you're unable to speak for yourself. Combined with a durable power of attorney for medical care, advance directives help ensure that your wishes will be adhered to.

For example, you may or may not want to be resuscitated in the event that your heart stops beating or you stop breathing. You may or may not want to be hooked up to a ventilator or other forms of life support under various circumstances. Or you may or may not want a feeding tube or certain interventions for failing organs, such as dialysis for kidney failure.

Discuss various scenarios with your doctors (and loved ones if you want). Then, complete the appropriate advance directive forms for your state and make sure all the important people in your life know about them.

Alternatively, in some states, you have the option of completing much more comprehensive orders for your end-of-life care. Known as Physician Orders for Life-Sustaining Treatment (POLST) or by similar names, this option can offer clear guidance to doctors and family members when medical situations aren't as well defined, such as whether to hospitalize you or provide certain treatments in the event that you get a serious infection like pneumonia.

Having advance directives can make things easier for your loved ones, lessening the guilt they feel and minimizing conflicts with each other. It can also help maximize the quality of your end-of-life care.

8. Enlist support.

If and when you feel comfortable enough to share your news with a wider audience, don't hesitate to ask for help. People are often eager to provide any support they can to those they know with terminal medical conditions. Even simple or routine tasks like doing laundry, getting groceries, caring for a pet, or cooking meals can make the people in your circle feel valued and useful. And soliciting that kind of support can enhance and maintain your social well-being as your illness progresses.Social media platforms like Facebook can help you reach out and keep your friends, acquaintances, and loved ones informed and connected. Or you can set up a free private website through CaringBridge for sharing updates, making requests, and receiving messages of encouragement.

9. Get everything else in order.

In addition to your care plans and medical directives, you need to start thinking about a variety of other practical issues. For example, what do you want to happen after you pass away? Consider questions such as:

•Do I want a traditional funeral or memorial service?
•Do I prefer burial or cremation?
•Should I make my own funeral arrangements?
•Am I covered by life or final expense insurance?
•Have I drawn up my will? Does it need any updates?
•Do I have the financial resources to pay for any out-of-pocket care expenses?
•Who should get my pets when I'm gone?
•How should I handle my social media accounts?
•Should I name a digital executor who can manage my online accounts when I'm gone?

The more you get in order now, the greater peace of mind you can enjoy during the rest of your remaining time. So it's wise to consult with a trusted attorney, financial planner, and any other professional who can help sort out your affairs.For instance, maybe you have questions about your life insurance or long-term care (LTC) insurance coverage. A trusted legal or financial professional can examine your existing policies and help you understand them. As an example, you can learn more about how, in term insurance, "terminal illness" is generally defined as one of the life-ending situations that is covered if you were diagnosed with it after activating your policy.

Or maybe you have critical illness insurance that you can tap into in order to help pay for various expenses that aren't covered through Medicare, Medicaid, or other means. Generally, critical illness covers most life-altering medical conditions, including terminal diseases. However, like most insurance policies, critical illness plans often come with some exclusions, so you need to read the fine print in order to make sure that your particular illness is one of the covered conditions.

Of course, some terminally ill seniors are still part of the workforce when they're diagnosed with their conditions. If you're one of them, you may wonder about things like your pension or employee disability benefits. Depending on your employer's particular plan, you can get your pension
if you are terminally ill and already at retirement age. Some pension programs also allow employees to access their funds early if they have a terminal illness and haven't yet reached their plan's defined retirement age.

Terminally ill seniors with employee disability benefits can often receive funds if they are unable to continue working for the remainder of their lives, a condition often termed "total permanent disability" (TPD). Usually, TPD covers cancer (at the late stages), dementia, advanced heart disease, and many other types of terminal medical conditions when they become debilitating and effective treatments are no longer available.

Stay active and engaged.

Having fun and staying socially connected—as much as possible—is essential for enhancing your quality of life. Regardless of whether you're getting treatments or just managing your symptoms, staying engaged in life's daily activities will help you feel like you still matter. A lot of seniors with terminal illnesses go about this by:

•Playing games
•Doing crafts
•Finding old friends
•Traveling while they're still able to
•Playing with their dogs
•Taking up yoga
•Gardening
•Bird-watching
•Learning new hobbies
•Writing letters or making videos for their friends and family
•Attending social gatherings
•Finishing creative projects

Incidentally, you can get travel insurance if you have terminal cancer or another terminal illness. However, under most policies, you generally can't make a claim for anything that is a direct result of your condition. For instance, you may not be covered for any costs arising from being treated or hospitalized for your terminal illness when traveling.
On another note, it can be useful to maintain a daily diary of your pain and other symptoms. That way, you and your doctors will be able to more accurately assess how quickly or slowly your illness is progressing. The practice of keeping a diary may also help you stay more mindful of the present moment and less inclined to look too far ahead.

How Can I Cope Emotionally With My Terminal Illness?

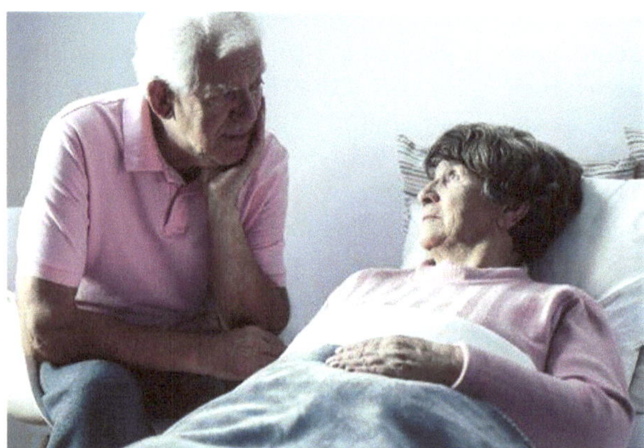

Fig.20.1 Husband is trying to console his wife who is suffering from terminal illness

Following the 10 steps above will go a long way toward helping you cope. Just keep in mind that it's normal and healthy to experience a full range of emotions, even the uncomfortable ones. In fact, effectively coping with terminal illness may require fully embracing the difficult emotions (at least temporarily) instead of trying to push them away When you're living with a terminal illness, inspirational words can certainly be nice to hear or read. But for some patients, a kind of "inspiration fatigue" can set in and eventually do more to lower their spirits than raise them. After all, with so much positivity coming at you, it can start to feel like you're doing things wrong—especially if your experience doesn't match the stories you read or see on TV about the most upbeat patients, some of whom have seemingly even cheated death. All of the inspiring and cheerful portrayals of terminally ill patients in the media can also make you feel like you have to constantly show a positive and hopeful attitude in order to get any sympathy. As a result, you may feel tempted to pretend that you're upbeat and optimistic, even when you don't feel that way. But, in most situations, your job isn't to prevent other people's uncomfortable feelings about your illness. Your job is to be fully you. Whether positive, negative, or somewhere in between, your emotions can help you and other people better understand your current reality. Pretending that your difficult emotions don't exist can become exhausting and lead to problems like depression. "Thinking positive" and "faking it 'til you make it" may work for some people, but you shouldn't feel bad if it doesn't work for you. We're all different

A lot of terminally ill seniors do best when they utilize a variety of coping tactics. For example, you might try:

•**Listening to your favorite music:** The songs and compositions you love most can provide a lot of comfort and therapeutic benefit. According to Harvard Health Publishing, research has shown that music therapy can benefit patients both physically and emotionally. So it may be worthwhile to find a certified music therapist in your area.

•**Getting acceptance and commitment therapy (ACT):** With this type of therapy, the emphasis is on helping you learn how to lessen the impact of your distressing emotions and troubling thoughts. Rather than trying to change or challenge them, you learn how to observe and accept them, as well as commit to actions that serve your values and best interests. You may be able to find an ACT therapist near you.

•**Having deep conversations with close friends and family:** Sometimes, you might just need to cry on the shoulder of a loved one or have an open, honest, and generous discussion with a friend in which you both listen intently and share your most intimate feelings. The more you help your loved ones understand what you're going through, the better they can comfort you and support your coping strategies.

•**Talking to your caregivers and/or a counselor:** When talking to your friends or loved ones feels too challenging, it can help to ask other people in your sphere of support to listen to your thoughts and share their own. Some of your nurses, care aides, doctors, or other people on your care team are likely good candidates for this. You may also want to ask for a referral to a good geriatric counselor who specializes in helping seniors cope with the emotional difficulties of medical problems.

•**Speaking with a spiritual advisor:** Having conversations with a clergyperson or leader of your faith can be very comforting, especially if you're feeling scared or confused about death or the purpose or meaning of your life. But you don't necessarily have to be a follower of any particular religion to benefit from this kind of discussion. If you want, you can simply take what sounds wise or useful to you and ignore the parts that don't align with your own spirituality.

•**Joining support groups:** For many terminally ill older adults, talking to other people who are in the same kind of situation is a powerful way to feel a little more normal and a lot less isolated. That's why, when you're trying to cope with a terminal illness, support groups can be invaluable. Some hospitals, charities, hospice organizations, and community centers offer in-person and/or online support groups. Your doctors, nurses, caregivers, counselor,or therapist should be able to recommend some options based on your particular situation.

•**Getting pet therapy:** You don't necessarily need a full-time animal companion in order to reap the emotional benefits of having one. If any of your friends or family have friendly, cuddly pets, see whether you can arrange to visit them or have them come to you. Or ask around for a local volunteer organization that can bring trained therapy animals to your home or care setting.

•**Maintaining a normal routine:** You might benefit from focusing on creating as much day-to-day stability as possible. Give yourself simple tasks that you can do at the same times each day. Combine practical tasks (such as making a basic breakfast) with some things you'll look forward to (such as playing a game, reading a book, or having a favorite drink). These simple pleasures will help remind you that every day that you're still alive can be a true gift.

•**Resolving personal conflicts:** Maybe you need to free yourself of the burdensome feelings that come from having unresolved problems with people from your past and/or present. By making an effort to forgive or apologize to those you've cared about, you may be able to lighten the emotional load you've been carrying.

•**Thinking about your best memories:** Your most positive experiences can still resonate and have a profound impact on your current feelings. You may just need a little help resurrecting them. For example, try looking through old photos, reading personal letters you've received, talking with old friends, or even traveling to some of the places that have a lot of significance for you.

•**Sharing your stories and the wisdom you've acquired:** Your younger friends and family members will likely appreciate learning more about your life and what you have learned along the way. But reflecting on your life and sharing your experiences and insights can benefit you as well by giving you a comforting sense of purpose, meaning, and satisfaction.

•**Reading profound or uplifting books:** The world is full of amazing writers, many of whom have shared their own truths, experiences, and insights in heartfelt memoirs or other books of wisdom. Plus, some books are available in audio format, which is useful if you have poor eyesight, have trouble focusing while reading, or simply prefer to listen to someone else's voice. Here are some of the books that are often recommended for terminally ill patients and their loved ones:

What Should I Do If My Friend or Loved One Is Terminally Ill?

First, don't panic. You can get through this. Many people like you are going through the same thing as they face the unwanted reality of their friends' or family members' terminal illnesses. In fact, it's a fairly common experience, especially among adult children of terminally ill seniors. So you aren't alone if you don't quite know how to talk to a parent with terminal cancer or any other kind of terminal condition.

Nobody wants the people they care about to die. Yet, in at least one way, a diagnosis of a terminal illness can be a gift for patients and their loved ones. After all, it gives you a little time to prepare yourselves and say goodbye in the way you both want. By contrast, a sudden, unexpected death would give you no chance at all to do that.

Still, this is not an easy experience. Even though your friend or family member is the one with the terminal illness, you'll likely be profoundly impacted. So it's essential to know how to navigate the experience in a way that helps foster the greatest possible well-being for you and the terminally ill person you care about. Here are some of the approaches that often work best:

1. Show up and just listen.

Your presence may be all that's necessary to comfort the person you love. You may not have to say or do anything except provide hugs and listen without judgment. You don't have to ask questions or offer advice or go out of your way to demonstrate your love or usefulness. And you don't have to play the role of therapist or spiritual counselor.

Let your friend or loved one choose when to share his or her thoughts and feelings with you. You can invite that kind of sharing, but don't try to force it. When the sharing does happen, stay open and allow it to take whatever form it wants to.

Even if a flood of confusing or distressing thoughts and emotions are being shared—such as fear or denial—let them come, without interrupting the flow or trying to offer solutions or a sunnier perspective. Simply provide a safe space for the person you care about to release and process those feelings.

2. Learn about the kind of care and support your friend or loved one needs.

By showing that you're open, nonjudgmental, and happy to listen, you create an atmosphere of trust in which the other person feels comfortable talking about what he or she really wants and needs. That's when you can discover how to best lend your support going forward.

Some terminally ill seniors want help deciding what to do about their treatments, care, or other affairs. But many others simply want to be supported in what they have already decided to do. Listen, learn, and figure out how to define your role in a way that aligns with your friend or family member's wishes.

It could be that you simply need to be present or help foster a sense of normalcy. Or, on the other end of the spectrum, perhaps you need to be more involved in handling practical matters or advocating for the best care possible on behalf of the person you love. Just remember that it's usually better to let him or her make that decision.

3. Nurture the best qualities of your relationship while keeping an open mind to potential changes.

Every relationship has its own special dynamics. In the face of a terminal illness, the most positive points of connection are needed more than ever. It's a time to build upon your existing bond with the other person, creating more bridges while finding gentle ways of working around any obstacles.

Through it all, remember that his or her personality may seem to change in ways that alter the relationship dynamic. But if you accept those changes, you might have the opportunity to deepen the relationship and make it stronger.

4. Find healthy ways to cope with your own grief.

There's no question about it: You will experience a range of emotions that may challenge your ability to handle the circumstances. But many of the tips above for coping emotionally with a terminal illness can help you just as much as your friend or loved one. It's vital to prioritize your own self-care so that you can provide the best support possible to the terminally ill senior in your life.

Remember that it's normal to feel guilt, worry, sadness, and other troubling emotions in this situation. But if the stress starts to feel overwhelming or you find it difficult to carry out your own day-to-day activities, it's imperative that you seek help from a professional counselor or therapist. Otherwise, you run the risk of becoming depressed or even physically unwell.

Prioritize getting enough sleep, eating healthy, and staying physically active. Daily exercise can help lower your stress and elevate your mood.

5. Seek unity with your family.

When someone is diagnosed with a terminal illness, the impact on his or her entire family can be immense. In fact, it can reignite long-held conflicts or resentments, causing extra turmoil at a time when the opposite is needed. After all, family members often have to work out who will take on various financial and caregiving issues. Plus, when everyone is feeling heightened stress and emotion, communication can break down, patience can wear thin, and misunderstandings can reign supreme.

That's why it can be useful to hire an objective third party, such as a family therapist and/or geriatric care manager—someone to help the family navigate the grieving process and any practical matters that must be handled. But even without the help of a professional, it's possible to work toward family unity.

Focus on communicating openly and honestly. Listen attentively. Remind each other that your loved one needs all of you to come together. And look at this time as an opportunity to heal old wounds and move forward in a generous spirit of unconditional love, perhaps in new or redefined roles.

6. Speak with care and compassion while avoiding common pitfalls.

Knowing what to say to someone with terminal cancer or another terminal illness can definitely be challenging. As previously mentioned, you may not have to say anything at all. But when you do speak, it's often essential to pay special attention to how you're saying something. Give your friend or loved one your full attention and keep your body language open and relaxed so that you don't appear defensive or aggressive.

In terms of what you say, always remember that the person you care about is going through a unique experience. Trying to relay a story about someone else's similar situation can make you seem uncaring or out of touch. Your friend or loved one wants you to understand his or her distinctive experience. By the same token, try to avoid implying that the person's terminal illness was somehow caused by his or her choices or brought about as part of some grand cosmic plan.

Sometimes, the best things to talk about are joyful memories or funny or fascinating current events, movies, or TV shows. Try to share some laughs. And if you want to offer words of hope and encouragement, always be sensitive to the reality of the situation. (Don't push the belief that a miracle will happen.)

7. Don't intervene or offer solutions unless it's requested or becomes absolutely necessary.

Your friend or family member may already have a solid plan in place. Respect it. You may not agree with all of his or her choices, but it isn't your life that's coming to an end.

You don't need to actively research potential cures or treatments. In fact, it's better if you don't—unless you're asked to. The person you care about may be putting a lot of effort toward accepting the reality of the situation and probably already knows about the various options. Allow the terminally ill senior you care about to choose his or her own final journey.

Only consider intervening if essential responsibilities aren't being handled or you see clear signs of self-neglect or elder abuse that run counter to your friend or loved one's wishes or that unnecessarily harm his or her remaining quality of life.

For instance, some terminally ill people (and/or well-meaning family members) fall victim to costly scams and misleading marketing for so-called "miracle" cures or treatments that aren't actually supported with substantial peer-reviewed scientific evidence. That's because the hope for a miracle can make terminally ill people and their loved ones more gullible than they otherwise would be.

Such scams can not only drain financial resources, but also cause medical harm that shortens a terminally ill patient's life even more or leads to new symptoms or complications that must be managed. For example, a lot of unproven treatments are related to things like essential oils, supplements, special diets, and energy-based therapies.

8. Ask about your friend or loved one's end-of-life preferences.

Don't assume that the person you care about will want you to be present at the time of his or her death. Some people prefer to pass away in private. So it's best to discuss this subject ahead of time, keeping in mind that terminally ill people sometimes change their minds as they get closer to the end.

9. Accept that the moment of death is out of your control.

Even if your friend or loved one wants you present at the end, it is unrealistic to be at his or her side on a constant basis. You'll need to take care of yourself, which includes eating, getting enough sleep, going for short walks, and taking care of your own basic bodily functions.

It's perfectly OK to take breaks and let other people maintain a presence in your place. Simply say "I love you" each time you take a break and leave the room.

Embrace the reality that the person you love may pass away while you're gone. If that's what happens, don't beat yourself up. You haven't let your friend or family member down. It's beyond your control.

But if you do happen to be present for the end, remember that the actual moment of death isn't always easy to detect. It may require confirmation from a nurse or physician.

10. Give your friend or loved one the space, comfort, and permission to let go.

Some terminally ill patients try to hang on as long as possible for the sake of their loved ones. They often don't feel right about giving up the struggle while those they care about are still hanging around and supporting them. That's why you and your family might need to give your terminally ill loved one the permission to move on.

Even if he or she is unconscious, your words may be heard, and your presence may be felt. So it doesn't hurt to say that it's OK to let go, perhaps while gently stroking your loved one's arm and holding his or her hand. And if you think or know that your loved one wants privacy in order to feel comfortable passing on, go ahead and provide it.

11. Get support when your friend or family member passes on.

If you're present for the moment of death, take the time you need to sit with your loved one. You don't have to notify anyone right away. But as soon as you're ready, be sure to let the appropriate professionals know so that the death can be medically confirmed.

You've likely done a lot of grieving up to this point, but you still may not feel prepared for the moment your friend or loved one actually passes on. So don't hesitate to reach out to others for emotional support. Many people find it helpful to talk with a grief counselor.

How Do I Make Difficult Decisions About End-of-Life Care?

The answer to this question usually comes down to the potential amount of additional suffering involved. However, a lot of people don't give this subject the deep consideration it deserves—until it's too late. In fact, in a survey by Pew Research Center, nearly a third of Americans said that "everything possible" should always be done to save someone's life. Yet, in a lot of situations, "everything possible" can greatly reduce a terminally ill patient's remaining quality of life.

That's why it helps to ask questions that can provide more clarity, such as:

•Should painful or uncomfortable medical interventions be carried out if they aren't likely to extend a person's life for any significant period of time?

•Might quality of life be more important than quantity of life?

Here's something you may not know: A lot of physicians who become terminally ill choose to forgo the kind of aggressive end-of-life care that many of their own patients expect to receive. They view a lot of treatments as futile, costly, excessive, and likely to cause unnecessary suffering and a less-than-peaceful death. For example, consider these common situations that are often caused by a "do everything possible" approach:

•When breathing stops: A tube may be put down a patient's windpipe and attached to a ventilator in order to force his or her lungs to function. But since having a tube down your throat can be a miserable experience when you're awake, sedation is often needed. And many patients need to have their arms restrained so that they don't try to rip the tube out.

•When the heart stops: If a defibrillator isn't immediately available, then CPR (cardiopulmonary resuscitation) might be performed. But the amount of effort that is required to perform effective chest compressions can cause painful injuries such as collapsed lungs or broken ribs. Plus, CPR is often unsuccessful when performed on seniors who are already battling other medical conditions.

•When eating or drinking stops: A feeding tube may be inserted in order to supply nutrition. But one kind of feeding tube comes with risks like nausea, infection, and pneumonia. And the other type of feeding tube can be so uncomfortable that restraints are required.

The most aggressive end-of-life interventions tend to take place in hospitals. That's why, on average, it costs about $32,000 to keep a terminally ill patient alive in a hospital during his or her final month, according to Arcadia. In a nursing home, it costs about $21,000. In contrast, care in a hospice facility costs less than $20,000, and home care costs less than $5,000. Choosing palliative care at home or in a hospice facility also tends to result in a more peaceful and comfortable death.

When a terminally ill patient is unconscious and put on a life-support system, such as a ventilator, decisions for his or her family members can become especially difficult. That's why it's essential to think about all of this ahead of time. If you are terminally ill, make sure you consider preparing advance directives so that you minimize the chances of your family members having to make these kinds of decisions on your behalf.Request an open and honest conversation with your doctors about all of the potential end-of-life interventions and the benefits and drawbacks of each one. And make sure you understand what each type of advance directive covers so that you can prepare them according to your wishes, leaving as few gaps as possible. (For example, many people don't realize that a feeding tube is not included in a do-not-resuscitate (DNR) order. Typically, a DNR only covers interventions such as CPR, defibrillation, breathing tubes, and certain medications.)

You should also know that, upon admission, all medical facilities in the U.S. are required to provide patients with information about their decision-making rights. They must ask you whether you have any advance directives. And they must comply with those directives.

You have the right to refuse any kind of medical intervention. Always make sure that your physicians, nurses, and family members know your wishes when it comes to the specific kinds of end-of-life interventions you do or do not want to receive.

If you are a family member of a terminally ill patient who is incapacitated and hard decisions need to be made in the absence of appropriate advance directives, then it's important to ask good questions. For example, depending on the situation, your questions may need to center on issues like:

•What may happen if certain treatments or interventions are started, continued, or stopped

•How long a certain course of action might realistically extend the person's life without reducing the quality of it

•Whether particular interventions will cause additional suffering or introduce new risks and side effects

•What could happen if a particular intervention doesn't work

It helps to have just one person in a family act as the point of contact for the medical team. It's also important to let medical staff know about any of your distinctive family traditions, preferences, or cultural beliefs related to dying.

But here's one of the most essential tips: Don't stop with this article. This subject is so nuanced, complex, and emotionally charged that you really should learn about it in a more in-depth way, from people with deep knowledge and relevant experience in these matters.

Bibliography and Acknowledgement

- Abdul - Razzak A, Sherifali D, You J, Simon J, Brazil K. 'Talk to me': a mixed methods study on preferred physician behaviours during end - of - life communication from the patient perspective. Health Expect. 2016;19:883 - 896. [PMC free article] [PubMed] [Google Scholar]
- Brumley R, Enguidanos S, Jamison P, et al. Increased satisfaction with care and lower costs: results of a randomized trial of in - home palliative care. J Am Geriatr Soc. 2007;55:993 - 1000. [PubMed] [Google Scholar]
- Cardona - Morrell M, Kim J, Anstey M, Mitchell I, Hillman K. Non - beneficial treatments in hospital at the end of life – A systematic review and meta - analysis on extent of the problem. Int J Qual Health Care. 2016;28:456 - 469. [PubMed] [Google Scholar]
- Duffield CM, Twigg DE, Pugh JD, Evans G, Dimitrelis S, Roche MA. The Use of unregulated staff: time for regulation? Policy Polit Nurs Pract. 2014;15:42 - 48. [PubMed] [Google Scholar]
- Epstein RM, Fiscella K, Lesser CS, Stange KC. Why the nation needs a policy push on patient - centered health care. Health Aff. 2010;29:1489 - 1495. [PubMed] [Google Scholar] Foreman LM, Hunt RW, Luke CG, Roder DM. Factors predictive of preferred place of death in the general population of South Australia. Palliat Med. 2006;20:447 - 453. [PubMed] [Google Scholar]
- Glass DC, Kelsall HL, Slegers C, et al. A telephone survey of factors affecting willingness to participate in health research surveys. BMC Public Health. 2015;15:1017. [PMC free article] [PubMed] [Google Scholar]
- Hillman K, Chen J. Conflict resolution in end of life treatment decisions: an Evidence Check rapid review brokered by the Sax Institute for the Centre for Epidemiology and Research. Sydney: The Sax Institute; 2008. [Google Scholar]
- Jeffs L, Saragosa M, Law MP, Kuluski K, Espin S, Merkley J. The role of caregivers in interfacility care transitions: a qualitative study. Patient Prefer Adherence. 2017;11:1443 - 1450. [PMC free article] [PubMed] [Google Scholar]
- Kelley AS, McGarry K, Fahle S, Marshall SM, Du Q, Skinner JS. Out - of - pocket spending in the last five years of life. J Gen Intern Med. 2013;28:304 - 309. [PMC free article] [PubMed] [Google Scholar]
- Lambert C, Jomeen J, McSherry W. Reflexivity: A review of the literature in the context of midwifery research. British Journal of Midwifery. 2010;18:321 - 326. [Google Scholar]
- Mold JW. Facilitating shared decision making with patients. Am Fam Physician. 2006;74(1209–1210):1212. [PubMed] [Google Scholar]
- Nyman DJ, Sprung CL. End - of - life decision making in the intensive care unit. Am J Respir Crit Care Med. 2000;26:1414 - 1420. [PubMed] [Google Scholar]
- Proulx K, Jacelon C. Dying with dignity: the good patient versus the good death. Am J Hosp Palliat Care. 2004;21:116 - 120. [PubMed] [Google Scholar]
- Poole M, Bamford C, McLellan E, et al. End - of - life care: a qualitative study comparing the views of people with dementia and family carers. Palliat Med. 2017;32:631 - 642. [PubMed] [Google Scholar]
- Rosenwax L, Spilsbury K, Arendts G, McNamara B, Semmens J. Community - based palliative care is associated with reduced emergency department use by people with dementia in their last year of life: a retrospective cohort study. Palliat Med. 2015;29:727 - 736. [PMC free article] [PubMed] [Google Scholar]

- Rosenwax L, Spilsbury K, Arendts G, McNamara B, Semmens J. Community - based palliative care is associated with reduced emergency department use by people with dementia in their last year of life: a retrospective cohort study. Palliat Med. 2015;29:727 - 736. [PMC free article] [PubMed] [Google Scholar]

- Rosenwax L, Spilsbury K, McNamara BA, Semmens JB. A retrospective population based cohort study of access to specialist palliative care in the last year of life: who is still missing out a decade on? BMC Palliative Care. 2016;15:46. [PMC free article] [PubMed] [Google Scholar]
- Sautter JM, Tulsky JA, Johnson KS, et al. Caregiver experience during advanced chronic illness and last year of life. J Am Geriatr Soc. 2014;62:1082 - 1090. [PMC free article] [PubMed] [Google Scholar]
- Seifart C, Hofmann M, Bar T, Riera Knorrenschild J, Seifart U, Rief W. Breaking bad news - what patients want and what they get: evaluating the SPIKES protocol in Germany. Ann Oncol. 2014;25:707 - 711. [PMC free article] [PubMed] [Google Scholar]
- Simon J, Porterfield P, Bouchal SR, Heyland D. 'Not yet' and 'Just ask': barriers and facilitators to advance care planning—a qualitative descriptive study of the perspectives of seriously ill, older patients and their families. BMJ Support Palliat Care. 2015;5:54 - 62. [PubMed] [Google Scholar]
- Smith S, Brick A, O'Hara S, Normand C. Evidence on the cost and cost - effectiveness of palliative care: a literature review. Palliat Med. 2014;28:130 - 150. [PubMed] [Google Scholar]
- Steinhauser KE, Clipp EC, McNeilly M, Christakis NA, McIntyre LM, Tulsky JA. In search of a good death: observations of patients, families, and providers. Ann Intern Med. 2000;132:825 - 832. [PubMed] [Google Scholar]
- Taylor C, Donoghue J. New ways to provide community aged care services. Australas J Ageing. 2015;34:199 - 200. [PubMed] [Google Scholar]
- Virdun C, Luckett T, Davidson PM, Phillips J. Dying in the hospital setting: a systematic review of quantitative studies identifying the elements of end - of - life care that patients and their families rank as being most important. Palliat Med. 2015;29:774 - 796. [PMC free article]
- Willmott L, White B, Smith MK, Wilkinson DJ. Withholding and withdrawing life - sustaining treatment in a patient's best interests: Australian judicial deliberations. Med J Aust. 2014;201:545 - 547. [PubMed] [Google Scholar]
- You JJ, Downar J, Fowler RA, et al. Barriers to goals of care discussions with seriously ill hospitalized patients and their families: a multicenter survey of clinicians. JAMA Intern Med. 2015;175:549 - 556. [PubMed] [Google Scholar]
- Zier LS, Burack JH, Micco G, Chipman AK, Frank JA, White DB. Surrogate decision makers' responses to physicians' predictions of medical futility. Chest. 2009;136:110 - 117. [PMC free article]

Management of Kidney Failure by Grad system and HWI Therapy An Alternative to Renal Dialysis

Kidney dialysis is a painful and stressful treatment for patients. Also, it can lead to side effects. Fatigue, low blood pressure, muscle cramps, itchy skin, joint pain, and insomnia are some of the common side effects caused due to dialysis. But, HIIMS has the best natural care service for kidney failure. With 360-degree postural therapy, hot water immersion therapy, and a dip diet, kidney functioning can be revived properly without any side effects. HIIMS believes to offer safe and effective kidney care services. The therapies offered to kidney patients can help in the natural recovery of the kidneys. Likewise, our services are safe, surgery-free, and painless to provide the best care to every patient.

An expert team of doctors who ensure to follow the pathway of Ayurveda to provide natural care to every patient. The natural methods of kidney treatment make sure that patients can recover completely without any requirement of surgery, dialysis, transplant, or pain. Also, we believe that diet plans can work excellently to improve the functioning of organs and the entire body perfectly to beat every health issue.

Why 360° Postural medicine to kidney patients?

Many reasons prove why kidney patients should go for 360° Postural medicine-

- This method takes less time than machinery based dialysis.
- It eliminates patients' dependency on machines.
- Each session of 360° Postural medication improves the patient's kidney health, whereas machinery-based dialysis makes the kidney even weaker.
- It costs zero, whereas hospitalized treatments cost you thousands.
- Once learnt this simple technique, it becomes a self-sustainable process for the person.
- Along with improving kidney health, it offers other health benefits also that support a person's overall health.
- This method is 100% safe and effective.

Now, let's have a look at what 360° Postural medication looks like. Let's take you through all the safe and effective medication steps.

How we stop dialysis: All about GRAD System-(Gravitational Resistance And Diet System)

Yes, you read it absolutely right, " STOP DIALYSIS". 360° Postural medicine aims to stop dialysis and to improve kidney health. It basically uses the earth's strongest force, the Gravitational force, as medicine. To treat dialysis, we use GRAD System, i.e. Gravitational Resistance And Diet System.

360° Postural medicine includes making a person lay down to certain degrees in specific postures and using gravitational force as a medicine. This doesn't use any machines, devices or ventilators but a person's own body to treat his health problem. The whole process includes various steps that includes:

HDT Therapy

HDT stands for Head Down Tilt. In this 360° Postural medication therapy, the patient is made to lie down to certain degrees to make the body self-corrections. The patient is made to lie down at 10 degrees, lifting up his lower body. This leads to an increase in sodium excretion from the body. Thus, it flushes out toxins through urine and sweat. The body's blood pressure decreases. In this way, with the help of HDT Therapy, kidney patients start self-dialysis within a few minutes of being tilted into this position.

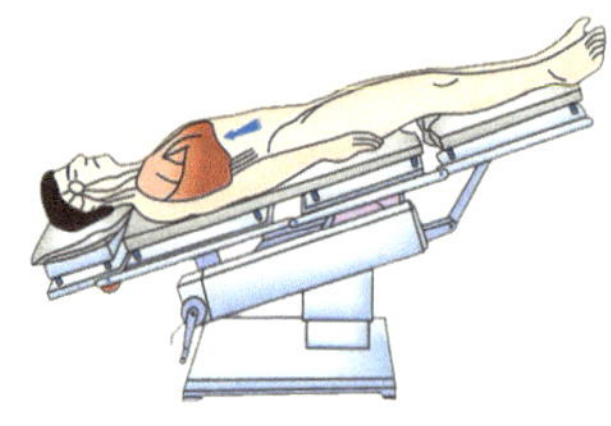

Fig 21.1 The patient is made to lie down at 10 degrees, lifting up his lower body. This leads to an increase in sodium excretion from the body. Thus, it flushes out toxins through urine and sweat.

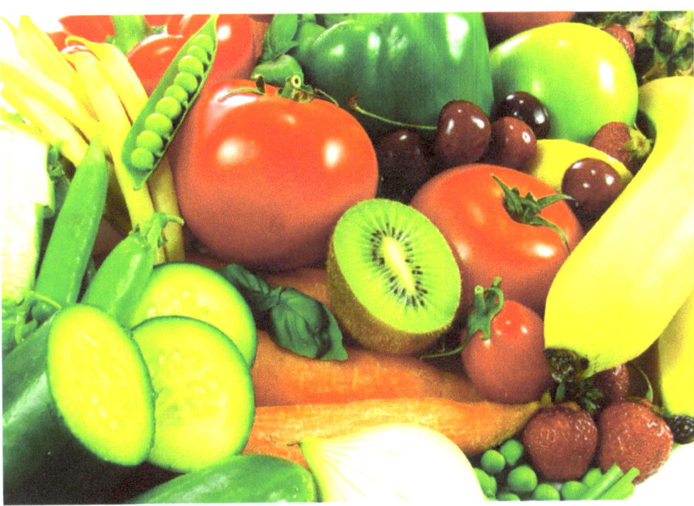

Fig 21.2 Showing fruit and vegetables which becomes the part of treating kidney failure by GRAD system

Kidneys are the most essential organs of the human body. It filters out blood while eliminating the harmful toxins to keep us healthy and active. But like our whole body, the Kidney is not immune from chronic diseases, which might also lead to organ failure if left untreated. While there are plenty of causes that trigger kidney issues, an unhealthy diet and a sedentary lifestyle are the primary ones that give birth to such life-threatening concerns. One should always remember that we are what we eat; hence, always intake nutrient-rich food items to keep your inner self happy and healthy. Since kidneys play a crucial role in our overall well-being, one should pay attention to all earliest symptoms indicating kidney trouble and opt for the best measure to root out the cause. If you are suffering from kidney diseases and want to cure them permanently, think no further than a DIP DIET and help your kidneys recover faster.

It is a special diet that lets the body cure itself on its own without any external machinery support. Want to know more? Our experts have compiled a comprehensive guide entailing all essential aspects of this special diet. Keep scrolling the page and find everything you must know before opting for the process.

What Is DIP Diet?

DIP Diet, also known as the Disciplined & Intelligent People's Diet, is introduced by Dr. Bishwaroop Roy Chowdhury, who is an internationally renowned medical nutritionist. This diet plan is all about adding naturally occurring food items to your daily diet to yield maximum benefits.

Dr. Bishwaroop Roy Chowdhary believes that when we eat food in its natural form, it behaves in a disciplined manner in our bodies. Such a diet contains live enzymes while boosting our metabolism rate. This special diet plan is ideal for all, be it a healthy person or someone who is suffering from any chronic disease.Following this pre-determine Basic diet ensures long-term health without any side effects. The best thing about this plan is that you can modify it in different ways to achieve the desired health goals. With the help of the special DIP DIET, you can get rid of all stubborn diseases that are incurable in allopathy, including kidney troubles, Diabetes, High BP, Cancer, and many more.

Research claims that 57% of Diabetes Type 1 Patients can get rid of insulin dependency while 100% of Diabetes Type 2 patients can maintain a good blood sugar level without medicine. Along with eliminating chronic health concerns, this diet is a sure-shot way for those suffering from obesity and other weight issues. You will be amazed to find out that a person can experience an average weight loss of 1.4kg within 72 hours of adopting the diet plan, thus letting you achieve your fitness goals in the minimum time.

A Complete Guide To The Benefits Of the DIP Diet

Still, wondering whether opting for DIP DIET is worth it or not? Here, we've pulled together some of the benefits that might change your perspective about this special diet plan. Let's have a look.

Healthy Weight Loss

Shedding those extra pounds has never been so easy, but this diet plan has completely changed the scenario. Since the diet is meant to cut off the extra calories from your body, it helps you achieve your weight loss goals without feeling lethargic. It also helps in reducing cholesterol levels in our blood, thus controlling obesity.

Keeps the digestive system strong

The DIP diet is all about eating nutrient-rich food items in their natural form, which further detoxifies the body and flushes out harmful toxins. It helps in increasing the metabolism of an individual and thus keeps the digestive system healthy and active. amount of proteins to the body that helps patients to recover fast.

Helps to get rid of chronic diseases

One of the best advantages of adopting this special diet plan is that it helps root out chronic diseases without causing further impacts. The diet provides the essential

A Step-by-Step Guide To Layout the DIP Diet

So now that you have made up your mind to adopt the DIP DIET plan, it's time to reveal the step-by-step process of layout the same. Remember that the diet only works if followed appropriately. Hence, follow the guide and get the best results.

Step 1: Morning Breakfast

You should eat only fruits till noon. Mix any 3 – 4 seasonal fruits to satiate your hunger. The minimum amount of fruits should be equal to your (body weight X 10) grams. For example, if your body weight is 50kg, then you must consume at least 500grams of fruits.

Step 2: Lunch/ Dinner

One should always eat lunch or dinner in two plates. It might sound surprising at once but has certain logic which really makes sense.

Plate 1 should include four types of greens, such as tomato, radis, cucumber, and carrot. Remember that you have to eat them in uncooked form. The minimum quantity for a plate is your (body weight X 5) grams.

Plate 2 includes homely cooked vegetarian meals with negligible oil and salt. First, you need to consume plate 1 and then turn to Plate 2 for maximum results.

While the guidelines for lunch and dinner are identical, one should complete his dinner before 7 pm. People who have adopted this diet can consume fresh coconut water, sprouts, dry fruits, and Hunza tea, if they crave snacking between lunch and dinner.

What should be avoided?

Below are mentioned some food items that you should avoid while following the DIP DIET at any cost; otherwise, it put all your efforts in vain and delivers no results.

- Animal food, including milk products
- Multivitamin capsules and tonic
- Refined and packed food items
- All dairy products
- Alcoholic beverages and cold drinks

How DIP Diet Helps Cure Kidney Disease?

Are you a kidney patient thinking about how a DIP DIET can cure kidney-related troubles? This diet plan helps in the regeneration of nephrons in the kidneys, thus allowing the patient's body to cure itself without any external support. Following the diet strictly can increase the metabolic rate, which in turn, helps in treating the kidney's ability to function.

That's all about this special diet plan!! We hope our in-depth guide will help you make an informed decision. Think no more!! Adopt for DIP Diet plan right away and keep your body fit and healthy.

HWI Therapy

HWI stands for Hot Water Immersion. In this therapy, we use a big tub filled with hot water and the patient is made to sit in that tub. When the patient's body is subjected to beingcovered up in hot water, within a few minutes, the body starts producing desirable chemicals. The sodium excretion increases five times, potassium excretion increases two times. Also, urine volume increases three times. Thus, the swelling and excessive weight due to accumulated waste in the body gets reduced. The body can flush out excessive waste loaded with toxins, providing relief to the patient. Along with dialysis, HWI Therapy relaxes the body, cures heart disease, hypertension, and diabetes, and improves overall health.

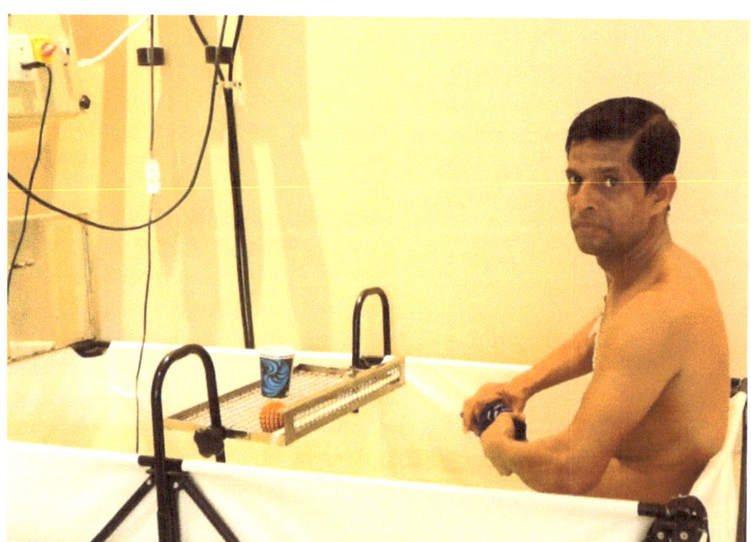

Fig.21.3 A Renal failure patient is seen immersed in hot water tub using HWI technique .

Bibliography and Acknowledgement

- Abdelbaqi-Salhab M, Shalhub S, Morgan MB. A current review of the cutaneous manifestations of renal disease. J Cutan Pathol. 2003;30(9):527–538
- Ahn YM, Kim SK, Lee SH, et al. Renoprotective effect of Tanshinone IIA, an active component of Salvia miltiorrhiza, on rats with chronic kidney disease. Phytother Res. 2010;24(12):1886–1892
- al-Tamer YY, Hadi EA, al-Badrani II. Sweat urea, uric acid and creatinine concentrations in uremic patients. Urol Res. 1997;25(5):337–340
- al-Tamer YY, Hadi EA. Age dependent reference intervals of glucose, urea, protein, lactate and electrolytes in thermally induced sweat. Eur J Clin Chem Clin Biochem. 1994;32(2):71–77
- Baron SE, Goodwin RG, Nicolau N, Blackford S, Goulden V. Use of complementary medicine among outpatients with dermatologic conditions within Yorkshire and South Wales, United Kingdom. J Am Acad Dermatol. 2005;52(4):589–594
- Baumann L. Botanical ingredients in cosmeceuticals. J Drugs Dermatol. 2007;6(11):1084–1088
- Bedi MK, Shenefelt PD. Herbal therapy in dermatology. Arch Dermatol. 2002;138(2):232–242
  Berger TG, Steinhoff M. Pruritus and renal failure. Semin Cutan Med Surg. 2011;30(2):99–100
- Canavan D, Yarnell E. Successful treatment of poison oak dermatitis treated with Grindelia spp. (Gumweed). J Altern Complement Med. 2005;11(4):709–710
- Chen JX, Hu LS. Traditional Chinese medicine for the treatment of chronic prostatitis in China: a systematic review and meta-analysis. J Altern Complement Med. 2006;12(8):763–769
- Cohen AD, Shalev R, Yaniv R, Shemer A. An open-label study of an herbal topical medication (QoolSkin) for patients with chronic plaque psoriasis. Scientific World J. 2007;7:1063–1069
- Cooper BA, Branley P, Bulfone L, et al. A randomized, controlled trial of early versus late initiation of dialysis. N Engl J Med. 2010;363(7):609–619
- Crinnion WJ. Sauna as a valuable clinical tool for cardiovascular, autoimmune, toxicant-induced and other chronic health problems. Altern Med Rev. 2011;16(3):215–225
- Dohm GL, Williams RT, Kasperek GJ, van Rij AM. Increased excretion of urea and N tau-methylhistidine by rats and humans after a bout of exercise. J Appl Physiol. 1982;52(1):27–33
- Dou C, Wan Y, Sun W, et al. Mechanism of Chinese herbal medicine delaying progression of chronic kidney disease. Zhongguo Zhong Yao Za Zhi. 2009;34(8):939–943
- Eisalo A, Luurila OJ. The Finnish sauna and cardiovascular diseases. Ann Clin Res. 1988;20(4):267–270
- Engle JE, Steele TH. Variation of urate excretion with urine flow in normal man. Nephron. 1976;16(1):50–56
- Falodun O, Ogunbiyi A, Salako B, George AK. Skin changes in patients with chronic renal failure. Saudi J Kidney Dis Transpl. 2011;22(2):268–272
- Feng Q, Wan Y, Jiang C, et al. Mechanisms and effects of Chinese herbal medicine delaying progression of chronic renal failure. Zhongguo Zhong Yao Za Zhi. 2011;36(9):1122–1128
- Gayda M, Paillard F, Sosner P, et al. Effects of sauna alone and postexercise sauna baths on blood pressure and hemodynamic variables in patients with untreated hypertension. J Clin Hypertens (Greenwich). 2012;14(8):553–
- Hajheydari Z, Makhlough A. Cutaneous and mucosal manifestations in patients on maintenance hemodialysis: a study of 101 patients in Sari, Iran. Iran J Kidney Dis. 2008;2(2):86–89
- Huang CT, Chen ML, Huang LL, Mao IF. Uric acid and urea in human sweat. Chin J Physiol. 2002;45(3):109–115
- Kanlayavattanakul M, Lourith N. Therapeutic agents and herbs in topical application for acne treatment. Int J Cosmet Sci. 2011;33(4):289–297
- Koban F, Hornak H, Schubert E, Rose W. Secretory performance of eccrine sweat glands from the nephrologic viewpoint. Z Gesamte Inn Med. 1987;42(9):242–245
- Koo J, Desai R. Traditional Chinese medicine in dermatology. Dermatol Ther. 2013;16(2):98–105
- Kuypers DR. Skin problems in chronic kidney disease. Nat Clin Pract Nephrol. 2009;5(3):157–170
- Li X, Wang H. Chinese herbal medicine in the treatment of chronic kidney disease. Adv Chronic Kidney Dis. 2005;12(3):276–281
- Luurila OJ. The sauna and the heart. J Intern Med. 1992;231(4):319–320
- Man in't Veld AJ, van Maanen JH, Schicht IM. Stimulated sweating in chronic renal failure. Br Med J. 1978;2(6131):172–173
- Mangos J. Transductal fluxes of Na, K, and water in the human eccrine sweat gland. Am J Physiol. 1973;224(5):1235–1240
- McIntyre CW, Rosansky SJ. Starting dialysis is dangerous: how do we balance the risk? Kidney Int. 2012;82(4):382–387
- Miao XH, Wang CG, Hu BQ, Li A, Chen CB, Song WQ. TGF-beta1 immunohistochemistry and promoter methylation in chronic renal failure rats treated with Uremic Clearance Granules. Folia Histochem Cytobiol. 2010;48(2):284–291
- Miyamoto H, Kai H, Nakaura H, et al. Safety and efficacy of repeated sauna bathing in patients with chronic systolic heart failure: a preliminary report. J Card Fail. 2005;11(6):432–436
- Narita I, Iguchi S, Omori K, Gejyo F. Uremic pruritus in chronic hemodialysis patients. J Nephrol. 2008;21(2):161–165
- Parker T 3rd, Hakim R, Nissenson AR, Steinman T, Glassock RJ. Dialysis at a crossroads: 50 years later. Clin J Am Soc Nephrol. 2011;6(2):457–461
- Parker TF 3rd, Straube BM, Nissenson A, Hakim RM, Steinman TI, Glassock RJ. Dialysis at a crossroads—Part II: a call for action. Clin J Am Soc Nephrol. 2012;7(6):1026–1032
- Peng A, Gu Y, Lin SY. Herbal treatment for renal diseases. Ann Acad Med Singapore. 2005;34(1):44–51
- Picó MR, Lugo-Somolinos A, Sánchez JL, Burgos-Calderón R. Cutaneous alterations in patients with chronic renal failure. Int J Dermatol. 1992;31(12):860–863
- Pruijm M, El-Housseini Y, Mahfoudh H, et al. Stimulated sweating as a therapy to reduce interdialytic weight gain and improve potassium balance in chronic hemodialysis patients: a pilot study. Hemodial Int. 2013;17(2):240–248
- Qian X, Zhu XX, Chen XY. Effect of Bufei Qingyu Granule in mollifying skin of mouse scleroderma model. Zhongguo Zhong Xi Yi Jie He Za Zhi. 2006;26(11):1018–1020
- Sato K, Feibleman C, Dobson RL. The electrolyte composition of pharmacologically and thermally stimulated sweat: a comparative study. J Invest Dermatol. 1970;55(6):433–438
- Sato K. The physiology, pharmacology, and biochemistry of the eccrine sweat gland. Rev Physiol Biochem Pharmacol. 1977;79:51–131
- Yosipovitch G, Reis J, Tur E, et al. Sweat electrolytes in patients with advanced renal failure. J Lab Clin Med. 1994;124(6):808–812
- Zhang H, Ho YF, Che CT, Lin ZX, Leung C, Chan LS. Topical herbal application as an adjuvant treatment for chronic kidney disease -- a systematic review of randomized controlled clinical trials. J Adv Nurs. 2012;68(8):1679–1691
- Zou C, Wu YC, Lin QZ. Effects of Chinese herbal enema therapy combined basic treatment on BUN, SCr, UA, and IS in chronic renal failure patients. Zhongguo Zhong Xi Yi Jie He Za Zhi. 2012;32(9):1192–1195

Health Implications of Human Body Earthing ToThe Earth's Surface Electrons

Environmental medicine focuses on interactions between human health and the environment, including factors such as compromised air and water and toxic chemicals, and how they cause or mediate disease. Omnipresent throughout the environment is a surprisingly beneficial, yet overlooked global resource for health maintenance, disease prevention, and clinical therapy: the surface of the Earth itself. It is an established, though not widely appreciated fact, that the Earth's surface possesses a limitless and continuously renewed supply of free or mobile electrons. The surface of the planet is electrically conductive (except in limited ultradry areas such as deserts), and its negative potential is maintained (i.e., its electron supply replenished) by the global atmospheric electrical circuit Mounting evidence suggests that the Earth's negative potential can create a stable internal bioelectrical environment for the normal functioning of all body systems. Moreover, oscillations of the intensity of the Earth's potential may be important for setting the biological clocks regulating diurnal body rhythms, such as cortisol secretion It is also well established that electrons from antioxidant molecules neutralize reactive oxygen species (ROS, or in popular terms, free radicals) involved in the body's immune and inflammatory responses. The National Library of Medicine's online resource PubMed lists 7021 studies and 522 review articles from a search of "antioxidant + electron + free radical" . It is assumed that the influx of free electrons absorbed into the body through direct contact with the Earth likely neutralize ROS and thereby reduce acute and chronic inflammation

Throughout history, humans mostly walked barefoot or with footwear made of animal skins. They slept on the ground or on skins. Through direct contact or through perspiration-moistened animal skins used as footwear or sleeping mats, the ground's abundant free electrons were able to enter the body, which is electrically conductive. Through this mechanism, every part of the body could equilibrate with the electrical potential of the Earth, thereby stabilizing the electrical environment of all organs, tissues, and cells. Modern lifestyle has increasingly separated humans from the primordial flow of Earth's electrons. For example, since the 1960s, we have increasingly worn insulating rubber or plastic soled shoes, instead of the traditional leather fashioned from hides. Rossi has lamented that the use of insulating materials in post-World War II shoes has separated us from the Earth's energy field . Obviously, we no longer sleep on the ground as we did in times past. During recent decades, chronic illness, immune disorders, and inflammatory diseases have increased dramatically, and some researchers have cited environmental factors as the cause . However, the possibility of modern disconnection with the Earth's surface as a cause has not been considered. Much of the research reviewed in this paper points in that direction. In the late 19th century, a back-to-nature movement in Germany claimed many health benefits from being barefoot outdoors, even in cold weather .

In the 1920s, White, a medical doctor, investigated the practice of sleeping grounded after being informed by some individuals that they could not sleep properly "unless they were on the ground or connected to

the ground in some way," such as with copper wires attached to grounded-to-Earth water, gas, or radiator pipes. He reported improved sleeping using these techniques . However, these ideas never caught on in mainstream society.
At the end of the last century, experiments initiated independently by Ober in the USA and K. Sokal and P. Sokal in Poland revealed distinct physiological and health benefits with the use of conductive bed pads, mats, EKG- and TENS-type electrode patches, and plates connected indoors to the Earth outside. Ober, a retired cable television executive, found a similarity between the human body (a bioelectrical, signal-transmitting organism) and the cable used to transmit cable television signals. When cables are "grounded" to the Earth, interference is virtually eliminated from the signal. Furthermore, all electrical systems are stabilized by grounding them to the Earth. K. Sokal and P. Sokal, meanwhile, discovered that grounding the human body represents a "universal regulating factor in Nature" that strongly influences bioelectrical, bioenergetic, and biochemical processes and appears to offer a significant modulating effect on chronic illnesses encountered daily in their clinical practices. Earthing (also known as grounding) refers to contact with the Earth's surface electrons by walking barefoot outside or sitting, working, or sleeping indoors connected to conductive systems, some of them patented, that transfer the energy from the ground into the body. Emerging scientific research supports the concept that the Earth's electrons induce multiple physiological changes of clinical significance, including reduced pain, better sleep, a shift from sympathetic to parasympathetic tone in the autonomic nervous system (ANS), and a blood-thinning effect.

Review of Earthing Papers

The studies summarized below involve indoor-testing methods under controlled conditions that simulate being barefootoutdoors

1. Sleep and Chronic Pain

In a blinded pilot study, Ober recruited 60 subjects (22 males and 28 females) who suffered from self-described sleep disturbances and chronic muscle and joint pain for at least six months . Subjects were randomly divided for the month-long study in which both groups slept on conductive carbon fiber mattress pads provided by Ober. Half the pads were connected to a dedicated Earth ground outside each subject's bedroom window, while the other half were "sham" grounded—not connected to the Earth. Most grounded subjects described symptomatic improvement while most in the control group did not. Some subjects reported significant relief from asthmatic and respiratory conditions, rheumatoid arthritis, PMS, sleep apnea, and hypertension while sleeping grounded. These results indicated that the effects of earthing go beyond reduction of pain and improvements in sleep.

2. Sleep, Stress, Pain, and Cortisol

A pilot study evaluated diurnal rhythms in cortisol correlated with changes in sleep, pain, and stress (anxiety, depression, and irritability), as monitored by subjective reporting.Twelve subjects with complaints of sleep dysfunction, pain, and stress were grounded to Earth during sleep in their own beds using a conductive mattress pad for 8 weeks. In order to obtain a baseline measurement of cortisol, subjects chewed Dacron salvettes for 2 minutes and then placed them in time-labeled sampling tubes that were stored in a refrigerator. Self-administered sample collections began at 8 AM and were repeated every 4 hours. After 6 weeks of being grounded, subjects repeated this 24-hour saliva test. The samples were processed using a standard radioimmunoassay.

Subjective symptoms of sleep dysfunction, pain, and stress were reported daily throughout the 8-week test period. The majority of subjects with high- to out-of-range nighttime secretion levels experienced improvements by sleeping grounded. This is demonstrated by the restoration of normal day-night cortisol secretion profiles
Eleven of 12 participants reported falling asleep more quickly, and all 12 reported waking up fewer times at night. Grounding the body at night during sleep also appears to positively affect morning fatigue levels, daytime energy, and nighttime pain levels. About 30 percent of the general American adult population complain of sleep disruption, while approximately 10 percent have associated symptoms of daytime functional impairment consistent with the diagnosis of insomnia. Insomnia often correlates with major depression, generalized anxiety, substance abuse, dementia, and a variety of pain and physical problems.

The direct and indirect costs of chronic insomnia have been estimated at tens of billions of dollars annually in the USA alone . In view of the burdens of personal discomfort and health care costs, grounding the body during sleep seems to have much to offer.

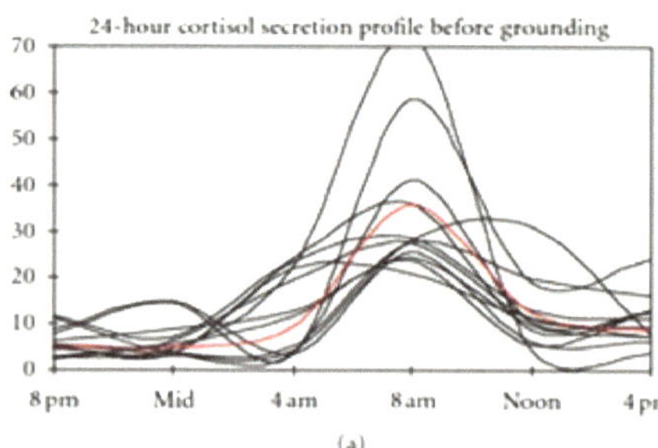

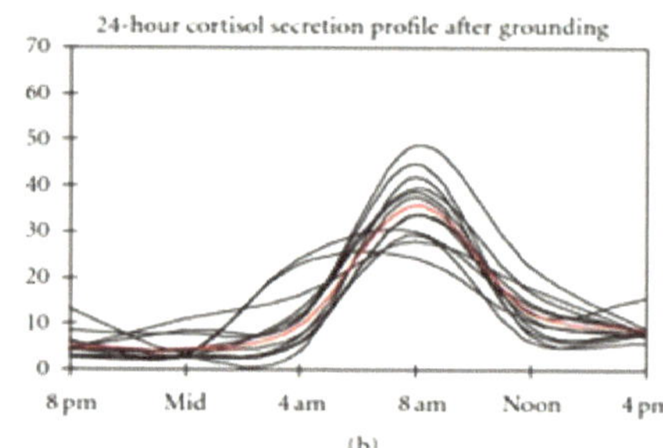

Fig.22.1 *Cortisol levels before and after grounding. In unstressed individuals, the normal 24-hour cortisol secretion profile follows a predictable pattern: lowest around midnight and highest around 8 a.m. Graph (a) illustrates the wide variation of patterns among study participants prior to grounding, while (b) shows a realignment and normalization trend of patterns after six weeks of sleeping grounded.*

3. Earthing Reduces Electric Fields Induced on the Body

Voltage induced on a human body from the electrical environment was measured using a high-impedance measurement head. Apple white, an electrical engineer and expert in the design of electrostatic discharge systems in the electronic industry, was both subject and author of the study . Measurements were taken while ungrounded and then grounded using a conductive patch and conductive bed pad. The author measured the induced fields at three positions: left breast, abdomen, and left thigh.

Each method (patch and sheet) immediately reduced the common alternating current (AC) 60 Hz ambient voltage induced on the body by a highly significant factor of about 70 on average. Figure 2 shows this effect.

The study showed that when the body is grounded, its electrical potential becomes equalized with the Earth's electrical potential through a transfer of electrons from the Earth to the body. This, in turn, prevents the 60 Hz mode from producing an AC electric potential at the surface of the body and from producing perturbations of the electric charges of the molecules inside the body. The study confirms the "umbrella" effect of earthing the body explained by Nobel Prize winner Richard Feynman in his lectures on electromagnetism . Feynman said that when the body potential is the same as the Earth's electric potential (and thus grounded), it becomes an extension of the Earth's gigantic electric system. The Earth's potential thus becomes the "working agent that cancels, reduces, or pushes away electric fields from the body."

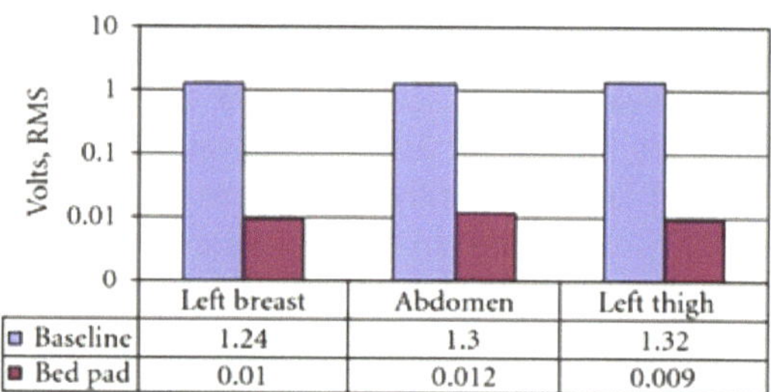

Fig.22.2 *Effect of bed pad grounding on 60 Hz mode.*

Apple white was able to document changes in the ambient voltage induced on the body by monitoring the voltage drop across a resistor. This effect clearly showed the "umbrella effect" described above. The body of the grounded person is not subject to the perturbation of electrons and electrical systems. Jamieson asks whether the failure to appropriately ground humans is a factor contributing to the potential consequences of electropollution in office settings.Considerable debate exists on whether electromagnetic fields in our environment cause a risk to health , but there is no question that the body reacts to the presence of environmental electric fields. This study demonstrates that grounding essentially eliminates the ambient voltage induced on the body from common electricity power sources.

4. Physiological and Electrophysiological Effects Reductions in Overall Stress Levels and Tension and Shift in ANS Balance

Fifty-eight healthy adult subjects (including 30 controls) participated in a randomized double-blind pilot study investigating earthing effects on human physiology .Earthing was accomplished with a conductive adhesive patch placed on the sole of each foot.Abio feed back system recorded electrophysiological and physiological parameters. Experimental subjects were exposed to 28 minutes in the unearthed condition followed by 28 minutes with the earthing wire connected. Controls were unearthed for 56 minutes

Upon earthing, about half the subjects showed an abrupt, almost instantaneous change in root mean square (rms) values of electroencephalograms (EEGs) from the left hemisphere (but not the right hemisphere) at all frequencies analyzed by the biofeedback system (beta, alpha, theta, and delta). All grounded subjects presented an abrupt change in rms values of surface electromyograms (SEMGs) from right and left upper trapezius muscles. Earthing decreased blood volume pulse (BVP) in 19 of 22 experimental subjects (statistically significant) and in 8 of 30 controls (not significant). Earthing the human body showed significant effects on electrophysiological properties of the brain and musculature, on the BVP, and on the noise and stability of electrophysiological recordings. Taken together, the changes in EEG, EMG, and BVP suggest reductions in overall stress levels and tensions and a shift in ANS balance upon earthing. The results extend the conclusions of previous studies.

Confirming Shift from Sympathetic to Parasympathetic Activation

A multiparameter double-blind study was designed to reproduce and expand on previous electrophysiological and physiological parameters measured immediately after grounding with an improved methodology and state-of-the-art equipment . Fourteen men and 14 women, in good health, ages 18–80, were tested while seated in a comfortable recliner during 2-hour grounding sessions, leaving time for signals to stabilize before, during, and after grounding (40 minutes for each period). Sham 2-hour grounding sessions were also recorded with the same subjects as controls. For each session, statistical analyses were performed on four 10-minute segments: before and after grounding (sham grounding for control sessions) and before and after ungrounding (sham ungrounding for control sessions). The following results were documented: 1. an immediate decrease (within a few seconds) in skin conductance (SC) at grounding and an immediate increase at ungrounding. No change was seen for the control (sham grounding) sessions.

2. respiratory rate (RR) increased during grounding, an effect that lasted after ungrounding. RR variance increased immediately after grounding and then decreased;

3. blood oxygenation (BO) variance decreased during grounding, followed by a dramatic increase after ungrounding;

4. pulse rate (PR) and perfusion index (PI) variances increased toward the end of the grounding period, and this change persisted after ungrounding.

The immediate decrease in SC indicates a rapid activation of the parasympathetic nervous system and corresponding deactivation of the sympathetic nervous system. The immediate increase in SC at cessation of grounding indicates an opposite effect. Increased RR, stabilization of BO, and slight rise in heart rate suggest the start of a metabolic healing response necessitating an increase in oxygen consumption.

Immune Cell and Pain Responses with Delayed-Onset Muscle Soreness Induction

Pain reduction from sleeping grounded has been documented in previous studies . This pilot study looked for blood markers that might differentiate between grounded and ungrounded subjects who completed a single session of intense, eccentric exercise resulting in delayed-onset muscle soreness (DOMS) of the gastrocnemius . If markers were able to differentiate these groups, future studies could be done in greater detail with a larger subject base. DOMS is a common complaint in the fitness and athletic world following excessive physical activity and involves acute inflammation in overtaxed muscles. It develops in 14 to 48 hours and persists for more than 96 hours . No known treatment reduces the recovery period, but apparently massage and hydrotherapyand acupuncture can reduce pain.

Eight healthy men ages 20–23 were put through a similar routine of toe raises while carrying on their shoulders a barbell equal to one-third of their body weight. Each participant was exercised individually on a Monday morning and then monitored for the rest of the week while following a similar eating, sleeping, and living schedule in a hotel. The group was randomly divided in half and either grounded or sham grounded with the use of a conductive patch placed at the sole of each foot during active hours and a conductive sheet at night.

Complete blood counts, blood chemistry, enzyme chemistry, serum and saliva cortisol, magnetic resonance imaging and spectroscopy, and pain levels (a total of 48 parameters) were taken at the same time of day before the eccentric exercise and at 24, 48, and 72 hours afterwards. Parameters consistently differing by 10 percent or more, normalized to baseline, were considered worthy of further study. Parameters that differed by these criteria included white blood cell counts, bilirubin, creatine kinase, phosphocreatine/inorganic phosphate ratios, glycerolphosphorylcholine, phosphorylcholine, the visual analogue pain scale, and pressure measurements on the right gastrocnemius. The results showed that grounding the body to the Earth alters measures of immune system activity and pain. Among the ungrounded men, for instance, there was an expected, sharp increase in white blood cells at the stage when DOMS is known to reach its peak and greater perception of pain This effect demonstrates a typical inflammatory response. In comparison, the grounded men had only a slight decrease in white blood cells, indicating scant inflammation, and, for the first time ever observed, a shorter recovery time. Brown later commented that there were “significant differences” in the pain these men reported . The rapid change in skin conductance reported in an earlier study led to the hypothesis that grounding may also improve heart rate variability (HRV), a measurement of the heart's response to ANS regulation. A double-blind study was designed with 27 participants [27]. Subjects sat in a comfortable reclining chair. Four transcutaneous electrical nerve stimulation (TENS) type adhesive electrode patches were placed on the sole of each foot and on each palm.

Participants served as their own controls. Each participant's data from a 2-hour session (40 minutes of which was grounded) were compared with another 2-hour sham-grounded session. The sequence of grounding versus sham-grounding sessions was assigned randomly. During the grounded sessions, participants had statistically significant improvements in HRV that went way beyond basic relaxation results (which were shown by the nongrounded sessions). Since improved HRV is a significant positive indicator on cardiovascular status, , it is suggested that simple grounding techniques be utilized as a basic integrative strategy in supporting the cardiovascular system, especially under situations of heightened autonomic tone when the sympathetic nervous system is more activated than the parasympathetic nervous system.

Reduction of Primary Indicators of Osteoporosis, Improvement of Glucose Regulation, and Immune Response

K. Sokal and P. Sokal, cardiologist and neurosurgeon father and son on the medical staff of a military clinic in Poland, conducted a series of experiments to determine whether contact with the Earth via a copper conductor can affect physiological processes . Their investigations were prompted by the question as to whether the natural electric charge on the surface of the Earth influences the regulation of human physiological processes.

Double-blind experiments were conducted on groups ranging from 12 to 84 subjects who followed similar physical activity, diet, and fluid intake during the trial periods. Grounding was achieved with a copper plate (30 mm × 80 mm) placed on the lower part of the leg, attached with a strip so that it would not come off during the night. The plate was connected by a conductive wire to a larger plate (60 mm × 250 mm) placed in contact with the Earth outside. In one experiment with nonmedicated subjects, grounding during a single night of sleep resulted in statistically significant changes in concentrations of minerals and electrolytes in the blood serum: iron, ionized calcium, inorganic phosphorus, sodium, potassium, and magnesium. Renal excretion of both calcium and phosphorus was reduced significantly. The observed reductions in blood and urinary calcium and phosphorus directly relate to osteoporosis. The results suggest that Earthing for a single night reduces primary indicators of osteoporosis

Earthing continually during rest and physical activity over a 72-hour period decreased fasting glucose among patients with non-insulin-dependent diabetes mellitus. Patients had been well controlled with glibenclamide, an antidiabetic drug, for about 6 months, but at the time of study had unsatisfactory glycemic control despite dietary and exercise advice and glibenclamide doses of 10 mg/day.K. Sokal and P. Sokal drew blood samples from 6 male and 6 female adults with no history of thyroid disease. A single night of grounding produced a significant decrease of free tri-iodothyronine and an increase of free thyroxin and thyroid-stimulating hormone. The meaning of these results is unclear but suggests an earthing influence on hepatic, hypothalamus, and pituitary relationships with thyroid function. Ober et al. have observed that many individuals on thyroid medication reported symptoms of hyperthyroid, such as heart palpitations, after starting grounding. Such symptoms typically vanish after medication is adjusted downward under medical supervision.

Through a series of feedback regulations, thyroid hormones affect almost every physiological process in the body, including growth and development, metabolism, body temperature, and heart rate. Clearly, further study of earthing effects on thyroid function is needed. In another experiment, the effect of grounding on the classic immune response following vaccination was examined. Earthing accelerated the immune response, as demonstrated by increases in gamma globulin concentration. This result confirms an association between earthing and the immune response, as was suggested in the DOMS study. K. Sokal and P. Sokal conclude that earthing the human body influences human physiological processes, including increasing the activity of catabolic processes and may be "the primary factor regulating endocrine and nervous systems."

Altered Blood Electrodynamics

Since grounding produces changes in many electrical properties of the body , a next logical step was to evaluate the electrical property of the blood. A suitable measure is the zeta potential of red blood cells (RBCs) and RBC aggregation. Zeta potential is a parameter closely related to the number of negative charges on the surface of an RBC. The higher the number, the greater the ability of the RBC to repel other RBCs. Thus, the greater the zeta potential the less coagulable is the blood.Ten relatively healthy subjects participated in the study . They were seated comfortably in a reclining chair and were grounded for two hours with electrode patches placed on their feet and hands, as in previous studies. Blood samples were taken before and after. Grounding the body to the earth substantially increases the zeta potential and decreases RBC aggregation, thereby reducing blood viscosity. Subjects in pain reported reduction to the point that it was almost unnoticeable. The results strongly suggest that earthing is a natural solution for patients with excessive blood viscosity, an option of great interest not just for cardiologists, but also for any physician concerned about the relationship of blood viscosity, clotting, and inflammation. In 2008, Adak and colleagues reported the presence of both hypercoagulable blood and poor RBC zeta potential among diabetics. Zeta potential was particularly poor among diabetics with cardiovascular disease

Until now, the physiological significance and possible health effects of stabilizing the internal bioelectrical environment of an organism have not been a significant topic of research. Some aspects of this, however, are relatively obvious. In the absence of Earth contact, internal charge distribution will not be uniform, but instead will be subject to a variety of electrical perturbations in the environment.

It is well known that many important regulations and physiological processes involve events taking place on cell and tissue surfaces. In the absence of a common reference point, or "ground," electrical gradients, due to uneven charge distribution, can build up along tissue surfaces and cell membranes.

We can predict that such charge differentials will influence biochemical and physiological processes. First, the structure and functioning of many enzymes are sensitive to local environmental conditions. Each enzyme has an optimal pH that favors maximal activity. A change in the electrical environment can alter the pH of biological fluids and the charge distribution on molecules and thereby affect reaction rates. The pH effect results because of critical charged amino acids at the active site of the enzyme that participate in substrate binding and catalysis. In addition, the ability of a substrate or enzyme to donate or accept hydrogen ions is influenced by pH. Another example is provided by voltage-gated ion channels, which play critical biophysical roles in excitable cells such as neurons. Local alterations in the charge profiles around these channels can lead to electrical instability of the cell membrane and to the inappropriate spontaneous activity observed during certain pathological states

Earthing research offers insights into the clinical potential of barefoot contact with the Earth, or simulated barefoot contact indoors via simple conductive systems, on the stability of internal bioelectrical function and human physiology. Initial experiments resulted in subjective reports of improved sleep and reduced pain . Subsequent research showed that improved sleep was correlated with a normalization of the cortisol day-night profile . The results are significant in light of the extensive research showing that lack of sleep stresses the body and contributes to many detrimental health consequences. Lack of sleep is often the result of pain. Hence, reduction of pain might be one reason for the benefits just described.Pain reduction from sleeping grounded has been confirmed in a controlled study on DOMS. Earthing is the first intervention known to speed recovery from DOMS . Painful conditions are often the result of various kinds of acute or chronic inflammation conditions caused in part by ROS generated by normal metabolism and also by the immune system as part of the response to injury or trauma. Inflammation can cause pain and loss of range of motion in joints. Inflammatory swelling can put pressure on pain receptors (nocireceptors) and can compromise the microcirculation, leading to ischemic pain. Inflammation can cause the release of toxic molecules that also activate pain receptors.

Modern biomedical research has also documented a close relationship between chronic inflammation and virtually all chronic diseases, including the diseases of aging, and the aging process itself. The steep rise in inflammatory diseases, in fact, has been recently called "inflamm-aging" to describe a progressive inflammatory status and a loss of stress-coping ability as major components of the aging process.Reduction in inflammation as a result of earthing has been documented with infrared medical imaging and with measurements of blood chemistry and white blood cell counts.

The logical explanation for the anti-inflammatory effects is that grounding the body allows negatively charged antioxidant electrons from the Earth to enter the body and neutralize positively charged free radicals at sites of inflammation Flow of electrons from the Earth to the body has been documented . A pilot study on the electrodynamics of red blood cells (zeta potential) has revealed that earthing significantly reduces blood viscosity, an important but neglected parameter in cardiovascular diseases and diabetes [29], and circulation in general. Thus, thinning the blood may allow for more oxygen delivery to tissues and further support the reduction of inflammation. Stress reduction has been confirmed with various measures showing rapid shifts in the ANS from sympathetic to parasympathetic dominance, improvement in heart rate variability, and normalization of muscle tension . Not reported here are many observations over more than two decades by Ober et al. and K. Sokal and P. Sokal indicating that regular earthing may improve blood pressure, cardiovascular arrhythmias, and autoimmune conditions such as lupus, multiple sclerosis, and rheumatoid arthritis. Some effects of earthing on medication are described by Ober et al. As an example, the combination of earthing and coumadin has the potential to exert a compounded blood thinning effect and must be supervised by a physician. Multiple anecdotes of elevated INR have been reported. INR (international normalized ratio) is a widely used measurement of coagulation. The influence of earthing on thyroid function and medication has been described earlier.From a practical standpoint, clinicians could recommend outdoor "barefoot sessions" to patients, weather, and conditions permitting. Ober et al. have observed that going barefoot as little as 30 or 40 minutes daily can significantly reduce pain and stress, and the studies summarized here explain why this is the case. Obviously, there is no cost for barefoot grounding. However, the use of conductive systems while sleeping, approach working, or relaxing indoors offer a more convenient and routine-friendly approach.

"Earthing" or "Grounding"
Direct physical contact of the human body with the surface of the earth
reduces blood viscosity
improves cardiovascular health
better sleep
reduces pain
feeling of well-being

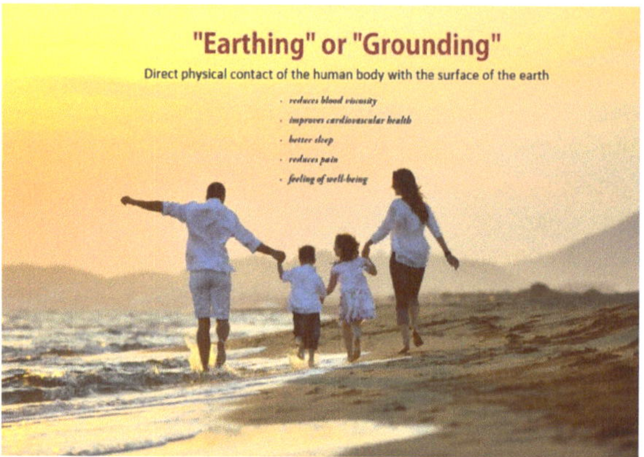

Fig.22.3 *Direct physical contactof the human body with the surface of the earth*

What Is Earthing?

The terms "earthing" and "grounding" are interchangeable. It is simply the act of placing your bare feet on the earth, or walking barefoot. When you do, free electrons are transferred from the earth into your body, and this grounding effect is one of the most potent antioxidants we know of. Unfortunately, few people ever walk barefoot anymore to experience it. Hopefully, as more and more people become aware of the importance of being grounded, this will change, or at the very least spawn a much needed change in the way most footwear is made. Synthetic rubber soles disconnect you from the earth. Leather soles do not. So you can still find shoes that allow you to remain grounded without going barefoot. Grounding has numerous benefits, aside from creating a general feeling of well-being. For example, walking barefoot can help ameliorate the constant assault of electromagnetic fields and other types of radiation from cell phones, computers and Wi-Fi. By getting outside, barefoot, touching the earth, and allowing the excess charge in your body to discharge into the earth, you can alleviate some of the stress put on your system. That is the grounding effect. I have personally prioritized grounding myself to the earth as much as possible for over 5 years.

Inflammation — The Root of Most Disease

One of the primary health benefits of grounding is its antioxidant effect. It helps alleviate inflammation throughout your body. Dr. Sinatra goes on to tell the inspiring story of a contractor he met about 23 years ago, who at one point worked with a group of Scandinavian carpenters who really understood the benefits of grounding and supported each other in maintaining this healthy habit:

According to Dr. Sinatra, inflammation thrives when your blood is thick and you have a lot of free radical stress, and a lot of positive charges in your body. Grounding effectively alleviates inflammation because it thins your blood and infuses you with negatively charged ions through the soles of your feet. But beware; not all surfaces allow you to ground.

What Surfaces Will Allow You to Properly Ground?

Good grounding surfaces include:

- Sand (beach)
- Grass (preferably moist)
- Bare soil
- Concrete and brick (as long as it's not painted or sealed)
- Ceramictile

The following surfaces will NOT ground you:

- Asphalt
- Wood
- Rubber and plastic
- Vinyl
- Tarortarmac

An interesting tidbit offered by Dr. Sinatra is how to ground while flying. I typically bring a grounding pad with me when I fly, but Dr. Sinatra claims that simply taking your shoes off and putting your feet (bare or with socks) on

The Earth Is a Rich Source of Healthful Electrons

The earth is struck by lightning thousands of time each minute, primarily around the equator. Subsequently, the earth carries an enormous negative charge. It's always electron-rich and can serve as a powerful and abundant supply of antioxidant free radical-busting electrons.

The human body appears to be finely tuned to "work" with the earth in the sense that there's a constant flow of energy between our bodies and the earth. When you put your feet on the ground, you absorb large amounts of negative electrons through the soles of your feet. In today's world, this is more important than ever, yet fewer people than ever actually connect with the earth in this way anymore. Free radical stress from exposure to mercury pollution, cigarettes, insecticides, pesticides, trans fats, and radiation, just to name a few, continually deplete your body of electrons.

Recharge Your 'Batteries' with Grounding

Dr. Sinatra, like myself, is a proponent for CoQ10, as it is a major electron donor and helps turn over ATP, which is the energy generated within each of your body's cells.

Amazingly, grounding can also enhance ATP, via another mechanism. How do dietary-derived, oral antioxidants compare to the electrons transferred from the earth through your skin? According to Dr. Sinatra:

Walking Barefoot Is a Valuable Aspect of a Healthy Lifestyle

Exercising barefoot outdoors is one of the most wonderful, inexpensive and powerful ways of incorporating Earthing into your daily life and will also help speed up tissue repair, as well as easing the muscle pain you sometimes get from strenuous exercise. A review of the available research, published January 2012 in the Journal of Environmental and Public Health, agrees with the concept of reaping health benefits when connecting to the Earth. According to the authors:

"Mounting evidence suggests that the Earth's negative potential can create a stable internal bioelectrical environment for the normal functioning of all body systems. Moreover, oscillations of the intensity of the Earth's potential may be important for setting the biological clocks regulating diurnal body rhythms, such as cortisol secretion.

It is also well established that electrons from antioxidant molecules neutralize reactive oxygen species (ROS, or in popular terms, free radicals) involved in the body's immune and inflammatory responses. The National Library of Medicine's online resource PubMed lists 7021 studies and 522 review articles from a search of 'antioxidant + electron + free radical.' It is assumed that the influx of free electrons absorbed into the body through direct contact with the Earth likely neutralize ROS and thereby reduce acute and chronic inflammation.

Throughout history, humans mostly walked barefoot or with footwear made of animal skins. They slept on the ground or on skins. Through direct contact or through perspiration-moistened animal skins used as footwear or sleeping mats, the ground's abundant free electrons were able to enter the body, which is electrically conductive. Through this mechanism, every part of the body could equilibrate with the electrical potential of the Earth, thereby stabilizing the electrical environment of all organs, tissues, and cells.

Modern lifestyle has increasingly separated humans from the primordial flow of Earth's electrons. For example, since the 1960s, we have increasingly worn insulating rubber or plastic soled shoes, instead of the traditional leather fashioned from hides. Rossi has lamented that the use of insulating materials in post-World War II shoes has separated us from the Earth's energy field. Obviously, we no longer sleep on the ground as we did in times past.

During recent decades, chronic illness, immune disorders, and inflammatory diseases have increased dramatically, and some researchers have cited

environmental factors as the cause. However, the possibility of modern disconnection with the Earth's surface as a cause has not been considered. Much of the research reviewed in this paper points in that direction.

How Grounding Changes Your Blood

Grounding helps thin your blood by improving its zeta potential, which means it improves the energy between your red blood cells. Research has demonstrated it takes about 80 minutes for the free electrons from the earth to reach your blood stream and transform your blood

Do you know what a high-sugar diet, smoking, radio frequencies and other toxic electromagnetic forces, emotional stress, anxiety, high cholesterol, and high uric acid levels do to your blood?All of these make your blood hypercoagulable, meaning it makes it thick and slow-moving, which increases your risk of having a blood clot or stroke. Hypercoagulable blood is the essence of inflammation, because when your blood does not flow well, oxygen can't get to your tissues. In fact, grounding's effect on blood thinning is so profound if you are taking blood thinners you must work with your health care provider to lower your dose otherwise you may overdose on the medication. Zeta potential is the electrical potential of solids and liquids, also referred to as electrokinetic potential. Your red blood cells repel each other and function at the speed of light, traveling through your body at an astounding 186,000 miles per second. Grounding actually increases zeta potential by an average of 280 percent. According to Dr. Sinatra

"This is the most incredible discovery, because if you can increase the thinning of your blood naturally by grounding, you can fight off disease. Not only heart disease and stroke, but I'm thinking cancer, Alzheimer's, multiple sclerosis, or any illness that requires good oxygenation to the tissues."

Similarly, anything that lowers zeta potential of your blood will promote disease. For example, early (and some current) birth control pills were notorious for causing heart attacks in women. One of the mechanisms that causes this increased risk is that synthetic estrogens and progesterones increase blood viscosity, i.e., they decrease the zeta potential of your blood. There are currently studies being performed at the University of Arizona which will objectively document grounding effect on the zeta potential. They are anticipated to be completed this year.

Other Beneficial Changes Caused By Grounding

Animal experiments have also shown that ungrounded rats had higher blood sugar compared to their grounded counterparts, despite being fed identical diets. If disconnecting from the earth disrupts human sugar metabolism, we may have identified yet another contributing cause for the dramatic rise of diabetes in children. Experiments in Poland, the U.S. and Canada, using both animal and human models, show that grounding improves the human physiology. Other biochemical alterations caused by grounding include changes in:

- Phosphorus
- Calcium metabolism
- Fibroid metabolism
- White blood cells

Grounding also calms your sympathetic nervous system, which supports your heart rate variability. And, when you support heart rate variability, this promotes homeostatis, or balance, in your autonomic nervous system. In essence, anytime you improve heart rate variability, you're improving the entire organism — in this case, your entire body and all its functions.

Contraindications and Other Warnings

While walking barefoot is clearly one of the most natural things you can possibly do to improve your health, there are still some contraindications and situations in which you may want to use caution. *"I don't like people to ground when they're taking Coumadin," Dr. Sinatra warns. "It's a relative contraindication because we have had people ground, taking Coumadin at the same time, and their blood became like water. It was like red wine and then it got really thin. That could be dangerous. If you have high blood pressure, [or]... if you had a stroke and you have thin blood, it's a disaster. We basically tell people that if you're on Coumadin, you must work with your doctor, because your doctor's going to have to reduce the Coumadin."*

Depending on your health status and toxic load, your health may also get worse before it gets better when you start grounding on a regular basis. This is a classic detox reaction, which you may also experience with other detox methods

"Some patients with polyneuropathy would get worsening of their limb pain on grounding, and some would get better. I want to make that clear that grounding is not a panacea," Dr. Sinatra says. "But what I've learned with grounding is that the sicker you are, the more you need to ground."

The traditionally core components of alternative, lifestyle, and preventive medicine include nutrition, exercise, stress management, and relationships. One key component that is missing from this overall formula is the practice of Earthing, which is commonly referred to as grounding.

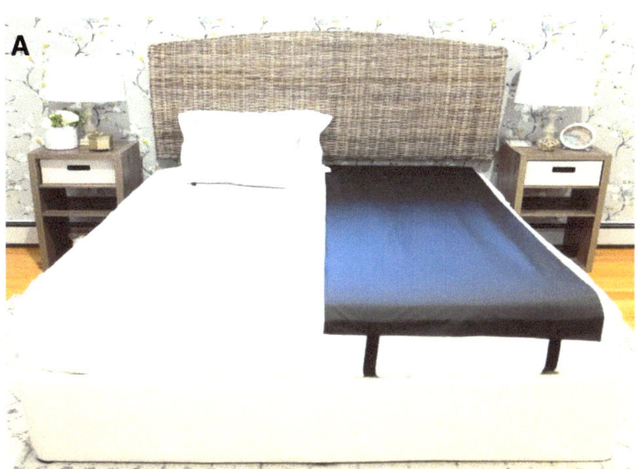

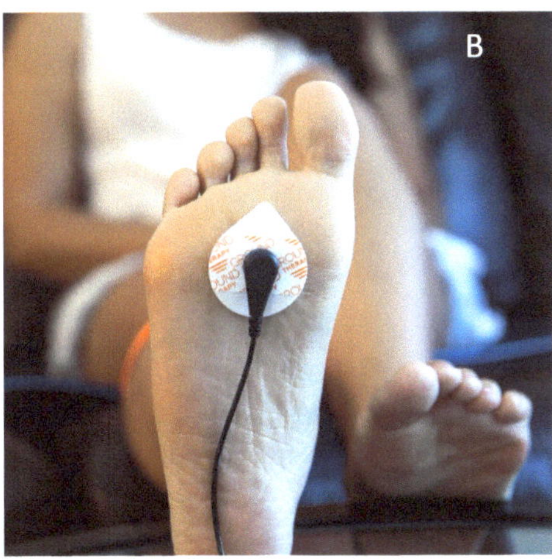

Fig.22.4 *Grounded sleep system. Notes: Grounded sleep system consists of a cotton sheet with conductive carbon or silver threads woven into it. The threads connect to a wire that leads out the bedroom window or through the wall to a metal rod inserted into the Earth near a healthy plant. Alternatively, it can be connected to the ground terminal of an electrical outlet. Sleeping on this system connects the body to the Earth. A frequent report from people using this system is that sleeping grounded improves the quality of sleep and reduces aches and pains from a variety of causes. B. Attachment of foot patch in body earthing.*

Grounding and the Cardiovascular System

In 1977, Steve Sinatra, MD became a board-certified cardiologist. After writing dozens of peer review articles, books, and chapters in medical text books over the past 40 years, I thought about my greatest discoveries as a physician. Indeed, it was the utilization of coenzyme Q10 in my patients as well as the cardiovascular implications of grounding, also known as Earthing the body. This chapter is a testimony to the incredible discovery of grounding to the natural electric charge of the planet

It was almost 15 years ago at an American College of Cardiology conference that I met Clint Ober in San Diego. He introduced to me the theory of grounding, and it made a lot of sense to me. I was excited about the entire concept, as well as trying to take it to a higher level. However, like anything else in medicine, the theory behind grounding needed intensive research. Ever since that encounter with Clint, more than 20 peer reviewed articles on the benefits of grounding have become available to mainstream medicine.

Over the past 4 decades, I have treated hundreds of patients with acute coronary syndrome and unstable angina, as well as acute myocardial infarction. Although the utilization of thrombolytic therapies, percutaneous transluminal coronary angioplasty, stents, and statin medications are crucial in the care of these patients, the grounding phenomena also needed to be recognized.

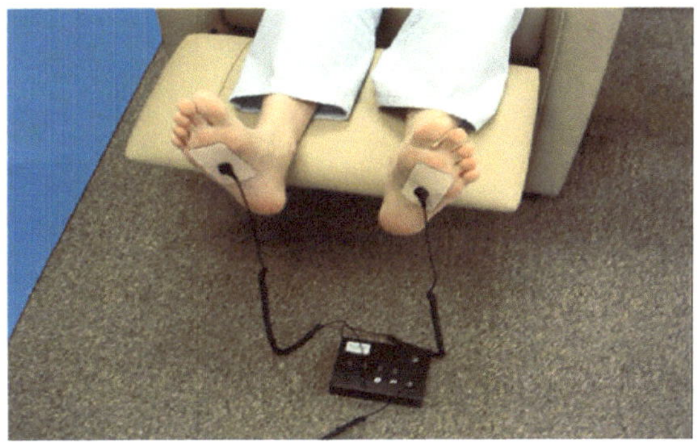

Fig 22.5 ***Grounding system showing patches, wires, and box connecting to a ground rod planted outside through a switch (not shown) and a fuse (not shown). Similar patches and wires from the hands were also connected to the box to ground the hands.***

Simply stated, when one grounds to the electron-enriched earth, an improved balance of the ANS occurs. Improvements in HRV can support patients with emotional stress, anxiety, fear, and any other symptoms of autonomic dystonia.A 2017 study performed at the Pennsylvania State University Children's Hospital Neonatal Intensive Care Unit in Hershey revealed that grounding premature infants produced immediate and significant improvements in measurements of the ANS. Grounding improves vagal tone and may support resilience to stress, which could lower the risk of neonatal mortality in preterm infants

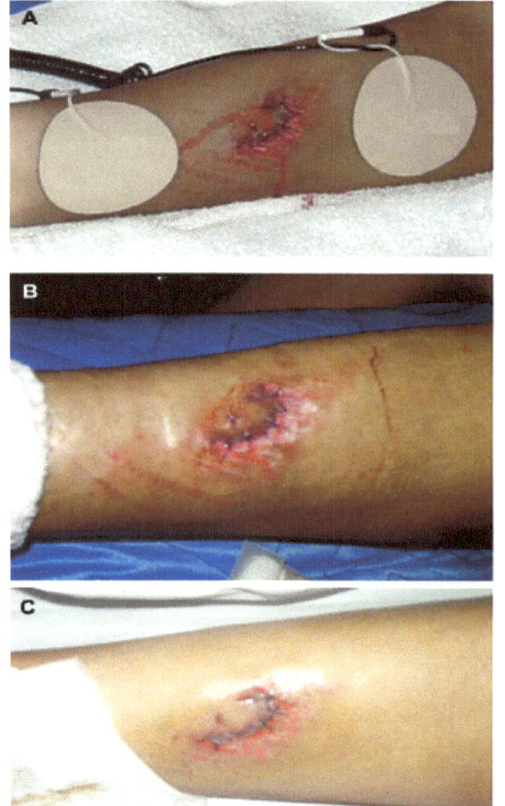

Fig. 22.6 *Rapid recovery from a serious wound with minimal swelling and redness expected for such a serious injury. Notes: Cyclist was injured in Tour de France competition – chain wheel gouged his leg. (A) Grounding patches were placed above and below wound as soon as possible after injury. Photo courtesy of Dr Jeff Spencer. (B) Day 1 after injury. (C) Day 2 after injury. There was minimal redness, pain, and swelling, and cyclist was able to continue the race on the day following the injury. (B and C) Copyright © 2014. Reprinted with permission from Basic Health Publications, Inc. Ober CA, Sinatra ST, Zucker M. Earthing: The Most Important Health Discovery Ever? 2nd ed. Laguna Beach: Basic Health Publications; 2014.*

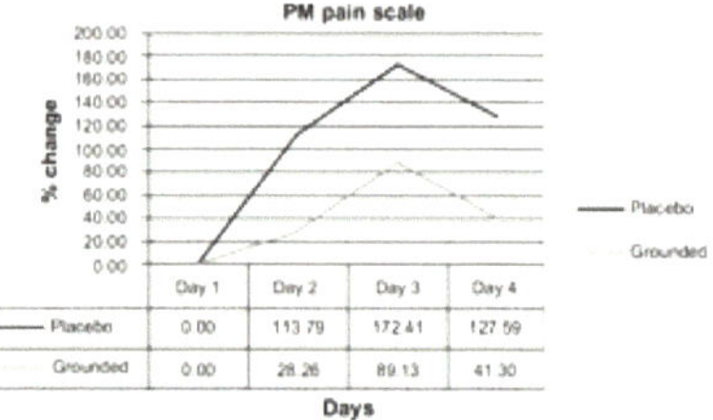

	Day 1	Day 2	Day 3	Day 4
Placebo	0.00	113.79	172.41	127.59
Grounded	0.00	28.26	89.13	41.30

Fig. 22.7 *Changes in afternoon (PM) visual analog pain scale was completely pain-free reports.*

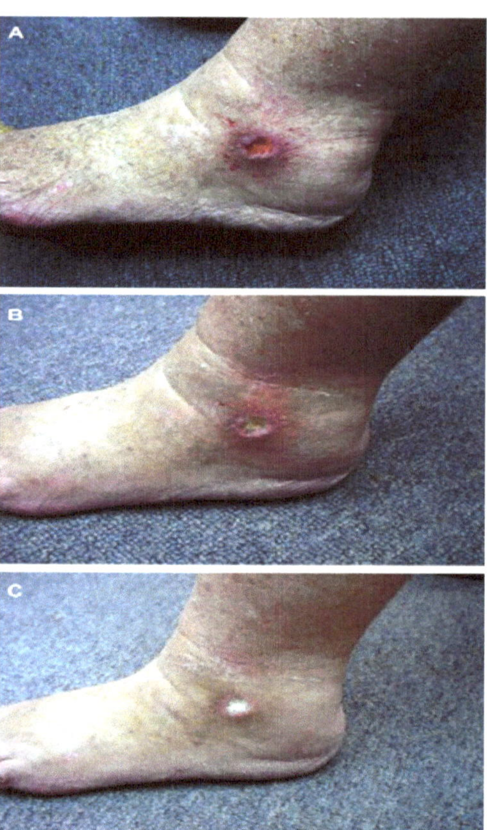

Fig.22.8 *Photographicimages documenting accelerated improvement of an 8-monthold, non-healing open wound suffered by an 84-year-old diabetic woman. Notes: (A) Shows the open wound and a pale-gray hue to the skin. (B) Taken after one week of grounding or earthing treatments, shows a marked level of healing and improvement in circulation, as indicated by the skin color. (C) Taken after 2 weeks of earthing treatment, shows the wound healed over and the skin color looking dramatically healthier. Treatment consisted of a daily 30-minute grounding session with an electrode patch while patient was seated comfortably. The cause of the wound adjacent to the left ankle was a poorly fitted boot. A few hours after wearing the boot, a blister formed, and then developed into a resistant open wound. The patient had undergone various treatments at a specialized wound center with no improvement. Vascular imaging of her lower extremities revealed poor circulation. When first seen, she had a mild limp and was in pain. After an initial 30 minutes of exposure to grounding, the patient reported a noticeable decrease in pain. After 1 week of daily grounding, she said her pain level was about 80% less. At that time, she showed no evidence of a limp. At the end of 2 weeks, she said she*

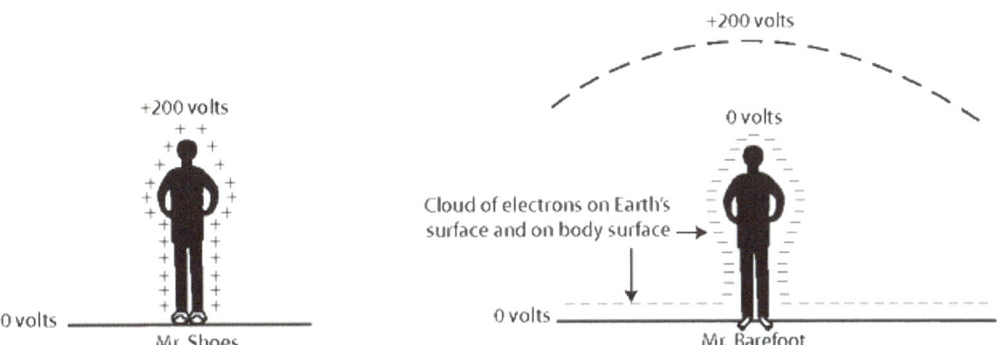

Fig.22.9 *The object is essentially residing within the protective "umbrella" of earth's natural electric field. This protective phenomenon also occurs inside your house or office if you are connected to the earth with an earthing device, such as a grounding wrist pad or a foot pad. Adapted from Richard Feynman's famous Berkeley Lectures on Physics. (From Ober C, Sinatra ST, Zucker M. Earthing: The Most Important Health Discovery Ever? Laguna Beach, CA: Basic Health Publications; Second Edition, 2014, p. 76.)*

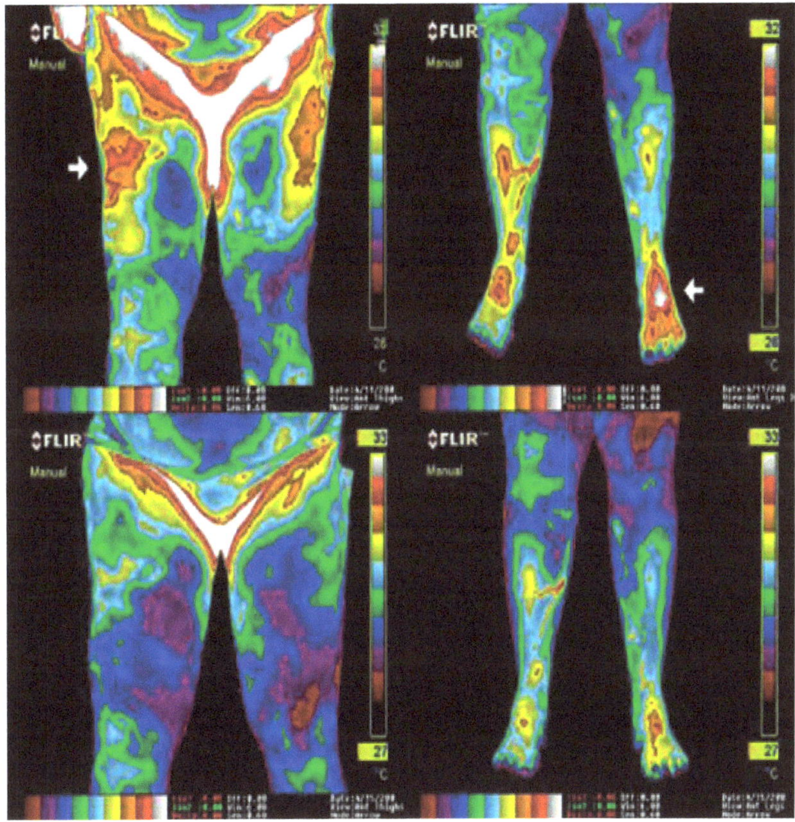

Fig.22.10 *Reduction in inflammation and pain after sleeping grounded for four nights. Medical infrared imaging shows warm and painful areas (arrows). Sleeping grounded for four nights resolved the pain and the hot areas cooled. (From Amalu W. Medical Thermography case studies. Clinical earthing application in 20 case studies.*

The traditionally core components of alternative, lifestyle, and preventive medicine include nutrition, exercise, stress management, and relationships. One key component that is missing from this overall formula is the practice of Earthing, which is commonly referred to as grounding. The simplicity and the multitude of benefits provided by Earthing are not understood by many people.

Before we proceed any further, let's examine exactly what Earthing means.

Earthing simply means reconnecting the conductive human body to the Earth's natural and subtle surface electric charge, an effortless lifestyle activity that systematically influences the basic bioelectrical function of the body Implementation of this simple lifestyle change surprisingly stabilizes the physiology, reduces inflammation, pain, and stress, enhances sleep, blood flow, and lymphatic/venous return to the heart, and produces greater well-being. People report very positive effects from a regular schedule of Earthing. They report that they feel and look healthier and younger. Those suffering from pain state that they feel less pain and their mood improves. Earthing is quite simple to implement and often achieves rapid results, particularly for individuals with chronicc health disorders

Our Lost Connection To The Earth

The Earth has long been recognized and utilized by the electrical industry as an essential source of stability and safety. All modern electrical systems, from large grids and power stations to homes, buildings, and factories, and the machinery and appliances powered by electricity, are all connected to the Earth for stability and safety. Essentially, electrical systems are "healthier" precisely because of their connection to the Earth

It is now time for the medical world to start recognizing that a body connected to the ground – a grounded body – is similarly more stable and healthier. It functions more naturally, a state lost over time because humans have become largely disconnected from the Earth

We obviously no longer sleep on the ground, rarely walk barefoot outdoors, and, for more than a half century, almost exclusively wear insulating synthetic soled shoes instead of traditional and conductive leather footwear. We live and work, and spend much or most of our time disconnected, often far above ground in high rises. This disconnection with the Earth may contribute to electrical imbalances, a build-up of disruptive static electricity (positive charges), and an unknown electron deficiency in the body, and with it, susceptibility to dysfunction, disorder, and disease .The electrical charge provided by Earth and its limitless supply of electrons and their diurnal frequencies, provides a form of "electric nutrition" so to speak Research supports the hypothesis that Earthing facilitates a significant transfer of free electrons into the body, a transfer resulting in rapid, sometimes instant, physiological changes Earthing restores and maintains a natural internal electrical environment. Research indicates that Earthing the human body represents a "universal regulating factor in Nature" strongly influencing bioelectrical, bioenergetics, and biochemical processes and appears to offer a significant modulating effect on chronic illnesses and dysfunction.

Earth ,the Original Anti-inflammatory

One of the most prevailing effects of Earthing, as documented over nearly 20 years of research, along with feedback from thousands of individuals around the world, is reduction and even elimination of chronic inflammation, a common cause or aggravating factor for chronic and aging-related diseases, as well as pain.

This finding suggests that the planet we live on is the original painkiller, the original anti-inflammatory: nature's way to counteract inflammation. Briefly, the hypothesis for this effect is as follows: Free radicals (also known as reactive oxygen species, ROS) are positively charged molecules produced normally, that strip electrons from healthy tissue, resulting in damage. Every cell produces billions of free radicals every day. Earthing allows huge numbers of free electrons to enter the body where they are believed to neutralize free radicals. The active mechanisms of electron transportation to a site of inflammation may encompass the nervous, meridian, and circulatory systems. It is indicated that the influx of free electrons absorbed into the body serves as a powerful anti-inflammatory reinforcement for the immune system.

Earthing typically reverses both acute and chronic inflammation, and does so rapidly. Interestingly, three studies based on a sports medicine research model called delayed onset muscular soreness (DOMS) documented clear evidence of pain relief and reduced inflammation from Earthing.. DOMS refers to the pain, tenderness, and stiffness felt in muscles several hours to days after unaccustomed or strenuous exercise.

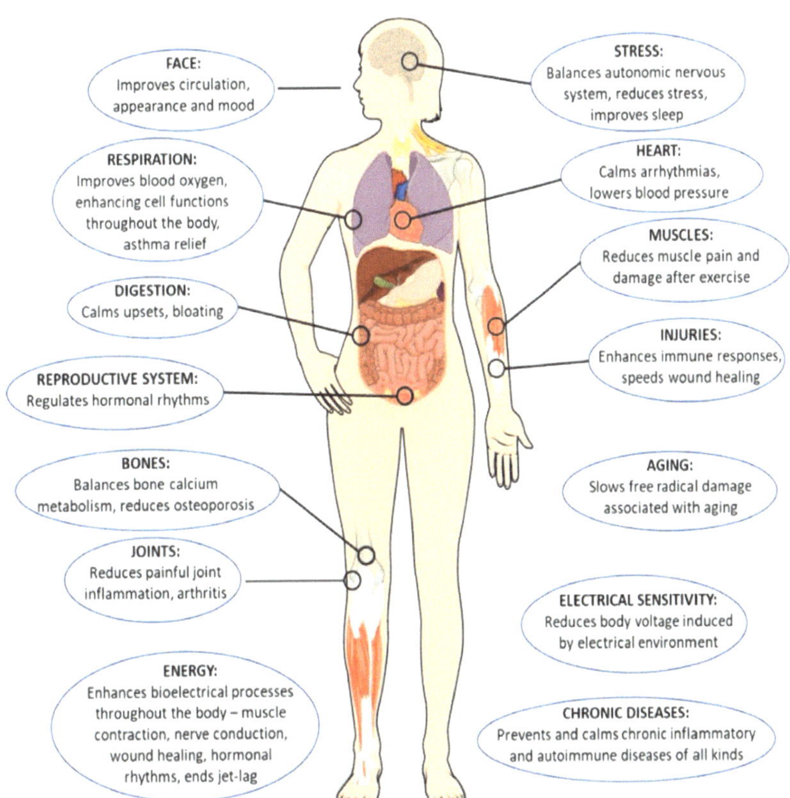

Fig.22.11 *Effects of earthing on our body system .*

Copper Plate Earthings

3E solutions supply the complete range of Copper Earthing Plates that are also used as a conventional earthing solution. We install Copper earthing plate installation as per IS:3043 in a 3 Feet Long x 3 Feet Wide x10 Deep earth hole with alternate layers of Salt and Charcoal. The salt helps to reduce the earthing resistance by creating an electrolytic environment surrounding earthing plate but over the time leach out deeper in the earth and need salt and water at more frequent intervals. Since salt also corrode the earthing plate and terminal strip that connect the copper plate with equipment and reduce the dependability, generally, chemical earthings are preferred. Earthing Copper Plate Size: As per Copper earthing Plate Design, Plates are available in 600mm x 600m (2 Feet x 2 Feet) and 300mm x 300mm (1 Feet x 1 Feet) dimensions with 3mm thickness or as per requirements. Earthing Plate is fixed with copper strip and GI Pipe. After digging 3 feet x 3 feet 10 feet hole, the earthing plate is inserted in and salt and charcoal added in alternate layers upto the level of the plate. Funnel / Wire mesh is used to avoid soil in water pipe.

The natural soil or 3E make backfill compound mixed with good quality (pref black cotton soil) to backfill till the top and a chamber is installed to measure the earthing resistance values once a year. After testing the earthing, the earthing is connected to the equipment through a test link. The test link is used to disconnect earthing with interconnection to equipotential bonding while testing of the earthings.

Table 22.1 *Following Items are used in installation as per Copper Plate Earthings Design*

1.Copper Earthing Plate
2.Copper Strip connected to GI Pipe at the bottom
3 GI Pipe for watering
4 Salt
5 Charcoal
6 Cast Iron Cover Brass Nut Bolts Washer

Conclusion

De Flora et al. wrote the following: "Since the late 20th century, chronic degenerative diseases have overcome infectious disease as the major causes of death in the 21st century, so an increase in human longevity will depend on finding an intervention that inhibits the development of these diseases and slows their progress".Could such an intervention be located right beneath our feet? Earthing research, observations, and related theories raise an intriguing possibility about the Earth's surface electrons as an untapped health resource—the Earth as a "global treatment table." Emerging evidence shows that contact with the Earth—whether being outside barefoot or indoors connected to grounded conductive systems—may be a simple, natural, and yet profoundly effective environmental strategy against chronic stress, ANS dysfunction, inflammation, pain, poor sleep, disturbed HRV, hypercoagulable blood, and many common health disorders, including cardiovascular disease. The research done to date supports the concept that grounding or earthing the human body may be an essential element in the health equation along with sunshine, clean air and water, nutritious food, and physical activity.

Summary

Environmental medicine generally addresses environmental factors with a negative impact on human health. However, emerging scientific research has revealed a surprisingly positive and overlooked environmental factor on health: direct physical contact with the vast supply of electrons on the surface of the Earth.

Modern lifestyle separates humans from such contact. The research suggests that this disconnect may be a major contributor to physiological dysfunction and unwellness. Reconnection with the Earth's electrons has been found to promote intriguing physiological changes and subjective reports of well-being. Earthing (or grounding) refers to the discovery of benefits—including better sleep and reduced pain—from walking barefoot outside or sitting, working, or sleeping indoors connected to conductive systems that transfer the Earth's electrons from the ground into the body. This paper reviews the earthing research and the potential of earthing as a simple and easily accessed global modality of significant clinical importance.

Bibliography ans Acknowledgement

Adak S, Chowdhury S, Bhattacharyya M. Dynamic and electrokinetic behavior of erythrocyte membrane in diabetes mellitus and diabetic cardiovascular disease. Biochimica et Biophysica Acta. 2008;1780(2):108–115. [PubMed] [Google Scholar]

Anisimov S, Mareev E, Bakastov S. On the generation and evolution of aeroelectric structures in the surface layer. Journal of Geophysical Research D. 1999;104(12):14359–14367. [Google Scholar]

Applewhite R. The effectiveness of a conductive patch and a conductive bed pad in reducing induced human body voltage via the application of earth ground. European Biology and Bioelectromagnetics. 2005;1:23–40. [Google Scholar]

Bobbert MF, Hollander AP, Huijing PA. Factors in delayed onset muscular soreness of man. Medicine and Science in Sports and Exercise. 1986;18(1):75–81. [PubMed]

Brown R, Chevalier G, Hill M. Pilot study on the effect of grounding on delayed-onset muscle soreness. Journal of Alternative and Complementary Medicine. 2010;16(3):265–273. [PMC free article] [PubMed] [Google Scholar]

Chahine M, Chatelier A, Babich O, Krupp JJ. Voltage-gated sodium channels in neurological disorders. CNS and Neurological Disorders—Drug Targets. 2008;7(2):144–158. [PubMed] [Google Scholar]

Chevalier G, Mori K, Oschman JL. The effect of Earthing (grounding) on human physiology. European Biology and Bioelectromagnetics. 2006;2(1):600–621. [Google Scholar]

Chevalier G, Sinatra S. Emotional stress, heart rate variability, grounding, and improved autonomic tone: clinical applications. Integrative Medicine: A Clinician's Journal. 2011;10(3) [Google Scholar]

Chevalier G, Sinatra ST, Oschman JL, Delany RM. Grounding the human body reduces blood viscosity—a major factor in cardiovascular disease. Journal of Alternative and Complementary Medicine. In press. [PMC free article] [PubMed] [Google Scholar]

Chevalier G. Changes in pulse rate, respiratory rate, blood oxygenation, perfusion index, skin conductance, and their variability induced during and after grounding human subjects for 40 minutes. Journal of Alternative and Complementary Medicine. 2010;16(1):1–7. [PubMed] [Google Scholar]

de Flora S, Quaglia A, Bennicelli C, Vercelli M. The epidemiological revolution of the 20th century. FASEB Journal. 2005;19(8):892–897. [PubMed] [Google Scholar]

Feynman R, Leighton R, Sands M. The Feynman Lectures on Physics. II. Boston, Mass, USA: Addison-Wesley; 1963. [Google Scholar]

Franceschi C, Bonafè M, Valensin S, et al. Inflamm-aging: an evolutionary perspective on immunosenescence. Annals of the New York Academy of Sciences. 2000;908:244–254. [PubMed] [Google Scholar]

Genuis SJ. Fielding a current idea: exploring the public health impact of electromagnetic radiation. Public Health. 2008;122(2):113–124. [PubMed] [Google Scholar]

Ghaly M, Teplitz D. The biologic effects of grounding the human body during sleep as measured by cortisol levels and subjective reporting of sleep, pain, and stress. Journal of Alternative and Complementary Medicine. 2004;10(5):767–776. [PubMed] [Google Scholar]

Holiday D, Resnick R, Walker J. Fundamentals of Physics, Fourth Edition. New York, NY, USA: John Wiley & Sons; 1993. [Google Scholar]

Hübscher M, Vogt L, Bernhörster M, Rosenhagen A, Banzer W. Effects of acupuncture on symptoms and muscle function in delayed-onset muscle soreness. Journal of Alternative and Complementary Medicine. 2008;14(8):1011–1016.

Jamieson KS, ApSimon HM, Jamieson SS, Bell JNB, Yost MG. The effects of electric fields on charged molecules and particles in individual microenvironments. Atmospheric Environment. 2007;41(25):5224–5235. [Google Scholar]

Just A. Return to Nature: The True Natural Method of Healing and Living and The True Salvation of the Soul. New York, NY, USA: B. Lust; 1903. [Google Scholar]

NIH State-of-the-Science Conference on Manifestations and Management of Chronic Insomnia in Adults. http://consensus.nih.gov/2005/insomniastatement.htm, June 13-15, 2005.

Ober C, Sinatra ST, Zucker M. Earthing: The Most Important Health Discovery Ever? Laguna Beach, Calif, USA: Basic Health Publications; 2010. [Google Scholar]

Ober C. Grounding the human body to neutralize bioelectrical stress from static electricity and EMFs. ESD Journal, http://www.esdjournal.com/articles/cober/ground.htm, January 2000.

Oschman JL. Can electrons act as antioxidants? A review and commentary. Journal of Alternative and Complementary Medicine. 2007;13(9):955–967. [PubMed] [Google Scholar]

Oschman JL. Charge transfer in the living matrix. Journal of Bodywork and Movement Therapies. 2009;13(3):215–228.

Oschman JL. Perspective: assume a spherical cow: the role of free or mobile electrons in bodywork, energetic and movement therapies. Journal of Bodywork and Movement Therapies. 2008;12(1):40–57. [PubMed] [Google Scholar]

Rossi W. The Sex Life of the Foot and Shoe. Vol. 61. Hertfordshire, UK: Wordsworth Editions; 1989. [Google Scholar]

Sokal K, Sokal P. Earthing the human body influences physiologic processes. Journal of Alternative and Complementary Medicine. 2011;17(4):301–308. [PMC free article] [PubMed] [Google Scholar]

Stein R. Is Modern Life Ravaging Our Immune Systems? Washington Post; 2008. [Google Scholar]

Tartibian B, Maleki B, Abbasi A. The effects of ingestion of Omega-3 fatty acids on perceived pain and external symptoms of delayed onset muscle soreness in untrained men. Clinical Journal of Sport Medicine. 2009;19(2):115–119. [PubMed] [Google Scholar]

Vaile J, Halson S, Gill N, Dawson B. Effect of hydrotherapy on the signs and symptoms of delayed onset muscle soreness. European Journal of Applied Physiology. 2008;102(4):447–455. [PubMed] [Google Scholar]

White G. The Finer Forces of Nature in Diagnosis and Therapy. Los Angeles, Calif, USA: Phillips Printing Company; 1929. [Google Scholar]

Williams E, Heckman S. The local diurnal variation of cloud electrification and the global diurnal variation of negative charge on the Earth. Journal of Geophysical Research. 1993;98(3):5221–5234. [Google Scholar]

Zainuddin Z, Newton M, Sacco P, Nosaka K. Effects of massage on delayed-onset muscle soreness, swelling, and recovery of muscle function. Journal of Athletic Training. 2005;40(3):174–180. [PMC free article] [PubMed] [Google Scholar]

Artificial Intelligence-Based Smart Comrade Robot for Elders Healthcare.

Technology is a trend that affects human existence in every part of the world. Robots are an exciting example of what the future of technology holds. Robotics has enhanced human life and industry significantly, thanks to the technology . Adults with autism are already a regular thing in many industries, including healthcare, military service, and domestic assistance. The global population is growing, therefore making the requirements of this demographic an increasingly significant issue for health providers, government officials, caretakers, and families. Due to these reasons, buddy robots (which serve as aids to elderly people) are often seen as having an authoritarian function in helping individuals do their caring duties without assistance. An increased old population is often brought up as a method of dealing with the rising number of senior persons. Actually, robots are becoming more prevalent in the senior care sector. We should have been aware of certain ethical issues that have recently been brought to light as a result of these advances. Artificial intelligence approaches are applicable for various fields of utility. Digital smart systems, medical data analysis, healthcare system, and other applications are possible with AI model. Specifically, disease diagnosis with deep learning, radiology model with ML, automatic systems, and so forth are the most utilized healthcare systems of AI.

A rising need for new technology has emerged for older adults because of the greying of our current generation. The primary reasons in favour of this are that there are too few hospital workers and many individuals want to live as independently as possible rather than be placed in an institution . Additionally, we will need an adequate supply of healthcare professionals together with the use of cutting-edge technology. Robotics is playing a significant role in helping older people these days. A household use robot that is particularly intended for use at home may be regarded as a level of service robot. The business of making robots specifically for the house is expanding from scientific and commercial standpoints. In order for Comrade robot to be the most effective in the house, it should be able to carry out several activities such as home monitoring, gadget management, personal assistance, and entertaining.

When more and more robots are developed to engage with a human being to give the sort of care that is often provided by a licensed therapist, the lack of healthcare and the standard of living for the elderly will both improve . Designing a providing assurance "robotic arm" to supervise the old person is the method being used. The overall aim is to create a low rental Comradeship robot to assist an elderly person with daily home automation.

In the end, the house robot could traverse the usual home settings without any human assistance, carrying out duties such as senior citizens monitoring devices, home gadget management, and security and stability sensing, as well as in the case of an attack. This document has two distinct sections. One is a Comrade robot, while the other is a health monitoring band. A Comrade robot does so in the form of "making itself helpful"; that is, it is capable of assisting people in a household setting. The old person is constantly being kept under constant supervision by the Comrade robot . With the sensors incorporated in the design, the leaving comments industrial vehicle ensures both safe and secure environment in the family environment. Trespassers, gas leaks, and fire are all on the list. In the creative and emotional realm, Comrade robots and emotional synthetic avatars have now been created for graduate training. It may be difficult to extract a ministry of planning from both materials; therefore, teams that want to build Comrade robots must create their own website from scratch. Of course, there are many representations of structure for Comrade robot, but it is also tough to locate how the actual ones operate. Most articles concern themselves with how well an overall behavior performs, with little emphasis on the detailed architecture needed for replication.

The RoboCare program is dedicated to creating distributed applications where programming and autonomous agents all work together to accomplish an overall objective, which is to provide a supply of services that are ready for use in settings where people may need help and direction.

While we are also interested in supporting endangered elderly individuals to enjoy an inclusive environment in their own homes, our primary focus is on bringing the concept to market. According to recent data, Europe and Japan are gradually growing older. In order to increase public attention to this matter of "independence" and "ageing at home," new ways of supporting the seniors and persons with disabilities have been created.

This is why when it comes to RoboCare, most of the study deals with two potential situations, which are referred to as the RoboCare Household Atmosphere and the Quality of Life Institution setting . Robotic frameworks, wearable devices, activity monitoring in complicated settings, and human relationships are the main components of strong reliance for the future of robotic care. Here we will give the reader a short summary of the key findings that we have discovered so far and many lessons we have learnt from those efforts to custom-tailor AI for assisted living. Remote sensing data-based applications, image processing, video and audio recognition system, security system, and so forth are the applications of this research field. The major objective is to improve the performance state of medical data analysis and the robot model construction with efficient analysis is designed. This research contributes to improving the robot technology and availability of AI in medical healthcare system. Comrade robot model with AI utility helps to obtain a better performance result.

Why Robotic Help Would Be Required In Future?

Lifespans across the globe are rising, and therefore the percentage of the people in retirement ages is growing (Moyle et al. As visual acuity in older adults diminishes, this necessitates the provision of more services and has a larger impact on budgets for healthcare provision. The older population needs more research to help them retain emotional human fellow. Robotic technology may be used to assist both rehabilitative and sociable robots in relieving strain on social care facilities. Large data processing, overlapping issue, and feature set analysis difficulties are the major problem of conventional work.You may also look into Comradeship robotics, which are little robots that are made to look and behave like animals (Pu et al]). They aid creatures during rodent therapy by decreasing the dangers for the mammals individually. In general, Schrödinger, the mechanical seal, is a famous example. The advantages of getting to know Paro, a simulated nursing care Comrade for elderly people, include decreased irritation as well as depressive disorder in cognitive impairment, better immune responses, less burden on care providers, and enhanced affect and information exchange among both elderly people and their day care providers.. Furthermore, paracetamol may help to minimize the need for hallucinogenic and analgesia medications and may help to lower cholesterol levels.

The authors in and others examine the main methodologies, including designation as well as learning algorithms, which are essential in the development of developing quantum computing, as well as designation and learning algorithms, and computational efficiency that are applicable in the field of growing artificial intelligence and intricate their use .Research methods employed in data security, personal computing, and cloud services provide better findings, as diverse assessment criteria are taken into consideration.

The impact of robot animals upon autonomous older adults was examined in a clinical trial (Abubshait et al.) and also the researchers reported that robotic dogs may offer social enjoyment and relationships. While practical assistance was very attractive, the fact that the robot looked and felt more like a human created a conflict. People preferred soft fur and recommended play elements, such as plush toys, as potential improvements for the Comrade robots that are presently available. When new, brightly colored, child-oriented dogs were used, this restricted the kind of impressions respondents might create. Note that although older persons and individuals with memory are incorporated throughout Comrade robot creation, they are seldom, if ever, offered the opportunity to be engaged. Interaction typically happens in the project design whenever healthcare services are engaged.

It was recommended that the construction of something like an everyone around collapse detection technique be undertaken (Celis et al.). Utilizing just one aeration rate, an innovative wearable gadget for the detection of falls was created. Ubiquitous computing Remote Monitoring for the Old capable of detecting an individual's fall as maintaining the health of the patients. An Intelligent Home Security System based on GSM and ARM Architectural design: Industrial robots have lately been created utilizing a range of technologies, including the Web, wireless communications, wirelessly, and speech recognition.

Robotic Over Review In General

The word robot was originally derived from the Czech word robot, which means forced labor. Karel Capek, the Czech writer, introduced the term robot in his play "R.U.R." Capek used the term robotic in a series called "Rossum's Universal Robots" that premiered in Prague in 1921. The robots in R.U.R were built by man, and they were supposed to work for humanity. Thus, from generations to generations, human people have made use of robots to do various jobs. However, there is just no generally accepted definition for robots Despite this disagreement, the University of the Robot Society still sees a robot as a multipurpose fully programmable tool that is used to transfer credible commitments, tools, or optical disks in various ways using preprogrammed movements. This concept differentiates robots from other automated machines, because they are programmable. A robot may be described as an upgradeable, complex nervous, sentient, and transportable machine that uses energy to do work. Regardless of its form and size, a robot has seven major elements. This collaboration serves a particular goal. Figure 1 depicts the parts of a robot.

1. Controller

The commander is in charge of coordinating the robot's movements. The operational environment refers to the area within which a robot may operate . The microcontroller is also in charge of collecting input first from surrounding environment via the use of its sensing.

2. Power Conversion Unit

The fusion reactor supplies the robot's controls. Electricity, combustible materials, and battery storage are all commonplace power stations in robots . Most of the electricity that is provided to a building comes from the grid, and, in order to power the building, the system uses an AC/DC electrical power converter to change the AC electricity into DC electricity.

• Sensors

Robots may now have the sensor take a specific measurements of the surroundings, with the sensing' data helping to shape the robot's behaviors. To guarantee the robot's security, this is often done. Devices utilize a robot to respond to environmental variations.

• Actuator

In most of the robots, the actuators are often known as the muscles of the robot. The conversion takes place by using the energy that drives your robot's mobility.

• Control and Task Program

A collection of commands from the manufacturers of the robot's controller are known as the management plan, while a sequence of questions typically supplied by the user are called the task programme . To accomplish a particular job, the manipulator must carry out the movements task programmed by the task programme.

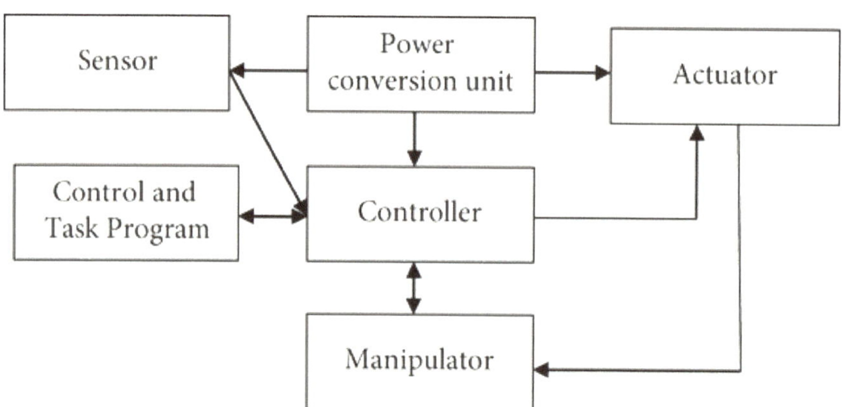

Fig. 23.1 *Components of a robot.*

3. Manipulator

The robotics have had the capacity to pick up, alter, and blow things up. The robot's manipulation imitates outstretched arm of something like a human individual. Manipulators typically refer to the joints connecting the arms with the upper arms, elbows, and wrists. Joints tend to be either rotational or sliding . Reaction kinetics refer to the way wherein the joints are arranged to define the potential stepper motor.

4. End Effector

The final part of the system, which connects to the input device, is known as the manipulation link. The instrument handle's link is known as an actuation. It imitates the mechanical arm, mimicking the results obtained.

Development Of Comrade Robot Structure

To develop up with a proper Comrade robot structure, we also must research the many needs that Comrade robots may have. Just one "perfect" Comrade robot might fulfill all these criteria. Meanwhile, theoretically speaking, the need of a Comrade robot does not quite apply; in reality, one is still required . The specifications for a given robot rely on a variety of different variables, including the kind of intended application and also the particular hardware components that are required.Here we provide a comprehensive list of all potential criteria an engineer should consider while designing a generic structure. The main task of the Comrade robot is to sense the environment around it, including hearing, seeing, and touching. Intercultural competence calls for synchronizing data; thus, various kinds of data need attention

In addition, inputs processing may be programmed to target specific sensor data, in response to predictions from a mixing process. Significance must be verified on every piece of data received, and all information collected must also be classified before it can be kept.

The Comrade robot was able to have a classroom discussion with the user. What this implies is not just to create effective sentences and also to take fundamental principles of communicating into consideration . A Comrade robot should constantly be likely to preserve the dialogue flowing in order to sustain a strong connection. The usage of live interaction also incorporates elements like this; for instance, in order to prevent boring or misunderstanding the user, lengthy pauses should not be present in a discussion. It should be able to communicate across all modalities and should do so in a logical and reasonable manner. Speech would overlap with proper lip motions, which have been prioritized about the present face animations and the robot dealing with the lips both of it. We illustrate the construction of a Comrade robot and address the specifications outlined above. However, observe that perhaps the design is abstracted from the specifics of various kinds of friend robotics, allowing its application to diverse kinds of robot Comrades. We are emphasizing again here that it was for a Comrade robot that also has an "overall" personality; nevertheless, you may build various parts without putting any content into them. Initial set of data processing uses dialogue engine and reasoning engine. Depending on the goals, rules, memory unit, and emotion recognitions are taken with heuristics approach. After that, the input and output processing states are determined with facial recognition with animation approach. Dataset uses source from camera, sound, and so forth and the speech recognition and facial recognition data are synchronized. With the low-level behavior, the animation controls are processed. Here this conflict scheduler, the performance of output state is determined.

AI and Robotic Technology in Elder Healthcare

By building a framework that incorporates current state-of-the-art AI technologies from an off way, RoboCare aims to help service providers fully appreciate the kind of assistance resources available . The difficult part is to find out whether the methods listed above might help create educational software parts that can be purchased off market. Robotic systems now provide us the ability to create robotic system with very accurate survival skills. We have effectively implemented these systems in both the home and hospital facility settings thanks to a variety of methods.

The professional diagnosis and management Comrade robot is able to provide guidance on prevention and prognosis by collecting data like clinical findings, a client's medical records, and previous medical instances. The robot was created by the robotics and artificial intelligence, that is, related to clinical texts, two million clinical data, and many individual instances The hospital is conducting a pilot programme in which people participate to evaluate the robot. When interacting with a client all through physical diagnosis, the robot "pays attention" to the dialogue and takes the sensor readings along with source information to help the clinician diagnose and prescribe medication . The clinician then collects information to interact with the clinician. It is anticipated that the robot would assist doctors to come to a conclusion about the cause of the patient's symptoms quicker and cut down on mistakes.

The Health System Mechanism, is made up of several AI industrial robots.

To arrive at a prognosis, the speech based EHR system and image natural antibiotic are both utilized. Comrade proposes a diagnosis and therapy in which all relevant information is collected.

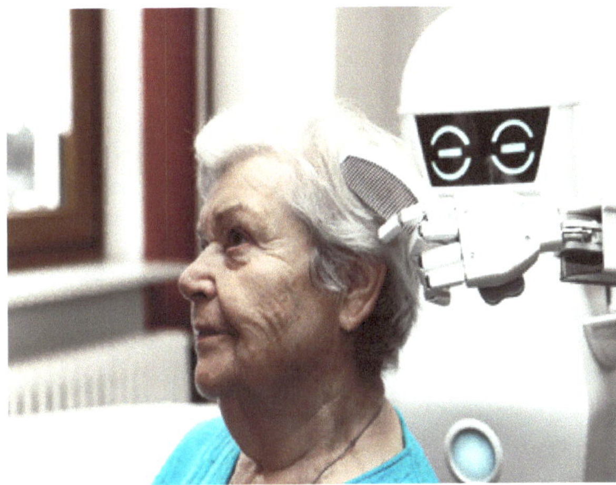

Fig.23.2 *AI chatbots can help fill the void by providing some companionship*

Thanks to advancements in technology, it is now possible to provide ambient independent living solutions to help seniors in their dwellings . The multidisciplinary approach that is required for robotics technology problems includes knowledge from fields like building, fashion, psychological, law, and ethics, as well as technology, computer programming, science, and medicine. In order to benefit everyone, robots and information and communication technology (ICT) must be made accessible across the populace at school, in hospitals, in home languages, and in smart neighborhoods. A high degree of acceptance and usefulness for the users may be achieved by integrating these approaches in the development of the surroundings.

Some basic suggestions for social order, together with technological and legal troubles, may be discovered through the applying load with actual customers in some kind of a contemporary context

Society Centered Design

Robotic technologies should be planned, manufactured, and

deployed to assist people in the day-to-day tasks in a societal architecture.The intelligent machines must be able to go from a user-centered design process to a social system design process, at which development process is properly considered and is further integrated with the society's requirements . Many of the ideas shown in the previous sections included users throughout the whole development process, starting with the study of end-users' requirements and leading all the way through the assessment of the prototype system for valuable suggestions..

Stakeholder Readiness

It is also essential to consider the speed to market in evaluating integrated services. That level of readiness indicates how soon the individuals and organizations are prepared to take and spread the technologies. The gap among study and implementation is the only problem with this topic.

Low Cost

Considering that personalized robotics are meant to be used by the individual, the price must be in line with their financial capability, in place to encourage for broad service usage. Robotic alternatives incur a reduced cost for the sake of a costing system , they are costly owing to the increased components they employ, but then on the other hand they are less costly for the public health system. Cloud automation solution models may enable a new breed of personalized robots for businesses.

Customizability, Flexibility, and Modularity

The requirements of the users will fluctuate. Having provided component services, it is essential to offer one that can respond to customer requirements and competences that vary.

Robustness, Dependability, Safety, and Security

Because the test equipment is expected to engage with those who are vulnerable and aged, it must have been secure and dependable.

Autonomy

Robotics institutions are expected to move independently and make choices based on the needs of consumers. They ought to be capable of identifying errors that users have made or they have made and make corrections on their own when required.

Social Informatics of Knowledge Embodiment

Our study has significance that are present in the system; it is applied to other comparable systems. Nonetheless, in order to validate our results, further research with healthcare practitioners in the field is required. In our research of AI-infused autonomous vehicles, we disregarded electronic archives, too. The usage of other things, like computers, may be affected by AI industrial robotics; however, in our research paper, we have not seen this. The possibility of further study includes research that compares cognitive manifestation in various entities in order to learn about how they support or replace one another.Lastly, we have not investigated the nature of senior executives' interest in, or usage of, AI machines. Understanding the four forms of information embodiment as a generative framework for finding motivators may be the most useful. Mechanistic explanation of cognitive immersion should rely on knowing the motive. From a social bioinformatics viewpoint, AI technology is relevant in the context.

It is vital to understand the sociospatial relationships AI has with people in order to fully comprehend its true worth. STIN analytic approach is particularly helpful, since it offers a paradigm for incorporating various social actors' perspectives while considering technologies. An excellent illustration of our findings is that, in contrast to the robots that were intended to make people's job and emphasizing, the AI humanoid systems that operate as rivals and magisters encounter greater opposition from economic systems than those that work as collaboration and guild mates.

This STIN study also showed that the automation technologies supplier has a minimal but nonetheless significant impact on the market. Requiring timely deployment of AI mobile robots for skilled employees, the supplier highlighted the technologies' complimentary and nonconfrontational character to help people gain confidence. This research confirms that our awareness of the use of AI industrial robotics in intellectual work requires a social information systems viewpoint.

By using powerful computers like AI robotic systems, researchers are showing that they can behave as an independent social actor in addition to just being a tool for humans. When humans and robots interact more naturally and intuitively, the difference between the humanity and the machine may become obsolete. Further refinement of the notion of interconnections in social bioinformatics as interpersonal relations and living organism connection converge may be required in order to help more people have social networks.

A manifestation of information changes understanding labor, and the introduction of new privacy practices is probable. Since making scientific have yet to comprehend the consequences of artificial intelligence, it is possible that the necessary training activities may need new methods of collecting, analyzing, and displaying data at employment. Social and community customers frequently need to work with machines, as well. Because of the resulting shift in the organization, in other words, the dissemination of materials is most likely to be caused. and shows major module utilizing expansion, emancipation, equipping, and expediting. Speech data with knowledge analysis, human cognition, augmentation, and AI robot are analyzed in expansion set. Actuation and competitor design of emancipation is determined. Assistance and automation model uses the procedural knowledge and final declaration.

Methodology Employed

Robotic systems that utilize the making plans, observation, concurrence, and successive cognitive orientations review process acquire questionnaire questions from guardians and carry out the intellectual orienting examination control and experimental group. The robot then engages in a discussion with the user and gathers feedback. When the robot has finished evaluating the responses, it reports back to those same caregivers with the results .This section describes the cognitive assessment method and the communication mechanisms platform. Our Friend Robotic, a 3D-printed desk device, is fitted with a cognition assessment process. The capacitive touch screen is linked to an ARM-based microcomputer executing Android platform, and the interaction is shown on it. In addition to having a 3D camera, this robot is equipped with a vision circuit composed of an RGB-D camera for image recognition and four loudspeakers that help with sound localization. We have also included voice and physical movement detection in our robot arm.The cognitive orientation assessment method has seven critical features: a development tool, inquiry and response creation, agreement between two parties, excessive screen, Internet computer vision, answer appraisal, and intelligence score .An online dataset and native databases are required for the relational database. In the public cloud, Q&A worksheets containing users' accounts and summaries of memory score are stored, along with cognitive orientations evaluations. These may be revised and checked by a caretaker. The personal dataset provides the user's focus strategy, test timetables, and Q&A answers.

Modeling and Formulations of Comrade Robots

The study of bending moment enables one to approach performs of large masses. According to the current motion, one may see the position, orientations, and higher incidence as having evolved through time. Dynamics in robotics are used to build up basic equations of controls, with the dynamic transfer function for deceivers acting as the explanation governing motion. Torque is the mechanism that is responsible for producing the dynamic movement of both manipulating arms in a robot's arm .. Dynamic modeling is involved in the development of the differential equations of the manipulation as a function of something like the displacements acting on it. In dynamic modeling, the robotics manipulator's components are constrained to a set of forces and; as a result, the locations, velocities, and deceleration are determined:(i)People who have torque needed to achieve certain end-effector movements are all determined by this calculation (the direct dynamic problem) (ii)The elastic scattering issue is modeled mathematically, and there are a variety of control methods which use the model(iii)It enables the calculation of the real manipulation to be done usinga control scheme equations and manipulate Lagrange's movement. Joint characteristics and characteristics of the manipulation define the motion. A communication model with overall energy K and gravitational potential V is shown as follows. Lagrange refers to. It is a simple procedure using the Lagrangian differential equation derived. The general force that corresponds to the generalized coordinate qi is referred to as Qi. Connection I has kinetic and potential energy provided. A second-order linear evolution equation may be used to describe the Lagrangian equations of motion for the n-th links manipulators.where

Evaluation Process

Google has published a new open software speech recognition processing framework, known as SyntaxNet, to the public. Syntax Net's main purpose is to find out the words and phrases, and each word is clearly shown in phrase. A parser is capable of determining the morphological purpose of any single phrase, including conjunctions, in the phrase. In addition to providing an also before the model named Parse McParseface, Goggling also offers a grammar models, known as Parsey McParseface, that is developed. No matter how complicated the root of a phrase may be, SyntaxNet is able to recognize it is able to trace out the connection between the word meaning and each individual word in the phrase. This study aimed to use SyntaxNet, so that the customer's voice communication may be processed genuinely.

To illustrate, a phrase will be spoken, at which point the voice activation component will transform textual content, which is then processed by SyntaxNet for deeper comprehension. To put a POS on a word, SyntaxNet examines the whole phrase as well as the word's semantics. Similarly, since SyntaxNet can correctly predict the calculated value used when a machine evaluates the provided response with the right answer, assessing answers that utilize math is quite simple. The capabilities of SyntaxNet may also be utilized to detect whether there is negativity in the word but when the phrase has a pejorative perception.The programming language we use to describe paragraph characteristics is called SyntaxNet. Step one is answering the question, and step two is evaluating the response. Next, the input is examined and processed using SyntaxNet to identify both user responses and right answers. Long computational network and right answer structure are created from the interpreted results. Those trees stand for the concept of a "pos" and how words relate to one other . The second step in the algorithm is to connect two trees, and the saplings are compared using a mating Canadian land. A compatibility score is given for these tree trunks, depending on their resemblance.

The robot gives a score of 1 to a right answer tree and a score of 0 to an erroneous solution tree. A partial number may be given if the answer matches both trees; however, the progress and achievement are used to evaluate the two trees. To determine the user's cognitive score, the participant's characteristics and a caregiver-determined criterion are utilized.

Recognition state of robot has various questionnaires, which translates the audio data to text data. Depending on the availability of given response, the NLP is performed and messages are taken with NLP analysis model. The parsed text is extracted with the feature set of given database. These correlated results are analyzed and desired answers are taken for the task accomplishment. Feedbacks are saved; then the respective description database assessment result is produced.

In conlusion ,Artificial intelligence is a rapidly expanding area of research, which has implications in many sectors, such as medical services, and to provide pharmaceutical aid. It is well established that the area of healthcare is a dynamic market for AI. In this article, a robotics framework is created which uses human messages between a human and a robot to carry out cognitive orientation evaluation. SyntaxNet, which enables the robots to comprehend programming knowledge naturally, helped carry out natural language processing. The Comrade robot was created from the ground up to handle this entire ecosystem. We do not need outside assistance in order to conduct a cognitive orientation evaluation, since the system is capable of doing it. This research sought to elicit tasks where a certain robot aids with increasing the quality of life (QoL) and assisting with an autonomous, healthy ageing. This research presents occupations that are an important component of the lives of older people in all the secondary classrooms. This study demonstrates that it is possible to use technologies with an eye on improving the quality of life for older people. At a profound level, elderly people need robots to do more complex tasks. In the future, the research work may be adopted with big data analysis, image processing, and statistical analysis reviewed with comparative analysis of machine learning approach.

AI Robots- the future of technology

Artificial intelligence (AI) is the simulation of human intelligence in machines that programmed to think and act like humans. The machine associated with a human mind such as learning and problem-solving. The ideal characteristic of artificial intelligence is its ability to take action for the best chance of achieving a specific goal. The goals of artificial intelligence are based on learning, reasoning, and perception. Machines use a cross-disciplinary approach based on mathematics, computer science, linguistics, psychology, and more. Key points are as;-

- AI is the simulation of human intelligence in machines.
- The aim of artificial intelligence includes learning, reasoning, and perception.
- AI is used across different industries including finance and healthcare.
- Weak AI tends to be single-task oriented and strong AI is more complex and human-like.

AI Robots

Robotics is a domain in artificial intelligence with the study of creating intelligent and efficient robots. Robots are the artificial agents for the real-world environment. Robots manipulate the objects by perceiving, picking, moving, modifying the physical properties of objects, destroying it, or having an effect thereby freeing manpower from doing repetitive functions without getting bored, distracted, or exhausted. It is a branch of AI composed of Electrical Engineering, Mechanical Engineering, and Computer Science for designing, construction, and application of robots. The robots have mechanical construction designed to accomplish a particular task with power and control of the machinery. They contain some level of a computer program that determines what, when, and how a robot doing things.

Difference in Robot System and AI Program

Here is the difference between the two –

- AI programs operate in computer-simulated worlds. The input of the AI program is in symbols and rules. They need general-purpose computers to operate the programs.
- Robots operate in the real physical world. The Inputs to robots is in analog signal in the form of speech waveform or images. They function with special hardware with sensors and effectors

Robot Locomotion

Locomotion is the mechanism where the robot is capable of moving in its environment. There are various types of locomotions

Legged

This type of locomotion consumes more power while doing walk, jump, trot, hop, climb up or down, etc. It requires several motors to accomplish a movement. It is suited for rough and smooth terrain wherein irregular or too smooth surface it consumes more power for wheeled locomotion. Sometimes it is a little difficult to implement because of stability issues. It comes with a variety of legs that is two, four, or six legs. Leg coordination is necessary for locomotion which has multiple legs. Gaits is a periodic sequence of lift and release events for each of the total legs. The total number of possible gaits where a robot travel depends upon the number of its legs. If a robot has k legs, then the number of possible events N = (2k-1)!. There are six possible different events –

- Lifting the Left leg
- Releasing the Left leg
- Lifting the Right leg

- Releasing the Right leg
- Lifting both the legs together
- Releasing both the legs together

In the case of k=6 legs, there are 39916800 possible events. Hence, the complexity of robots is directly proportional to the number of legs.

Wheeled Locomotion

It requires fewer number of motors to complete a movement. It is easy to implement with less stability issues in case if there is more number of wheels. It is more efficient as compared to legged locomotion. The Standard wheel rotates around the wheel axle and the contact. The Castor wheel rotates around the wheel axle and the offset steering joint. Swedish 45o and Swedish 90o wheels rotate around the contact point, around the wheel axle, and the rollers. Ball or spherical wheel is the Omnidirectional wheel which is difficult to implement technically.

Slip/Skid Locomotion

The robot is steered by moving the tracks with different speeds in the same or opposite direction. It has stability because of the large contact area of track and ground.

Components of a Robot

Robots are constructed with the following –

- Power Supply – The robots are powered by batteries, solar power, hydraulic
- Actuators – It converts energy into movement.
- Electric motors (AC/DC) – Motors are required for rotational movement.
- Pneumatic Air Muscles contract almost 40% when air is sucked in them.
- Muscle Wires contract by 5% when an electric current is passed through them.
- Piezo Motors and Ultrasonic Motors are the best for industrial robots.
- Sensors provide knowledge of the real-time information on the task environment

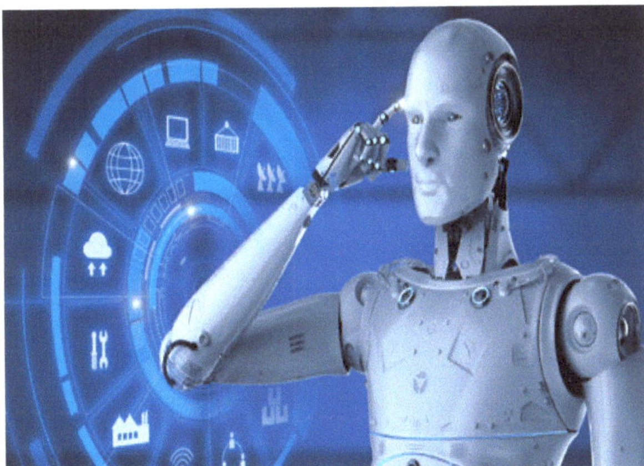

Fig.23.3 *Showing the features of a Robot in use*

Computer Vision

This is a technology of AI in which the robots can see. Vision plays a crucial role in the domains of safety, security, health, access, and entertainment. It automatically extracts, analyzes, and comprehends useful information from a single image or an array of images. This process accomplishes automatic visual comprehension.

Hardware of Computer Vision System

This involves Power supply, Image acquisition devices such as camera, processor, software, a Display device, accessories such as camera stands, cables, and connectors

Tasks of Computer Vision

- Optical Character Reader is a software to convert scanned documents into editable text, which accompanies a scanner.
- Face Detection comes with this feature, which enables to read the face and take the picture of perfect expression.
- Object Recognition is installed in supermarkets, cameras, high-end cars such as BMW, GM, and Volvo.
- Estimating the Position of an object to the camera as in the position of the tumor in the human body.

Application of Computer Vision

- Agriculture
- Autonomous vehicles
- Biometrics
- Character recognition
- Forensics, security, and surveillance
- Industrial quality inspection
- Face recognition
- Gesture analysis
- Geoscience
- Medical imagery
- Pollution monitoring
- Process control
- Remote sensing
- Robotics
- Transport

Applications of Robotic. The robotics has been instrumental in the various domains such as –

- Industries – Robots are used for handling material, cutting, welding, color coating, drilling, polishing, etc.
- Military – It reaches inaccessible and hazardous zones during the war. A robot named Daksh, developed by DRDO used to destroy life-threatening objects safely.
- Medicine – These robots carry hundreds of clinical tests simultaneously, rehabilitating permanently disabled people, and performing complex surgeries such as brain tumors.
- Exploration – These robots used for space exploration, underwater drones used for ocean exploration.
- Entertainment – Disney's have created hundreds of robots for animated movies.

Using AI to Help Care for Senior Citizens

- Providing Companionship
- Helping Seniors Live Securely and Independently in Their Homes
- Pose Detection for Preventive Care
- Trust Mindy Support for Your Medical Data Annotation Needs

As the world's population gradually becomes older, there is an increasing need to develop new technology to help provide better care for them. In fact, according to a report by the United Nations, there are 703 million people aged 65 and older, a number that is expected to more than double by 2050. Since the population of older adults is growing at such a rapid speed, there are various social, economic, and health challenges that must be addressed. This is an area where AI can be of great assistance since it can help the healthcare system deal with the increased demand for senior healthcare services. In this article, we will take a look at some of the ways AI is helping senior citizens take better care of themselves and maintain their independence.

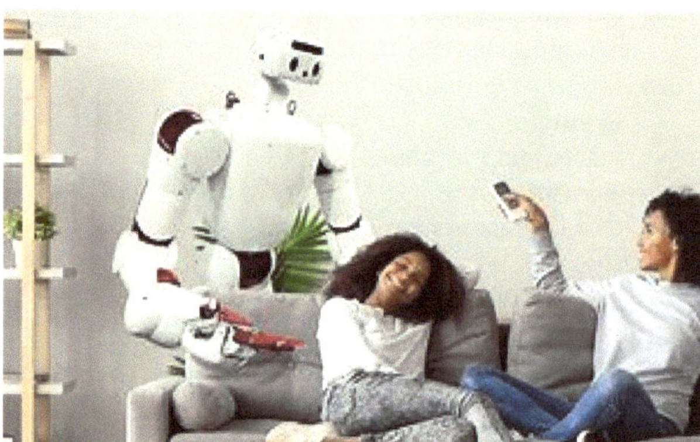

Fig.23.4 *Personal AI-based robots as lifetime human companions*

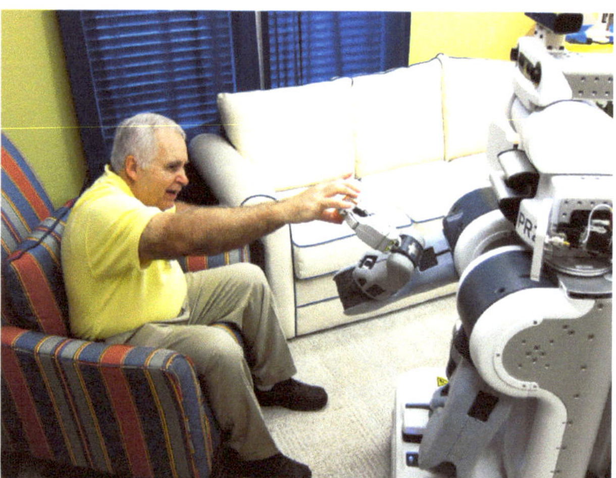

Fig, 23 5 *Scientists have created a robot that could help elderly people with dementia and other limitations live independently in their own homes*

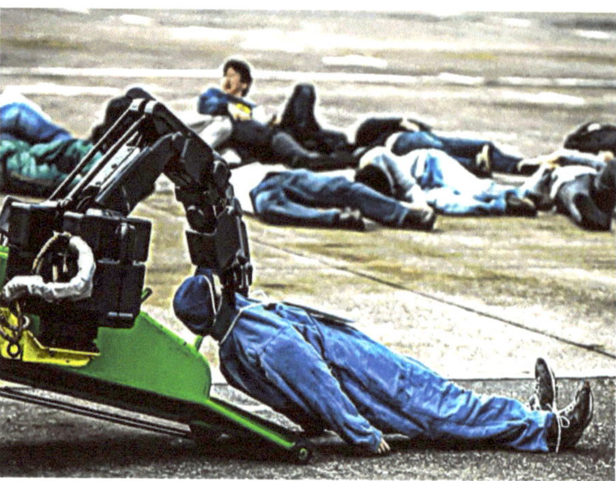

Fig. 23.6 *Robot is doing rescue-job*

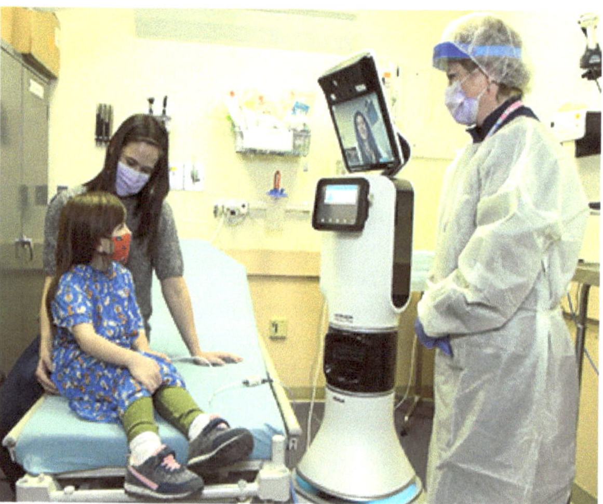

Fig.23 .7 *New robot helps care for kids in the emergency room*

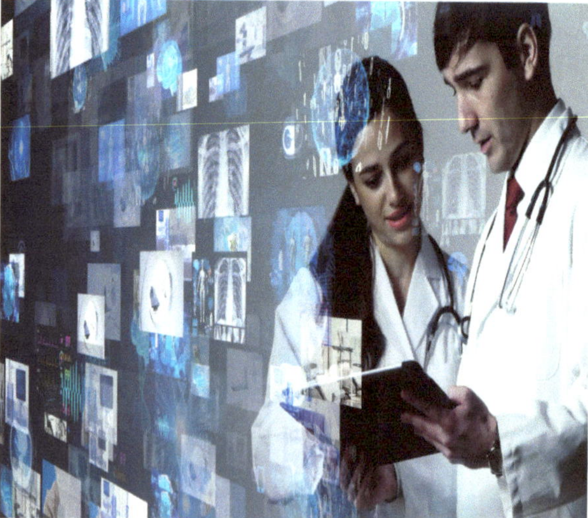

Fig. 23.8 *Using AI to Efficiently Diagnose and Reduce Medical Errors*

Pose Detection for Preventive Care

Falls are a leading cause of unintentional injuries and can result in devastating disabilities and fatalities when left undetected and not treated in time. In fact, worldwide, falls are a leading cause of unintentional injuries in adults older than 65 years old, with 37.3 million falls requiring medical attention and 646,000 resulting in deaths annually. Human pose detection can play a key role in elderly care for fast responses and preventing seniors from falling. A lot of studies have been done in Japan to create such pose detection software. For example, researchers at the Toyohashi University of Technology have done extensive research into estimating human poses using deep learning with depth data from twin camera systems in elderly care robots. The technology was able to generate data using computer graphics and motion capture technologies various poses that could signal a potential fall within acceptable reliability levels.

While fall prevention products are still being perfected, there are other products on the market, such as For example, in Canada there is a very useful tool called the AltumView's Cypress Smart Home Care Alert System that can call for help if a fall does occur. It can also provide a heat map of an area where falls have frequently occurred. This allows the caregiver to take measures, such as removing certain obstacles or blocking access to that location, to prevent similar accidents from happening again.

Trust Mindy Support for Your Medical Data Annotation Needs

Regardless of whether or not your dataset requires trained medical professionals to do the annotation or such work can be done without a medical background, Mindy Support can assemble a team for you to get the job done. Thanks to our skills and expertise, we can help you actually even the most daring and imaginative products. Contact us today to learn more about how we can help you.

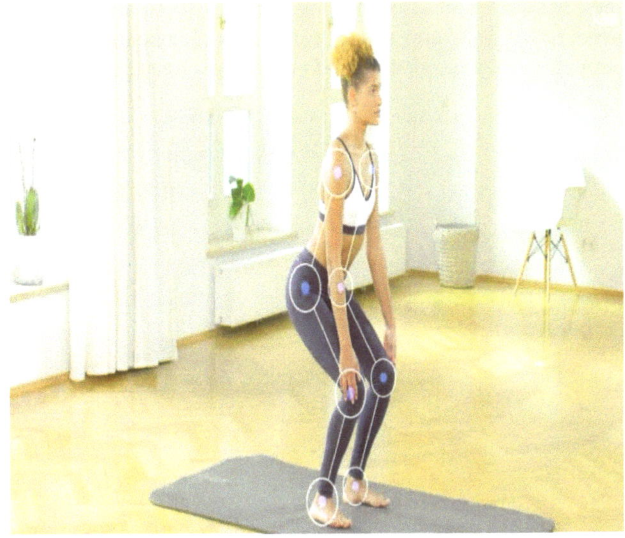

Fig. 23.9 *AI Pose Estimation Technology and How You Can Use It*

Helping Seniors Live Securely and Independently in Their Homes

According to a report from the AARP, 90% of seniors want to stay in their homes as they age. However, the homes of senior citizens often cannot accommodate their individual needs, posing many risks to their safety and wellness. This is why a lot of seniors in the US us various smart home devices to maintain their independence. This includes activity-based sensors that are connected to a smart security system and can trigger alarms and send help for potential break-ins, fires, and unsafe levels of carbon monoxide.

Another interesting feature is using machine learning to understand a senior's patterns and behaviors. If the system detects a change in their routine, such as the sensor on a medicine cabinet not being triggered when it's time to take a scheduled prescription, the AI spots this break in the pattern and notifies interested parties via email, text, and/or push notifications.

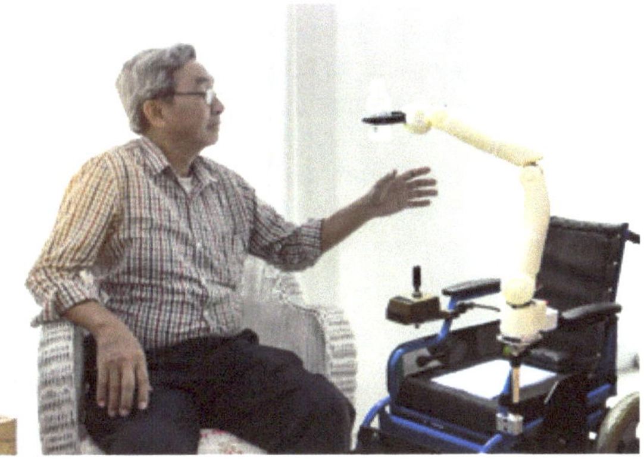

Fig.23.10 *AI helping seniors lve securely and independently in their homes*

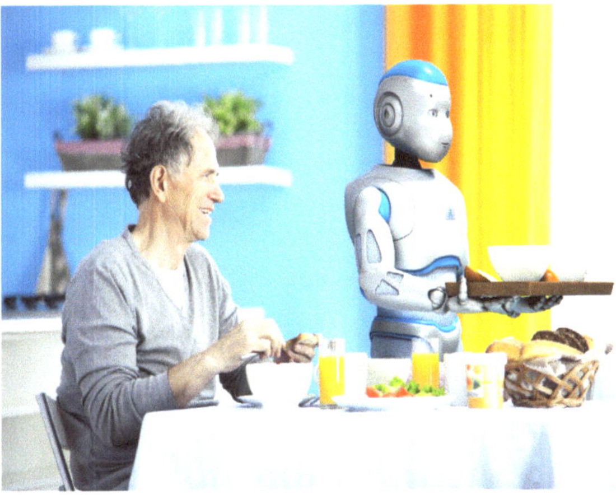

Fig. 23.11 *AI Romeo-An Intelligent French Robot To Help Elderly With Daily Tasks*

It won't be long before robots become a normal part of our everyday lives. Soon, our mobile companions will provide everything from coaching to communication to companionship, keeping us independent as we grow older. The era of human and robot interaction has begun, and it is changing the way we experience ageing.Can robots solve the problems of an ageing society? Ongoing research suggests they can. Today's robots can take out the trash, help you walk and do the shopping

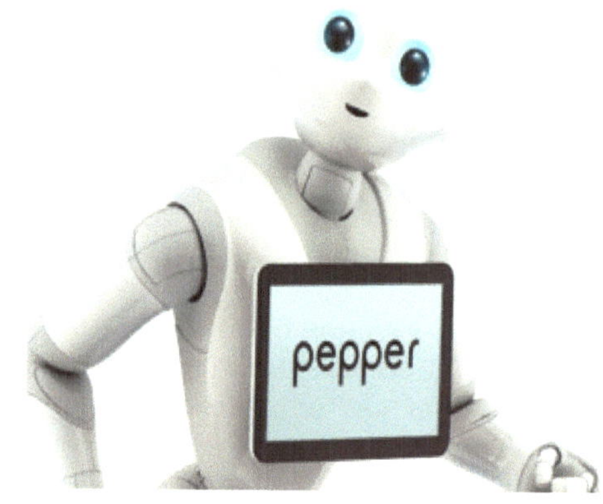

Fig.23.12 SoftBank's personal robot 'Pepper' will go on sale in Japan starting today. Initially, only 1,000 units of the robot will be available for purchase. Pepper is an intelligent humanoid robot that is capable of reading people's , basic human emotions and hold a conversation

How Robots Can Help The Elderly

The main reasons robots have been developed for elderly people are:

•To aid them with small tasks such eating or fetching things
•To help with mobility and transport, including getting out of bed or moving around
•To reduce loneliness and help them with social and emotional needs
•To set reminders for medicines, meals, and appointments

Robots can also be programmed to learn an elderly person's preferences and habits and detect changes in behaviour, including alerting caregivers or emergency services in the event of a fall. From small tasks to more significant help, the overall aim is to improve elderly people's quality of life, making them feel more independent, happier and more confident living alone or with reduced support.

1. Social Interaction - Pepper The Social Robot

Unfortunately a side effect of getting old is often loneliness, as people lose partners and friends and are no longer as physically able to go outside. In fact, according to Age UK, more than a million elderly people in the UK say that they go for over a month without speaking to anyone.

Enter Pepper, the world's first social humanoid robot. Pepper was created specifically for human interaction and can recognise faces, basic human emotions and hold a conversation. Pepper has been successfully trialled in care homes in both the UK and Japan, with residents' mental health found to improve after spending time with the robot across two weeks

Pepper and other robots like Cruzr have also been equipped with sensors to monitor blood pressure, oxygen saturation and body temperature, allowing caregivers to provide the proper care and treatments on a flexible basis.

2. Robotic Therapy Pets

In the wake of the pandemic, visitation restrictions and social distancing guidelines meant that many elderly people experienced feelings of isolation, as they were unable to see family and friends.In order to help them cope, robotics companies created a robotic 'pet' to give to residents in nursing homes, hospitals and assisted living facilities. These robotic pets register touch, light and sound, can respond to being stroked, recognise words, bark or purr and even have a heartbeat.

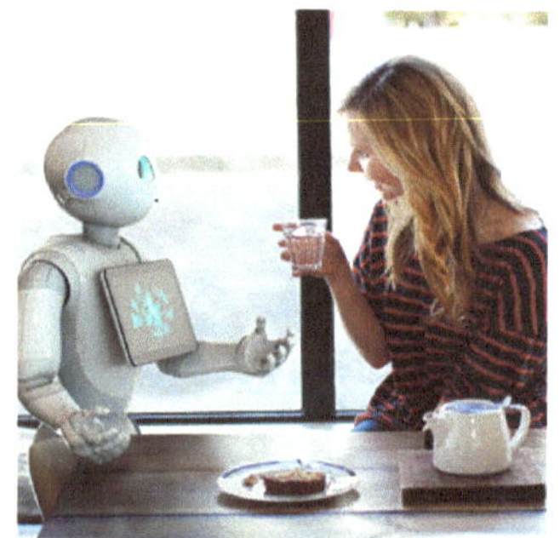

Fig.23.13 HERB stands for Home Exploring Robot Butler and is an autonomous robot that can learn to perform tasks such as putting books on a bookshelf, loading a dishwasher, offering tea ,clearing a table and fetching drinks from the fridge

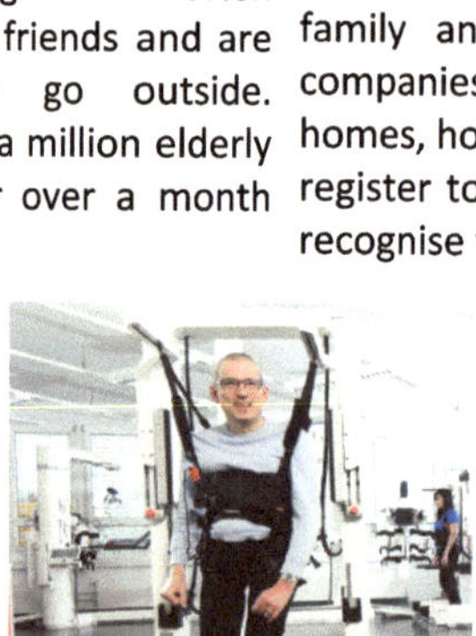

Fig.23.14 Andago is a mobile robot for body-weight supported gait training that allows upright, hands-free walking without spatial limitations.

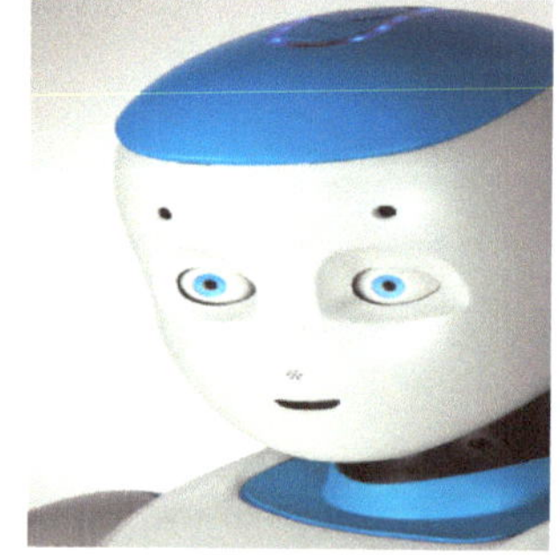

Fig.23 15 A robot called Romeo to do just that. Tall for a service robot at 1.40 m, he can keep track of your schedule, remind you to buy milk and tell you how much medicine to take. He'll offer advice to help you through your daily activities while making sure you didn't leave the stove on.

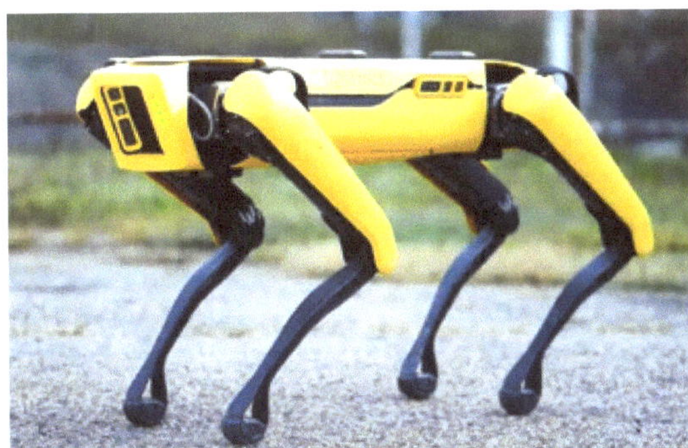

Fig.23.16 Here's how Boston Dynamics' robot dog encourages social distancing [video]The policing of social distancing and general citizen behaviour during the pandemic has been the subject of much controversy. Have you met Spot the Dog?

therapy pets have similar effects to real life therapy pets, including reduced stress, increased wellbeing, comfort and companionship - similar to that of companionship care.

3. Feeding Robots

When we get older, tasks we used to find easy often become more difficult, including washing, dressing and eating. There are now several types of robot available to help elderly people eat and drink, such as the My Spoon robot from Robotarm.

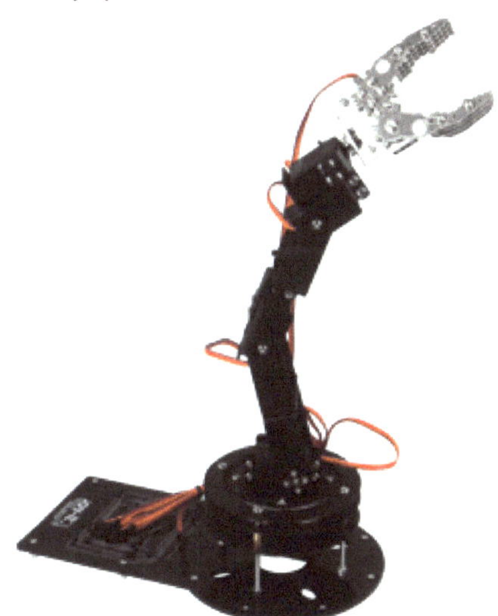

Fig.23.17 Robotarm. to help elderly people eat and drink, such as the my Spoon robot

My Spoon helps those with limitations in arm and hand function by bringing food from a plate or a bowl to their mouth.

4. Futuristic Baths

Baths are great - not only do they keep us clean, but they're also good for relaxing, promoting blood circulation and wellbeing. However, when you get to a certain age, having a bath may no longer be an option if you don't have someone to help you. At the World Expo in 1970, Sanyo unveiled their 'Ultrasonic Bath', otherwise known as 'The Human Washing Machine', which used a combination of water jets, wave generators and driers to wash and dry people.

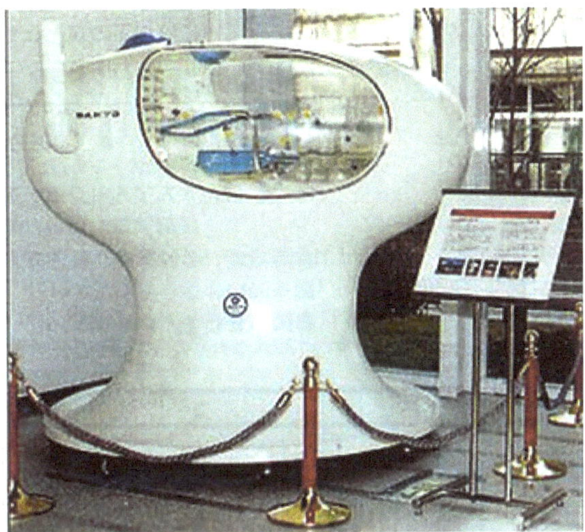

Fig.23.18 Sanyo Ultrasonic Bath: Human In Roll-lo Bathing

Robotics companies are still working on bath robots that can lift elderly people safely in and out of a bathtub and provide assistance with washing.

5. Lifting And Carrying

Elderly people tend to be less able to get up and move around than younger people, so several robots have been developed to help with this aspect of life

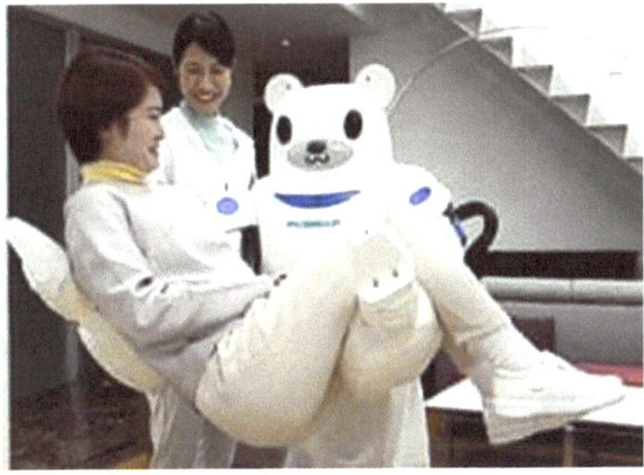

Fig.23.19 Japanese robot can lift patients from beds into wheelchairs or help them to stand up, promising 'powerful yet gentle care' for the elderly

The Robear robot was an experimental nursing care robot developed by the RIKEN-SRK Collaboration Center for Human-Interactive Robot Research and Sumitomo Riko Company in Japan. Robear aimed to lift people out of bed, help them into wheelchairs and even offer assistance with standing. Other models like the RIBA (Robot for Interactive Body Assistance) are capable of moving residents in and out of bed and wheelchair.

6. Independence - ElliQ

Next on our list is ElliQ, an interactive robot that promotes independence to help older adults feel more comfortable doing things for themselves. ElliQ provides companionship, entertainment and fun, as well as helping people reach their health and wellness goals

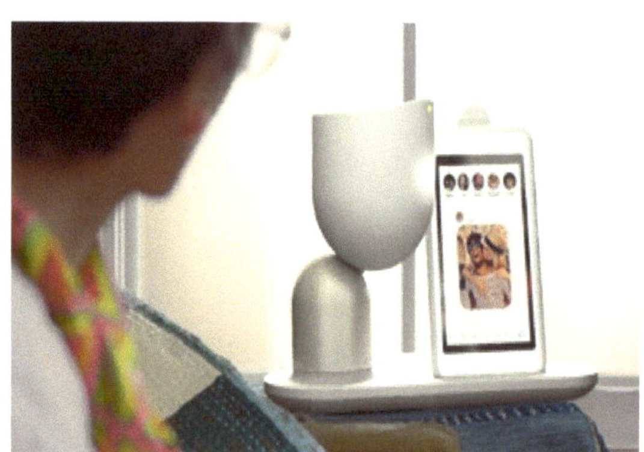

Fig.23.20 Elli.Q, a small but extremely advanced companion robot, has been designed to use speech tones, lights and 'body' language to convey emotions. An adorable talking robot 'friend' designed to keep elderly people company has been launched in London.The many features offered by ElliQ include conversation, music streaming, news, sports and weather, cognitive games, health check-ins, mindfulness exercises, messaging with family members, interesting facts and general health info, plus physical exercise! As users spend more time with ElliQ, the robot adapts its approach to tailor suggestions to their unique needs and preferences, personalising the experience to make it more genuine.

7. Cleaning Robots

Inventions like the Roomba, the robotic vacuum cleaner, can really help elderly people with daily housework. Instead of the person having to lift a heavy hoover around and potentially hurt their back bending over, the Roomba automatically travels through the home to hoover up dust and dirt in no time at all. Special cameras and sensors enable the Roomba to avoid obstacles and return to a 'base' after cleaning to stop them from getting underfoot. Some models even self empty into a self-sealing bag.

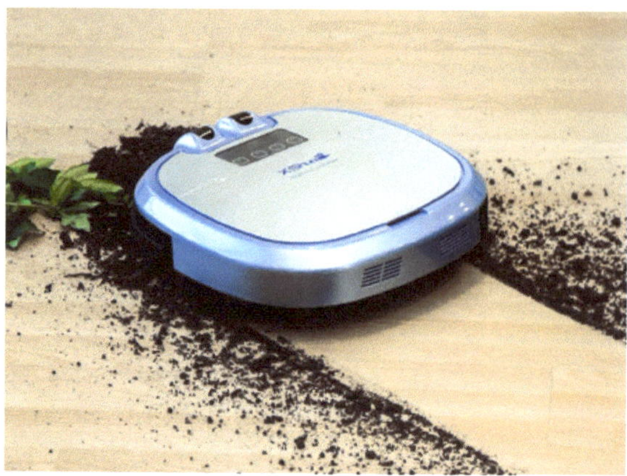

Fig.23.21 The Roomba automatically travels through the home to hoover up dust and dirt in no time at all.

8. Medical Assistance - Moxi The Medical Robot

The use of medical robots in elderly care is a growing industry. One example of this is Moxi, a one-armed robot that can travel around a hospital, picking up and delivering medicines, equipment, patient samples or bedding Moxi was invented by Andrea Thomaz and Vivian Chu in Austin, Texas and during studies, was found to save clinicians several hours a day by creating its own internal map and following delivery orders through an app.

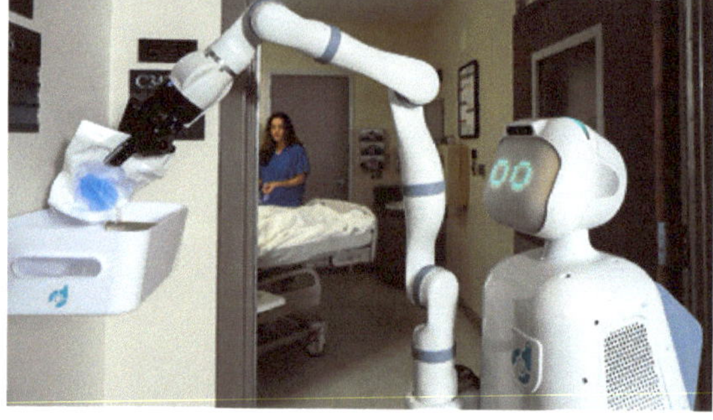

Fig.23.22 Moxi, a one-armed robot that can travel around a hospital, picking up and delivering medicines, equipment, patient samples or bedding

9. General Assistance - HERB The Robot Butler

HERB stands for Home Exploring Robot Butler and is an autonomous robot that can learn to perform tasks such as putting books on a bookshelf, loading a dishwasher, clearing a table and fetching drinks from the fridge - pretty impressive! Designed in Japan as part of the Carebotsinitiative, HERB effectively maps out its environment in order to navigate safely around without crashing into things or knocking them over.

Bibliography and Acknowledgement

- Abubshait, E. Wiese, and Y. L. Human, "You look human, but act like a machine: agent appearance and behavior modulate different aspects of Human-Robot interaction," Frontiers in Psychology, vol. 8, 2017.
- B. Kartal, E. Nunes, J. Godoy, and M. Gini, "Monte Carlo tree search with branch and bound for multi-robot task allocation symposium conducted at the meeting of the the IJCAI-16 workshop on autonomous mobile service robots," vol. 30, no. 1, 2016.
- B. Zohuri and M. Moghaddam, "Neural network driven supper artificial intelligence based on internet of things and big data," Business Resilience System (BRS), vol. 1, 2018.
- D. SverreSyrdal, J. Saunders, and K. DautenhahnK. L. Koay and N. Burke, ""Teach me–show me""'—"end-user personalization of a smart home and comrade robot"," IEEE transactions on Human Machine Systems, vol. 46, no. 1, 2016.
  Davison, Introduction to Robotics, Department of Computing, Imperial College, London, UK, 2016.
- F. Al-Turjman and J. P. Lemayian, "Intelligence, security, and vehicular sensor networks in internet of things (IoT)-enabled smart-cities: an overview," Computers & Electrical Engineering, vol. 87, Article ID 106776, 2020.
- G. Viejo, D. D. Torrico, F. R. Dunshea, and S. Fuentes, "Development of artificial neural network models to assess beer acceptability based on sensory properties using a robotic pourer: a comparative model approach to achieve an artificial intelligence system," Beverages, vol. 5, 2019.
- G. Yang, Z. Pang, M. J. Deen et al., "Homecare robotic systems for healthcare 4.0: visions and enabling technologies," IEEE Journal of Biomedical and Health Informatics, vol. 24, pp. 2535–2549, 2020.
- H. Ashrafian, A. Darzi, and T. Athanasiou, "A novel modification of the Turing test for artificial intelligence and robotics in healthcare," International Journal of Medical Robotics and Computer Assisted Surgery, vol. 11, pp. 38–43, 2015.
- H. BozU. Kose, "Emotion extraction from facial expressions by using artificial intelligence techniques," Broad Research in Artificial Intelligence and Neuroscience, vol. 8, pp. 5–16, 2017.
- H. Manoharan, Y. Teekaraman, P. R. Kshirsagar, S. Sundaramurthy, and A. Manoharan, "Examining the effect of aquaculture using sensor-based technology with machine learning algorithm," Aquaculture Research, vol. 51, no. 11, pp. 4748–4758, 2020.
- J. Celis, S. Castro, and D. Guevara, "Voice processing with Internet of Things for a home automation system," in Proceedings of the International conference on Electronics, Electricalengineering and computing, pp. 8–10, IEEE, Lima, Peru, August 2018.
- J.Cowie, "Evaluation of a digital consultation and self-care advice tool in primary care: a multi-methods study," Inter. Jour.of Environ Res Public Health, vol. 15, 2018.Sensmeier, "Harnessing the power of artificial intelligence," Nursing Management, vol. 48, no. 11, pp. 14–19, 2017.
- Hameed, I. S. Bajwa, S. Ramzan, W. Anwar, and A. Khan, "An intelligent IoT based healthcare system using fuzzy neural networks," Scientific Programming, vol. 2020, Article ID 8836927, 15 pages, 2020.
- Pu, W. Moyle, C. Jones, and M. Todorovic, "The effectiveness of social robots for older adults: a systematic review and meta-analysis of randomized controlled studies," Gerontologist Jan, vol. 59, no. 1, pp. e37–51, 2019.
- M. M. A. D. Graaf, S. B. Allouch, and J. A. G. M. V. Dijk, "Why would I use this in my home? a model of domestic social robot acceptance," Human-Computer Interaction, vol. 34, pp. 115–173, 2019.
- M. Mortazavi, F. Aminiazad, H. Parsaei, and M. A. Mosleh-Shirazi, "An artificial neural network-based model for predicting annual dose in healthcare workers occupationally exposed to different levels of ionizing radiation," Radiation Protection Dosimetry, vol. 189, 2020.
- M. Sg, T. Ak, A. St, S. Sv, and O. Mj, "Role of artificial intelligence in health care," Biochemistry Ind Journal, vol. 11, no. 5, pp. 1–14, 2017. Mesko, "The role of artificial intelligence in precision medicine," Expert Rev Precis Med Drug Dev, vol. 2, pp. 239–241, 2017.
- P. R. Kshirsagar, H. Manoharan, F. Al-Turjman, and K. Kumar, "Design and testing of automated smoke monitoring sensors in vehicles," IEEE Sensors Journal, vol. 1, p. 1, 2020.
- P.-P. C. F. Rudzicz and S. Raimondo, "Ludwig: a conversational robot for people with alzheimer's," The Journal of the Alzheimer's Association, vol. 13, 2017.
- R. Bhatnagar and D. Batra, "Robotic process automation in healthcare-a review," International Robotics & Automation Journal, vol. 5, 2019.
  S. Montani, R. Bellazzi, A. Riva, C. Larizza, L. Portinale, and M. Stefanelli, "Artificial intelligence techniques for diabetes management: the T-IDDM project. ECAI," in Proceedings of the 14th European conerence on Artificial Intelligence, pp. 1–5, Berlin, Germany, August 2000.
- W. Moyle, C. Jones, L. Pu, and S. C. Chen, "Applying user-centred research design and evidence to develop and guide the use of technologies, including robots, in aged care," Contemporary Nurse, vol. 54, pp. 1–3, 2018.
- W. Yu, A. Kapusta, J. Tan, C. C. Kemp, G. Turk, and C. K. Liu, "Haptic simulation for robot-assisted dressing," in Proceedings of the IEEE International Conference on Robotics and Automation, pp. 6044–6051, Singapore, May 2017

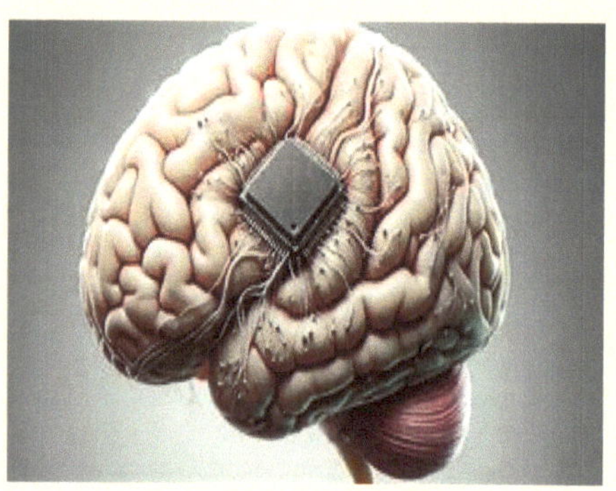

Implantable Cardiac And Non- Cardiac Electronic Devices in Elderly Population

The number of cardiac implantable electronic devices (CIED) has been increasing year-on-year. This, coupled with improvements in life expectancy,means that more elderly patients will meet the criteria for a CIED. National and international guidelines set out clear criteria and make recommendations for CIED use based on available evidence. However, the majority of clinical trials include few, if any, elderly patients (>80 years), with supposed benefits in the elderly population extrapolated from data derived from younger patients. The aim of this review is to give an overview of the different types of CIEDs and to discuss our approach on their use in the elderly population (>75 years) going beyond guideline recommendations.

1.Implantable Loop Recorders

Falls are a common presentation among elderly patients admitted to hospitals. These include mechanical falls or those resulting from a transient loss of consciousness. In the majority of cases, a detailed history, physical examination (including lying and standing blood pressure) and simple investigations such as an ECG may help determine the cause. The challenge lies with patients in whom a cause is not apparent but an arrhythmia is suspected either clinically or epidemiologically. Given the short duration of Holter monitoring, there is often a low yield in correlating arrhythmia with clinical symptoms. In contrast, implantable cardiac monitors can be useful in determining any correlation between symptoms and rhythms, aiding in the diagnosis of a clinically relevant arrhythmia. They are particularly helpful for patients whose initial investigations have been negative with a normal baseline ECG.

The elderly population are much more likely than younger patients to have brady-arrhythmia as a cause of their syncope. Understanding the background to the fall or loss of consciousness is also critical to the decision-making process, and the following characteristics are typical of an event that may be bradycardia related:

- Sudden loss of consciousness without any preceding symptoms.
- The patient is unconscious before they hit the floor (and may have facial injury as they have not put their hands out to save themselves).
- The patient feels better almost as soon as they regain consciousness.
- The loss of consciousness occurs while sitting or lying (slumping over while have a meal with friends or family is a classic warning that the patient has a cardiac rhythm problem).

In patients with some degree of underlying conduction disease on ECG (bifascicular or trifascicular block, marked first-degree atrio-ventricular [AV] block) then this, combined with a compelling clinical history of syncope, may warrant implantation of a pacemaker without evidence of higher-degree block correlating with symptoms.5 However, the obvious disadvantage of the loop recorder is the necessity of another syncopal episode for its diagnostic utility, minimising its suitability for high-risk patients.

Although loop recorders are often used to investigate infrequent palpitations, in a patient with preserved ejection fraction (EF) and no evidence of inherited arrhythmogenic tendency, palpitations will usually represent a benign symptomatic problem. In such mildly symptomatic patients, implantation of a loop recorder is unlikely to change the management plan. Alternatives such as the hand-held, smartphone-based ECG recording devices can instead be offered to the patient or they can purchase them themselves. These may yield similar results without the need for invasive monitoring. Loop recorders can be useful to screen for asymptomatic AF, particularly in high CHA2DS2-VASc score patients who have had cryptogenic stroke.

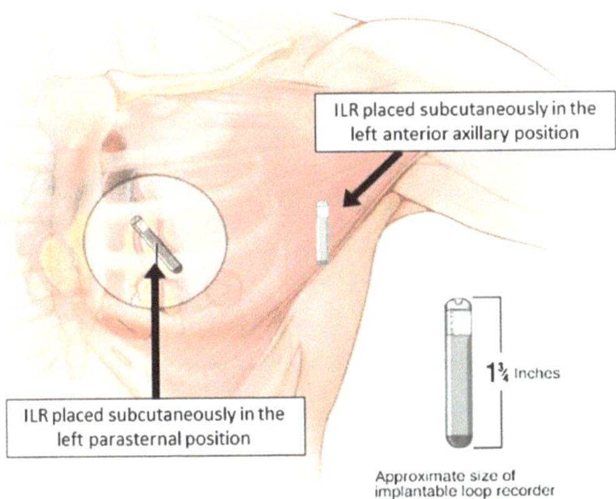

Fig.24.1 Implantable loop recorder (ILR) in the left parasternal and left anterior axillary positions. Both devices are placed subcutaneously

2.Pacemakers

Over 80% of pacemakers are implanted in the elderly patient (mean age 75±10 years). The most common indication is AV block and sinus node disease. All patients with complete heart block and type 2 second-degree AV block should be implanted with a pacemaker regardless of symptoms as this has prognostic significance. Beyond this, pacing is generally only carried out if bradycardia is accompanied by symptoms.Elderly patients are more prone to complications. A meta-analysis by Armaganijan et al. showed that elderly patients undergoing device implantation are at increased risk of complications, in particular pneumothorax and lead dislodgements. Pneumothorax conveys significant morbidity in older patients, with prolonged hospital stays and a risk of developing infections. To reduce the risk of pneumothorax, a traditional 'blind' subclavian puncture should be avoided wherever possible. Implantation using the cephalic vein, the use of ultrasound-guided punctures or extra-thoracic punctures with fluoroscopic guidance have been shown to reduce the risk of pneumothorax and should be used when possible. The higher incidence of lead dislodgement in the elderly is often related to an increase in venous tortuosity as well as reduced cardiac mass for lead attachment. Additional redundancy should be left on the lead during the implant. Data from the Pacemaker Selection in the Elderly (PASE) trial demonstrated that older age is a risk factor for lead perforation. Furthermore, a study by Sterlinski et al. demonstrated that – compared with passive leads – active leads were more likely to result in perforation.Therefore, to minimise the risk of perforation we recommend either using a passive fixation lead or an active fixation lead to the interventricular septum avoiding the right ventricular apex.

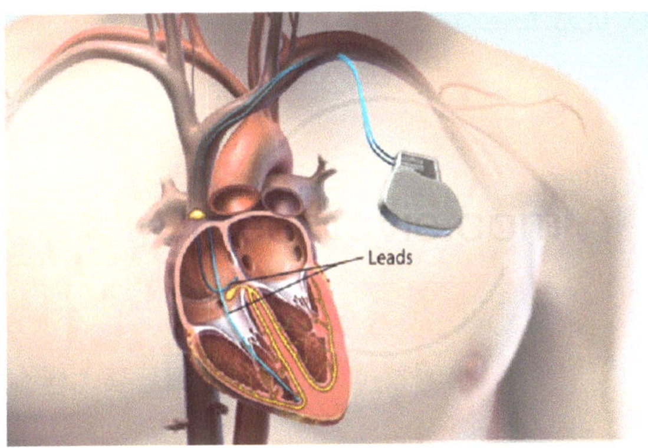

Fig.24.2 The pacemaker is implanted beneath the skin, usually below the left collarbone. The area is cleaned with a sterile solution. You will be given an antibiotic for protection against microbes and a sedative through an intravenous line. A large sterile sheet will cover your body and will partially cover your face.One or two leads will be threaded through a vein and positioned in your heart under X-ray guidance. These are then connected to the pacemaker which is positioned under the skin before the incision is sewn over and dressed.

While there are data demonstrating that dual-chamber may be superior to single-chamber pacemakers in the elderly regarding symptoms related to the pacemaker syndrome,17 there may be circumstances when a single-chamber system is appropriate. In frail, unstable, agitated patients presenting in complete heart block, it would be reasonable to reduce the procedure time and implant a single-lead device to render the patient safe and to avoid a more prolonged procedure that could be distressing.

It is important to offer an individual, tailored approach when pacing is considered in the elderly. These patients are more likely to have multiple co-morbidities that could affect the decision-making process. For example, in a bed-bound patient with an incidental finding of sinus node disease who is having fleeting dizzy spells, any benefit may not outweigh the risk and inconvenience of pacemaker implantation. Therefore, when discussing therapy with any patient – but particularly the elderly where the trauma of intervention may have a bigger impact than the existing symptoms –

3.Implantable Cardioverter Defibrillator (ICD)

ICDs are implanted either for secondary prevention in patients who have a survived cardiac arrest or as primary prevention therapy.5,6 The evidence for the use of ICDs in these situations is well established but, as in many clinical trials, the elderly (>75 years) are poorly represented in these studies with a mean age of 63 in published randomised controlled trials (RCTs).

Healey et al. first highlighted the issue on the overall benefit of ICDs as secondary prevention by pooling data from published RCTs. They found that elderly patients had a higher incidence of non-arrhythmic deaths, minimising the benefit of an ICD. However, the modest sample of 252 elderly patients (aged ≥75 years) in this study may not reflect modern-day practice. Other observational studies from the Ontario database highlighted that age alone cannot be the sole

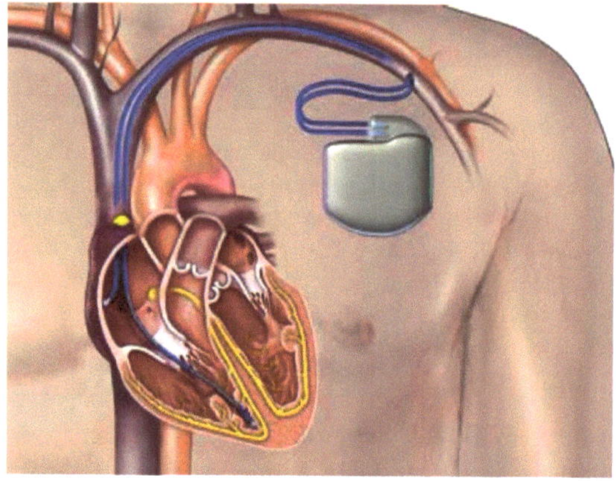

Fig.24.3 The conventional approach to implanting an ICD is similar to that for implanting a pacemaker, and the procedural risks are very similar. The ICD device is larger than a pacemaker, so can be more prominent. In people with a low body mass index, it is occasionally preferable to position the device underneath, rather than in front of the pectoral muscle.

predictor of mortality but rather that other co-morbidities like chronic renal failure, heart failure and chronic obstructive pulmonary disease are significant predictors of mortality.

An analysis of real-world data on the impact on ICD for secondary prevention involving over 12,000 patients over the age of 65 years showed that, while the rates of death increased with age, four in five older patients survived beyond 2 years. However, the study did not demonstrate the mode of death. Interestingly, beyond mortality, older patients have significant morbidity following an ICD implantation with higher rates of admission to special nursing facilities and re-admission to hospitals.While offering an ICD as secondary prevention seems like a logical choice and in line with current guidelines, it should be noted that – although it can prolong life – ICD implantation carries certain risk of increased morbidity. In the elderly population, some patients would value quality of life rather than longevity and therefore an open and honest discussion needs to take place prior to embarking on an implant. It is important to recognise that the ICD may simply change the mode of death from a sudden one to a longer, protracted and ultimately more distressing one, with no impact upon quality of life in the intervening period. This is likely in conflict with the end-of-life expectations of most – if not all – patients.

Primary prevention ICDs are indicated in patients with heart failure with a left ventricular EF <35% except those in New York Heart Association (NYHA) class IV and who have been on optimal medical therapy for a minimum of 3 months and expected to live more than a year. Mode of death in patients with heart failure can either be driven by a life-threatening arrhythmia or pump failure. Data from the ALTITUDE registry showed that the frequency of ICD therapy in the older age group is lower and other observational studies show that the mode of death in the elderly is more likely to be pump failure.

Elderly patients are also more likely to have multiple co-morbidities that could impact on 1-year survival. Ferretto et al. studied patients aged >75 years who had an ICD implanted for primary prevention. The authors concluded that age alone was not a predictor of 1-year mortality but rather EF <25% and moderate to severe renal failure predicted a high 1-year non-arrhythmia death of up to 45.5%.The use of ICDs in heart failure patients changes the mode of death from an arrhythmia cause to one of progressive pump failure. Furthermore, although older patients have been found to be less likely to have ICD shocks, both appropriate and inappropriate shocks are likely to have a significant impact on physical and mental wellbeing.

A clear plan for disabling anti-tachycardia therapy when approaching end-of-life care should be discussed with all patients having an ICD implanted so that they are able to make their wishes clear, ideally well in advance of any potential incapacity. It is important to ensure that the patient understands the distinction between bradycardia and tachycardia therapies when having this discussion.

Generally, if one has not had the potentially uncomfortable, albeit necessary discussion with the elderly patient about how they 'want to die' then it is likely that one has not really given them all the information they need to decide whether an ICD is right for them.

4. Cardiac Resynchronisation Therapy

Cardiac resynchronisation therapy (CRT) either alone (CRT-P) or in combination with a defibrillator (CRT-D) is well established in the treatment of patients with heart failure. Its use in the elderly is increasing, with up to 40% of CRT being implanted in patients over the age of 80 years.

Although clinical trials do not exclude elderly patients, the major trials that influence our clinical practice have a predominantly younger population making results derived from these trials unrepresentative of the older age group.

Killu et al. conducted a retrospective analysis to determine the outcomes of CRT in patients aged >80 years. They demonstrated that although overall survival was worse when compared to their younger counterparts, CRT resulted in improvement in NYHA class, EF and mitral regurgitation severity.

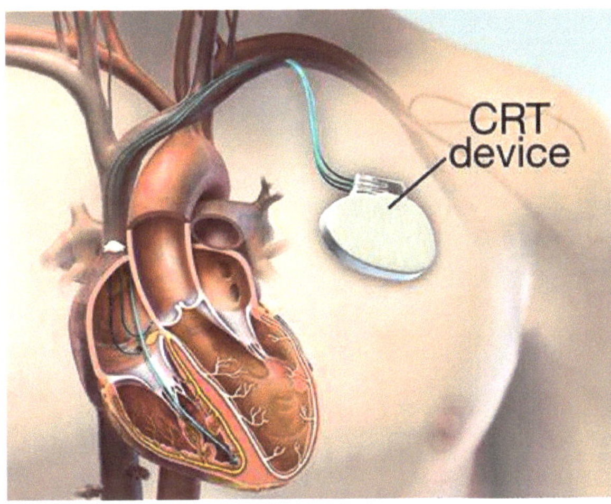

Fig.24.4 The CRT device goes under your skin, beneath your collarbone and is connected to your heart by wires called leads. A CRT device can detect when the heart is not beating in a coordinated manner . The CRT device then sends electrical signals to the heart to help the ventricles contract at the same time. This strengthens the heartbeat and increases the amount of blood pumped out of the heart

Martens et al. investigated the impact of CRT on both morbidity and mortality. Their findings were similar to those of Killu et al., with improvements in NYHA class and EF compared with younger counterparts. They also showed that elderly patients had higher all-cause mortality but this was no different to age-matched controls who had no heart failure. In addition, they demonstrated that elderly patients had a similar rate of heart-failure-related admissions compared to younger patients. The mode of death in octogenarians was mainly non-cardiac. When a death had a cardiac cause it was because of worsening heart failure rather than malignant arrhythmia. Aktas et al. analysed data from the multicentre automatic defibrillator trial and showed that elderly patients (>75 years) had a lower risk of ventricular tachy-arrhythmias compared with their younger counterparts (<75 years) providing further evidence to support the notion that malignant arrhythmias are less frequent in the elderly.

5.Remote Monitoring

Remote monitoring has been shown to be easy to use and well accepted in the elderly population. There are two areas where this could have a significant impact in this population group. The first is in AF detection as elderly patients tend to have a high CHA2DS2-VASc score and remote

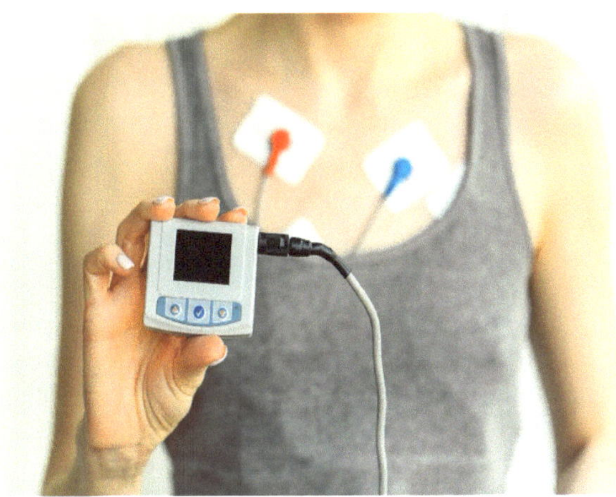

Fig.24.5 These devices allow healthcare professionals to remotely monitor patients' heart conditions, provide prompt consultations, and modify treatment plans as necessary. The adoption of remote monitoring devices is being driven by the accessibility and convenience of telehealth services.

Decision making for device implantation in elderly people should not be driven by guidelines alone. These patients may have complex co-morbidities and personal wishes that cannot be accommodated by guidelines. It is important to have a clear, open discussion with patients about the reasons for device therapy and to ensure this meets their expectations and wishes. This sometimes can be challenging in the presence of other family members where their wishes and views may not be aligned with the patient's. Therefore there may be times when one has to ensure that the patient has a genuine opportunity to individually assess their treatment options, albeit keeping in mind that having the family engaged and involved is crucial.

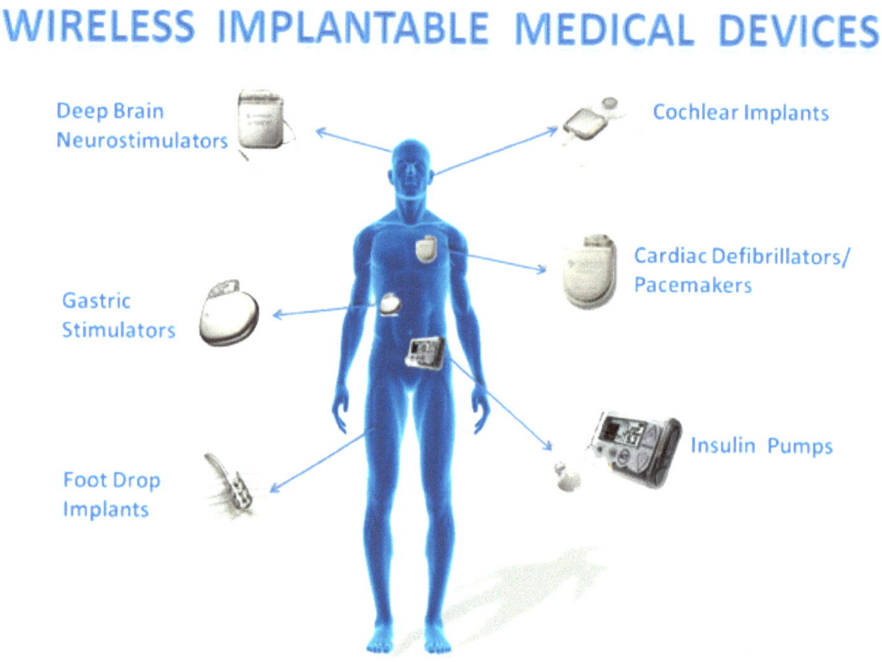

WIRELESS IMPLANTABLE MEDICAL DEVICES

Deep Brain Neurostimulators

Cochlear Implants

Cardiac Defibrillators/ Pacemakers

Gastric Stimulators

Insulin Pumps

Foot Drop Implants

Fig.24.6 Illustration showing different types of wireless implantable medical devices in the management of diseases .

6. Deep brain stimulation (DBS)

Deep brain stimulation (DBS) involves implanting electrodes within areas of the brain. The electrodes produce electrical impulses that affect brain activity to treat certain medical conditions. The electrical impulses also can affect cells and chemicals within the brain that cause medical conditions.

The amount of stimulation in deep brain stimulation is controlled by a pacemaker-like device placed under the skin in the upper chest. A wire that travels under the skin connects this device to the electrodes in the brain.

Deep brain stimulation is commonly used to treat a number of conditions, such as:

- Parkinson's disease.
- Essential tremor.
- Conditions that cause dystonia, such as Meige syndrome.
- Epilepsy.
- Tourette syndrome.
- Obsessive-compulsive disorder.
- Deep brain stimulation also is being studied as a potential treatment for:
- Chorea, such as Huntington's disease.
- Chronic pain.
- Cluster headache.
- Dementia.
- Depression.
- Addiction.
- Obesity.

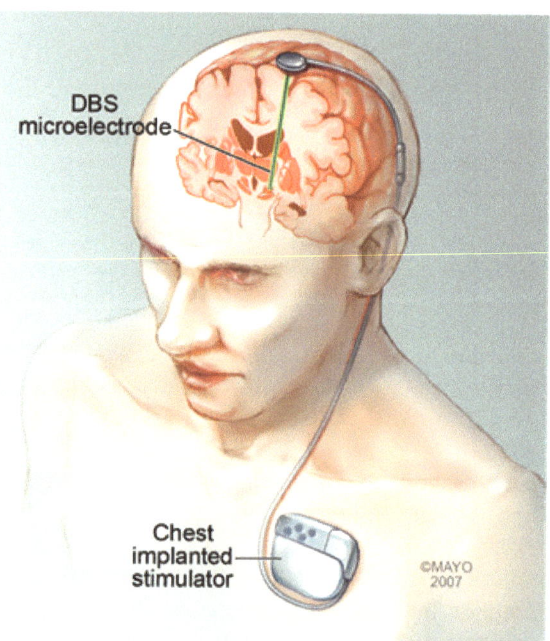

Fig. 24.7 Showing connections in Deep brain stimulation technique

7.Cochlear implants

Cochlear implants are complex medical devices that work differently than hearing aids. Rather than amplifying sound—which helps a person with residual hearing ability—a cochlear implant provides the sense of sound by stimulating the auditory nerve directly. Cochlear implants do not cure hearing loss or restore hearing, but they do provide an opportunity for the severely hard of hearing or deaf to perceive the sensation of sound by bypassing the damaged inner ear. Unlike hearing aids, they require surgical implantation.

Older adults and cochlear implants: What are the guidelines?

Senior citizens are generally candidates if:

- You have moderate to profound sensorineural hearing loss in both ears
- You receive limited benefit from hearing aids, measured by how well you perform on a hearing test in noise
- You are in reasonably good health and can withstand surgery

However, your doctors may or may not recommend an implant in other circumstances.

A.

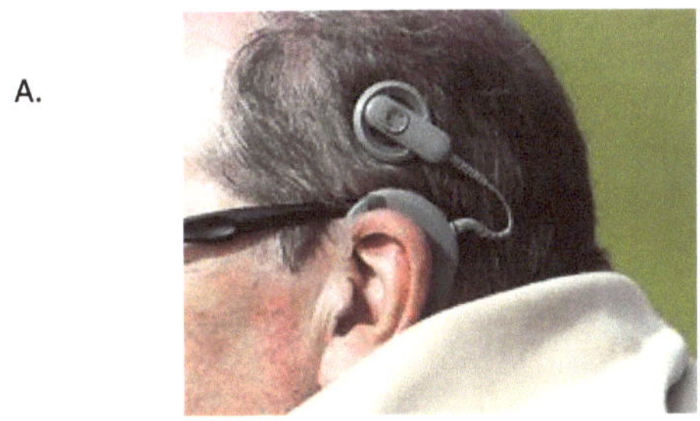

B.

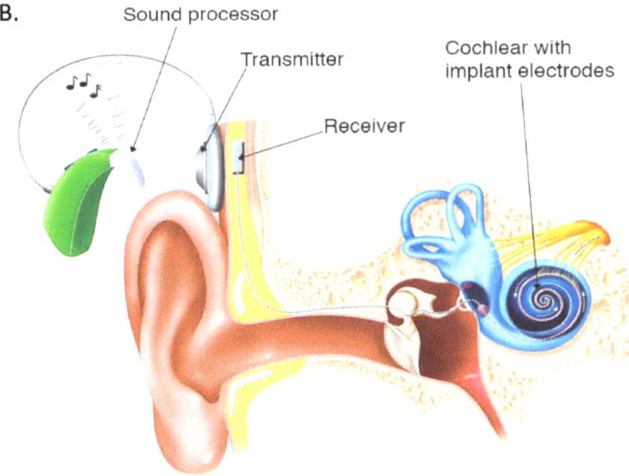

Fig 24.8 (A) old man is fitted with cochlear implant . (B) Various components of cochlear implant as shown o

What will my hearing be like with a cochlear implant?

A cochlear implant can give you the ability to pick up a variety of ordinary sounds, speak on the phone and enjoy music. According to the Food and Drug Administration (FDA), the benefits of a cochlear implant range widely. For people with implants, the FDA states:

"Hearing ranges from near normal ability to understand speech to no hearing benefit at all .Adults often benefit immediately and continue to improve for about 3 months after the initial tuning sessions. Then, although performance continues to improve, improvements are slower. Cochlear implant users' performances may continue to improve for several years.

Most perceive loud, medium and soft sounds. People report that they can perceive different types of sounds, such as footsteps, slamming of doors, sounds of engines, ringing of the telephone, barking of dogs, whistling of the tea kettle, rustling of leaves, the sound of a light switch being switched on and off, and so on. Many understand speech without lip-reading. However, even if this is not possible, using the implant helps lip-reading.

Many can make telephone calls and understand familiar voices over the telephone. Some good performers can make normal telephone calls and even understand an unfamiliar speaker. However, not all people who have implants are able to use the phone.Many can watch TV more easily, especially when they can also see the speaker's face. However, listening to the radio is often more difficult as there are no visual cues available.Some can enjoy music. Some enjoy the sound of certain instruments (piano or guitar, for example) and certain voices. Others do not hear well enough to enjoy music.

How does a Cochlear implant work?

An Implant works by bypassing non-functioning parts of the inner ear (Cochlea) and providing electrical stimulation directly to auditory nerve fibres in the cochlea. A Cochlear implant consists of two parts: an externally worn audio processor, which sits behind or over the ear, and an internal cochlear implant, which is surgically placed under the skin. Here is the process:

- The audio processor captures sounds and turns them into digital codes.
- These digital codes are transmitted to the internal implant through the coil, which is placed outside of the head.
- The implant converts the digitally-coded sound into electrical impulses and sends them along the electrode array placed inside the inner ear.
- These electrodes stimulate the cochlear nerve, which then transmits the electrical signals to the brain where they are interpreted as sounds.

8.Gastric Stimulators

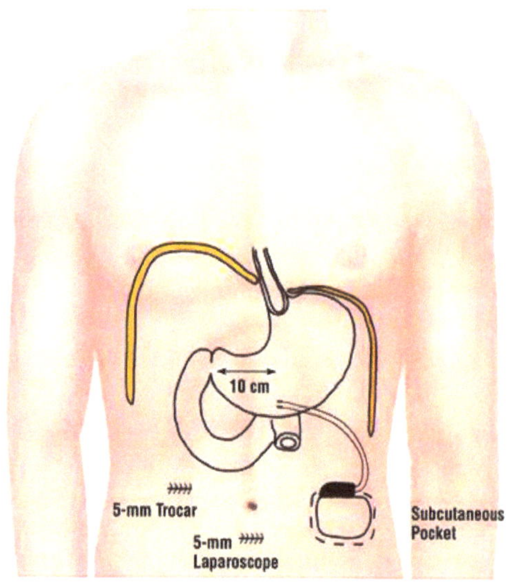

Fig 24.9 Gastric connections in gastric stimulation technique

Gastric electrical stimulation (GES) is a bioelectric therapy[1] first used in humans over 30 years ago.[2] Since its inception, GES, as currently performed, has been used in over 10,000 patients worldwide. This review provides a brief history, methods, indications, mechanisms of action, clinic data, future developments and possible new applications.

These types of settings for GES are widely used including increasing the current up to a maximum of about 20 milliamps (assuming an impedance of 500 Ohms) and increasing the on time to a maximum of 4 seconds on with 1 seconds off (still providing pulse bursts every 5 seconds). Changes to burst rate and pulse width are usually done as later steps as they will decrease battery life in accordance with how much energy is used. Changes in device settings are often made based on patients' symptoms and sometimes related to gastric emptying or electrogastrogram values at regular intervals. Based on current practice,

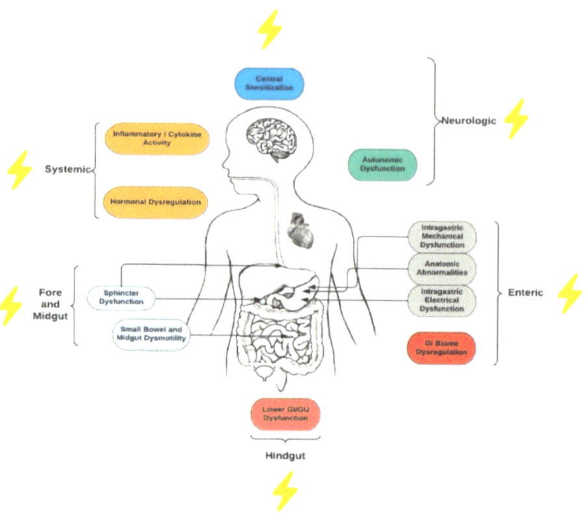

Fig 24.10 Some of the known pathophysiologic areas for gastroparesis syndromes as well as possible mechanisms of action/effects of GES as noted with the symbol. Adapted from Management of Gastroparesis in 2022.[10] GI: gastrointestinal; GES: gastric electrical stimulation; GU: genitourinary.

many patients end up with settings of about 15 milliamps with 2 seconds on and 3 seconds off.in conclusion,Gastric electrical stimulation is a proven bioelectric therapy that is FDA-approved for gastroparesis. Gastric electrical stimulation's mechanisms of action are increasingly being determined and validated. The bioelectric therapy of gastric electrical stimulation, which is still evolving, may have the potential for helping more patients with gastroparesis and other related illnesses in the future.

9.Insulin Pump Therapy for the Managementof Diabetes

Continuous subcutaneous insulin infusion (CSII), more commonly referred to as insulin pump therapy, is one of the most notable advancements in diabetes technology in the past 50 years. The first commercial insulin pumps were on the market as early as the 1970s; however, rapid uptake of insulin pump technology did not occur until the early 2000s, after the conclusion of the landmark Diabetes Control and Complications Trial (DCCT) in the early 1990s. The DCCT demonstrated the importance of intensive insulin therapy to maintain tight glycemic control and prevent diabetes complications such as retinopathy, neuropathy, nephropathy, and cardiovascular disease Since the conclusion of the DCCT, insulin pump technology has advanced rapidly in an attempt tomore closely mimic physiologic insulin secretion and help patients achieve tight glycemic control while minimizing the risk of hypoglycemia. As a result, use of insulin pumps has increased dramatically in the United States from <7,000 users in 1990 to nearly 100,000 users in 2000 and >350,000 users today . The majority of insulin pump users have type 1 diabetes, although 10% have type 2 diabetes . According to the T1D Exchange registry, >60% of individuals within the T1D Exchange use an insulin pump instead of a multiple daily injection (MDI) regimen for intensive insulin therapy. Additionally, the use of insulin pump therapy for individuals with type 2 diabetes is increasing

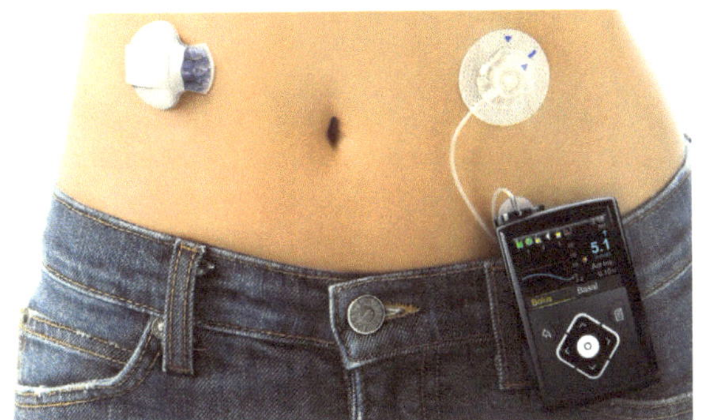

Fig. 24.11 An insulin pump can help you manage your diabetes. By using an insulin pump, you can match your insulin to your lifestyle,

There are many advantages to using an insulin pump compared to an MDI regimen. Insulin pump therapy allows for more precise and flexible insulin dosing with fewer injections. Many individuals with type 1 diabetes report using insulin pumps because they want improved glycemic control and a more flexible lifestyle than is afforded with MDI therapy, especially around meals and social situations . Many studies and systematic reviews have demonstrated improved glycemic control and a reduction in hypoglycemia with insulin pump therapy compared to MDI in pediatric and adult populations with type 1 diabetes . Although some randomized controlled trials have shown no difference in glycemic control in young children (<7 years of age) when comparing insulin pump therapy to MDI , parental satisfaction with insulin pump therapy is high . Further, insulin pumps offer many advantages in managing unpredictable eating habits and low insulin requirements in the youngest children, suggesting that insulin pump therapy may be an ideal option for many young children with type 1 diabetes and their families.Overall, insulin pump technology is evolving at an extraordinary rate, with new technologies becoming available every year. The integration of insulin pumps with continuous glucose monitoring (CGM) systems has drastically expanded the insulin pump market with "smarter" insulin pumps that suspend insulin for hypoglycemia or even automate some insulin delivery, all with the goal of helping individuals meet glycemic targets with less burden. However, this rapid technological progression can be overwhelming for individuals with diabetes and their health care providers. Thus, the purposes of this to provide an overview of insulin pump technologies, from simple, disposable pumps designed for those with type 2 diabetes to complex automated insulin delivery systems and 2) to discuss the clinical implications of these insulin pump technologies.

Conventional Insulin Pump Therapy

An insulin pump is a small, digital device that continuously delivers rapid-acting insulin through a small catheter inserted into the subcutaneous tissue and secured in place on the skin with adhesive (referred to as an "infusion set" or "infusion cannula"). In most insulin pumps, the infusion set connects to the pump by plastic tubing, and insulin infuses from the pump through the tubing to the infusion set cannula and into the subcutaneous tissue.. Some pumps, referred to as "patch pumps," do not use tubing and instead adhere directly to the skin. Patch pumps deliver insulin through the infusion cannula and are programmed from a remote device using wireless technologyInsulin pumps generally use rapid-acting insulin formulations (i.e., insulin lispro, aspart, or glulisine). Lispro and aspart are approved by the U.S. Food and Drug Administration (FDA) for use in a pump insulin reservoir for up to 144 hours, but glulisine should be replaced every 48 hours due to a risk of crystallization. Regular insulin is also FDA-approved for use in pumps and is sometimes used instead of rapid-acting formulations because of its lower cost. Concentrated insulins (e.g., U200 or U500), dilute insulin (e.g., U50 or U10), and ultra-rapid-acting insulin analogs (e.g., Fiasp) are undergoing studies but are not yet FDA-approved for use in pumps.

Insulin pumps deliver insulin in two primary ways: a continuous infusion of rapid-acting insulin throughout the day and night (basal), and discrete, one-time doses of rapid-acting insulin given by the user for meals or high blood glucose correction (bolus). Basal insulin delivery replaces the use of the longer-acting exogenous insulin formulations used in MDI regimens.

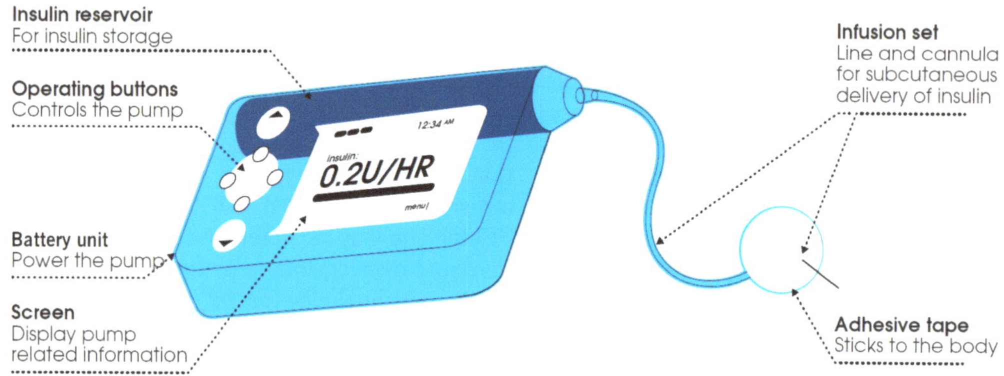

Fig24.12. showing various functional elements of insulin pump with small battery-operated electronic device (computerized syringe)

What is an insulin pump

An insulin pump is a small battery-operated electronic device (computerized syringe) about the size of a mobile phone that delivers tiny amounts of fast acting insulin into the blood throughout the day and night. An insulin pump is worn 24 hours a day. Research has shown that insulin pump therapy can reduce the frequency of severe hypoglycaemia as well as improve quality of life. Using an insulin pump may also improve suboptimal blood glucose control. Only fast acting insulin is used in the insulin pump. Whenever food is eaten the insulin pump is programmed to deliver a surge of insulin into the body similar to the way the pancreas does in people without diabetes. Between meals a small and steady rate of insulin is delivered.

Insulin pumps can deliver insulin in two ways:

- In a steady measured and continuous dose (the "basal" insulin)
- As a surge ("bolus") dose, at your direction, around mealtime.

The insulin pump is not an artificial pancreas (because you still have to monitor your blood glucose level), but pumps can help some people achieve better control, and many people prefer this continuous system of insulin delivery over injections.

Insulin pump therapy may especially be of assistance if any of the following applies to you:

- hypoglycemia unawareness (inability to detect 'hypos')
- severe and frequent hypoglycemia
- frequent night time hypoglycemia
- gastroparesis (delayed emptying of the stomach)
- an unpredictable lifestyle or daily routine (e.g. working nightshifts)
- extreme insulin sensitivity
- dawn phenomenon (rising blood glucose early in the morning)
- planning for, and during, pregnancy.
- Pumps can be programmed to releases small doses of

insulin continuously (basal), or a bolus dose close to mealtime to control the rise in blood glucose after a meal. This delivery system most closely mimics the body's normal release of insulin.

Using an insulin pump may:

- reduce large fluctuations in blood glucose levels
- improve blood glucose (diabetes) levels
- increase your flexibility in the quantity and timing of meals
- decrease your risk of hypoglycemia during exercise while maintaining optimal blood glucose levels
- improve your quality of life.

Insulin pump therapy may especially be of assistance if any of the following applies to you:

- hypoglycemia unawareness (inability to detect 'hypos')
- severe and frequent hypoglycemia
- frequent night time hypoglycemia
- gastroparesis (delayed emptying of the stomach)
- an unpredictable lifestyle or daily routine (e.g. working nightshifts)
- extreme insulin sensitivity
- dawn phenomenon (rising blood glucose early in the morning)
- planning for, and during, pregnancy.
- Pumps can be programmed to releases small doses of insulin continuously (basal), or a bolus dose close to mealtime to control the rise in blood glucose after a meal. This delivery system most closely mimics the body's normal release of insulin.

Using an insulin pump may:

- reduce large fluctuations in blood glucose levels
- improve blood glucose (diabetes) levels
- increase your flexibility in the quantity and timing of meals
- decrease your risk of hypoglycemia during exercise while maintaining optimal blood glucose levels
- improve your quality of life.

You attach the insulin pump to your skin. Insulin flows into your body through a tiny flexible plastic tube called a catheter under your skin. With the aid of a small needle, the catheter is inserted through the skin into the fatty tissue and is taped in place. The tube (catheter) is replaced every 2 to 3 days and the insulin pump moved to another part of your body.

An insulin pump delivers a set amount of background insulin. You then add your extra mealtime insulin using the pump.

Advantages of using a diabetes insulin pump

Some advantages of using an insulin pump instead of insulin injections are:

- Using an insulin pump means eliminating individual insulin injections
- Insulin pumps deliver insulin more accurately than injections
- Insulin pumps often improve HbA1C. HbA1c is a measure of long-term blood glucose levels. Research investigating the efficacy of insulin pump therapy in relation to blood glucose levels suggests that it can improve HbA1c, especially in those with an elevated HbA1c and in those who have been unable to reduce their HbA1c with multiple daily injections.
- Using an insulin pump usually results in fewer large swings in your blood glucose levels
- Using an insulin pump makes delivery of bolus insulin easier
- Insulin pumps allow you to be flexible about when and what you eat
- Using an insulin pump reduces severe low blood glucose episodes
- Using an insulin pump eliminates unpredictable effects of intermediate- or long-acting insulin
- Insulin pumps allow you to exercise without having to eat large amounts of carbohydrate

It is important that you have realistic expectations regular contact with your diabetes educator or endocrinologist for review and adjustment of pump rates.

about insulin pump therapy. It is not a cure for people who require insulin to manage their diabetes but a way of delivering insulin that may offer increased flexibility, improved glucose levels and improved quality of life.

Insulin pump therapy requires motivation, regular blood glucose checking, the ability to learn insulin pump technology and the willingness to keep in regular contact with your diabetes educator or endocrinologist for review and adjustment of pump rates.

How does an insulin pump work

An insulin pump can provide all the insulin requirements of a person with type 1 diabetes.

The pump contains a reservoir or cartridge filled with insulin. A microcomputer built into the pump allows you to program the pump to deliver a dose of insulin according to your needs. A small motor inside the pump controls the delivery of insulin. Insulin is delivered from the reservoir/cartridge through flexible tubing fitted with a small Teflon® (or metal) cannula that is inserted subcutaneously (under the skin) and held in place with special adhesive tape. Together, the tubing and cannula are called an infusion set. The cannula is easily inserted and removed by you; it is not surgically implanted. An introducer needle allows the cannula to be inserted under the skin. The needle is then removed leaving behind the cannula only. For those who do not want to insert the needles manually, there are disposable and reusable devices to assist with cannula insertion.

The cannula must be changed every two to three days. Metal cannulas may need to be changed every one to two days. The most common site to place infusion sets is in the abdomen (easy to access) but they can also be placed in the upper buttock, upper outer thigh, hip or upper arm.

Insulin pumps deliver rapid- or short-acting insulin 24 hours a day through a catheter placed under the skin. Your insulin doses are separated into:

- Basal rates
- Bolus doses to cover carbohydrate in meals
- Correction or supplemental doses

Basal insulin is delivered continuously over 24 hours, and keeps your blood glucose levels in range between meals and overnight. It delivers the insulin in two ways (basal and bolus), therefore replacing the need for long-acting insulin. Often, you program different amounts of insulin at different times of the day and night.

An insulin pump delivers rapid-acting insulin such as NovoRapid® and Humalog®. This insulin starts working within 10 to 15 minutes of delivery, peaks within one to three hours and ceases working after three to five hours. A lack of insulin can lead to the rapid development of ketones and diabetic ketoacidosis (DKA) which is a life-threatening condition. For this reason, it is important to never disconnect from the pump for more than two hours without using an alternative method of insulin delivery (e.g. insulin injections) and to regularly check that the pump is delivering insulin. Prompt attention to rising blood glucose levels is essential in order to prevent diabetic ketoacidosis (DKA).

Disadvantages of using a diabetes insulin pump

Although there are many good reasons as to why using an insulin pump can be an advantage, there are some disadvantages.

The disadvantages of using an insulin pump are that it:

- Can cause weight gain
- Can cause diabetic ketoacidosis (DKA) if your catheter comes out and you don't get insulin for hours
- Can be expensive
- Can be bothersome since you are attached to the pump most of the time
- Can require a hospital stay or maybe a full day in the outpatient center to be trained
- There are pluses and minuses to using an insulin pump. Even though using an insulin pump has disadvantages, most pump users agree the advantages outweigh the disadvantages.

10.What Is Neuralink? What We Know So Far.

Neuralink is a neurotechnology company founded by Elon Musk that's building an implantable, brain-computer interface capable of translating thought into action. Launched in 2016, the private venture claims its neural device will allow people with paraplegia to regain movement and restore vision to those born blind.

Neuralink implanted its first device in a patient's brain in January 2024. The patient, who is paralyzed below the shoulders, played chess on his laptop using the Neuralink device.

Neuralink is a technology company building a device "designed to connect human brains directly to computers," said Ramses Alcaide, CEO of Neurable, a neurotech company developing non-invasive, brain-computer interfaces in the form of headphones. "[Neuralink's technology] is capable of recording and decoding neural signals and then transmitting information back to the brain using electrical stimulation."

The implant itself is called "the Link." This coin-sized brain chip is surgically embedded under the skull, where it receives information from neural threads that fan out into different sections of a subject's brain in control of motor skills. Each wire contains sensors capable of recording and emitting electrical currents that are "so fine and flexible that they can't be inserted by the human hand," according to Neuralink's website. That's why Neuralink has built a neurosurgical robot that's designed to become fully automated.

The company is also developing an app that would allow a person to manipulate a keyboard and mouse using only their mind.

"Neuralink is really at the vanguard of creating the commercialized, scalable versions of what has been pioneered in academia," said Sumner Norman, a scientist at nonprofit startup Convergent Research and former chief brain-computer interface scientist at software firm AE Studio.

How Does Neuralink Work?

Neuralink's underlying technology works in the same way as electrophysiology, Norman explained.

The electrical chemical signals in our nervous system spark as neurons communicate with one another across gaps between nerve cells known as synapses. This brain activity is captured by electrodes, or sensors that detect voltages, measuring the change in "spikes" of when these voltages fire (or potentially fire).

In other words, our brain activity data is captured not only when we take action, but also if we think about taking action.

That's not to say the brain-computer interfacing that Neuralink does is on the same level as mind reading.

"It simply measures the brain activity and interprets it as an action," said Sonal Baberwal, a Dublin City University-based researcher developing machine learning algorithms built into brain computer interface wearables.

Baberwal likened this procedure to how blood pressure interprets a patient's level of stress or relaxation.

"Similarly with your brain signals — eyes closed or opened, a relaxed or deep-sleep state, an action or focus state — all of these aspects can be detected,"

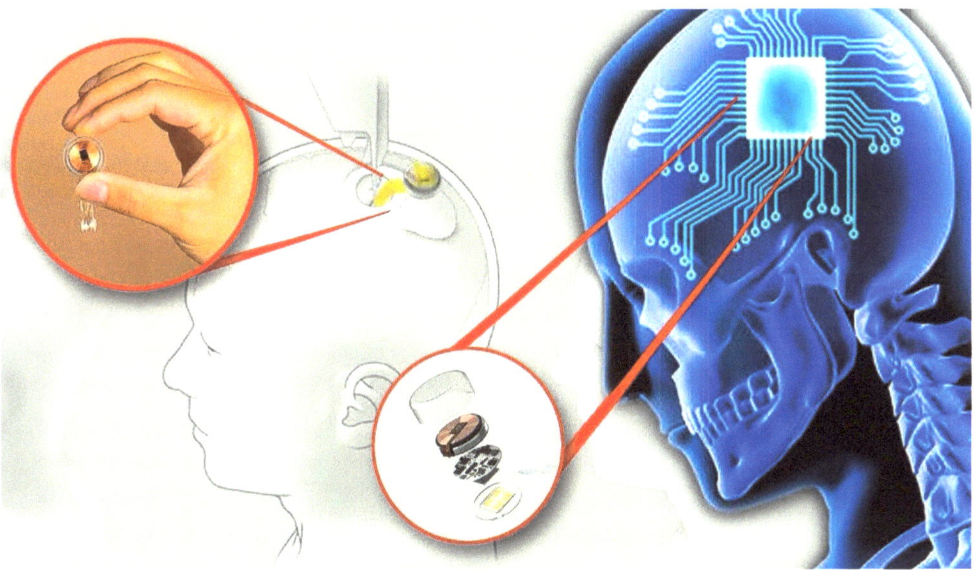

Fig. 24.13 Elon Musk Neuralink Brain Chip

What Will Neuralink Do?

According to Neuralink's website, the company's initial goal is to help those immobilized by paralysis regain lost skills of communication. Down the line, it intends to pursue restoring motor, sensory and visual functions as well as treatment of neurological disorders.

"A Neuralink-like device has the potential to enhance human memory, processing speed and cognitive abilities by creating a direct interface between the human brain and digital devices," Alcaide said.

Restore Mobility

Brain-computer interfaces can be used to control prosthetics or exoskeletons. This use case would enable people with paralysis or amputations to regain a certain level of mobility and independence, according to Alcaide.

Improve Communication for Non-verbal Individuals

Neuralink's main focus is to help people who are unable to speak or write communicate with others by allowing them to control a virtual mouse, keyboard or send messages by thought.

For example, someone with paraplegia would be able to manipulate a computer or mobile device using speech or text synthesis to surf the web and create digital art.

Treat Neurological Conditions

By monitoring brain activity, brain-computer interfaces can also detect changes that may indicate neurological conditions such as epilepsy, bipolar disorder, obsessive-compulsive disorder, Alzheimer's or Parkinson's disease, Alcaide said. They can also be used to monitor mental health symptoms. Electrical stimulation could b delivered to targeted areas in the brain as a treatment for burnout, fatigue, anxiety and depression, which, unlike motor skills that are localized to one area, are spread throughout the brain, Norman noted.

"Treating or curing paralysis, neurological disorders and injuries could make the world a substantially nicer place, where very few people have untreatable forms of depression or anxiety," said Norman, who has spent a decade developing brain-computer interfaces and neuroprosthetics for people with neurological injury or disease. "Giving agency back to those who've lost it — that's an undeniable benefit."

Enhance Cognitive Abilities

This tech can also help people improve their focus, memory and attention by allowing them to train their brain using real-time biofeedback and other techniques. In Musk's words, the Link is a sort of "Fitbit in your skull" with "all the sensors you'd expect to see in a smartwatch."

"If suddenly you could get every neuron in the human brain and sense them all at once, what would you actually do with that data?" We don't know," Norman said. "There's 80 billion neurons in the brain with about 1,000 synapses in between them — how do you interpret that kind of data?"

Neuralink's technology is currently detecting up to 10,000 of these connections — a big step up from the hundreds being studied in academic trials, Norman said.

Is Neuralink FDA Approved?

Yes. Neuralink announced on May 25, 2023 that it has received U.S. Food and Drug Administration clearance for an in-human clinical trial. The company has not yet opened recruitment for the trial, but shared in a tweet that the company would "announce more information on this soon."

Is Neuralink Being Used on Humans?

A human patient, 29-year-old Noland Arbaugh, received the first Neuralink implant on January 28, 2024. In a May 2024 blog post, Neuralink reported that, in the weeks following the surgery, Arbaugh had been successfully using the implant to control his laptop while lying down in bed. The company also reported that multiple threads retracted from Arbaugh's brain, reducing the number of effective electrodes.

Previously, the neural implant had only been tested on rats, mice, monkeys, sheep and pigs.

Frequently Asked Questions

Q. What does Neuralink actually do?

ANS. Neuralink is an implant that can monitor and stimulate brain activity using electrical currents.

Neuralink aims to help people with paralysis communicate by allowing them to remotely control devices using brain activity. In the future, Neuralink may help enhance user memory and cognitive abilities, restore a user's motor, sensory and visual functions as well as treat neurological disorders.

Q.What are the risks of Neuralink?

ANS. The potential risks of Neuralink include:

- Brain injury or infection
- Physical side effects like bleeding, headaches, nausea or seizures
- Psychological side effects like mood changes
- Allergic reaction to implanted materials
- Movement of implanted threads and wires to other parts of the brain
- Cybersecurity, hacking and privacy vulnerabilities
- Unknown long-term effects of use

Q.Who is eligible for Neuralink?

ANS. Those eligible for participating in future Neuralink clinical trials must:

- Be a U.S. citizen or permanent resident in the United States.
- Be at least 18 years old and the age of majority in their state.
- Have quadriplegia, paraplegia, visual impairment or blindness, hearing impairment or deafness and/ or aphasia or the inability to speak.
- Be able to consent to participation.

Bibliography and Acknowledgement

- Aktas MK, Goldenberg I, Moss AJ, et al. Comparison of age (<75 years versus >75 years) to risk of ventricular tachyarrhythmias and implantable cardioverter defibrillator shocks (from the Multicentre Automatic Defibrillator Implantation Trial With Cardiac Resynchronization Therapy). Am J Cardiol;2014:114:1855–60. Crossref| PubMed
- Betz JK, Katz DF, Peterson PN, et al. Outcomes among older patients receiving implantable cardioverter-defibrillators for secondary prevention: From the NCDR ICD Registry. J Am Coll Cardiol 2017;69:265–74. Crossref| PubMed
- Cleland JG, Daubert JC, Ermann E, et al. The effect of cardiac resynchronisation on morbidity and mortality in heart failure. N Eng J Med 2005;352:1539–49.Crossref| PubMed
- Döring M, Ebert M, Dagres N, et al. Cardiac resynchronisation therapy in the ageing population – with of without an implantable defibrillator? Int J Cardiol 2018:263:48–53. Crossref| PubMed
- Elming MB, Nielsen JC, Haarbo J, et al. Age and outcome of primary prevention implantable cardioverter defibrillators in patients with nonischaemic systolic heart failure. Circulation 2017;136:1772–80. Crossref| PubMed
- Gale CR, Cooper C, Sayer AA. Prevalence and risk factor for falls in older men and woman: The English Longitudinal study of Ageing. Age Aging 2016;45;789–94.
- Lamas GA, Orav EJ, Stambler BS, et al. Quality of life and clinical outcomes in elderly patients treated with ventricular pacing as compared with dual-chamber pacing. Pacemaker Selection in the Elderly Investigators. N Engl J Med 1998;338:1097–104.Crossref| PubMed
- Marijon E, Leclercq C, Narayanan K, et al. Causes of death analysis of patients with cardiac resynchronisation therapy:

  An analysis of the CeTuDe cohort study. Eur Heart J 2015;36:2767–76. Crossref| PubMed
- National Institute for Health and Care Excellence. Dual chamber pacemaker for symptomatic bradycardia due to sick sinus syndrome without atrioventricular block. London: NICE, 2014.
- Priori S, Blomström-Lundqvist C, Mazzanti A et al. 2015 ESC guidelines for the management of patients with ventricular arrhythmias and the prevention of sudden cardiac death: The task force for management of patients with ventricular arrhythmias and the prevention of sudden cardiac death. Eur Heart J 2015;36:2793–867. Crossref| PubMed Ricci
- RP, Morichelli L, Varma N. Remote monitoring for follow-up patients with cardiac implantable electronic devices. Arrhythm Electrophysiol Rev 2014;3:123–8.
- Saxon LA, Hayes DL, Gilliam FR, et al. Long-term outcome after ICD and CRT implantation and influence of remote device follow-up: the ALTITUDE survival study. Circulation 2010;122:2359–67.
- Theuns DA, Schaer BA, Soliman OI, et al. The prognosis of implantable defibrillator patients treated with cardiac resynchronisation therapy: comorbity burden as predictor of mortality. Europace 2011;13:62–9.Crossref| PubMed
- Yung D, Birnie D, Dorian P, et al. Survival after implantable cardioverter - defibrillator implantation in the elderly. Circulation 2013;127:2383–92. Crossref| PubMed
- A human patient, 29-year-old Noland Arbaugh, received the first Neuralink implant on January 28, 2024. In a May 2024 blog post,

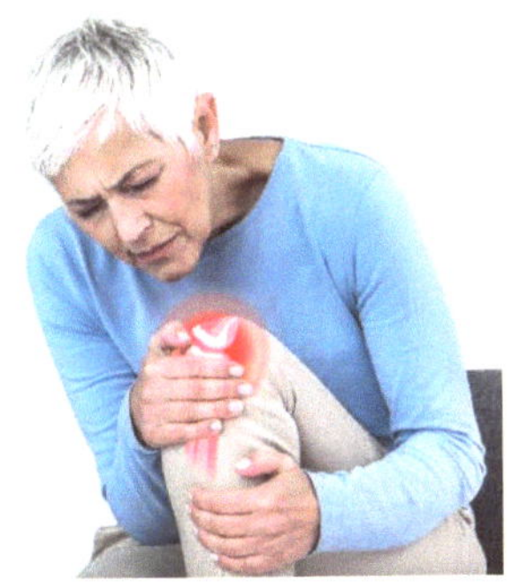

Common Diseases In The Elderly

Older adults are at high risk for developing chronic illnesses that require ongoing medical attention and limit their daily activities. In fact, an estimated 80% of adults aged 65 and older have at least one chronic condition, while close to 70% have two or more. Physiological processes such as inflammation, exposure to environmental pollutants and lifestyle factors like smoking, poor eating habits, and lack of physical activity can accelerate the progression of these diseases in the elderly. Below, we explain the most common age-related illnesses and conditions, their symptoms, and available treatments.

1. HEART DISEASE

Heart disease, also referred to as cardiovascular disease, is a range of conditions that affect the heart, such as coronary heart disease, heart rhythm problems (arrhythmia), and heart infections. Heart disease is the leading cause of death among men and women of all ethnic groups in the United States.

Coronary heart disease (CHD)

Coronary heart disease, also known as ischemic heart disease, is caused by plaque buildup in the arteries that lead to the heart. Narrow or blocked arteries decrease the amount of blood delivered to the heart and may cause complications such as blood clots, angina pectoris, or heart attack. Certain medical conditions and lifestyle choices increase the risk of developing coronary heart disease, for example, smoking, high blood pressure, high cholesterol, obesity, and diabetes.

Heart arrhythmia

A heart arrhythmia is an abnormal heartbeat where the heart beats too fast, too slowly, or with an irregular pattern. A variety of factors such as stress, smoking, congenital heart defects, a previous heart attack, using substances or medications can affect the heart's rhythm.

The most common type of heart arrhythmia is atrial fibrillation that causes an irregular, fast heartbeat. The condition usually occurs in older adults. It increases the risk of a stroke by around 5 times and is of particular concern to people with high blood pressure (hypertension), heart failure, diabetes, and a previous history of blood clots.

Heart failure

Heart failure is a serious condition where the heart doesn't pump enough blood either because it can't fill up with blood or if it is too weak to pump properly. Heart failure can damage the liver or kidneys, cause heart valve disease, and sudden cardiac arrest. It is typically caused by other conditions that damage the heart such as coronary artery disease, high blood pressure, and previous cases of a heart attack.

Symptoms

- Heart attack
- Chest pain or discomfort
- Upper back or neck pain
- Indigestion
- Heartburn
- Nausea or vomiting
- Extreme fatigue
- Upper body discomfort
- Dizziness
- Shortness of breath

Arrhythmia

- Fluttering feelings in the chest (palpitations)
- Racing heartbeat (tachycardia)
- Slow heartbeat (bradycardia)
- Anxiety
- Fatigue
- Sweating
- Lightheadedness
- Dizziness
- Fainting

Heart failure

- Shortness of breath
- Fatigue
- Swelling of the feet, legs, abdomen, or neck veins

Treatment

In order to prevent and manage heart disease, the senior should make the following lifestyle changes:

•Stop smoking
•Limit the intake of saturated and trans fats, sugar, and salt
•Lower high blood pressure
•Exercise regularly
•Maintain a healthy weight
•Manage diabetes
•Reduce stress
•Limit alcohol intake
•Use medication if necessary
•Know when and if they are at risk of a heart attack.

2. ARTHRITIS

Arthritis is a joint disease that causes joint pain and inflammation which can restrict movement. Arthritis typically occurs together with other chronic diseases, such as diabetes and heart disease. This is one of the most common medical conditions among older people, affecting approximately one in five American adults. Arthritis is particularly dangerous for the elderly as it increases the risk of a fall and subsequent injury.

There are more than a hundred types of arthritis. The most common ones in older adults are osteoarthritis and rheumatoid arthritis.

Osteoarthritis

Osteoarthritis is a condition where the joint cartilage gradually breaks down over time, causing swelling and inflammation which lead to pain and stiffness of the joints. It is caused by wear and tear and therefore affects mostly older people. Unfortunately, this condition is often left undiagnosed until a fall causes a bone fracture.

Factors such as obesity, prior joint injury, as well as genetics can make the elderly susceptible to osteoarthritis. Women are somewhat more likely to have osteoporosis because they lose bone density more rapidly than men.

Rheumatoid arthritis

Unlike osteoarthritis, rheumatoid arthritis is an autoimmune disorder. It damages the lining of the small joints in hands and feet, causing a painful swelling that can result in the deformity of the joints. In addition to restricting joint mobility, rheumatoid arthritis may affect the entire body with fevers and fatigue.

Symptoms

•Joint pain, tenderness, and stiffness
•Inflammation in and around the joints
•Warm, red skin over the affected joint
•Weakness and muscle wasting
•Restricted movement of the joints.

Treatment

Although there is no cure for arthritis, the condition is successfully treated with pain-relieving or anti-inflammatory medications, in addition to occupational or physiotherapy and lifestyle changes such as weight loss and exercise. In some cases, surgery may be necessary to correct joint damage and reduce the functional limitations due to arthritis.

3. OSTEOPOROSIS

Osteoporosis, also known as brittle bone disease, is another common medical condition that affects older people, particularly Caucasian and Asian women. Having osteopenia, or low bone density, is among the risk factors for developing osteoporosis. Osteoporosis weakens the bones, making them more likely to break. According to the National Osteoporosis Foundation, around 50% of women and 27% of men over the age of 50 suffer hip and wrist fractures due to osteoporosis. This condition represents a serious problem for older adults as it may result in a loss of mobility and independence.

Symptoms

•A stooped posture
•Loss of height over time
•Bones that break much more easily than expected
•Back pain caused by a fractured or collapsed vertebra.

Treatment

Certain medications, dietary supplements such as calcium and vitamin D, and weight-bearing muscle-strengthening exercises can help maintain bone health and combat osteoporosis.

Furthermore, to prevent and manage osteoporosis in the elderly, it is important to:

•Have knowledge about the condition and the existing treatments
•Undergo regular screening for osteoporosis
•Eat a healthy, balanced diet
•Exercise regularly
•Maintain correct posture.

4. CANCER

Cancer is a disease where cells grow uncontrollably to form a tumor. They may either cause the tumor to grow or spread through the body. Some types of cancer are more common in the elderly, for example, skin, breast, lung, colorectal, prostate, bladder, non-Hodgkin's lymphoma, and stomach cancers.

One of the biggest risk factors for developing many types of cancer is age. According to the American Cancer Society, over two-thirds of all cancer cases are diagnosed in adults over the age of 55. Although cancer survival rates have been on the rise for many years, they are generally lower for older people. That's why it is very important to notice symptoms and begin treatment as early on as possible.

Symptoms

•Fatigue or extreme tiredness that doesn't get better with rest
•Weight gain or loss of more than 10 pounds without a known reason
•Lack of appetite, trouble swallowing, stomach pain
•Nausea and vomiting
•Swelling or lumps anywhere in the body
•Pain, especially new or for an unknown reason, that doesn't go away or that gets worse
•Skin changes such as a lump that bleeds or turns scaly
•A new mole or a change in a mole
•A sore that doesn't heal
•Yellowish color to the skin or eyes (jaundice)
•Cough or hoarseness that doesn't go away
•Unusual bruising or bleeding for no known reason
•Change in bowel habits, such as constipation or diarrhea, that doesn't go away
•Change in how the stool looks
•Bladder changes such as pain when passing urine, blood in the urine, or needing to pass urine more or less often
•Fever or night sweats
•Headaches
•Vision or hearing problems
•Mouth changes such as sores, bleeding, pain, or numbness.

Treatment

Current cancer treatments include:

•Surgery to remove as much of the cancer as possible
•Chemotherapy, a procedure that uses drugs to kill cancer cells
•Radiation therapy that uses high doses of radiation to kill cancer cells
•Bone marrow transplant
•Immunotherapy
•Hormone therapy
•Targeted drug therapy
•Cryoablation, a treatment to kill cancer cells with extreme cold
•Radiofrequency ablation, a pain relief procedure where an electric current is used to heat a small area of nerve tissue to stop it from sending pain signals
•Clinical trials or research studies of new drugs, procedures, and other cancer treatments.

5.ALZHEIMER'S DISEASE

Alzheimer's disease is the most common type of dementia or the loss of cognitive functioning. This progressive disease is characterized by memory decline and difficulty thinking and problem-solving that interfere with everyday life. Older people living with Alzheimer's disease and other dementias are at greater risk for developing disability and experiencing injury from falls.

Experts estimate that around five million Americans aged 65 years and older suffer from Alzheimer's disease. In addition to age, the biggest risk factors are family history of the disease. People who have a parent or sibling with Alzheimer's are more likely to develop the disease themselves.

Incorporating the following habits into the senior's lifestyle may slow or prevent the onset of Alzheimer's:

•Eating a healthy, balanced diet
•Getting good quality sleep
•Exercising regularly, both the body and the brain
•Maintaining social connections.

Symptoms

•Memory loss
•Poor judgment leading to bad decisions
•Loss of spontaneity
•Lacking a sense of initiative
•Taking longer to complete normal daily tasks
•Repeating questions
•Trouble handling money and paying bills
•Wandering and getting lost
•Losing and misplacing things
•Mood and personality changes
•Increased anxiety and aggression.

Treatment

Aducanumab is the only FDA-approved medication that is currently used to treat Alzheimer's disease. This is an intravenous drug that works by sticking to and removing a protein that builds up in the brain and causes Alzheimer's.

6. DIABETES MELLITIS

Diabetes is a chronic disease that occurs when the level of glucose in the blood or blood sugar is too high. This happens either because the pancreas doesn't produce enough insulin or the body is resistant to the insulin it produces.

Over time, high blood sugar may damage the eyes, kidneys, nerves, heart, and blood vessels. It may lead to health conditions like blindness, kidney disease, and nerve problems. People with diabetes are also more likely to have heart disease or a stroke at an earlier age.

The two most common types of diabetes are type 1 and type 2 diabetes. Type 1 diabetes is an autoimmune disease usually diagnosed in children and young adults, although it can occur at any age. Type 2 diabetes usually affects older people and is a combination of genetics and lifestyle factors.

Symptoms

•Frequent urination, especially at night
•Extreme thirst
•Unexplained weight loss
•Blurry vision
•Numb or tingling hands or feet
•Sores and wounds take longer to heal
•Extreme fatigue.

Treatment

Although there is no cure for diabetes, it is possible to take steps to manage the disease and stay healthy. The main treatment for type 1 diabetes is taking insulin to replace the hormone that the body is not able to produce. A healthy diet and exercise can usually help control and manage type 2 diabetes. However, in some cases where lifestyle changes alone aren't enough to lower blood sugar, medications and insulin therapy may be necessary.

7. RESPIRATORY DISEASES

Respiratory diseases are a range of conditions affecting the lungs that make it difficult to breathe. These diseases are often more complex and more dangerous for seniors with weakened immune systems than they are for younger people. Around 15% of older adults suffer from a respiratory disorder such as asthma or chronic obstructive pulmonary disease (COPD).

Asthma

Asthma is one of the most common respiratory diseases in seniors. It occurs when the airways become inflamed as the result of an allergic reaction to a trigger such as pollen or smoke, making it difficult to breathe. Asthma usually starts in childhood, but adult-onset asthma affects people above the age of 60.

COPD

Chronic compulsive pulmonary disease (COPD) is common in older adults who smoke. The condition causes shortness of breath, coughing, chest tightness, and difficulty breathing. The best way to prevent COPD or slow its progression is to quit smoking and to avoid exposure to anything that can irritate the lungs, for example, secondhand smoke, chemical fumes, and dust.

Symptoms

Asthma

•Chest tightness or pain
•Shortness of breath
•Wheezing when exhaling
•Coughing attacks

COPD

•Coughing that produces mucus
•Wheezing
•Shortness of breath
•Trouble taking a deep breath
•Frequent respiratory infections
•Lack of energy.

Treatment

Depending on the type of respiratory disease, treatments may consist of taking medications, using inhalers to facilitate breathing, and undergoing intravenous therapy.

8.INFLUENZA AND PNEUMONIA

Influenza, commonly known as the flu, is a respiratory illness caused by viruses that infect the nose, throat, and lungs. Older adults with weakened immune systems are at higher risk of developing serious influenza-related complications such as pneumonia.

Pneumonia is a condition where the lungs can't function properly because of the presence of fluid in the air sacs (alveoli). This disease is particularly dangerous for the elderly who are at higher risk for hospitalization, complications, and death due to pneumonia.

Symptoms

Influenza

•High fever
•Chills
•Fatigue
•Shortness of breath
•A productive cough with phlegm
•Chest pain when breathing or coughing
•Urinary incontinence
•Lack of appetite
•Confusion or delirium.

Pneumonia

•Symptoms of pneumonia are similar to that of the flu, but they usually last longer and are more severe.

Treatment

Antibiotics can treat the most common forms of bacterial pneumonia, but the best approach for the elderly is to try to avoid infection in the first place. Essential preventive measures for people over the age of 65 with chronic illnesses include getting a pneumococcal pneumonia vaccine along with flu shots, hand washing, and extra care during cold and flu season

9. DEPRESSION

Depression is a mental illness that causes persistent feelings of sadness, hopelessness, difficulty making decisions, and a loss of interest in activities that the person usually enjoys. Seniors who require home care and those who are hospitalized are at a greater risk of developing clinical depression. It is important to keep in mind that despite being prevalent among the aging population, depression is not a normal part of aging.

Symptoms

- Feelings of sadness and emptiness
- Anxiety, agitation, and restlessness
- Feelings of worthlessness, guilt, and self-blame
- Angry outbursts
- Irritability and frustration over small matters
- Loss of interest in normal everyday activities
- Lack of energy and fatigue
- Unexplained physical problems, such as back pain or headaches
- Reduced appetite
- Weight loss or increased cravings for food and weight gain
- Slowed thinking, speaking, and body movements
- Sleep issues, for example, insomnia or sleeping too much
- Trouble thinking and concentrating
- Difficulty making decisions
- Memory issues
- Frequent or recurrent thoughts of death
- Suicidal thoughts and suicide attempts.

Treatment

Depression is a serious condition but a highly treatable one. Antidepressant medications and psychotherapy (also called talk therapy), or a combination of both, are effective for most people with depression. Hospitalization may be necessary in more severe cases.

To prevent or manage depression, it is important that the elderly:

- Stay connected with others
- Practice self-care
- Eat a healthy diet without artificial sweeteners and highly processed foods
- Limit the intake of alcohol and caffeine
- Exercise regularly
- Talk to the doctor about treatment options like therapy or medications.

10. SHINGLES

Shingles is a skin condition triggered by the varicella zoster virus that causes chickenpox. The virus remains dormant in the body and may get reactivated years later. Anyone who has had chickenpox can develop shingles, but it is more common among seniors aged 60 and above. The infection typically causes a painful and very itchy rash on the face or body.

Symptoms

- An itchy rash
- Fluid-filled blisters
- Sensitivity to the touch
- Burning or tingling sensation on the skin
- Fever
- Headache
- Chills
- Upset stomach.

Treatment

The treatment for shingles include:

- Antiviral medication
- Pain medication
- Anticonvulsant medication (commonly used to prevent seizures)
- Calamine lotion with a cooling effect on the skin that can relieve the itchy feeling
- Mindful meditation.

It is recommended that everyone above the age of 60 get the shingles vaccine (Shingrix) as the most efficient way of preventing the condition and avoiding complications.

11. ORAL HEALTH

Medications and age-related chronic illnesses such as diabetes and heart disease increase the risk of oral health problems in seniors. The most common issues include untreated tooth decay, tooth loss, oral cancer, and gum disease.

Untreated tooth decay

Statistics show that over 96% of adults aged 65 years or older have had a cavity and 20% suffer from untreated tooth decay. In addition, most older Americans take prescription and over-the-counter medications that may cause dry mouth and increase the risk of cavities

Tooth loss

Approximately one in five American adults over the age of 65 have lost all of their teeth. Dentures can affect nutrition because the elderly who wear them often prefer eating soft food that is easy to chew instead of fresh fruits and vegetables.

Oral cancer

Cancers of the mouth (oral and pharyngeal cancers) primarily affect older adults due to lack of dental care and not following regular oral hygiene practices.

Gum (periodontal) disease

Elderly people with chronic diseases such as arthritis, diabetes, heart diseases, and chronic obstructive pulmonary disease are more likely to develop gum disease, an inflammatory condition affecting the tissues surrounding the teeth.

Symptoms

- Tooth pain
- Deteriorating gums
- Bleeding or swollen gums
- Alterations in gum color
- Alterations to the tongue
- Growths within the mouth.

Treatment

It is essential for seniors to brush twice a day with fluoride toothpaste, floss regularly, and clean their dentures daily.

Regular dentist appointments can help keep teeth healthy and prevent dental problems. Unfortunately, dental care is often difficult to access for older adults due to loss of dental insurance after retirement or economical disadvantages, making it more difficult to maintain good oral health.

12. EAR HEALTH AND HEARING

Poor ear health and poor hearing can have implications for communication, social participation, independent living and employment (AIHW 2016). Middle-age hearing loss can also be linked to an increased risk of later developing dementia (Livingston et al. 2017). Ear disease and the associated hearing loss can develop over time for many reasons (such as injury, infection or genetic causes) but, for the most part, these are preventable (AIHW 2018).

In 2017–18, an estimated 1 in 3 (34%) people aged 65 and over reported complete or partial deafness as a long-term health condition (ABS 2018b). The 2018 ABS Survey of Disability Ageing and Carers also estimated that among older people, 7.7% (300,000 people) had a main long-term health condition of the ear (diseases of the ear and mastoid process), with a higher proportion of older men affected (11%) than older women (4.7%) (ABS 2019).

13. EYE HEALTH AND SIGHT

Chronic eye conditions vary in their presentation, treatment and consequences, but many are commonly experienced by older people. In 2017–18, the majority of people aged 65 and over reported a chronic eye condition (93%, 3.4 million people). The most common chronic eye condition was long-sightedness (62%), followed by short-sightedness (41%), presbyopia (9.6%) – a type of long-sightedness – and cataracts (9.1%) (ABS 2018b).

The prevalence of long-term eye conditions was broadly similar for both older men and women (AIHW 2021b). Looking at selected eye conditions among older Australians between 2007–08 and 2017–18, the prevalence by sex remained relatively stable

14. CHRONIC KIDNEY DISEASE

Chronic kidney disease (CKD) refers to dysfunctional or damaged kidneys. At the earlier stages of the disease, people may not feel ill, but in the end stages of the disease, people require dialysis or transplants to stay alive. For various reasons, not all people with end-stage kidney disease receive dialysis or transplant, particularly in the older age groups (AIHW 2020a).

Measured data from the 2011–12 Australian Health Survey – which takes into account biomedical signs as well as self-reporting – showed that the prevalence of biomedical signs of CKD increased rapidly in older ages. The prevalence of CKD was twice as high for people aged 75 and over as for those aged 65–74 (42% and 21%, respectively) and around 7 times as high as for those aged 18–44 (5.5%) and 45–54 (5.6%) (AIHW 2020d). The incidence rate (meaning newly diagnosed cases) similarly increased with age.In 2017–18, 7 in 10 (70%) of hospitalisations where kidney disease was identified as the principal or additional diagnosis were for people aged 65 and over (AIHW 2020d). The rates of hospitalisations also increased with age.

This can reflect the repeated nature of dialysis treatment: older people are more likely to have kidney disease, and people with kidney disease may visit hospital very regularly. The rates of CKD-related hospitalisations for both men and women were highest in those aged 85 and over (19,100 and 11,000 per 100,000 population, respectively) – at least 1.6 times as high as for those aged 75–84 (11,100 and 6,900 per 100,000, respectively) (AIHW 2020d).

Bibliography and Acknowledgement

- Chaurasia H, Srivastava S. Abuse, Neglect, and Disrespect against Older Adults in India. Population Ageing. 2020;13: 497–511. doi: 10.1007/s12062-020-09270-x [CrossRef] [Google Scholar]
- Chokshi M, Patil B, Khanna R, Neogi SB, Sharma J, Paul VK, et al. Health systems in India. J Perinatol. 2016;36: S9–S12. doi: 10.1038/jp.2016.184 [PMC free article] [PubMed] [CrossRef] [Google Scholar]
- Cockerham WC, Hamby BW, Oates GR. The Social Determinants of Chronic Disease. Am J Prev Med. 2017;52: S5–S12. doi: 10.1016/j.amepre.2016.09.010 [PMC free article] [PubMed] [CrossRef] [Google Scholar]
- Dandona L, Dandona R, Kumar GA, Shukla DK, Paul VK, Balakrishnan K, et al. Nations within a nation: variations in epidemiological transition across the states of India, 1990–2016 in the Global Burden of Disease Study. The Lancet. 2017;390: 2437–2460. doi: 10.1016/S0140-6736(17)32804-0 [PMC free article] [PubMed] [CrossRef] [Google Scholar]
- Dey S, Nambiar D, Lakshmi JK, Sheikh K, Reddy KS. Health of the Elderly in India: Challenges of Access and Affordability. Aging in Asia: Findings From New and Emerging Data Initiatives. National Academies Press (US); 2012. Available: https://www.ncbi.nlm.nih.gov/books/NBK109208/. [PubMed] [Google Scholar]
- Directorate General of Health Services, Ministry of Health & Family welfare, Government of India. National Programme for the Health Care of the Elderly (NPHCE): An approach towards active and healthy ageing. New Delhi: Ministry of Health &
- Family welfare, Government of India.2011. http://mohfw.nic.in/WriteReadData/l892s/26126565260 perational_Guidelines_NPHCE_final.pdf.
- Ewing R, Schmid T, Killingsworth R, Zlot A, Raudenbush S. Relationship between Urban Sprawl and Physical Activity, Obesity, and Morbidity. Am J Health Promot. 2003;18: 47–57. doi: 10.4278/0890-1171-18.1.47 [PubMed] [CrossRef] [Google Scholar]
- Geldsetzer P, Manne-Goehler J, Theilmann M, Davies JI, Awasthi A, Vollmer S, et al. Diabetes and Hypertension in India. JAMA Intern Med. 2018;178: 363–372. doi: 10.1001/jamainternmed.2017.8094 [PMC free article] [PubMed] [CrossRef] [Google Scholar]
- Gupta R. Convergence in urban–rural prevalence of hypertension in India. Journal of Human Hypertension. 2016;30: 79–82. doi: 10.1038/jhh.2015.48 [PubMed] [CrossRef] [Google Scholar]
- Hellström Y, Hallberg IR. Perspectives of elderly people receiving home help on health, care and quality of life. Health & Social Care in the Community. 2001;9: 61–71. doi: 10.1046/j.1365-2524.2001.00282.x [PubMed] [CrossRef]
- Jones DA, Peters TJ. Caring for elderly dependants: effects on the carers' quality of life. Age and ageing. 1992. Nov 1;21(6):421–8. doi: 10.1093/ageing/21.6.421 [PubMed]
- Lahariya C. 'Ayushman Bharat' Program and Universal Health Coverage in India. Indian Pediatr. 2018;55: 495–506. doi: 10.1007/s13312-018-1341-1 [PubMed] [CrossRef] [Google Scholar]
- Liu S, Yan Z, Liu Y, Yin Q, Kuang L. Association between air pollution and chronic diseases among the elderly in China. Nat Hazards. 2017;89: 79–91. doi: 10.1007/s11069-017-2955-7
- Marttila A, Johansson E, Whitehead M, Burström B. Living on social assistance with chronic illness: Buffering and undermining features to well-being. BMC Public Health. 2010;10: 754. doi: 10.1186/1471-2458-10-754 [PMC free article] [PubMed] [CrossRef] [Google Scholar]
- Ng R, Sutradhar R, Yao Z, Wodchis WP, Rosella LC. Smoking, drinking, diet and physical activity—modifiable lifestyle risk factors and their associations with age to first chronic disease. Int J Epidemiol. 2020;49: 113–130. doi: 10.1093/ije/dyz078 [PMC free article] [PubMed] [CrossRef]
- Parmar MC, Saikia N. Chronic morbidity and reported disability among older persons from the India Human Development Survey. BMC Geriatr. 2018;18. doi: 10.1186/s12877-018-0979-9 [PMC free article] [PubMed] [CrossRef]
- [Google Scholar]
  Rajan I, Risseeuw C, Perera M, editors. Institutional Provisions and Care for the Aged. Anthem Press; 2009. doi: 10.7135/UPO9781843317777 [CrossRef] [Google Scholar]
- Samanta T, Chen F, Vanneman R. Living Arrangements and Health of Older Adults in India. The Journals of Gerontology: Series B. 2015;70: 937–947. doi: 10.1093/geronb/gbu164 [PubMed] [CrossRef] [Google Scholar]
- Shannawaz M. Overweight Obesity An Emerging Epidemic in India. -. 2018 [cited 8 Dec 2021]. Available: http://shodhganga.inflibnet.ac.in:8080/jspui/handle/10603/287932.
- Singh L, Goel R, Rai RK, Singh PK. Socioeconomic inequality in functional deficiencies and chronic diseases among older Indian adults: a sex-stratified cross-sectional decomposition analysis. BMJ Open. 2019;9: e022787. doi: 10.1136/bmjopen-2018-022787 [PMC free article] [PubMed]
- Singh PK, Singh L, Dubey R, Singh S, Mehrotra R. Socioeconomic determinants of chronic health diseases among older Indian adults: a nationally representative cross-sectional multilevel study. BMJ Open. 2019;9: e028426. doi: 10.1136/bmjopen-2018-028426 [PMC free article] [PubMed]
- Tripathy JP, Thakur JS, Jeet G, Chawla S, Jain S, Prasad R. Urban rural differences in diet, physical activity and obesity in India: are we witnessing the great Indian equalisation? Results from a cross-sectional STEPS survey. BMC Public
- Health. 2016;16: 816. doi: 10.1186/s12889-016-3489-8 [PMC free article] [PubMed] [CrossRef] [Google Scholar]
  Verma R, Khanna P. National Program of Health-Care for the Elderly in India: A Hope for Healthy Ageing. Int J Prev Med. 2013;4: 1103–1107. [PMC free article] [PubMed] [Google Scholar]
- World Health Organization. World Health Statistics 2012. Geneva, Switzerland: World Health Organization. 2012. [Google Scholar]
- Yadav K, Krishnan A. Changing patterns of diet, physical activity and obesity among urban, rural and slum populations in north India. Obesity Reviews. 2008;9: 400–408. doi: 10.1111/j.1467-789X.2008.00505.x [PubMed]
- Yadav S, Arokiasamy P. Understanding epidemiological transition in India. Glob Health Action. 2014;7. doi: 10.3402/gha.v7.23248 [PMC free article] [PubMed]
  Yuan S-C, Weng S-C, Chou M-C, Tang Y-J, Lee S-H, Chen
- D-Y, et al. How family support affects physical activity (PA) among middle-aged and elderly people before and after they suffer from chronic diseases. Archives of Gerontology and
- Geriatrics. 2011;53: 274–277. doi: 10.1016/j.archger.2010.11.029

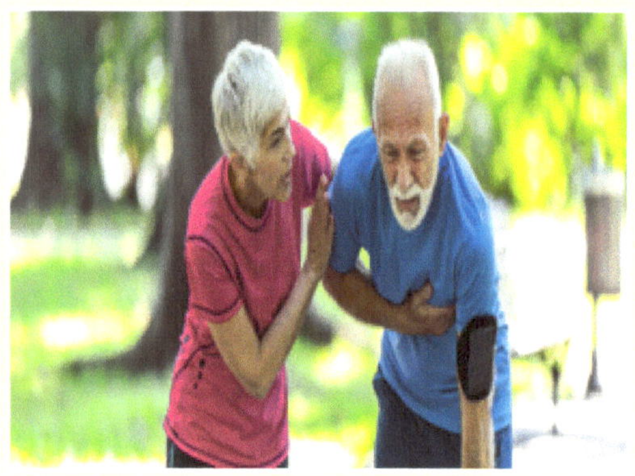

Cardiovascular Diseases In The Elderly

Seniors are at risk of developing heart diseases, such as coronary artery disease (CAD), cardiomyopathy, and arrhythmia. Older loved ones must undergo regular screening to detect cardiovascular diseases.

What is "cardiovascular disease"?

"Cardiovascular disease" refers to a group of disorders that affect both the heart and the blood vessels. These diseases can have an impact on your heart, blood vessels, and other components of your cardiovascular system. A person can be symptomatic (physically experiencing the condition) or asymptomatic (not feeling anything at all).

Cardiovascular disease refers to problems with the heart or blood arteries, and it includes:

- Constriction of the blood arteries in the heart
- Problems with the heart and blood vessels are evident from birth.
- Heart valves that aren't functioning as they should be.
- Abnormalities in heartbeat

What causes cardiovascular disease?

There are many different types of cardiovascular disease, each with its own set of risk factors. For example, both coronary artery disease and peripheral artery disease are caused by atherosclerosis, often known as the formation of plaque in the arteries. Arrhythmias can be caused by coronary artery disease, scarring of the heart muscle, genetic problems, or severe drug reactions. Valve diseases can be caused by ageing, infections, or rheumatic problems

What are some of the risk factors for cardiovascular disease?

If you have any of the following risk factors, your chance of getting cardiovascular disease may be higher:

- Unhealthy levels of blood pressure (hypertension).
- Poor cholesterol management (hyperlipidemia).
- Tobacco use (including vaping).
- Type 2 diabetes.
- A history of coronary artery disease in the family.
- Insufficient amount of physical activity.
- Struggling with obesity.
- Consumption of a lot of sodium, sugar, and fat in one's diet.
- Consumption of alcohol in excess.
- Abuse of either legally prescribed or illegally obtained medicines.
- Preeclampsia or toxemia.
- Diabetes mellitus in pregnancy
- Conditions characterized by persistent inflammation or autoimmunity.
- Kidney illness that persists over time

What are signs of heart problems in the elderly?

There is a wide range of possible symptoms that can be brought on by various forms of heart disease.

1. Arrhythmias

Arrhythmias are any anomalies in the heart's normal rhythm. The symptoms you're experiencing could be related to the sort of arrhythmia you have, which refers to irregular heartbeats that are either too fast or too slow. Some of the signs of an arrhythmia are as follows:

- Lightheadedness
- A heart that is either fluttering or beating very quickly
- A slow heartbeat
- Fainting spells
- Dizziness
- Chest pain

2.Atherosclerosis

When you have atherosclerosis, the blood circulation to your extremities can be diminished. Atherosclerosis causes a number of symptoms, the most prevalent of which are:

•Chest pain and shortness of breath.

•Discomfort caused by cold, especially in the limbs

- Numbness, most prominently in the extremities
- Strange or unexplained pain
- A lack of strength in both of your legs and arms

3.Heart conditions present at birth

Congenital heart defects are cardiac disorders that occur while the baby is still in the womb. Certain cardiac problems are never discovered. Others might be identified if any of the following signs are exhibited:

- Blue-tinged skin
- Edema of the limbs and extremities
- Discomfort in the chest or the inability to breathe normally
- Lack of energy and feelings of tiredness
- An uneven beat of the heart

4.Coronary Artery Disease (CAD)

Coronary artery disease is caused by plaque formation in the arteries that deliver oxygen-rich blood through the heart and lungs (CAD). CAD symptoms include the following:

- Ache or discomfort in the chest
- A sensation similar to that of chest compression or pressure
- A feeling of difficulty breathing
- Nausea
- A sensation similar to that of indigestion or gas

5.Cardiomyopathy

Cardiomyopathy is a disease that causes the heart muscles to grow and become inflexible, thick, or otherwise compromised. The following are some instances of this condition's symptoms:

- Fatigue
- Bloating
- Legs that are swollen, especially the ankles and feet
- A feeling of difficulty breathing
- Thumping or frenetic heartbeat

6.Infections of the heart:

The term "heart infections" refers to illnesses such as endocarditis and myocarditis that affect the heart. Some symptoms of a heart infection include:

Chest pain

- Congested chest or persistent coughing
- Fever
- Chills
- Skin rash

The age structure of the world population is expected to change dramatically over the next several decades with a nearly two-fold increase in the size of the population aged ≥65 years by 2050 .While adults aged 65-84 years accounted for 10.9% of the total population in the year 2000, this proportion is estimated to increase to approximately 16% by 2050. Moreover, it is anticipated that individuals ≥85 years of age will account for 4.3% of the population in the 2050, representing a more than two-fold increase from 2010 .In absolute terms, and considering the projected growth of the overall population, the number of adults aged ≥85 years is estimated to increase from approximately 5.8 million in 2010 to 19 million by 2050, a 228% increase. These projected changes in the U.S. age distribution translate into a significant burden in terms of morbidity, mortality, and costs related to cardiovascular diseases (CVD).

The age-related increase in CVD morbidity and mortality can be appreciated by consideration of the population-based disease-specific incidence and prevalence rates of CVD, including coronary heart disease (CHD), peripheral arterial disease (PAD), heart failure (HF), valvular heart disease, and stroke. Similarly insightful is a review of the associations between age and several measures of subclinical CVD, such as coronary artery calcification and the ankle brachial index (ABI). The impact of CVD on successful aging versus frailty, hospitalization rates, and cost will provide an important additional perspective.

Data presented in this review are derived primarily from population-based epidemiologic studies of community-dwelling U.S. adults, including those focusing on older adults, such as the Cardiovascular Health Study (CHS) .

MORBIDITY AND MORTALITY

Cardiovascular Disease

In 2005 CVD was the underlying cause of death in 864,480 of the approximately 2.5 million total deaths in the U.S., and adults aged ≥65 years accounted for 82% of all deaths attributable to CVD. In terms of morbidity, an estimated 80 million Americans have at least one form of CVD, and nearly one-half of these are aged ≥60 years.reflecting a marked increase in the incidence and prevalence of CVD with advancing age. The prevalence of CVD, including hypertension, CHD, HF, and stroke, increases from about 40% in men and women 40-59 years of age, to 70-75% in persons 60-79 years of age, and to 79-86% among those aged 80 years or older . Similarly, the incidence of CVD, including CHD, HF, and stroke or intracerebral hemorrhage, increases from 4-10 per 1,000 person-years in adults aged 45-54 years to 65-75 per 1,000 person-years in adults aged 85-94 years.

1.Coronary Heart Dsease (CHD)

CHD accounts for more than half of all CVD-related deaths. In 2005, CHD was the primary cause of 445,687 deaths, of which nearly 82% were in individuals aged ≥65 years . The prevalence of CHD increases markedly with age in both men and women Similarly, the incidence of CHD increases with age among older adults, irrespective of race or gender. Even at the age of 70 years, the lifetime risk of a first CHD event is 34.9% in men and 24.2% in women

Coronary artery disease is a condition in which there is an inadequate supply of blood and oxygen to the myocardium. It results from occlusion of the coronary arteries and results in a demand-supply mismatch of oxygen. It typically involves the formation of plaques in the lumen of coronary arteries that impede blood flow. It is the major cause of death in the US and worldwide. At the beginning of the 20th century, it was an uncommon cause of death. Deaths due to CAD peaked in the mid-1960s and then decreased however, it still is the leading cause of death worldwide.

Etiology

Coronary artery disease is a multifactorial phenomenon. Etiologic factors can be broadly categorized into non-modifiable and modifiable factors. Non-modifiable factors include gender, age, family history, and genetics. Modifiable risk factors include smoking, obesity, lipid levels, and psychosocial variables. In the Western world, a faster-paced lifestyle has led people to eat more fast foods and unhealthy meals which has led to an increased prevalence of ischemic heart diseases. In the US, better primary care in the middle and higher socioeconomic groups has pushed the incidence towards the later part of life. Smoking remains the number one cause of cardiovascular diseases. In 2016, the prevalence of smoking among the United States among adults was found to be at 15.5 %. The male gender is more predisposed than the female gender. Hypercholesterolemia remains an important modifiable risk factor for CAD. Increased low-density lipoproteins (LDL) increased the risk for CAD and elevated high-density lipoproteins (HDL) decrease the incidence of CAD. An individual's 10-year risk of atherosclerotic cardiovascular disease can be calculated using the ASCVD equation available online on the American Heart Association portal. Markers of inflammation are also strong risk factors for coronary artery disease. High sensitivity CRP (hsCRP) is thought to be the best predictor of coronary artery disease in some studies although uses for it in a practical setting are controversial.

Prevalence

The aging of the population in combination with improved survival in patients with CVD, particularly CHD and hypertension, has led to an increase in both the prevalence and incidence of HF. HF is relatively uncommon in individuals age 20-39 (0.1-0.2%), but the prevalence increases progressively with age to 5-10% in persons age 60-79 years and 12-14% in those ≥80 years . In CHS, the prevalence of HF increased from 12% in men and 6% in women 65-69 years of age to 18% in men and 14% in women age 85 or older .

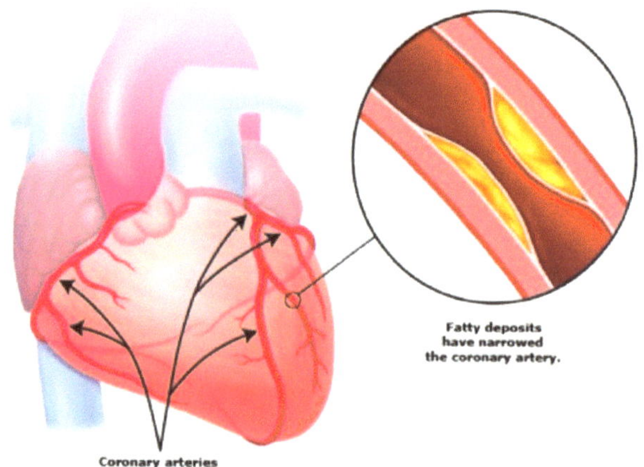

Fig.26.1Thickening of coronary artery in patient with angina pectoris

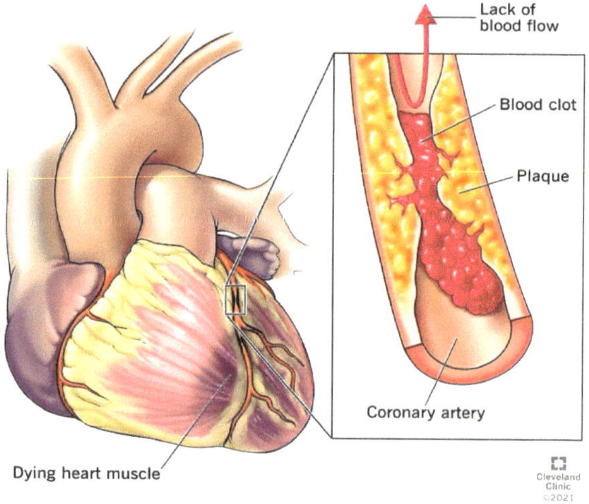

Fig 26.2 Illustration showing almost complete blockage of coronary artery in the genesis of myocardial infarction (heart attack

Pathophysiology

The hallmark of the pathophysiology of CAD is the development of atherosclerotic plaque. Plaque is a build-up of fatty material that narrows the vessel lumen and impedes the blood flow. The first step in the process is the formation of a "fatty streak." Fatty streak is formed by subendothelial deposition of lipid-laden macrophages, also called foam cells. When a vascular insult occurs, the intima layer breaks, and monocytes migrate into the subendothelial space where they become macrophages. These macrophages take up oxidized low-density lipoprotein (LDL) particles, and foam cells are formed. T cells get activated, which releases cytokines only to aid in the pathologic process. Growth factors released activate smooth muscles, which also take up oxidized LDL particles and collagen and deposit along with activated macrophages and increase the population of foam cells. This process leads to the formation of subendothelial plaque.

Over time, this plaque could grow in size or become stable if no further insult occurs to the endothelium. If it becomes stable, a fibrous cap will form, and the lesion will become calcified over time. As time passes, the lesion can become hemodynamically significant enough that not enough blood would reach the myocardial tissue at the time of increased demands, and angina symptoms would occur. However, symptoms would abate at rest as the oxygen requirement comes down. For a lesion to cause angina at rest, it must be at least 90% stenosed. Some plaques can rupture and lead to exposure of tissue factor, which culminates in thrombosis. This thrombosis could cause subtotal or total occlusion of the lumen and could result in the development of acute coronary syndrome (ACS) in the form of unstable angina, NSTEMI, or STEMI, depending on the level of insult.

Classification of coronary artery disease is typically done as under:

1. Stable ischemic heart disease (SIHD)
2. Acute coronary syndrome (ACS)
    (a) ST-elevation MI (STEMI)
    (b) Non-ST elevation MI (NSTEMI)
    (c) Unstable angina

History and Physical

It is very important to take a detailed history and physical examination before proceeding towards further workup. Coronary artery disease could manifest as stable ischemic heart disease (SIHD) or acute coronary syndrome (ACS). It can further progress into congestive heart failure (CHF) if not controlled. Patients should be asked about chest pain, its relation to physical activity, and radiation of the pain into the jaw, neck, left arm, or into the back. Dyspnea should be evaluated for rest and also on activity. The patient should also be asked about syncope, palpitations, tachypnea, lower extremity edema, orthopnea, and exercise capacity. A family history of ischemic heart diseases should be obtained along with dietary, smoking, and lifestyle habits.

Physical examination should include inspection, palpation, and auscultation. One should inspect for any acute distress, jugular venous distention, and peripheral edema. In palpation, one should palpate for fluid thrill and heave. The extent of peripheral edema if present should be evaluated. The distension of the jugular vein should be measured. In auscultation, the heart should be auscultated in all four locations and lungs should also be auscultated with a special focus on the lower zones.

Evaluation

There are several modalities to evaluate for coronary artery disease including EKG, Echo, CXR, Stress test, cardiac catheterization, and blood work to name the main ones. These tests are done depending on the context in which patients are presenting. The following are details on different diagnostic modalities we have available for the evaluation of coronary artery disease:

Electrocardiogram (EKG)

EKG is a very basic yet enormously helpful test in the evaluation of coronary artery disease. It measures electrical activity in the cardiac conduction system and is measured by 10 leads attached to the skin at standardized locations. It provides information about both the physiology and anatomy of the heart. It typically has 12 leads on the paper that is printed once the test is performed and each lead correlates with the specific location of the heart. Important information to notice on an EKG is a heart's rate, rhythm, and axis. After that, information regarding acute and chronic pathologic processes can be obtained. In acute coronary syndrome, one can see ST-segment changes and T wave changes. If an ACS has degenerated into arrhythmias, that can also be seen. In chronic settings, EKG can show information like axis deviation, bundle branch blocks, and ventricular hypertrophy. EKG is also a cost-effective and readily available testing modality that is not user-dependent.

Echocardiography

Echocardiography is an ultrasound of the heart. It is a useful and non-invasive mode of testing that is performed in both acute and chronic and inpatient and outpatient settings. In acute settings, it could tell about wall motion, valvular regurgitation and stenosis, infective or autoimmune lesions, and chamber sizes. It also is useful in the diagnosis of acute pulmonary pathologies like pulmonary embolism. It also evaluates the pericardial cavity. In chronic settings, it can be done to see the same information mentioned above and also a response to the therapy. It also is used in an outpatient setting as part of stress testing. In addition to diagnostics, it also has a role in therapeutics for example, pericardiocentesis could be performed with the needle-guided by echocardiography. This test is user-dependent and could be costly compared to EKG.

Stress Test

The stress test is a relatively non-invasive test to evaluate for coronary artery disease. It is used in the setting of suspected angina or angina equivalent and is helpful in ruling in or out coronary pathology when interpreted in an appropriate setting. During the test, the heart is artificially exposed to stress and if the patient gets certain abnormal EKG changes in ST segments or gets symptoms of angina, the test is aborted at that point and coronary artery disease is diagnosed. EKGs are obtained before, during, and after the procedure, and the patient is continuously monitored for any symptoms. There are mainly two types of stress tests; exercise stress test and pharmacologic stress test. In exercise stress tests, the patient has to run on a treadmill until he achieves 85% of the age-predicted maximal heart rate. If a patient develops exertional hypotension, hypertension (>200/110 mmHg), ST-segment elevations or depression, or ventricular or supraventricular arrhythmias.

Chest X-ray

Chest X-ray is an important component of the initial evaluation of cardiac disease. The standard imaging films include standing posteroanterior (PA) and left lateral decubitus. Sometimes, anteroposterior (AP) projection is obtained especially in inpatient settings with the patient lying down, however, this interpretation of AP films is significantly limited. Proper analysis of PA and AP views provides useful and cost-effective information about the heart, lungs, and vasculature. Interpretation should be done in a stepwise pattern so that important information is not overlooked.

Blood Tests

Blood work aids in establishing the diagnosis and assessing therapeutic responses. In acute settings, cardiac enzymes and B-type natriuretic peptides are often done along with complete blood counts and metabolic panels. BNP provides information about volume overload of cardiogenic origin however it has its limitations. It can be falsely elevated in kidney diseases and falsely low in obesity. Cardiac enzymes like CK and troponin provide information about an acute ischemic event. In chronic settings, lipid panel provides important prognostic information. C-reactive protein (CRP) and erythrocyte sedimentation rate (ESR) aid in assessing disease like acute pericarditis. Liver function tests (LFT) can be done to evaluate for an infiltrative process that can affect the liver and heart simultaneously like hemochromatosis. Liver tests are also done to assess increased right heart pressures, especially in chronic settings.

Cardiac Catheterization

Cardiac catheterization is the gold standard and most accurate modality to evaluate ischemic coronary heart disease. It is however an invasive procedure with associated complications. Not everyone is a candidate for the procedure. In non ACS settings, patients with intermediate pretest probability for CAD are usually the right candidates for it. In the ACS setting, all STEMI patients and selected NSTEMI patients get an emergent cardiac catheterization. This procedure is done in a cardiac catheterization lab, is expertise dependent, and is done under moderate sedation. There is contrast exposure in the procedure which could cause serious allergic reactions and kidney injury.

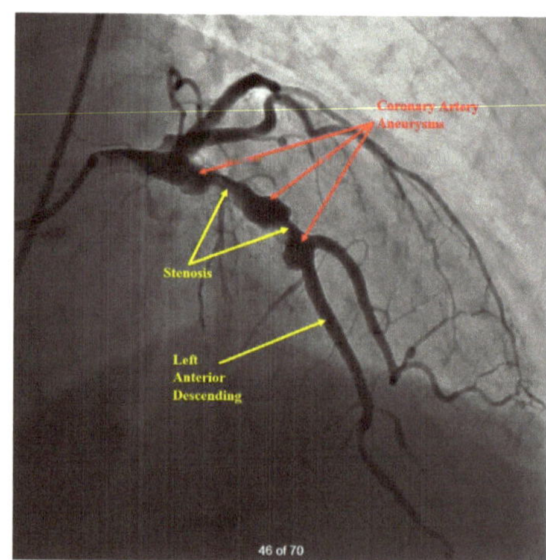

Fig.26.3 Coronary angiography. Left coronary artery injection demonstrating saccular aneurysms with associated stenoses involving 3 separate regions of the LAD.

Treatment / Management

Coronary artery disease could present either as stable ischemic heart disease (SIHD) or acute coronary syndrome (ACS). The former present in a chronic setting while the latter presents more in an acute setting. The management depends on the particular disease type. We will discuss the management of each subtype separately:

Stable Ischemic Heart Disease

Stable ischemic heart disease presents as stable angina. Stable angina typically presents as substernal chest pain or pressure that worsens with exertion or emotional stress and gets relieved with rest or nitroglycerin and is of 2 months duration. It is important to know that classic anginal symptoms could be absent and it could present differently with atypical symptoms and exertional dyspnea instead in certain demographic groups including women, elderly age, and diabetics. Management of SIHD includes both non-pharmacologic and pharmacologic interventions.Lifestyle modifications include smoking cessation, regular exercise, weight loss, good control of diabetes and hypertension, and a healthy diet.

Pharmacologic interventions include cardioprotective and antianginal medications.

Every patient should get guideline-directed medical therapy (GDMT) which includes low dose aspirin, beta-blocker, as-needed nitroglycerin, and moderate to high-intensity statin. If symptoms are not controlled with this, beta-blocker therapy should be titrated up to heart rates 55-60, and the addition of calcium channel blocker and long-acting nitrates should be considered. Ranolazine could also be added to relieve refractory anginal symptoms. If maximal GDMT has failed to relive angina, cardiac catheterization should be done to visualize the coronary anatomy and a decision should be made for percutaneous coronary intervention (PCI) or coronary artery bypass graft (CABG) based on the patient profile

Acute Coronary Syndrome

The acute coronary syndrome presents as sudden onset substernal chest pain or pressure typically radiating to the neck and left arm and may be accompanied by dyspnea, palpitations, dizziness, syncope, cardiac arrest, or new-onset congestive heart failure. Prompt EKG is necessary for all patients with ACS to assess for STEMI and typically is done pre-hospital by an emergency medical services crew. STEMI is recognized by the presence of ST elevation in contiguous leads of 1 mm in limb leads or precordial leads excepting V2 and V3. In V2 and V3, men need to have 2 mm elevations and women 1.5 mm to qualify for STEMI diagnosis.

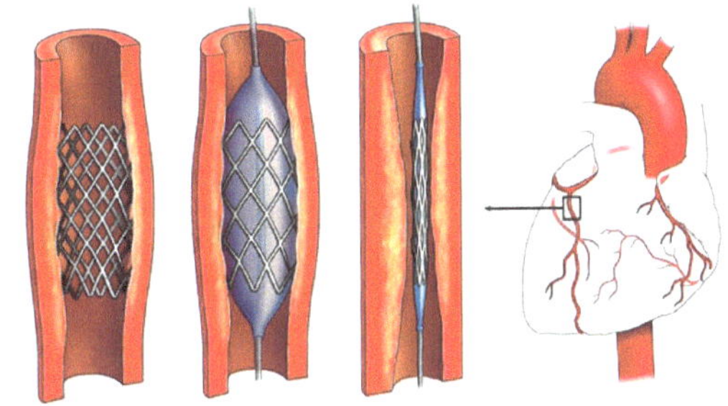

Fig. 26.4 Illustrations showing opening of the narrowed coronary artery by stentoplasty

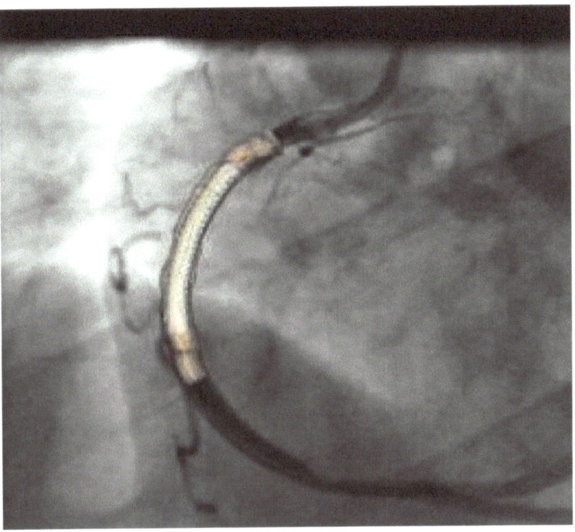

Fig.26.5 A 28mm stent deployment in a patient specific right coronary artery- The expansion is projected to the angiographic image.

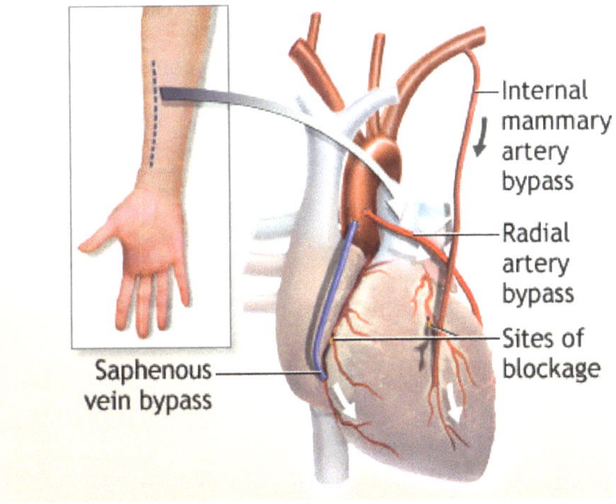

Fig.26.6 Coronary artery bypass surgery can be done with internal mammarya rtery,radial artery and sephenous vein bypass..

New-onset left bundle branch block (LBBB) is also considered a STEMI equivalent. If STEMI is present,

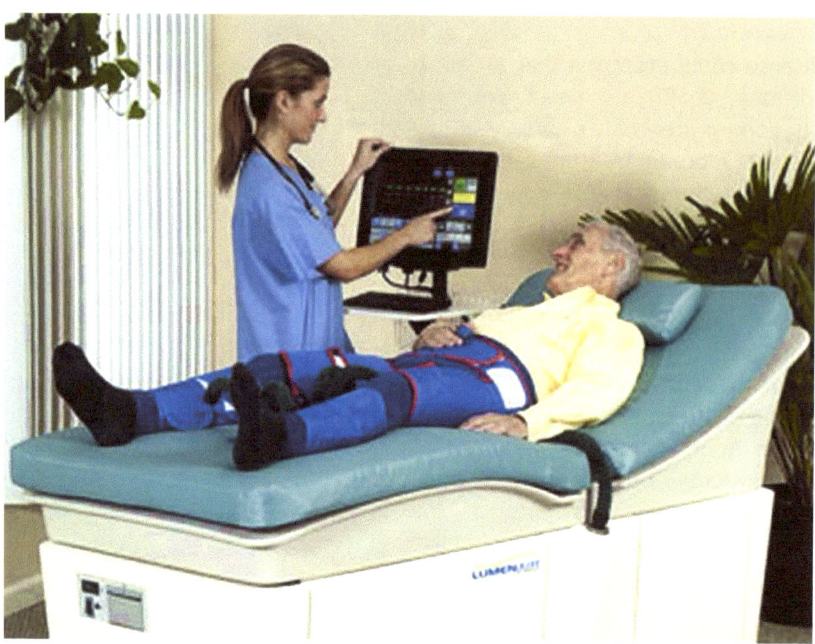

Fig.26.7 The EECP™ machine pumps between heartbeats. This counterpulsation to your own heartbeat increases blood flow to the heart muscle, decreases the heart's workload and creates greater oxygen supply while lowering oxygen demand.

emergency PCI is warranted in a PCI capable facility or if a PCI facility is available within 2 hours distance. If the PCI capable facility is more than 2 hours away, intravenous thrombolytic therapy is indicated after making sure there are no contraindications to it.

It is important to differentiate a true STEMI from other conditions that mimic STEMI on EKG like acute pericarditis, Brugada syndrome, early repolarization changes, and LVH associated changes. All patients should get a full dose of sublingual aspirin (324 mg) upon presentation. Nitrates should be given for pain relief after making sure there are no contraindications to nitrates like hypotension, RV failure, and consumption of phosphodiesterase inhibitors in the past 24-48 hours. High-dose statin therapy and beta-blockers should also be initiated early. P2Y12 inhibitors (prasugrel, ticagrelor, or prasugrel) should be started based on the patient profile. Patients who have NSTE ACS should get anticoagulation, typically heparin or enoxaparin are used. For NSTEMI, early invasive therapy within 24 hours is advised for patients with intermediate to high TIMI scores (>2).

Regular visits with cardiologists and family physicians are key to good long term management of coronary artery disease. Medication adherence and lifestyle modification are important.

EECP for Angina and Heart Failure

A non-invasive option to better health

Many people suffer from heart failure and angina, making simple activities challenging. Many think that the only option is heart bypass surgery or the placement of stents in the arteries to increase blood flow. However, for some this invasive medical treatment is not an option or desirable. For those there is a therapy called Enhanced External Counterpulsation (EECP). This therapy has been shown to be effective and safe. Studies show that 80% of the patients who finish the 35-hour course of treatment have significant relief of their symptoms that lasts for up to three years.The EECP therapy is done on an outpatient basis. Treatments usually last for an hour each day, five days a week, for a total of 7 weeks or 35 hours. The patient lies on a treatment table with large blood pressure-like cuffs wrapped around their legs and upper thighs. These cuffs inflate and deflate at intervals matching the heart beat of the patient. A continuous electro cardiogram (ECG) is used to set the intervals so the cuffs inflate while the heart is at rest, when it normally gets its supply of blood and oxygen. The cuffs deflate at the end of that rest period, just before the next heart beat. Oxygen levels in the blood are monitored using a special sensor applied to the finger. This also monitors the pressure waves created by the inflating/deflating cuffs.

Differential Diagnosis

Coronary artery disease has a wide range of differential diagnoses because of the proximity of the heart with adjacent organs, including the lungs, stomach, big vessels, and musculoskeletal organs. Acute anginal chest pain could mimic acute pericarditis, myocarditis, prinzmetal angina, pericardial effusion, acute bronchitis, pneumonia, pleuritis, pleural effusion, aortic dissection, GERD, peptic ulcer disease, esophageal motility disorders, and costochondritis. Stable ischemic heart disease could also mimic GERD, Peptic ulcer disease, costochondritis, and pleuritis. History, physical examination, and diagnostic studies should be carefully carried out to narrow down the differential diagnosis and reach an accurate diagnosis.

Toxicity and Adverse Effect Management

Both medical and surgical management for ischemic heart disease is associated with their side effects and complications. These undesirable effects could be mitigated by careful selection, physician expertise, and patient education. Aspirin therapy is associated with bleeding, idiosyncratic, and allergic drug reactions. Statin therapy can cause myalgias, diarrhea, and arthralgias among side effects.

Beta-blockers could cause bradycardia and hypotension. ACEIs could result in hypotension, dizziness, creatinine elevation, cough, and allergic reactions including angioedema. PCI can possibly cause coronary artery perforation, stent thrombosis in an acute setting, and in-stent restenosis on chronic basis. CABG can have its own complications including but not limited to arrhythmias, cardiac tamponade, post-op bleeding, infection, renal impairment, and phrenic nerve injury.

Prognosis

The prognosis of the disease depends on multiple factors some of which could be modified while others are non-modifiable. Patient's age, gender, family history and genetics, ethnicity, dietary and smoking habits, medication compliance, availability of healthcare and financial status, and the number of arteries involved are some of the factors. Comorbid conditions including diabetes mellitus, hypertension, dyslipidemia, and chronic kidney disease also have a role in the overall outcome

Complications

Arrhythmias, acute coronary syndrome, congestive heart failure, mitral regurgitation, ventricular free wall rupture, pericarditis, aneurysm formation, and mural thrombi are the main complication associated with coronary artery disease

High Blood Pressure

High blood pressure, also known as hypertension, is essentially when the force of your blood pushing against your artery walls is consistently too high, and it is a common concern among elderly people as well as younger adults

In fact, around one in three adults in the UK suffers from high blood pressure, with the first signs often appearing as early as in the early thirties.

Causes of high blood pressure

So, what is the main cause behind high blood pressure? As we age, our blood vessels tend to lose their flexibility and become less elastic, which can lead to increased blood pressure. High blood pressure is usually measured by a reading of 140/90mmHg or above, but if you have other health conditions, this can sometimes mean that lower readings might be considered high. Blood pressure is usually tested with an arm cuff and gauge

Lifestyle factors such as having a poor diet, being overweight, lack of exercise or stress can have a big impact on this condition. For instance, foods high in sugar or saturated fats can increase your blood pressure and cause heart damage over time. Similarly, salty foods, like processed meats or canned soups, can contain an excessive amount of sodium, causing your body to retain more fluids and raising your blood volume and pressure.

Symptoms of blood pressure

One of the dangerous facts about high blood pressure is that it often goes unnoticed and doesn't present any obvious symptoms, earning the nickname "silent killer". Therefore, regularly measuring blood pressure is the only reliable way to detect any issues and take proactive steps to manage the condition effectively. Very high pressure can, however, cause

- Dizziness
- Fatigue
- Nosebleed
- Headache
- Nausea
- Blurred vision
- Breathlessness
- Chest pain

When it comes to hypertension, it's important to remember that when it's not regulated by lifestyle changes and medication, it can lead to serious, life-threatening health risks including heart attacks, strokes or heart failure. You can also read our blog on Common elderly blood pressure issues to learn more about blood pressure fluctuations and its management.

Guidelines for BP Goals and Therapeutic Strategies in Older Patients With High BP

Blood Pressure Goals

The 2013 European guidelines based on the HYVET criteria recommend initiating an antihypertensive strategy in individuals ≥80 years with an SBP >160 mm Hg, and targeting SBP to <150 mm Hg.99 The more recent North American Guidelines propose not to modify therapeutic targets based on age and frailty level.101,102 It is, however, very difficult to find common BP goals in the different National and International guidelines:

The Canadian 2017 guidelines propose to target an SBP of <120 mm Hg for all individuals aged over 75 years.101 The 2017 American College of Cardiology/ American Heart Association guidelines indicate that a BP <130/80 mm Hg should be targeted after the age of 65 years.102 The 2018 guidelines propose a BP goal of <140/90 mm Hg for individuals older than 65 years.109 Finally, the 2017 American College of Physicians/ American Association of Family Physicians guidelines propose to target a BP <150/90 mm Hg.110

One can also observe important discrepancies in the definition of elderly or older adults. In the clinical studies during the 80s on the Hypertension in the elderly subjects over 60 or 65 years old were included, whereas presently this definition is mainly used for subjects >75 or >80 years old. This diversity is also found in the above-mentioned guidelines with variable age thresholds between 65 and 80 years old. We recognize that although these discrepancies are highly confusing, they reflect the dramatic demographic, cultural, and biomedical changes of the last few decades and the vast heterogeneity in functionality among older subjects. For this reason, we think that functionality/frailty/autonomy criteria for the potential adaptation of therapeutic strategies. We use often the age threshold of 80 years to define older individuals because, currently, the percentage of people with severe loss of functionality and loss of autonomy dramatically increases after that age. For this reason, the specific diagnostic and therapeutic strategies discussed in this article mainly apply to individuals aged ≥80 years.

Therapeutic Strategies

With regard to nonpharmacological interventions for lowering BP, although benefits have been shown in younger populations, there is little evidence from controlled studies in hypertensive patients aged 80 plus. Some of the proposed lifestyle changes, including weight reduction, Dietary Approaches to StopHypertension/Mediterranean diet, dietary sodium reduction, physical activity, and moderate alcohol consumption may, however, not be appropriate or relevant and may even bedetrimental. Thus, a weight reduction in patients >80 years easily induces a loss of muscle mass (sarcopenia) and can even cause cachexia, unless an intensive physical training program and adequate protein supplementation are concomitantly applied. Equally, an excessive salt reduction might induce hyponatremia, malnutrition, and orthostatic hypotension with increased risk of falls. Physical activity adapted to the functional capacities of the older person and to his or her preferences is of major importance, even if not meeting the amount recommended by current guidelines, which is similar for older and younger adult subjects. Finally, excessive alcohol intake should be discouraged, not only because of its pressor effect but also mainly because of increased risk of falls and confusion.In older individuals, in which polypharmacy (including antihypertensive agents) is a frequent phenomenon, drug-related problems are directly correlated with the number of drugs and, therefore, starting with monotherapy should be the rule.Most international guidelines propose the same *5 antihypertensive drug classes as for younger subjects: thiazide diuretics, calcium channel blockers, angiotensin-converting enzyme (ACE) inhibitor, angiotensin receptor blockers (ARB), and beta blockers (BB).* The American guideline on antihypertensive treatment in patients >60 years lists the adverse effects of drug classes but does not specifically advocate a particular drug class.110 The British NICE guidelines (National Institute for Health Care Excellence) do not include BB as a first line treatment in older adults.The European guidelines mostly favor a calcium channel blocker or a thiazide diuretic in the absence of a compelling disease-specific indication, in addition to lifestyle change recommendations when the latter is insufficient to achieve BP control. We have furthermore recently proposed that in patients > 80 years, ACE inhibitors should be among the first line medications because these represented 1 of the 2 drug classes used in HYVET However, the findings of some clinical studies argue against the use of ACE inhibitor as the first choice in older adults and propose replacing them by ARBs. It is important to regularly check for all potential clinical and biological side effects and the impact of these treatments on the functional status and quality of life of the older patients.However, we should always bear in mind that in this population, medication-induced side effects are more frequent, more severe, and less specific than in younger adults.Hence, all antihypertensive drugs can be responsible for certain common clinical manifestations and conditions such as fatigue, confusion / delirium, orthostatic hypotension, and falls.

Myocardial Infarction

Myocardial infarction also called acute myocardial infarction, is a medical term for a "heart attack" that happens when the flow of blood to your heart suddenly becomes blocked. The blockage is most often a buildup of fat, cholesterol and other substances, which form a plaque in the arteries that feed the heart (coronary arteries). The plaque eventually breaks away and forms a clot. The interrupted blood flow can damage or destroy part of the heart muscle. If not treated quickly, the heart muscle begins to die. But if you do get quick treatment, you may be able to prevent or limit damage to the heart muscle. That's why it's important to know the symptoms of a myocardial infarction and call your local emergency services number if you or someone else is having them. You should call your local emergency services number, even if you are not sure that it is a myocardial infarction. The current 2018 clinical definition of myocardial infarction requires the confirmation of the myocardial ischemic injury with abnormal cardiac biomarkers.Myocardial infarction is a clinical syndrome involving myocardial ischemia, ECG changes and chest pain

Myocardial infarction may be "silent" and go undetected, or it could be a catastrophic event leading to hemodynamic deterioration and sudden death 3). Most myocardial infarctions are due to underlying coronary artery disease, the leading cause of death in the United States. With coronary artery occlusion, the myocardium is deprived of oxygen. Prolonged deprivation of oxygen supply to the myocardium can lead to myocardial cell death and necrosis . Patients can present with chest discomfort or pressure that can radiate to the neck, jaw, shoulder, or arm. In addition to the history and physical exam, myocardial ischemia may be associated with ECG changes and elevated biochemical markers such as cardiac troponins .

Incidence

Nearly one-half million persons aged ≥75 years are diagnosed with an MI each year, accounting for more than one-third of all MIs in the U.S. Relative to individuals 35-44 years old, men and women 65-74 years old have an approximately ten-fold greater MI incidence rate. This represents an increase from approximately 1.0 to nearly 10 per 1,000 person-years in men and from 0.3-0.7 to 5.1-7.2 per 1,000 person-years in women. Data from CHS indicate that the age-related increase in MI incidence continues into the oldest age groups, with 2-3 fold increases in persons ≥80 years of age compared to those age 65-69 .

Factors associated with increased risk of a heart attack include:

- Age - increase in age weakens the heart muscles or build-up of plagues
- High cholesterol levels
- Diabetes
- Genetics - family history increases the risk
- Heart surgery
- High blood pressure
- Obesity
- Consumption of tobacco in any form, either chewable or smoked
- Extreme stress

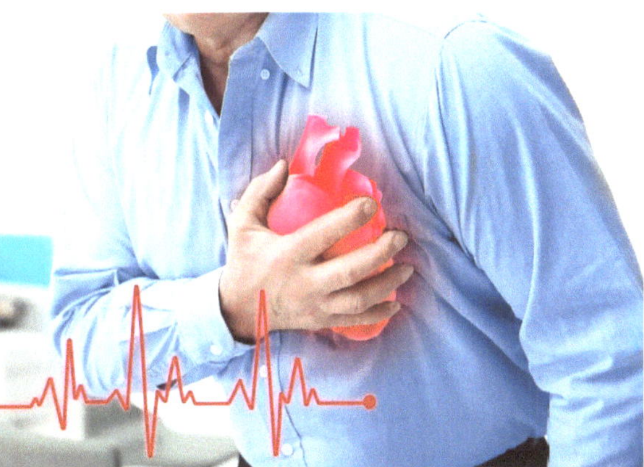

Fig. 26.8 older person has been shown to have chest pain during heart attack

Symptoms of Myocardial Infarction

A heart attack occurs when one or more coronary arteries get blocked. Over time, a coronary artery can narrow due to the build-up of various substances, including cholesterol (atherosclerosis). This condition is called coronary artery disease. During a heart **Chest discomfort.** It is often in center or left side of the chest. It usually lasts more than a few minutes. It may go away and come back. It can feel like pressure, squeezing, fullness, or pain. It also can feel like heartburn or indigestion.

Shortness of breath. Sometimes this is your only symptom. You may get it before or during the chest discomfort. It can happen when you are resting or doing a little bit of physical activity.

Discomfort in the upper body. You may feel pain or discomfort in one or both arms, the back, shoulders, neck, jaw, or upper part of the stomach.

You may also have other symptoms, such as nausea, vomiting, dizziness, and lightheadedness. You may break out in a cold sweat. Sometimes women will have different symptoms then men. For example, they are more likely to feel tired for no reason.

The most common cause of myocardial infarctions is coronary artery disease (coronary heart disease). With coronary artery disease, there is a buildup of cholesterol and other material, called plaque, on their inner walls or the arteries. This is atherosclerosis. It can build up for years. Eventually an area of plaque can rupture (break open). A blood clot can form around the plaque and block the artery.

A less common cause of myocardial infarction is a severe spasm (tightening) of a coronary artery. The spasm cuts off blood flow through the artery.

At the hospital, your doctor make a diagnosis based on your symptoms, blood tests, and different heart health tests. Treatments may include medicines and medical procedures such as coronary angioplasty. After a myocardial infarction, cardiac rehabilitation and lifestyle changes can help you recover.

Types of myocardial infarction

Myocardial infarction in general can be classified from Type 1 to Type 5 myocardial infarction based on the cause and pathogenesis .

Type 1 myocardial infarction is due to acute coronary atherothrombotic myocardial injury with plaque rupture. Most patients with ST-segment elevation myocardial infarction (STEMI) and many with non-ST-segment elevation myocardial infarction (NSTEMI) comprise this category.

Type 2 myocardial infarction is the most common type of myocardial infarction encountered in clinical settings in which is there is demand-supply mismatch resulting in myocardial ischemia. This demand supply mismatch can be due to multiple reasons including but not limited to presence of a fixed stable coronary obstruction, tachycardia, hypoxia or stress. However, the presence of fixed coronary obstruction is not necessary.

Other potential etiologies include coronary Vasospasm, coronary embolus, and spontaneous coronary artery dissection (SCAD). Sudden cardiac death patients who succumb before any troponin elevation comprise

Type 3 myocardial infarction. Types 4 and 5 myocardial infarctions are related to coronary revascularization procedures like Percutaneous Coronry Intervention (PCI) or Coronary artery Bypass Grfting (CABG).

For the sake of immediate treatment strategies such as reperfusion therapy, it is usual practice to designate myocardial infarction in patients with chest discomfort or other ischemic symptoms, who develop new ST-segment elevations in two contiguous leads or new bundle branch blocks with ischemic repolarization patterns as an ST-elevation myocardial infarction (STEMI). In contrast, patients without ST-segment elevation at presentation are usually designated non-ST-elevation myocardial infarction (NSTEMI). The categories of patients with STEMI, NSTEMI, or unstable angina are customarily included in the concept of acute coronary syndrome (ACS) 15). Unstable angina is similar to NSTEMI. However, cardiac markers are not elevated 16). In addition to these categories, myocardial infarction may be classified into various types based on pathological, clinical, and prognostic differences, along with different treatment strategies.

There is no universal consensus on the cardiac troponin (cTn) or high-sensitivity cardiac troponin (hs-cTn) cut-off points that clearly distinguish cardiac procedural myocardial injury from myocardial infarction 17). The distinction is made on the basis of an injury created by a flow-limiting complication during the procedure that results in sufficient myocardial ischemia to generate a procedure-related myocardial infarction. The size of the insult will determine the magnitude of the cardiac troponin release. Various groups have used multiples of the 99th percentile upper reference limit and set thresholds to diagnose periprocedural myocardial infarctions for clinical trials 18). Unless a standard assay is used for all analyses, given the heterogeneity of cardiac troponin assays, this approach could lead to very different values depending on the assay used locally. The Academic Research Consortium-2 (ARC-2) suggests a post-procedural cardiac troponin value ≥ 35 times the 99th percentile upper reference limit for both PCI and CABG in patients that have a normal baseline cardiac troponin value or in patients with elevated pre-procedure cardiac troponin values in whom the cardiac troponin levels are stable or falling. ARC-2 proposes that one ancillary criterion be required in addition to the ≥ 35 cardiac troponin rise to fulfill the definition of periprocedural myocardial infarction. The ancillary criteria are one or more of the following: new significant Q waves (or equivalent), flow-limiting angiographiccomplications in a major epicardial vessel or > 1.5 mm diameter branch, or a substantial new loss of viable myocardium on echocardiography related to the procedure. Furthermore, the Academic Research Consortium-2 (ARC-2) has defined stand-alone criteria for significant procedural myocardial injury if the rise in cardiac troponin is ≥ 70 times the 99th percentile upper reference limit (where the baseline is lower than the upper reference limit, elevated and stable, or falling)

Non-ST-segment elevation myocardial infarction (NSTEMI)

Acute coronary syndrome (ACS) is simply a mismatch in the myocardial oxygen demand and myocardial oxygen consumption. While the cause of this mismatch in ST-elevation myocardial infarction (STEMI) is nearly always coronary plaque rupture resulting in thrombosis formation occluding a coronary artery, there are several potential causes of this mismatch in non-ST-elevation myocardial infarction (NSTEMI). There may be a flow-limiting condition such as a stable plaque, vasospasm as in Prinzmetal angina, coronary embolism, or coronary arteritis. Non-coronary injury to the heart such as cardiac contusion, myocarditis, or presence of cardiotoxic substances can also produce NSTEMI . Finally, conditions relatively unrelated to the coronary arteries or myocardium itself such as hypotension, hypertension, tachycardia, aortic stenosis, and pulmonary embolism lead to NSTEMI because the increased oxygen demand cannot be met . NSTEMI is diagnosed in patients determined to have symptoms consistent with ACS and troponin elevation but without ECG changes consistent with STEMI. Unstable angina and NSTEMI differ primarily in the presence or absence of detectable troponin leak.

The "typical" presentation of NSTEMI is a pressure-like substernal pain, occurring at rest or with minimal exertion. The pain generally lasts more than 10 minutes and may radiate to either arm, the neck, or the jaw 25). The pain may be associated with shortness of breath (dyspnea), nausea or vomiting, syncope (fainting), fatigue, or excess sweatiness (diaphoresis). Sudden onset of unexplained shortness of breath (dyspnea) with or without associated symptoms is also a common presentation. Risk factors for acute coronary syndrome (ACS) include male sex, older age, family history of coronary artery disease, diabetes, personal history of coronary artery disease, and renal insufficiency. Atypical symptoms may include a stabbing or pleuritic pain, epigastric or abdominal indigestion, and isolated dyspnea. While all patients presenting with acute coronary syndrome (ACS) are more likely to present with typical symptoms than atypical symptoms, the likelihood of atypical presentations increases with age over 75, women and those with diabetes, renal insufficiency, and dementia.

Physical exam for acute coronary syndrome (ACS) and NSTEMI is often nonspecific. Clues such as back pain with aortic dissection or pericardial friction rub with pericarditis may point to an alternative diagnosis for a patient's chest pain, but no such exam finding exists that indicates acute coronary syndrome (ACS) as the most likely diagnosis. Signs of heart failure should increase concern for acute coronary syndrome (ACS) but are, again, nonspecific findings

ST-segment elevation myocardial infarction (STEMI)

ST-segment elevation myocardial infarction (STEMI) also known as acute ST-elevation myocardial infarction occurs due to occlusion of one or more coronary arteries, causing transmural myocardial ischemia (full thickness heart muscle ischemia) which in turn results in myocardial injury or necrosis . An ST-elevation myocardial infarction (STEMI) occurs from occlusion of one or more of the coronary arteries that supply your heart with blood. The cause of this abrupt disruption of blood flow is usually plaque rupture, erosion, fissuring or dissection of coronary arteries that results in an obstructing thrombus. The major risk factors for ST-elevation myocardial infarction (STEMI) are dyslipidemia, diabetes mellitus, hypertension, smoking, and family history of coronary artery disease

Type 1 myocardial infarction

Myocardial infarction caused by atherothrombotic coronary artery disease (coronary heart disease) and usually precipitated by atherosclerotic plaque disruption (rupture or erosion) is designated as a type 1 myocardial infarction . The relative burden of atherosclerosis and thrombosis in the culprit lesion varies greatly and the dynamic thrombotic component may lead to distal coronary embolization resulting in myocyte necrosis . Plaque rupture may not only be complicated by intraluminal thrombosis but also by hemorrhage into the plaque through the disrupted surface

Criteria for type 1 myocardial infarction:

Detection of a rise and/or fall of cardiac troponin values with at least one value above the 99th percentile upper reference limit and with at least one of the following:

- Symptoms of acute myocardial ischemia;
- New ischemic ECG changes;
- Development of pathological Q waves;

- Imaging evidence of new loss of viable myocardium or new regional wall motion abnormality in a pattern consistent with an ischemic atiology;
- Identification of a coronary thrombus by angiography including intracoronary imaging or by autopsy.

Post-mortem demonstration of an atherothrombus in the artery supplying the infarcted myocardium, or a macroscopically large circumscribed area of necrosis with or without intramyocardial hemorrhage, meets the type 1 myocardial infarction criteria regardless of cardiac troponin values.

It is essential to integrate the ECG findings with the aim of classifying type 1 myocardial infarction into STEMI or NSTEMI in order to establish the appropriate treatment according to current Guidelines

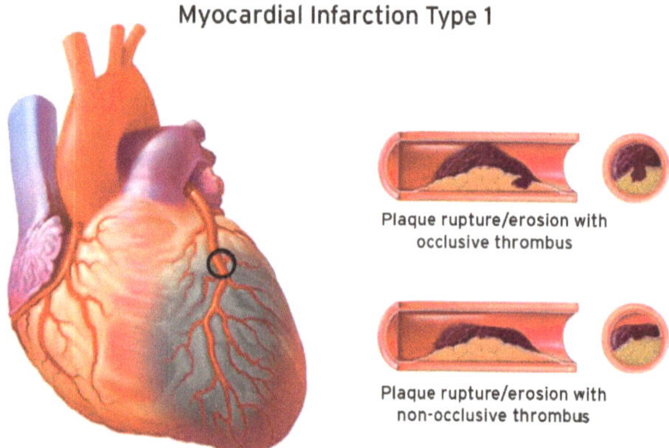

Fig. 26.9 Illustrations showing rupture of plaque with occlusive thrombosis in type 1 myocardial infarction.

Type 2 myocardial infarction

The pathophysiological mechanism leading to ischemic myocardial injury in the context of a mismatch between oxygen supply and demand has been classified as type 2 myocardial infarction 35). By definition, acute atherothrombotic plaque disruption is not a feature of type 2 myocardial infarction. In patients with stable known or presumed coronary artery disease (coronary heart disease), an acute stressor such as an acute gastrointestinal bleed with a precipitous drop in hemoglobin, or a sustained tachyarrhythmia with clinical manifestations of myocardial ischemia, may result in myocardial injury and a type 2 myocardial infarction 36). These effects are due to insufficient blood flow to the ischemic myocardium to meet the increased myocardial oxygen demand of the stressor. Ischemic thresholds may vary substantially in individual patients depending on the magnitude of the stressor, the presence of non-cardiac comorbidities, and the extent of underlying coronary artery disease and cardiac structural abnormalities.

Criteria for type 2 myocardial infarction :

Detection of a rise and/or fall of cardiac troponin values with at least one value above the 99th percentile upper reference limit, and evidence of an imbalance between myocardial oxygen supply and demand unrelated to acute coronary atherothrombosis, requiring at least one of the following:

- Symptoms of acute myocardial ischaemia;
- New ischemic ECG changes;
- Development of pathological Q waves;
- Imaging evidence of new loss of viable myocardium or new regional wall motion abnormality in a pattern consistent with an ischemic etiology.

All of the clinical information available should be considered in distinguishing type 1 myocardial infarction from type 2 myocardial infarction. The context and mechanisms of type 2 myocardial infarction should be considered when establishing this diagnosis. The myocardial oxygen supply/demand imbalance attributable to acute myocardial ischemia may be multifactorial, related either to: reduced myocardial perfusion due to fixed coronary atherosclerosis without plaque rupture, coronary artery spasm, coronary microvascular dysfunction (which includes endothelial dysfunction, smooth muscle cell dysfunction, and the dysregulation of sympathetic innervation), coronary embolism, coronary artery dissection with or without intramural hematoma, or other mechanisms that reduce oxygen supply such as severe bradyarrhythmia, respiratory failure with severe hypoxaemia, severe anaemia, and hypotension/shock; or to increased myocardial oxygen demand due to sustained tachyarrhythmia or severe hypertension with or without left ventricular hypertrophy.In patients who undergo timely coronary angiography, description of a ruptured plaque with thrombus in the infarct-related artery may be helpful in making the distinction between type 2 myocardial infarction vs. type 1 myocardial infarction, but angiography is not always definitive, clinically indicated, or required to establish the diagnosis of type 2 myocardial infarction.Studies have shown variable occurrences of type 2 myocardial infarction depending on criteria used for diagnosis.

Some reports rely on specific predetermined oxygen mismatch criteria 38), whereas others apply more liberal criteria. Most studies show a higher frequency of type 2 myocardial infarction in women. The short- and long-term mortality rates for patients with type 2 myocardial infarction are generally higher than for type 1 myocardial infarction patients in most but not all studies due to an increased prevalence of comorbid conditions . Coronary atherosclerosis is a common finding in type 2 myocardial infarction patients selected for coronary angiography. In general, these patients have a worse prognosis than those without coronary artery disease . Prospective evaluations of the importance of coronary artery disease with type 2 myocardial infarction using consistent definitions and approaches are needed.

It has been shown that the frequency of ST-segment elevation in type 2 myocardial infarction varies from 3–24% 42). In some cases, coronary embolism caused by thrombi, calcium or vegetation from the atria or ventricles, or acute aortic dissection may result in a type 2 myocardial infarction. Spontaneous coronary artery dissection with or without intramural hematoma is another non-atherosclerotic condition that may occur, especially in young women. It is defined as spontaneous dissection of the coronary artery wall with accumulation of blood within the false lumen, which can compress the true lumen to varying degrees

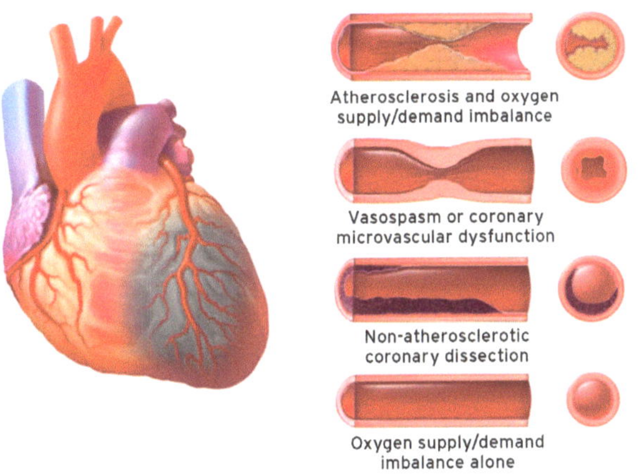

Fig. 26.10 Illustrations showing undergoing various changes in the coronary artery before causing type 2 myocardial infarction

Type 3 myocardial infarction

The detection of cardiac biomarkers in the blood is fundamental for establishing the diagnosis of myocardial infarction 45). However, patients can manifest a typical presentation of myocardial ischemia or myocardial infarction, including presumed new ischemic ECG changes or ventricular fibrillation, and die before it is possible to obtain blood for cardiac biomarker determination; or the patient may succumb soon after the onset of symptoms before an elevation of biomarker values has occurred. Such patients are designated as having a type 3 myocardial infarction, when suspicion for an acute myocardial ischaemic event is high, even when cardiac biomarker evidence of myocardial infarction is lacking 46). This category allows the separation of fatal myocardial infarction events from the much larger group of sudden death episodes that may be cardiac (non-ischemic) or non-cardiac in origin. When a type 3 myocardial infarction is diagnosed and a subsequent autopsy reveals recent evidence of an myocardial infarction, with a fresh or recent thrombus in the infarct-related artery, the type 3 myocardial infarction should be reclassified to a type 1 myocardial infarction. Original investigations addressing the incidence of type 3 myocardial infarction are sparse, but a study showed an annual incidence below 10/100,000 person-years and a frequency of 3–4% among all types of myocardial infarction Criteria for type 3 myocardial infarction :

Patients who suffer cardiac death, with symptoms suggestive of myocardial ischemia accompanied by presumed new ischemic ECG changes or ventricular fibrillation, but die before blood samples for biomarkers can be obtained, or before increases in cardiac biomarkers can be identified, or myocardial infarction is detected by autopsy examination

Type 4a myocardial infarction (myocardial infarction

It is associated with percutaneous coronary intervention) Stand-alone post-procedural increases of cardiac troponin (cTn) values are sufficient to establish a diagnosis of procedural myocardial injury but not for the diagnosis of type 4a myocardial infarction 49). Type 4a myocardial infarction requires an elevation of cardiac troponin values greater than five times the 99th percentile upper reference limit in patients with normal baseline values or, in patients with elevated pre-procedure cardiac troponin inwhom the cardiac troponin levels are stable (≤ 20% variation) or falling, the post-procedure cardiac troponin must rise > 20% to an absolute value more than five times the 99th percentile upper reference limit. In addition, there should be evidence of new myocardial ischaemia, either from ECG changes, imaging evidence, or from procedure-related complications associated with reduced coronary blood flow such as coronary dissection, occlusion of a major epicardial artery or a side branch occlusion/thrombus, disruption of collateral flow, slow flow or no-reflow, or distal embolization. The use of high-sensitivity cardiac troponin (hs-cTn) assays to diagnose type 4a myocardial infarction (and type 5 myocardial infarction) is an area of active research. Many high-sensitivity cardiac troponin (hs-cTn) assays are available, which have wide dynamic ranges. Different criteria may be required for different assays. However, it has recently been shown that the optimal hs-cTnT thresholds to predict cardiovascular events at 30 days and 1 year were very close to the five-fold increase suggested by the Third Universal Definition of Myocardial infarction 50). These criteria are therefore retained because of a lack of new scientific evidence that identifies superior criteria for defining this myocardial infarction subtype. Other criteria that meet the definition of type 4a myocardial infarction, regardless of hs-cTn or cTn values, are the development of new pathological Q waves or autopsy evidence of recent procedure-related thrombus in the culprit artery.

Criteria for percutaneous coronary intervention-related myocardial infarction ≤ 48 hours after the index procedure (type 4a myocardial infarction) :

Coronary intervention-related myocardial infarction is arbitrarily defined by an elevation of cardiac troponin (cTn) values more than five times the 99th percentile upper reference limit in patients with normal baseline values. In patients with elevated pre-procedure cTn in whom the cTn level are stable (≤ 20% variation) or falling, the post-procedure cTn must rise by > 20%. However, the absolute post-procedural value must still be at least five times the 99th percentile upper reference limit. In addition, one of the following elements is required:

- New ischemic ECG changes;
- Development of new pathological Q waves;
- Isolated development of new pathological Q waves meets the type 4a myocardial infarction criteria if cTn values are elevated and rising but less than five times the 99th percentile upper reference limit
- Imaging evidence of new loss of viable myocardium or new regional wall motion abnormality in a pattern consistent with an ischaemic etiology;
- Angiographic findings consistent with a procedural flow-limiting complication such as coronary dissection, occlusion of a major epicardial artery or a side branch occlusion/

thrombus, disruption of collateral flow, or distal embolization. hemorrhage meets the type 4a myocardial infarction criteria.

- Post-mortem demonstration of a procedure-related thrombus in the culprit artery, or a macroscopically large circumscribed area of necrosis with or without intra-myocardial

Type 4b myocardial infarction (stent/scaffold thrombosis associated with percutaneous coronary intervention)

Type 4b myocardial infarction, is a subcategory of percutaneous coronary intervention (PCI)-related myocardial infarction due to stent/scaffold thrombosis, as documented by angiography or autopsy using the same criteria utilized for type 1 myocardial infarction . It is important to indicate the time of the occurrence of the stent/scaffold thrombosis in relation to the timing of the percutaneous coronary intervention (PCI) procedure. The following temporal categories are suggested: acute, 0–24 hours; subacute, > 24 hours to 30 days; late, > 30 days to 1 year; and very late > 1 year after stent/scaffold implantation.

Type 4c myocardial infarction (restenosis associated with percutaneous coronary intervention)

Occasionally myocardial infarction occurs and—at angiography, in-stent restenosis, or restenosis following balloon angioplasty in the infarct territory—is the only angiographic explanation since no other culprit lesion or thrombus can be identified 54). This percutaneous coronary intervention (PCI)-related myocardial infarction type is designated as type 4c myocardial infarction, defined as focal or diffuse restenosis, or a complex lesion associated with a rise and/or fall of cardiac troponin values above the 99th percentile upper reference limit applying, the same criteria utilized for type 1 myocardial infarction.

Type 5 myocardial infarction (myocardial infarction associated with coronary artery bypass grafting)

Numerous factors can lead to procedural myocardial injury during a coronary artery bypass grafting (CABG) procedure. Many of them are related to the details of the cardiac preservation, the extent of the direct traumatic injury to the myocardium, as well as any potential ischemic injury. For that reason, increases in cardiac troponin values should be expected after all CABG procedures 55), which need to be taken into account when comparing the extent of procedural myocardial injury after cardiac surgery with that associated with less invasive approaches. Depending on whether it is off-pump or on-pump surgery, procedural myocardial injury is observed among 32–44% of CABG patients when quantified by late gadolinium enhancement cardiac magnetic resonance .

Criteria for CABG-related myocardial infarction ≤ 48 hours after the index procedure (type 5 myocardial infarction):

CABG-related myocardial infarction is arbitrarily defined as elevation of cardiac troponin values > 10 times the 99th percentile upper reference limit in patients with normal baseline cardiac troponin values. In patients with elevated pre-procedure cardiac troponin in whom cardiac troponin levels are stable (≤ 20% variation) or falling, the post-procedure cardiac troponin must rise by > 20%. However, the absolute post-procedural value still must be > 10 times the 99th percentile upper reference limit. In addition, one of the following elements is required:

- Development of new pathological Q waves;
- Isolated development of new pathological Q waves meets the type 5 myocardial infarction criteria if cardiac troponin values are elevated and rising but < 10 times the 99th percentile upper reference limit.
- Angiographic documented new graft occlusion or new native coronary artery occlusion;
- Imaging evidence of new loss of viable myocardium or new regional wall motion abnormality in a pattern consistent with an ischemic etiology.

Marked isolated elevation of cardiac troponin values within the 48 hours post-operative period, even in the absence of ECG/angiographic or other imaging evidence of myocardial infarction, indicates prognostically significant cardiac procedural myocardial injury 58). The presence of significant procedural myocardial injury in patients with operative problems (e.g. difficulty coming off bypass, technically difficult anastomoses in a heavily calcified aorta, of perioperative evidence of myocardial ischaemia, etc.) should prompt clinical review of the procedure and/or consideration of additional diagnostic testing for possible type 5 myocardial infarction.The area under the curve (AUC) and routine cardiac troponin sampling has demonstrated an excellent linear relationship with the mass of the new injury as defined by lategadolinium enhancement cardiac magnetic resonance.The area under the curve for creatine kinase MB isoform (CK-MB) is also good, although clearly inferior to cardiac troponin I (cTnI) 59). However, these relationships vary depending on the nature of the procedure, the nature of the cardioplegia, and the specific assay used to measure cardiac troponin. Very high cardiac troponin values are most often associated with coronary artery-related events 60). Thus, although cardiac biomarkers and especially cardiac troponin appear robust for the detection of procedural myocardial injury and also, in the presence of new myocardial ischaemia, for the detection of type 5 myocardial infarction, a specific cut-off value for all procedures and all cardiac troponin assays is difficult to define. However, in order to ensure consistency with the analogous standards of the preceding definition of type 5 myocardial infarction and because of the lack of new scientific evidence that identifies superior criteria for defining this myocardial infarction subtype, it is suggested that a cardiac troponin value > 10 times the 99th percentile upper reference limit is applied as the cut-off point during the first 48 hours following CABG, occurring from a normal baseline cardiac troponin value (≤ 99th percentile upper reference limit), for diagnosing type 5 myocardial infarction. It is important that the post-procedural elevation of cardiac troponin values is accompanied by ECG, angiographic, or imaging evidence of new myocardial ischaemia/new loss of myocardial viability.71 The higher cut-off of myocardial infarction after CABG than after PCI (10 times vs. 5 times the 99th percentile upper reference limit) has been arbitrarily selected due to the occurrence of more unavoidable myocardial injury during surgery than during PCI.

It should be recognized that ST-segment deviation and T wave changes are common after CABG due to epicardial injury, and are not reliable indicators of myocardial ischaemia in this setting. However, ST-segment elevation with reciprocal ST-segment depression or other specific ECG patterns may be a more reliable finding of a potential ischemic event

What is acute myocardial infarction?

Acute myocardial infarction is another term for a heart attack, which is caused by decreased coronary blood flow 63). The available oxygen supply cannot meet oxygen demand, resulting in cardiac ischemia. If blood flow Isn't restored quickly, the section of heart muscle begins to die. Decreased coronary blood flow is multifactorial. Atherosclerotic plaques classically rupture and lead to thrombosis, contributing to acute decreased blood flow in the coronary. Other etiologies of decreased oxygenation/ myocardial ischemia include coronary artery embolism, which accounts for 2.9% of patients, cocaine-induced ischemia, coronary dissection, and coronary vasospasm .

Acute myocardial infarction is one of the leading causes of death in the developed world. The prevalence of acute myocardial infarction approaches three million people worldwide with more than one million deaths in the United States, annually

Myocardial infarction prevention

It's never too late to take steps to prevent a myocardial infarction — even if you've already had one. Here are ways to prevent a myocardial infarction.

Medications. Taking medications can reduce your risk of a subsequent myocardial infarction and help your damaged heart function better. Continue to take what your doctor prescribes, and ask your doctor how often you need to be monitored.

Lifestyle factors. You know the drill: Maintain a healthy weight with a heart-healthy diet, don't smoke, exercise regularly, manage stress and control conditions that can lead to myocardial infarction, such as high blood pressure, high cholesterol and diabetes.Some preventive measures to overcome heart attack risks include:

- Quit smoking
- Eat a balanced and healthy diet
- Stay active: get plenty of exercise
- Get plenty of good quality sleep
- Keep diabetes under control
- Keep alcohol intake down
- Maintain blood cholesterol at optimum
- levels Keep blood pressure in control
- Maintain a healthy body weight
- Avoid stress and learn how to manage stress

Myocardial infarction complications

Potential complications from a myocardial infarction can vary widely, from mild to life threatening. Some people experience a "minor" myocardial infarction (although it can still be very serious) with no associated complications. This is also known as an uncomplicated myocardial infarction.

Other people experience a major myocardial infarction, which has a wide range of potential complications and may require extensive treatment. Complications are often related to the damage done to your heart during an attack. Some common complications of a myocardial infarction are discussed in more detail below:

- Abnormal heart rhythms (arrhythmias). Electrical "short circuits" can develop, resulting in abnormal heart rhythms, some of which can be serious, even fatal.
- Heart failure. An attack might damage so much heart tissue that the remaining heart muscle can't pump enough blood out of your heart. Heart failure can be temporary, or it can be a chronic condition resulting from extensive and permanent damage to your heart.
- Sudden cardiac arrest. Without warning, your heart stops due to an electrical disturbance that causes an arrhythmia. myocardial infarctions increase the risk of sudden cardiac arrest, which can be fatal without immediate treatment.

Arrhythmia

An arrhythmia is an abnormal heartbeat – this includes:

- beating too quickly (tachycardia)
- beating too slowly (bradycardia)
- beating irregularly (atrial fibrillation)
- Arrhythmias can develop after a myocardial infarction as a result of damage to the muscles. Damaged muscles disrupt electrical signals used by the body to control the heart.

Some arrhythmias, such as tachycardia, are mild and cause symptoms such as:

- palpitations – the sensation of your heart racing in your chest or throat
- chest pain
- dizziness or lightheadedness
- fatigue (tiredness)
- breathlessness

Other arrhythmias can be life threatening, such as:

- complete heart block, where electrical signals are unable to travel from one side of your heart to the other, so your heart cannot pump blood properly
- ventricular arrhythmia, where the heart begins beating faster before going into a spasm and stops pumping altogether; this is known as sudden cardiac arrest

These life-threatening arrhythmias can be a major cause of death during the 24-48 hours after a myocardial infarction.

However, survival rates have improved significantly since the invention of the portable defibrillator –

an external device that delivers an electric shock to the heart and "resets" it to the right rhythm.

Mild arrhythmias can usually be controlled with medication such as beta-blocrs.

More troublesome bradycardias that cause repeated and prolonged symptoms may need to be treated with a pacemaker. This is an electric device surgically implanted in the chest, which is used to help regulate the heartbeat.

Heart failure

Heart failure happens when your heart is unable to effectively pump blood around your body. It can develop after a myocardial infarction if your heart muscle is extensively damaged. This usually occurs in the left side of the heart (the left ventricle).

Symptoms of heart failure include:

- shortness of breath
- fatigue
- swelling in your arms and legs due to a build-up of fluid
- Heart failure can be treated with a combination of medications and, in some cases, surgery.

Cardiogenic shock

Cardiogenic shock is similar to heart failure, but more serious. It develops when the heart muscle has been damaged so extensively it can no longer pump enough blood to maintain many of the body's functions. Cardiogenic shock symptoms include:

- mental confusion
- cold hands and feet
- decreased or no urine output
- rapid heartbeat and breathing
- pale skin
- difficulty breathing

A type of medication called vasopressors (or inotropes) may be used. Vasopressors help constrict (squeeze) the blood vessels, which increases the blood pressure and improves blood circulation.

Once the initial symptoms of cardiogenic shock have been stabilised, surgery may be required to improve the functioning of the heart. This may still include PCI, alongside the insertion of a small pump, known as an intra-aortic balloon pump. This can help improve the flow of blood away from the heart.

Another option is a coronary artery bypass graft (where a blood vessel from another part of your body is used to bypass any blockage).

Heart rupture

A heart rupture is an extremely serious but relatively uncommon complication of myocardial infarctions where the heart's muscles, walls or valves rupture (split apart).

It can occur if the heart is significantly damaged duringa myocardial infarction and usually happens 1 to 5 days afterwards.

Symptoms are the same as those of cardiogenic shock. Open heart surgery is usually required to repair the damage.

The outlook for people who have a heart rupture isn't good, and it's estimated that half of all people die within five days of the rupture occurring.

Myocardial infarction diagnosis

Ideally, your doctor should screen you during regular physical exams for risk factors that can lead to a myocardial infarction.

If you're in an emergency setting for symptoms of a myocardial infarction, you'll be asked about your symptoms and have your blood pressure, pulse and temperature checked. You'll be hooked up to a heart monitor and have tests to see if you're having a myocardial infarction. Tests include:

Electrocardiogram (ECG). This first test done to diagnose a myocardial infarction records the electrical activity of your heart via electrodes attached to your skin. Impulses are recorded as waves displayed on a monitor or printed on paper. Because injured heart muscle doesn't conduct electrical impulses normally, the ECG may show that a myocardial infarction has occurred or is in progress.

Blood tests. Certain heart proteins slowly leak into your blood after heart damage from a myocardial infarction. Emergency room doctors will take samples of your blood to test for the presence of these enzymes.

Cardiac troponin-I (cTnI) and cardiac troponin-T (cTnT) are components of the contractile apparatus of myocardial cells and are expressed almost exclusively in the heart. Increases in cardiac troponin-I (cTnI) values have not been reported to occur following injury to non-cardiac tissues. Cardiac troponin-I (cTnI) and cardiac troponin T (cTnT) are the preferred biomarkers for the evaluation of myocardial injury) and high-sensitivity (hs)-cardiac troponin assays are recommended for routine clinical use . Other biomarkers, e.g. creatine kinase MB isoform (CK-MB), are less sensitive and less specific . Myocardial injury is defined as being present when blood levels of cTn are increased above the 99th percentile upper reference limit (URL) The injury may be acute, as evidenced by a newly detected dynamic rising and/or falling pattern of cardiac troponin values above the 99th percentile upper reference limit (URL) or chronic, in the setting of persistently elevatedcardiac troponin levels. Although elevated cardiac troponin values reflect injury to myocardial cells, they do not indicate the underlying pathophysiological mechanisms, and can arise following preload-induced mechanical stretch or physiological stresses in otherwise normal hearts . Various causes have been suggested for the release of structural proteins from the myocardium, including normal turnover of myocardial cells, apoptosis, cellular release of cardiac troponin degradation products, increased cellular wall permeability, the formation and release of membranous blebs, and myocyte necrosis . Yet, it is not clinically possible to distinguish which increases of cTn levels are due to which mechanisms . However, regardless of the mechanism, acute myocardial injury, when associated with a rising and/or falling pattern of cardiac troponins values with at least one value above the 99th percentile upper reference limit and caused by myocardial ischaemia, is designated as an acute myocardial infarction .

Histological evidence of myocardial injury with myocyte death can be detected in clinical conditions associated with non-ischaemic mechanisms of myocardial injury as well . mechanisms, and can arise following preload-induced mechanical stretch or physiological stresses in otherwise normal hearts . Various causes have been suggested for the release of structural proteins from the myocardium, including normal turnover of myocardial cells, apoptosis, cellular release of cardiac troponin degradation products, increased cellular wall permeability, the formation and release of membranous blebs, and myocyte necrosis . Yet, it is not clinically possible to distinguish which increases of cTn levels are due to which mechanisms . However, regardless of the mechanism, acute myocardial injury, when associated with a rising and/ or falling pattern of cardiac troponins values with at least one value above the 99th percentile upper reference limit and caused by myocardial ischaemia, is designated as an acute myocardial infarction . Histological evidence of myocardial injury with myocyte death can be detected in clinical conditions associated with non-ischaemic mechanisms of myocardial injury as well .

Additional tests

If you've had or are having a myocardial infarction, doctors will take immediate steps to treat your condition. You might also have these additional tests.

Chest X-ray. An X-ray image of your chest allows your doctor to check the size of your heart and its blood vessels and to look for fluid in your lungs.

Echocardiogram. Sound waves directed at your heart from a wandlike device(transducer) held on your chest bounce off your heart and are processed electronically to provide video images of your heart. An echocardiogram can help identify whether an area of your heart has been damaged and isn't pumping normally.

Coronary catheterization (angiogram). A liquid dye is injected into the arteries of your heart through a long, thin tube (catheter) that's fed through an artery, usually in your leg or groin, to the arteries in your heart. The dye makes the arteries visible on X-ray, revealing areas of blockage.

Exercise stress test. In the days or weeks after your myocardial infarction, you might also have a stress test to measure how your heart and blood vessels respond to exertion. You might walk on a treadmill or pedal a stationary bike while attached to an ECG machine. Or you might receive a drug intravenously that stimulates your heart similar to the way exercise does. Another possibility is a nuclear stress test, which is similar to an exercise stress test, but uses an injected dye and special imaging techniques to produce detailed images of your heart while you're exercising.

Cardiac CT or MRI. These tests can be used to diagnose heart problems, including the extent of damage from myocardial infarctions. In a cardiac CT scan, you lie on a table inside a doughnut-shaped machine. An X-ray tube inside the machine rotates around your body and collects images of your heart and chest. In a cardiac MRI, you lie on a table inside a long tubelike machine that produces a magnetic field. The magnetic field aligns atomic particles in some of your cells. When radio waves are broadcast toward these aligned particles, they produce signals that vary according to the type of tissue they are. The signals create images of your heart. The three components in the evaluation of the myocardial infarction are clinical features, ECG findings, and cardiac biomarkers.

ECG

The resting 12 lead ECG is the first-line diagnostic tool for the diagnosis of an acute coronary syndrome (ACS). It should be obtained within 10 minutes of the patient's arrival in the emergency room. Acute myocardial infarction is often associated with dynamic changes in the ECG waveform. Serial ECG monitoring can provide important clues to the diagnosis if the initial EKG is non-diagnostic at initial presentation. Serial or continuous ECG recordings may be helpful in determining reperfusion or re-occlusion status. A large and prompt reduction in ST-segment elevation is usually seen in reperfusion

ECG findings suggestive of ongoing coronary artery occlusion (in the absence of left ventricular hypertrophy and bundle branch block)

ST-segment elevation in two contiguous lead (measured at J-point) of:

- Greater than 5 mm in men younger than 40 years, greater than 2 mm in men older than 40 years, or greater than 1.5 mm in women in leads V2-V3 and/or
- Greater than 1 mm in all other leads

ST-segment depression and T-wave changes:

- New horizontal or down-sloping ST-segment depression greater than 5 mm in 2 contiguous leads and/or T inversion greater than 1 mm in two contiguous leads with prominent R waves or R/S ratio of greater than 1

The hyperacute T-wave amplitude, with prominent symmetrical T waves in two contiguous leads, may be an early sign of acute myocardial infarction that may precede the ST-segment elevation. Other ECG findings associated with myocardial ischemia include cardiac arrhythmias, intraventricular blocks, atrioventricular conduction delays, and loss of precordial R-wave amplitude (less specific finding)

ECG findings alone are not sufficient to diagnose acute myocardial ischemia or acute myocardial infarction as other conditions such as acute pericarditis, left ventricular hypertrophy (LVH), left bundle branch block (LBBB), Brugada syndrome, Takatsubo syndrome and early repolarization patterns also present with ST deviation.

ECG changes associated with prior myocardial infarction (in the absence of left ventricular hypertrophy and left bundle branch block):

- Any Q wave in lead V2-V3 greater than 0.02 s or QS complex in leads V2-V3
- Q wave > 03 s and greater than 1 mm deep or QS complex in leads I, II, aVL, aVF or V4-V6 in any two leads of contiguous lead grouping (I, aVL; V1-V6; II, III, aVF)
- R wave > 0.04 s in V1-V2 and R/S greater than 1 with a concordant positive T wave in the absence of conduction defect

Biomarker Detection of myocardial infarction

Cardiac troponins (I and T) are components of the contractile apparatus of myocardial cells and expressed almost exclusively in the heart. Elevated serum levels of cardiac troponin are not specific to the underlying mode of injury (ischemic vs. tension) .The rising and/or falling pattern of cardiac troponins (cTn) values with at least one value above the 99 percentile of upper reference limit (URL) associated with symptoms of myocardial ischemia would indicate an acute myocardial infarction. Serial testing of cTn values at 0 hours, 3 hours, and 6 hours would give a better perspective on the severity and time course of the myocardial injury. Depending on the baseline cardiac troponins value the rising/falling pattern is interpreted. If the cardiac troponins baseline value is markedly elevated, a minimum change of greater than 20% in follow up testing is significant for myocardial ischemia. Creatine kinase MB isoform can also be used in the diagnosis of myocardial infarction, but it is less sensitive and specific than cTn level .

Imaging

Different imaging techniques are used to assess myocardial perfusion, myocardial viability, myocardial thickness, thickening and motion, and the effect of myocyte loss on the kinetics of para-magnetic or radio-opaque contrast agents indicating myocardial fibrosis or scars Some imaging modalities that can be used are echocardiography, radionuclide imaging, and cardiac magnetic resonance imaging (cardiac MRI). Regional wall motion abnormalities induced by ischemia can be detected by echocardiography almost immediately after the onset of ischemia when greater than 20% transmural myocardial thickness is affected. Cardiac MRI provides an accurate assessment of myocardial structure and function.

Myocardial infarction treatment

Each minute after a myocardial infarction, more heart tissue deteriorates or dies. Restoring blood flow quickly helps prevent heart damage.

The treatment options for a myocardial infarction depend on whether you've had an ST segment elevation myocardial infarction (STEMI), or another type of myocardial infarction.

A STEMI is the most serious form of myocardial infarction and requires emergency assessment and treatment. It's important you're treated quickly to minimise damage to your heart.

If you have symptoms of a myocardial infarction and an electrocardiogram (ECG) shows you have a STEMI, you'll be assessed for treatment to unblock the coronary arteries. The treatment used will depend on when your symptoms started and how soon you can access treatment:

- If your symptoms started within the past 12 hours – you'll usually be offered primary percutaneous coronary intervention (PCI).
- If your symptoms started within the past 12 hours but you can't access percutaneous coronary intervention quickly – you'll be offered medication to break down blood clots.
- If your symptoms started more than 12 hours ago – you may be offered a different procedure, especially if symptoms have improved. The best course of treatment will be decided after an angiogram and may include medication, percutaneous coronary intervention or bypass surgery.

Medications

Medications given to treat a myocardial infarction might include:

- **Aspirin.** The emergency services operator might tell you to take aspirin, or emergency medical personnel might give you aspirin immediately. Aspirin reduces blood clotting, thus helping maintain blood flow through a narrowed artery.
- **Thrombolytics.** These drugs, also called clotbusters, help dissolve a blood clot that's blocking blood flow to your heart. The earlier you receive a thrombolytic drug after a myocardial infarction, the greater the chance you'll survive and have less heart damage.
- Antiplatelet agents. Emergency room doctors may give you other drugs known as platelet aggregation inhibitors to help prevent new clots and keep existing clots from getting larger.
- Other blood-thinning medications. You'll likely be given other medications, such as heparin, to make your blood less "sticky" and less likely to form clots. Heparin is given intravenously or by an injection under your skin.
- Pain relievers. You might be given a pain reliever, such as morphine.
- Nitroglycerin. This medication, used to treat chest pain (angina), can help improve blood flow to the heart by widening (dilating) the blood vessels.
- Beta blockers. These medications help relax your heart muscle, slow your heartbeat and decrease blood pressure, making your heart's job easier. Beta blockers can limit the amount of heart muscle damage and prevent future myocardial infarctions.
- ACE inhibitors. These drugs lower blood pressure and reduce stress on the heart.
- Statins. These drugs help control your blood cholesterol.

Thrombolytics

Medications used to break down blood clots, known as thrombolytics or fibrinolytics, are usually given by injection.

Thrombolytics or fibrinolytics, target and destroy a substance called fibrin. Fibrin is a tough protein that makes up blood clots by acting like a sort of fibre mesh that hardens around the blood.

Some examples of thrombolytics include:

- reteplase
- alteplase
- streptokinase

You may also be given an additional medication called a glycoprotein IIb/IIIa inhibitor if it is thought you have an increased risk of experiencing another myocardial infarction at some point in the near future.

Glycoprotein IIb/IIIa inhibitors don't break up blood clots, but they prevent blood clots from getting bigger. They're an effective method of stopping your symptoms getting worse.

Surgical and other procedures

In addition to medications, you might have one of these procedures to treat your myocardial infarction:

Coronary angioplasty and stenting.

In this procedure, also known as percutaneous coronary intervention (PCI), doctors insert a long, thin tube (catheter) that's passed through an artery in your groin or wrist to a blocked artery in your heart. If you've had a myocardial infarction, this procedure is often done immediately after a cardiac catheterization, a procedure used to find blockages. This catheter has a special balloon that, once in position, is briefly inflated to open a blocked coronary artery. A metal mesh stent might then be inserted into the artery to keep it open long term, restoring blood flow to the heart. Depending on your condition, you might get a stent coated with a slow-releasing medication to help keep your artery open.

Coronary artery bypass surgery also known as a coronary artery bypass graft (CABG). In some cases, doctors perform emergency bypass surgery at the time of a myocardial infarction. If possible, however, you might have bypass surgery after your heart has had time — about three to seven days — to recover from your myocardial infarction. Bypass surgery involves sewing veins or arteries in place beyond a blocked or narrowed coronary artery, allowing blood flow to the heart to bypass the narrowed section. Once blood flow to your heart is restored and your condition is stable, you're likely to remain in the hospital for several days.

Percutaneous coronary intervention

Primary percutaneous coronary intervention (PCI) or coronary angioplasty and stenting, is the term for emergency treatment of ST segment elevation myocardial infarction (STEMI), using a procedure to widen the coronary artery (coronary angioplasty).

Coronary angiography is performed first to assess your suitability for percutaneous coronary intervention (PCI). You may also be given blood-thinning medication to prevent further clots from developing, such as:

- aspirin
- heparin
- clopidogrel
- prasugrel
- ticagrelor
- bivalirudin

Some of these medications may be continued for some time after percutaneous coronary intervention (PCI).

Coronary angioplasty

Coronary angioplasty is a potentially complex type of procedure that requires specialist staff and equipment, and not all hospitals have the facilities.

This means you'll need to be taken urgently, by ambulance, to one of the specialist centers (myocardial infarction centers) that now serve most of the US's regions.

During coronary angioplasty, a tiny tube known as a balloon catheter, with a sausage-shaped balloon at the end, is put into a large artery in your groin or arm. The catheter is passed through your blood vessels and up to your heart, over a fine guide wire, using X-rays to guide it, before being moved into the narrowed section of your coronary artery.

Once in position, the balloon is inflated inside the narrowed part of the coronary artery to open it wide. A stent (flexible metal mesh) is usually inserted into the artery to help keep it open afterwards.

Coronary artery bypass graft

A coronary angioplasty may not be technically possible sometimes if the anatomy of your arteries is different from normal. This may be the case if there are too many narrow sections in your arteries or if there are lots of branches coming off your arteries that are also blocked.In such circumstances, an alternative surgical operation, known as a coronary artery bypass graft (CABG), may be considered. A CABG involves taking a blood vessel from another part of your body, usually your chest or leg, to use as a graft.

The graft bypasses any hardened or narrowed arteries in the heart. A surgeon will attach the new blood vessel to the aorta and the other to the coronary artery beyond the narrowed area or blockage.

Treating non-ST segment elevation myocardial infarction (NSTEMI) or unstable angina

If the results of your ECG show you have a "less serious" type of heart attack (known as a non-ST segment elevation myocardial infarction (NSTEMI) or unstable angina), then blood-thinning medication, including aspirin and other medications, is usually recommended. In some cases, further treatment with coronary angioplasty or coronary artery bypass graft may be recommended in cases of NSTEMI or unstable angina, after initial treatment with these medications.

Myocardial infarction recovery

Recovering from a myocardial infarction can take several months, and it's very important not to rush your rehabilitation.

During your recovery period, you'll receive help and support from a range of healthcare professionals, which may include:

- nurses
- physiotherapists
- dietitians
- pharmacists
- exercise specialists

These healthcare professionals will support you physically and mentally to ensure your recovery is conducted safely and appropriately.

The recovery process usually takes place in stages, starting in hospital, where your condition can be closely monitored and your individual needs for the future can be assessed.

After being discharged, you can continue your recovery at home.

The 2 most important aims of the recovery process are:

- to gradually restore your physical fitness so you can resume normal activities (known as cardiac rehabilitation)
- to reduce your risk of another myocardial infarction

Cardiac rehabilitation

Your cardiac rehabilitation program will begin when you're in hospital. Most hospitals offer programs that might start while you're in the hospital and continue for weeks to a couple of months after you return home. Cardiac rehabilitation programs generally focus on four main areas:

- medications,
- lifestyle changes,
- emotional issues and
- a gradual return to your normal activities.

It's extremely important to participate in this program. People who attend cardiac rehab after a myocardial infarction generally live longer and are less likely to have another myocardial infarction or complications from the myocardial infarction. If cardiac rehab is not recommended during your hospitalization, ask your doctor about it.

You should also be invited back for another session taking place within 10 days of leaving hospital.

A member of the cardiac rehabilitation team will visit you in hospital and provide detailed information about:

- your state of health and how the heart attack may have affected it
- the type of treatment you received
- what medications you'll need when you leave hospital
- what specific risk factors are thought to have contributed to your heart attack
- what lifestyle changes you can make to address those risk factors
- They can also answer any questions you have about finance, welfare rights, housing and social care.

Lifestyle and home remedies

To improve your heart health, take the following steps:

Avoid smoke. The most important thing you can do to improve your heart's health is to not smoke. Also, avoid being around secondhand smoke. If you need to quit, ask your doctor for help.

Control your blood pressure and cholesterol levels. If one or both of these is high, your doctor can prescribe changes to your diet and medications. Ask your doctor how often you need to have your blood pressure and cholesterol levels monitored.

Get regular medical checkups. Some of the major risk factors for myocardial infarction — high blood cholesterol, high blood pressure and diabetes — cause no symptoms early on. Your doctor can test for these conditions and can help you manage them, if necessary.Exercise. Regular exercise helps improve heart muscle function after a myocardial infarction and helps prevent a myocardial infarction. Walking 30 minutes a day, five days a week can improve your health.

Maintain a healthy weight. Excess weight strains your heart and can contribute to high cholesterol, high blood pressure and diabetes.

Eat a heart-healthy diet. Saturated fat, trans fats and cholesterol in your diet can narrow arteries to your heart, and too much salt can raise blood pressure. Eat a heart-healthy diet that includes lean proteins, such as fish and beans, and fruits and vegetables and whole grains.

Manage diabetes. Regular exercise, eating well and losing weight all help to keep blood sugar levels at more-desirable levels. Many people also need medication to manage their diabetes.

Control stress. Reduce stress in your day-to-day activities. Rethink workaholic habits and find healthy ways to minimize or deal with stressful events in your life.

If you drink alcohol, do so in moderation. That means up to one drink a day for women and men older than age 65, and up to two drinks a day for men age 65 and younger.

Exercise

Once you return home, it's usually recommended that you rest and only do light activities, such as walking up and down the stairs a few times a day or taking a short walk.

Gradually increase the amount of activity you do each day over several weeks. How quickly you can do this will depend on the condition of your heart and your general health.

Your care team can provide more detailed advice about a recommended plan to increase your activity levels.

Your rehabilitation program should contain a range of different exercises, depending on your age and ability.

Most of the exercises will be aerobic. These are designed to strengthen the heart, improve circulation and lower blood pressure.

Examples of aerobic exercises include riding an exercise bike, jogging on a treadmill and swimming.

Regular physical activity

Once you have made a sufficient physical recovery from the effects of a heart attack, it's recommended that you do regular physical activity.

Adults should do at least 150 minutes (2 hours and 30 minutes) of moderate-intensity aerobic activity such as cycling or fast walking every week.

The level of activity should be strenuous enough to leave you slightly breathless.

If you find it difficult to achieve 150 minutes of activity a week, start at a level that you feel comfortable with (for example, 5 to 10 minutes of light exercise a day) and gradually increase the duration and intensity of your activity as your fitness begins to improve.

Returning to work

Most people can return to work after having a myocardial infarction, but how quickly will depend on your health, the state of your heart and the kind of work you do.

If your job involves light duties, such as if you work in an office, you may be able to return to work in as little as 2 weeks.

But if your job involves heavy manual work or your heart was extensively damaged, it may be several months before you can return to work.

Your care team will provide a more detailed prediction of how long it'll take for you to return to work.

Sex after a myocardial infarction

Some people worry about having sex after a myocardial infarction, but most people can safely return to sexual activity after recovery. When you can resume sexual activity will depend on your physical comfort, psychological readiness and previous sexual activity. Ask your doctor when it's safe to have sex.According to the British Heart Foundation, you're usually able to start having sex again once you feel well enough, usually about 4 to 6 weeks after having a myocardial infarction.

Having sex won't put you at further risk of having another myocardial infarction.

Following a myocardial infarction, about 1 in 3 men have erectile dysfunction, which may make having sex difficult.

- This is most commonly due to anxiety and the emotional stress associated with having a myocardial infarction.
- Less commonly, erectile dysfunction is a side effect of beta blockers.
- If you experience erectile dysfunction, speak to your doctor. They may be able to recommend treatment.
- For example, you may be prescribed medication that stimulates the flow of blood to your penis, which makes it easier to get an erection.
- Some heart medications can affect sexual function. If you're having problems with sexual dysfunction, talk to your doctor.

Driving

If you drive a car or motorcycle and you have a myocardial infarction, you don't have to inform the Driver and Vehicle Licensing Agency (DMV).

Many people can now return to driving 1 week after a myocardial infarction, as long you don't have any other condition or complication that would disqualify you from driving.

But in more severe cases, you may need to stop driving for 4 weeks.

Your doctor or rehabilitation team should advise how long you must wait before driving after your myocardial infarction.

If you drive a large goods vehicle or passenger-carrying vehicle, you must inform the DMV if you have a myocardial infarction.

Your licence will be temporarily suspended, for a minimum of 6 weeks, until you have adequately recovered.

Your licence will be reissued if you can pass a basic health and fitness test, and don't have any other condition that would disqualify you from driving.

Depression

Having a myocardial infarction can be frightening and traumatic, and it's common to have feelings of anxiety afterwards.

For many people, the emotional stresses can cause them to feel depressed and tearful for the first few weeks after returning home from hospital.

If feelings of depression persist, speak to your doctor as you may have a more serious form of depression.

It's important to seek advice as serious types of depression often don't get better without treatment.

Your emotional state could also have an adverse effect on your physical recovery.

Reducing your risk for another myocardial infarction

Reducing your risk of having another myocardial infarction involves making lifestyle changes and taking a long-term course of different medications.

Diet

Making changes to your diet can help reduce your risk of having another myocardial infarction.

Other lifestyle changes, such as drinking less alcohol, taking regular exercise, giving up smoking (if you smoke) and maintaining a healthy weight can also help.

You should aim to follow a Mediterranean-style diet. This means eating more bread, fruit, vegetables and fish, and less meat.

Replace butter and cheese with products based on vegetable and plant oil, such as olive oil.

Oily fish, like herring, sardines and salmon, can form

part of a Mediterranean-style diet, but there's no need to eat this type of fish specifically to try to prevent another myocardial infarction.

Also, omega-3 fatty acid capsules or foods fortified with omega-3 fatty acids haven't been found to help prevent another myocardial infarction.

Never take a food supplement without first consulting your doctor. Some supplements, such as beta-carotene, are potentially harmful.

Mediterranean diet

There's evidence to show that eating a Mediterranean-style diet can reduce your risk of having another myocardial infarction.

To make your diet more Mediterranean you can:

- eat more fruit, salad and vegetables
- eat more wholegrains, nuts and seeds
- eat more fish
- eat less meat

choose products made from vegetable and plant oils, such as olive oil, rather than dairy products, such as butter and cheese

Oily fish

You should eat at least 2 portions of fish a week, including a portion of oily fish.

Oily fish is a rich source of omega-3 fatty acids, which help prevent heart disease.

Examples of oily fish include:

- herring
- sardines
- mackerel
- salmon
- trout

One portion is about 140g, which is equivalent to a small tin of oily fish or a small fillet of fresh fish.

Healthier ways to cook

Don't fry or roast food in fat. Instead, prepare and cook your food using healthy methods such as:

- steaming
- poaching
- baking
- stir-frying
- making a casserole
- using the microwave

Buttery, cheesy or creamy sauces tend to be high in fat. Instead, try adding flavour to your sauces using spices, herbs and lemon juice.

Foods to avoid

Avoid foods that are high in:

- saturated fat (this is the current guidance, although further studies on saturated fat are needed)
- salt
- sugar

Foods containing high amounts of fat, salt or sugar include:

- fried foods
- sweets and confectionery
- takeaways
- processed foods
- pre-packaged foods
- Supplements to avoid

Don't take beta-carotene supplements (beta-carotene is a type of vitamin A). Research has shown that taking these supplements may increase your risk of having another myocardial infarction.

Also, taking vitamin C, vitamin E or folic acid supplements won't help prevent another myocardial infarction. There's no evidence to suggest that taking any of these supplements will have any benefit.

Prognosis

MI in the elderly is associated with poor short- and long-term prognosis in terms of both morbidity and mortality [3, 9]. The proportion of patients ≥70 years with recurrent MI, stroke, or HF within 5 years following a first MI is 1.5 to 3-fold greater than in those aged 40-69 years. Likewise, the proportion of individuals aged ≥70 years that die within one year following a first MI is 2 to 3-fold higher than in those aged 40-69 years

Prognosis

MI in the elderly is associated with poor short- and long-term prognosis in terms of both morbidity and mortality. The proportion of patients ≥70 years with recurrent MI, stroke, or HF within 5 years following a first MI is 1.5 to 3-fold greater than in those aged 40-69 years. Likewise, the proportion of individuals aged ≥70 years that die within one year following a first MI is 2 to 3-fold higher than in those aged 40-69 years

HEART FAILURE

In 2005, HF, which is predominantly a disorder of the elderly, was the primary cause of approximately 59,000 deaths and was listed as a primary or contributory cause of death on nearly 300,000 U.S. death certificates

Prevalence

The aging of the population in combination with improved survival in patients with CVD, particularly CHD and hypertension, has led to an increase in both the prevalence and incidence of HF. HF is relatively uncommon in individuals age 20-39 (0.1-0.2%), but the prevalence increases progressively with age to 5-10% in persons age 60-79 years and 12-14% in those ≥80 years . In CHS, the prevalence of HF increased from 12% in men and 6% in women 65-69 years of age to 18% in men and 14% in women age 85 or older

Incidence

Older adults without HF have an approximately 1 in 5 lifetime risk for developing HF At age 80, men without HF have a 20.2% risk for developing HF, which is close to the 21.0% lifetime risk for 40 year old men. However, relative to younger adults, the short-term risk of HF is much greater in the elderly. For example, the 5-year risk of incident HF for an 80 year old person is about 8%, whereas the risk for a 40 year old is only 0.2% (i.e., a 40-fold difference).

In the CHS, the 10-year incidence of HF increased by up to 6-fold across age strata with similar increases in men and women and in Caucasians and African-Americans. In both Caucasians and African-Americans, men had a higher 10 year incidence of HF than women. While the overall incidence rate of HF was higher in Caucasian men than in African-American men, the reverse was true in women.

Symptoms of heart failure

Heart failure may be symptomless or range from mild to severe. Symptoms may be constant or infrequent and may include:

- Congested lungs – Fluid filled lungs resulting in shortness of breath, dry cough, or wheezing
- Fluid and water retention – Results from reduced blood supply to kidneys, in turn leading to swollen ankles, legs, and abdomen (body swelling), weight gain, increased frequency of urination at night, loss of appetite, and/or nausea
- Reduced blood supply to vital organs – Results in dizziness, tiredness, weakness, and confusion
- Rapid or irregular heartbeats
- Weight gain
- Chest pain
- Fainting in severe cases

Causes

Causes include:

- Coronary artery disease (CAD) – Reduced blood supply to heart muscles because of blocked or narrowed arteries
- Heart attack – Completely stopped blood supply to heart muscles, permanently damaging them
- Cardiomyopathy – Damaged heart muscles because of infection, alcohol or drug abuse
- Overworking of heart – because of high blood
- Uncontrolled high blood pressure
- Uncontrolled Diabetes
- Certain medications, such as nonsteroidal anti-inflammatory drugs (NSAIDs), antiarrhythmic drugs
-
- Sleep disorders
- Viral infection to the heart muscles
- Obesity
- Excessive alcohol consumption
- Irregular heart beat

Common tests & procedures

Blood test:

- Kidney and thyroid functions
- Cholesterol levels
- Blood cell count
- B-type natriuretic peptide (BNP) levels, a substance indicative of heart failure

X-ray: Chest X-ray detects enlarged heart and fluid filled lungs.

Magnetic resonance imaging (MRI): MRI of chest detects any damages to the heart muscles, blockages in the heart.

Echocardiogram: Helps in evaluating heart muscles and valves.

Electrocardiogram (ECG or EKG): To assess how well the heart pumps blood.

Ejection fraction (EF): To measure the amount of blood released during contraction of the heart.

Stress test: Measures the health of the heart and amount of stress it can sustain.

Cardiac catheterisation: To check for coronary artery disease.

Medication

- Angiotensin-converting enzyme (ACE) inhibitors: Converting enzyme inhibitors (ACE inhibitors)helps to open narrowed blood vessels.
- Benazepril . Captopril . Enalapril
- Beta blockers: To reduce blood pressure and slow down heart rate.
- Acebutolol . Atenolol . Bisoprolol
- Diuretics: To reduce fluid content in the body.
- Metolazone . Indapamide . Hydrochlorothiazide

Procedures

Coronary artery bypass graft (CABG): Correcting blocked coronary arteries using arteries from other areas of the body.

Heart valve surgery: Damaged valve is replaced or repaired. It could be either an invasive or a non-invasive procedure.

Implantable left ventricular assist device (LVAD) placement: Surgically inserting a battery-operated, mechanical pump-like device into the left ventricle.
Heart transplant: Advised in extreme cases when all other treatment options fail.

Nutrition

Foods to eat:

- Eat a healthy and nutritious diet
- Include fibre-rich food
- Limit fatty and sugary foods
- Include low fat or fat-free foods
- Limit your salt and sodium intake
- Quit alcohol

Foods to avoid:

- High cholesterol foods
- Foods rich in salty and sugary

STROKE

Stroke is the third leading cause of death and a leading cause of long-term disability in the U.S. While the prevalence of stroke is below 3% in adults aged 20-59 years, it increases to approximately 8% by age 60-79 years, and reaches 13-17% among persons aged ≥80 years

Symptoms

If you or someone you know is exhibiting symptoms of Stroke, seek medical attention immediately.
As different parts of brain control different parts of the body, symptoms will depend on the part of brain affected and the extent of damage. The main symptoms are:

- Paralysis or numbness or inability to move parts of The face, arm, or leg - particularly on one side of The body
- Confusion- including trouble with speaking
- Headache with vomiting
- Trouble seeing in one or both eyes
- Metallic taste in mouth
- Difficulty in swallowing
- Trouble in walking (impaired coordination)
- Dystonia
- Alexia
- Agnosia

Causes

Some people may experience only a temporary disruption of blood flow to the brain.
Stroke occurs when blood supply to brain is interrupted or reduced. This deprives oxygen and nutrients supplied to the brain, causing brain cells to die.
Stroke may be caused by the following:

Ischaemic stroke: The obstruction to blood flow is usually due to a thrombus or an embolism within The blood vessel
Haemorrhagic stroke: Haemorrhagic stroke is a type of stroke that follows bleeding in The brain
Transient Ischaemic attack: TIA is caused by same conditions that cause an Ischaemic stroke like thrombosis, embolism, or other conditions like arterial dissection, arteries or hypercoagulable states. TIA does not leave lasting symptoms because blockage is temporary

The risk factors include:

- Overweight
- Sedentary life
- Binge Drinking
- Diabetes
- Smoking
- High blood pressure
- High cholesterol
- Family history of stroke
- Cardiovascular diseases
- Age - people above age 55 are at higher risk
- Gender - men are at high risk of stroke than women

Common tests & procedures

Physical examination: Patient's symptoms, medical history, blood pressure and blood vessels at the back of the eyes are checked.
Blood test: To find out time taken for clotting of blood.
CT scan: Images of brain can show a haemorrhage, tumour, stroke or other medical conditions.
Ultrasound: To check the blood flow in the carotid arteries and to check for plaque, if any.
Magnetic resonance imaging (MRI): MRI of brain tissue to diagnose ischaemic stroke or brain haemorrhages.
Cerebral angiogram: Dyes is injected to get detailed view of brain and neck blood vessels visible under X-ray.
Echocardiogram: To check for any sources of clots that could have travelled to the brain and lead to stroke.

Medication

Clot dissolver: To dissolve clots and reopen arteries. Plasminogen activator (tPA)
Anticoagulants: Has the effect of retarding or inhibiting the coagulation of blood.
Aspirin . Clopidogrel

Procedures

Catheter mediated intra-arterial thrombolysis: To attain reperfusion in case of ischaemic stroke or transient ischemic attack.

Angioplasty and stent placement: Widens the blocked artery and a stent is placed.

Aneurysm clipping: To treat a balloon-like bulge of an artery wall known as an aneurysm.

Coil embolisation: To treat aneurysm that may have caused haemorrhagic stroke.

Carotid endarterectomy: To correct stenosis (narrowing) in the common carotid artery or internal carotid artery.

AVM removal: Carried out in case of haemorrhagic stroke.

Therapy

Rehabilitation:The rehabilitation is advised to start as early as possible upon recovery. Rehabilitation program will be decided as per the necessity and usually focuses on speech therapy; cognitive therapy; sensory and motor skills; and physical therapy.

Nutrition

Foods to eat:

- Fruits and vegetables: eat plenty of fruit and vegetables; between 5-7 servings per day
- Whole grain breads and cereals containing fiber and vitamins: They may reduce the risk of stroke
- Lean protein: Limiting the amount of cholesterol is another important step in reducing the risk of another stroke
- Choose low-fat meats or other protein
- Limit salt: Eating too much salt/sodium may cause you to retain water and raise your blood pressure

Foods to avoid:

- Heavy cholesterol foods
- foods rich in salt and sugar
- Alcoho

PERIPHERAL ARTERIAL DISEASE

PAD is a significant predictor of cardiovascular and overall mortality. In addition, PAD is associated with limitations in physical function and with reduced health-related quality of life . PAD, diagnosed by an ankle brachial index (ABI) <0.9, was present in 12.4% of 5,084 CHS participants [14]. In CHS, the prevalence of an ABI <0.9 among men without clinical CVD increased almost 3-fold from age 65-69 to age ≥85, reaching approximately 30% in the latter age group In women, the increase in prevalence of PAD with age was even more striking, with nearly 40% of women ≥85 having an abnormal ABI, representing an 8-fold increase relative to the 65-69 year age group.

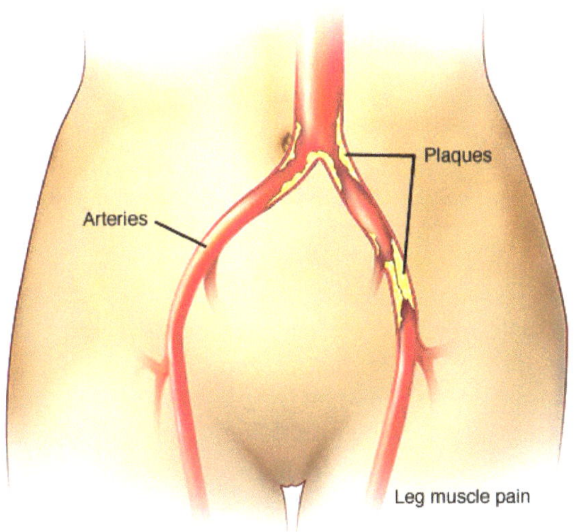

Fig.26.11 Claudication is pain in the legs or arms that occurs while walking or using the arms.

Peripheral artery disease (also called peripheral arterial disease) is a common condition in which narrowed arteries reduce blood flow to the arms or legs.

In peripheral artery disease (PAD), the legs or arms — usually the legs — don't receive enough blood flow to keep up with demand. This may cause leg pain when walking (claudication) and other symptoms.

Peripheral artery disease is usually a sign of a buildup of fatty deposits in the arteries (atherosclerosis). Atherosclerosis causes narrowing of the arteries that can reduce blood flow in the legs and, sometimes, the arms.Peripheral artery disease treatment includes exercising, eating a healthy diet and not smoking or using tobacco.

Symptoms

Many people with peripheral artery disease have mild or no symptoms. Some people have leg pain when walking (claudication).Claudication symptoms include muscle pain or cramping in the legs or arms that begins during exercise and ends with rest. The pain is most commonly felt in the calf. The pain ranges from mild to severe. Severe leg pain may make it hard to walk or do other types of physical activity.

Other peripheral artery disease symptoms may include:

- Coldness in the lower leg or foot, especially when compared with the other side
- Leg numbness or weakness
- No pulse or a weak pulse in the legs or feet
- Painful cramping in one or both of the hips, thighs or calf muscles after certain activities, such as walking or climbing stairs
- Shiny skin on the legs
- Skin color changes on the legs
- Slower growth of the toenails
- Sores on the toes, feet or legs that won't heal
- Pain when using the arms, such as aching and cramping when knitting, writing or doing other manual tasks
- Erectile dysfunction
- Hair loss or slower hair growth on the legs

If peripheral artery disease gets worse, pain may occur during rest or when lying down. The pain may interrupt sleep. Hanging the legs over the edge of the bed or walking may temporarily relieve the pain.

Causes

- Peripheral artery disease is often caused by a buildup of fatty, cholesterol-containing deposits (plaques) on artery walls. This process is called atherosclerosis. It reduces blood flow through the arteries.
- Atherosclerosis affects arteries throughout the body. When it occurs in the arteries supplying blood to the limbs, it causes peripheral artery disease.

Less common causes of peripheral artery disease include:

- Blood vessel inflammation
- Injury to the arms or legs
- Changes in the muscles or ligaments
- Radiation exposure

Risk factors

Smoking or having diabetes greatly increases the risk of developing peripheral artery disease.Other things that increase the risk of peripheral artery disease include:

- A family history of peripheral artery disease, heart disease or stroke
- High blood pressure
- High cholesterol
- High levels of an amino acid called homocysteine, which increase the risk for coronary artery disease
- Increasing age, especially after 65 (or after 50 if you have risk factors for atherosclerosis)
- Obesity (a body mass index over 30)

Complications

Complications of peripheral artery disease caused by atherosclerosis include:

Critical limb ischemia. In this condition, an injury or infection causes tissue to die. Symptoms include open sores on the limbs that don't heal. Treatment may include amputation of the affected limb.

Stroke and heart attack. Plaque buildup in the arteries can also affect the blood vessels in the heart and brain.

Prevention

The best way to prevent leg pain due to peripheral artery disease is to maintain a healthy lifestyle. That means:

- Don't smoke.
- Control blood sugar.
- Eat foods that are low in saturated fat.
- Get regular exercise — but check with your care provider about what type and how much is best for you.
- Maintain a healthy weight.
- Manage blood pressure and cholesterol.

Diagnosis

To diagnose peripheral artery disease, a health care provider will examine you. You'll usually be asked questions about your symptoms and medical history.

If you have peripheral artery disease, the pulse in the affected area may be weak or missing.

Tests

Tests that may be done to diagnose peripheral artery disease include:

Blood tests. Blood tests are done to check for conditions related to PAD such as high cholesterol, high triglycerides and diabetes.

Ankle-brachial index (ABI). This is a common test used to diagnose PAD. It compares the blood pressure in the ankle with the blood pressure in the arm. You may be asked to walk on a treadmill. Blood pressure readings may be taken before and immediately after exercising to check the arteries during walking.

Ultrasound of the legs or feet. This test uses sound waves to see how blood moves through the blood vessels. Doppler ultrasound is a special type of ultrasound used to spot blocked or narrowed arteries.

Angiography. This test uses X-rays, magnetic resonance imaging (MRI) scans or computerized tomography (CT) scans to look for blockages in the arteries. Before the images are taken, dye (contrast) is injected into a blood vessel. The dye helps the arteries show up more clearly on the test images.

Treatment

The goals of treatment for peripheral artery disease are:

- Manage symptoms, such as leg pain, so exercise isn't uncomfortable
- Improve artery health to reduce the risk of heart attack and stroke

Treatments for peripheral artery disease includes lifestyle changes and sometimes, medication.

Lifestyle changes can help improve symptoms, especially early in the course of peripheral artery disease. If you smoke, quitting is the single most important thing you can do to reduce the risk of complications. Walking or doing other exercise on a regular, scheduled basis (supervised exercise training) can improve symptoms dramatically.

Medications

If peripheral artery disease (PAD) is causing symptoms, your provider may prescribe medicine. Medications for PAD may include:

Cholesterol drugs. Medications called statins are commonly prescribed for people with peripheral artery disease. Statins help lower bad cholesterol and reduce plaque buildup in the arteries. The drugs also lower the risk of heart attacks and strokes. If you have PAD, ask your provider what your cholesterol numbers should be.

Blood pressure drugs. Uncontrolled high blood pressure can make arteries stiff and hard. This can slow the flow of blood. Ask your health care provider what blood pressure goal is best for you. If you have high blood pressure, your provider may prescribe medications to lower it.

Medications to control blood sugar. If you have diabetes, controlling your blood sugar levels becomes even more important. Talk with your provider about your blood sugar goals and how to reach them.

Medications to prevent blood clots. Peripheral artery disease is related to reduced blood flow to the limbs. So, medicines may be given to improve blood flow. Aspirin or another medication, such as clopidogrel (Plavix), may be used to prevent blood clotting.

Medications for leg pain. The drug cilostazol thins the blood and widens blood vessels. It increases blood flow to the limbs. The drug specifically helps treat leg pain in people who have peripheral artery disease. Common side effects of this medication include headache and diarrhea. An alternative medication is pentoxifylline. Side effects are rare with this medication, but it generally doesn't work as well as cilostazol.

Surgeries or other procedures

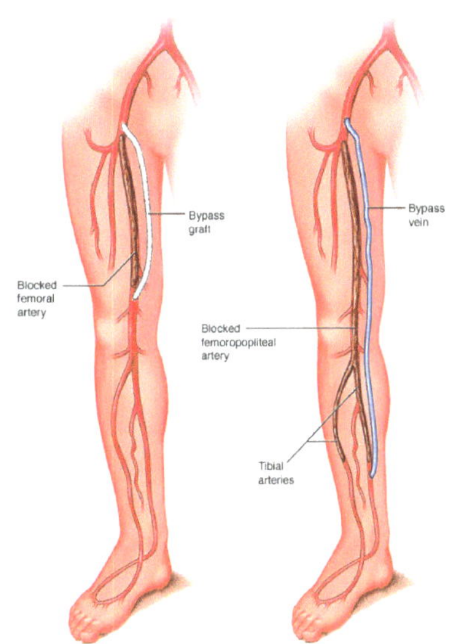

Fig.26.12 Graft bypassA graft is used to redirect blood flow around a blocked or narrowed artery. A graft can be a blood vessel from another part of the body or a synthetic substitute.

In some cases, angioplasty or surgery may be necessary to treat peripheral artery disease that's causing claudication:

Angioplasty and stent placement. This procedure is done to open clogged arteries. It can diagnose and treat a blocked vessel at the same time. The health care provider guides a thin, flexible tube (catheter) to the narrowed part of the artery. A tiny balloon is inflated to widen the blocked artery and improve blood flow. A small wire mesh tube (stent) may be placed in the artery to keep the artery open.

Bypass surgery. The surgeon creates a path around the blocked artery using either a healthy blood vessel from another part of the body or a synthetic one.

Thrombolytic therapy. If a blood clot is blocking an artery, a clot-dissolving drug may be given directly into the affected artery.

Lifestyle and home remedies

Making healthy lifestyle changes can help you manage peripheral artery disease symptoms and prevent them from getting worse. Try these tips:

Don't smoke. Smoking damages the arteries. It

increases the risk for peripheral artery disease (PAD). If you have PAD, smoking can make thecondition worse. If you need help quitting smoking, ask your care provider about strategies and medications that can help.

Eat a healthy diet. A heart-healthy diet low in saturated fat helps control blood pressure and cholesterol levels.

Avoid certain cold and sinus medications. Products that contain pseudoephedrine (Advil Cold and Sinus, Sudafed, others) tighten blood vessels and may increase PAD symptoms.

Exercise

Exercise is an important part of PAD treatment. Regular exercise helps the body use oxygen better and improves symptoms of PAD. Sometimes, the exercise that will help you get better may cause pain. But don't get discouraged. As you continue exercising, you'll be able to walk longer without pain. Your health care provider likely will prescribe supervised exercise therapy to increase the distance you can walk pain-free.

Careful foot care

In addition to lifestyle changes, take good care of your feet. People with PAD, especially those who also have diabetes, are at risk of poor healing of sores and injuries on the lower legs and feet.

Poor blood flow can delay or prevent proper healing. It also increases the risk of infection. Follow this advice to care for your feet:

- Wash your feet every day. Dry them completely. Use moisturizer to prevent cracks that can lead to infection. Don't moisturize between the toes, however, as this can help fungus grow.
- Wear well-fitting shoes and thick, dry socks.
- Promptly treat any fungal infections of the feet, such as athlete's foot.
- Take care when trimming your nails.
- Inspect your feet daily for injuries.
- Have a foot doctor (podiatrist) treat bunions, corns or calluses.
- See your care provider as soon as you notice a sore or injury to your skin.

Also, try sleeping with the head of the bed raised a few inches. Keeping the legs below the level of the heart usually reduces pain.

VALVULAR HEART DISEASE IN ELDERLY

Cardiac calcification

Cardiac calcification, a marker of increased CVD risk, is commonly detected in the elderly For example, a necropsy study of 490 patients aged ≥80 years found that 91% had calcified deposits involving the coronary arteries, aortic valve cusps, mitral valve annulus, and/or the left ventricular papillary muscles .

Mitral Annular Calcification

Mitral annular calcification (MAC), a degenerative condition of the mitral valve support ring, has been shown to be independently associated with 1.5- to two-fold increases in the risk of stroke and other CVD events, as well as CVD- and all-cause mortality .The prevalence of MAC increases with age. In the CHS, the overall prevalence of MAC was 42%, increasing from approximately 35% in 65-74 year olds to nearly 60% by age ≥85 years . Using different criteria for diagnosing MAC, the Framingham Heart Study reported an overall prevalence of 2.8% among 5694 adults. However, the prevalence of MAC increased with age in both genders, reaching 6.0% in men and 22.4% in women ≥80 years of age.

Aortic Valve Thickening and Calcification

Calcification of the aortic valve is a common finding in advanced age. In one study, calcification was present in 53% of adults over the age of 55 years, and the proportion increased with advancing age, from 28% at age 55-71 years to 75% in individuals aged 85-86 years .In addition, the prevalence of severe aortic valve calcification increased from 7% in 55-71 year-olds to 19% in persons aged 85-86 years.

Aortic valve sclerosis, defined as increased echogenicity and leaflet thickness without restriction of leaflet motion, is associated with an approximately 50% increase in the risk of CVD death and incident MI. Aortic valve sclerosis was present in 26% of CHS participants, increasing from 20% in 65-74 year-olds, to 35% in 75-84 year-olds, and to 48% in those aged ≥85 years .

Aortic Stenosis

In 2005, diseases of the heart valves accounted for 93,000 hospital discharges and nearly 21,000 deaths, of which approximately 13,000 were due to aortic valve disease .In CHS, the prevalence of aortic stenosis (AS), defined as an increased systolic velocity across the aortic valve (≥2.5 m/s by Doppler echocardiography), increased from 1.3% in participants aged 65-74 years, to 2.4% in those age 75-84, and to 4% among those ≥85 years . The Helsinki Ageing Study reported the prevalence of moderate or severe AS among 197 participants aged 75-76 years, 155 participants aged 80-81 years, and 124 participants aged 85-86 years .Moderate and severe AS were defined as calculated aortic valve areas ≤1.2 cm2 and ≤0.8 cm2, respectively. The overall prevalence rates of moderate and severe AS were 4.8% and 2.9%. The prevalence of at least moderate AS increased from 2.5% in subjects aged 75-76 years, to 3.9% in 80-81 year-olds, and to 8.1% by age 85-86. Prevalence rates for severe AS for these age categories were 0.5%, 2.6%, and 5.6%, respectively.

Valvular Regurgitation

In the Framingham Heart Study, the prevalence of valvular regurgitation involving the mitral, tricuspid, and aortic valves was determined in participants aged 26 to 83 years using Doppler echocardiography. In men, the prevalence of at least mild severity mitral regurgitation increased more than 4-fold from 8.9% in subjects aged 26-39 years to 39.3% in those aged 70-83 years. The prevalence of at least mild tricuspid regurgitation increased from 13.0% in participants aged 26-39 years to 27.3% in those aged 70-83 years. Similarly, the prevalence of aortic valve regurgitation increased from 0% in 26-39 year-olds to 14.4% in 70-83 year-olds. In women, the prevalence of at least mild mitral, tricuspid, and aortic valve regurgitation in those aged 26-39 years was 9.7%, 14.4%, and 0%, respectively. By ages 70-83 years, prevalence rates increased to 23.6%, 29.5%, and 16.9%, respectively. The age-related increase in prevalence of valvular heart disease has also been confirmed by a pooled analysis of echocardiographic data from 11,911 participants in three epidemiologic studies representing various age groups, including the Coronary Artery Risk Development in Young Adults (CARDIA) study, Atherosclerosis Risk in Communities (ARIC) study, and the Cardiovascular Health Study.In contrast to most other forms of valvular heart disease, the prevalence of mitral valve prolapse (MVP) has not been observed to vary significantly with Among 3491 Framingham Heart Study participants with a mean age of 54.7 years (range: 26 to 84 years), the overall prevalence of MVP was 2.4%. MVP prevalence rates were similar across age decades from 30 to 80 years.

ELECTROCARDIOGRAPHIC ABNORMALITIES AND ARRHYTHMIAS

Resting Electrocardiogram

Abnormalities on the resting electrocardiogram (ECG) are quite common in older adults. Evaluation of ECGs from 5,150 CHS participants revealed that theoverall prevalence of any ECG abnormality was 28.7%

Prevalence rates of specific ECG abnormalities were 8.7% for ventricular conduction defects, 5.3% for first-degree atrioventricular block, 3.2% for AF, 6.3% for isolated major ST-T wave abnormalities, 4.2% for left ventricular hypertrophy, and 5.2% for major Q/QS waves.

The prevalence of ECG abnormalities in men and women with known coronary artery disease (CAD) and hypertension (HTN) was 44.5% and 31.3%, respectively. In comparison, the prevalence of ECG abnormalities in men and women free of CAD and HTN was lower at 25.0% and 14.3%. In men free of CAD and HTN, the prevalence of ECG abnormalities increased from 16.0% in those aged 65-69 years, to 27.5% by age 75-79 years, and 45.9% by age ≥85 years. Likewise, in women free of CAD and HTN, the prevalence of ECG abnormalities increased from 10.5% at age 65-69 years, to 20.2% by age 75-79 years, and 31.6% by age ≥85 years.

Ambulatory Electrocardiogram

Twenty-four hour ambulatory electrocardiography was performed in 1,372 CHS participants and revealed that supraventricular ectopic beats and minor supraventricular arrhythmias were extremely common, occurring in approximately 97% of older adults . Similarly, ventricular ectopic activity was present in 82% of the CHS population. Frequent ectopic beats, defined as ≥15 beats per hour, were recorded in nearly half of men and women and were more commonly of supraventricular origin. Supraventricular arrhythmias were observed in 57.1% and 55.5% of men and women, respectively. There was an age-related increase in the prevalence of supraventricular arrhythmias, such that by age ≥80 years more than three-quarters of subjects manifested supraventricular arrhythmias.

Supraventricular tachycardia (SVT) of at least 3 beats was seen in 47.7% of men and 49.9% women. Ventricular arrhythmias were observed in 28.5% of men and 15.6% of women. Prevalence rates for ventricular tachycardia, defined as ≥3 consecutive complexes, were 13% and 4.3% in men and women, respectively. Conversely, serious arrhythmias, such as sustained ventricular tachycardia (≥15 complexes) and complete atrioventicular block, were rarely detected (≤0.5%) in CHS participants.

Atrial Fibrillation

Prevalence

In 2005, atrial fibrillation (AF) was estimated to affect 2.2 million Americans, but it is projected that by 2050 the number of individuals with AF will exceed 10 million, primarily due to population aging [3, 30]. In CHS, the overall prevalence rates of AF in men and women were 6.2% and 4.8%, respectively. The prevalence of AF varied by CVD status such that the prevalence in women with clinical CVD was 8.7%, compared to 4.5% in those with subclinical CVD, and 1.1% in women without evidence for CVD. The prevalence of AF in men was 9.4% in those with clinical CVD, 4.7% in those with subclinical CVD, and 2.7% in those without CVD. Regardless of CVD status, the overall prevalence of AF increased with age, from 5.9% in men and 2.8% in women aged 65-69 years, to 8.0% in men and 6.7% in women aged ≥80 years.

Incidence

The lifetime risk for AF in persons without HF or MI is approximately 15% at age 40 as well as at age 80 [32]. Overall incidence rates of AF in CHS men and women were 26.4 and 14.1 per 1,000 person-years, respectively [33]. There is an age-associated increase in the incidence of AF in both genders, such that the incidence increases from 12.3 per 1000 person-years in men aged 65-69 years to 58.7 per 1,000 person-years by age ≥80 years. Similarly, the incidence in women increases from 10.9 per 1,000 person-years in the 65-69 year age group to 25.1 per 1,000 person-years in women aged ≥80 years.

FRAILTY and SUCCESSFUL AGING

CVD is the second leading cause of disability among older adults (after arthritis), and it is an important cause of a decline in self-reported health. Certain features of aging are in part a reflection of not only clinical but also subclinical atherosclerotic burden. As with clinical CVD, the burden of subclinical CVD, evidenced by low ABI or high coronary artery calcium score, increases progressively with age in both men and women .

Data from the CHS also implicate CVD, both clinical and subclinical, as contributing to dementia and functional decline, manifested by loss of independence and the ability to perform routine activities of daily living. Further, there is a growing body of evidence linking CVD with frailty, a clinical syndrome associated with marked loss of physiologic reserve and an increased risk for disability, institutionalization, and death . In CHS, for example, compared to people 65 years of age or older with a normal ABI (i.e., ≥ 0.9), those with an ABI < 0.8 had a 3.5-fold increased risk of frailty . Viewed another way, the presence of subclinical CVD among participants in CHS was associated with a loss of approximately 6.5 years of "successful" life (i.e. with good health and function) in women and 5.6 years in men

MORTALITY

In the U.S., CVD accounts for more deaths than any other major cause, and CHD and stroke account for approximately two-thirds of CVD deaths . The remaining CVD deaths are due to HF (7%), high blood pressure (7%), diseases of the arteries (4%), and miscellaneous causes (14%) . As noted earlier, in 2005 approximately 80% of the 864,000 CVD deaths occurred in individuals aged ≥65 years and nearly 40% occurred in persons aged ≥85 years Furthermore, mortality rates from CHD, HF, and stroke are nearly 2-fold higher in the 75-84 year age group compared to the 65-74 year age group .

In 2004, 48% of all deaths in Americans aged ≥85 years were ascribed to CVD, compared to only 20% in those aged 35-44 years [40]. Among women, more than 200,000 of the 454,613 total CVD deaths occurred in the ≥85 year age group. In men, approximately 100,000 of the 409,867 total CVD deaths were in those ≥85 years . Thus, CVD exacts an exceptionally high toll in the very elderly, particularly among women.

HOSPITALIZATIONS

CVD accounted for 6.2 million hospital discharges in 2006, more than any other disease category [3]. Approximately 75% of admissions for HF occur in people 65 years of age or older, with more than half occurring in people age 75 or older. Persons over age 65 also account for more than 60% of admissions for acute MI and 75% of admissions for heart rhythm disorders. Likewise, in 2006, persons aged ≥65 years accounted for more than half of hospital discharges listing a major cardiac-related procedure as the principal procedure for the hospitalization. More specifically, persons aged ≥65 years accounted for 85% of pacemaker insertions, 61% of implantable defibrillators, 53% of coronary bypass operations, 51% of percutaneous coronary interventions, 60% of cardiac valve procedures, and 75% of endarterectomies

In light of the high prevalence rates and substantial morbidity associated with CVD among older adults, it is not surprising that the costs attributable to CVD in the elderly are extremely high. Most of the total expenditures for circulatory diseases, nearly three-quarters, are for persons aged ≥65 years .

Bibliography and Acknowledgement

- Agency for Healthcare Research and Quality, Healthcare Cost and Utilization Project HCUPnet. [Accessed March 15, 2009]. Available at: http://www.hcup.ahrq.gov/HCUPnet.jsp. Arnold AM, Psaty BM, Kuller LH, et al. Incidence of cardiovascular disease in older Americans: the cardiovascular health study. J Am Geriatr Soc. 2005 Feb;53(2):211–218. [PubMed] [Google Scholar]
- Barasch E, Gottdiener JS, Larsen EK, Chaves PH, Newman AB, Manolio TA. Clinical significance of calcification of the fibrous skeleton of the heart and aortosclerosis in community dwelling elderly. The Cardiovascular Health Study (CHS) Am Heart J. 2006 Jan;151(1):39–47. [PubMed] [Google Scholar
- Benjamin EJ, Plehn JF, D'Agostino RB, et al. Mitral annular calcification and the risk of stroke in an elderly cohort. N Engl J Med. 1992;327:374–379. [PubMed] [Google Scholar]
- Breek JC, Hamming JF, De Vries J, Aquarius AE, van Berge Henegouwen DP. Quality of life in patients with intermittent claudication using the World Health Organisation (WHO) questionnaire. Eur J Vasc Endovasc Surg. 2001 Feb;21(2):118–122. [PubMed] [Google Scholar]
- Bryan RN, Wells SW, Miller TJ, et al. Infarctlike lesions in the brain: prevalence and anatomic characteristics at MR imaging of the elderly-- data from the Cardiovascular Health Study. Radiology. 1997 Jan;202(1):47–54. [PubMed] [Google Scholar]

- Barasch E, Gottdiener JS, Larsen EK, Chaves PH, Newman AB, Manolio TA. Clinical significance of calcification of the fibrous skeleton of the heart and aortosclerosis in community dwelling elderly. The Cardiovascular Health Study (CHS) Am Heart J. 2006 Jan;151(1):39–47. [PubMed] [Google Scholar]
- Benjamin EJ, Plehn JF, D'Agostino RB, et al. Mitral annular calcification and the risk of stroke in an elderly cohort. N Engl J Med. 1992;327:374–379. [PubMed] [Google Scholar]

- Fox CS, Vasan RS, Parise H, et al. Mitral annular calcification predicts cardiovascular morbidity and mortality. Circulation. 2003;107:1492–1496.
- Freed LA, Levy D, Levine RA, et al. Prevalence and clinical outcome of mitral-valve prolapse. N Engl J Med. 1999 Jul 1;341(1):1–7. [PubMed] [Google Scholar]
- Hodgson TA, Cohen AJ. Medical care expenditures for selected circulatory diseases: opportunities for reducing national health expenditures. Med Care. 1999 Oct;37(10):994–1012. [PubMed] [Google Scholar]
- Izquierdo-Porrera AM, Gardner AW, Bradham DD, et al. Relationship between objective measures of peripheral arterial disease severity to self-reported quality of life in older adults with intermittent claudication. J Vasc Surg. 2005 Apr;41(4):625–630. [PubMed] [Google Scholar]
- Kuller L, Borhani N, Furberg C, et al. Prevalence of subclinical atherosclerosis and cardiovascular disease and association with risk factors in the Cardiovascular Health Study. Am J Epidemiol. 1994 Jun 15;139(12):1164–1179.
- Lindroos M, Kupari M, Heikkila J, Tilvis R. Prevalence of aortic valve abnormalities in the elderly: an echocardiographic study of a random population sample. J Am Coll Cardiol. 1993 Apr;21(5):1220–1225. [PubMed]
- Lloyd-Jones DM, Larson MG, Beiser A, et al. Lifetime risk of developing coronary heart disease. Lancet. 1999;353:89–92. [PubMed] [Google Scholar
- Manolio TA, Furberg CD, Rautaharju PM, et al. Cardiac arrhythmias on 24-h ambulatory electrocardiography in older women and men: the Cardiovascular Health Study. J Am Coll Cardiol. 1994 Mar 15;23(4):916–925. [PubMed] [Google
- National Center for Health Statistics. Centers for Disease Control and Prevention . Compressed Mortality File: Underlying Cause of Death. Centers for Disease Control and Prevention; Atlanta, GA: Available at: https://wonder.cdc.gov/mortSQL.html. [Google Scholar]
- Newman AB, Arnold AM, Naydeck BL, et al. "Successful aging": effect of subclinical cardiovascular disease. Arch Intern Med. 2003 Oct 27;163(19):2315–2322. [PubMed]
- Otto CM, Lind BK, Kitzman DW, et al. Association of aortic-valve sclerosis with cardiovascular mortality and morbidity in the elderly. N Engl J Med. 1999;341:142–147. [PubMed] [Google Scholar]
- Psaty BM, Manolio TA, Kuller LH, et al. Incidence of and risk factors for atrial fibrillation in older adults. Circulation. 1997 Oct 7;96(7):2455–2461. [PubMed] [Google Scholar]
- Rich MW, Bosner MS, Chung MK, Shen J, McKenzie JP. Is age an independent predictor of early and late mortality in patients with acute myocardial infarction? Am J Med. 1992 Jan;92(1):7–
- Roberts WC. The senile cardiac calcification syndrome. Am J Cardiol. 1986 Sep 1;58(6):572–574. [PubMed] [Google Scholar]
- Savage DD, Garrison RJ, Castelli WP, et al. Prevalence of submitral (anular) calcium and its correlates in a general population-based sample (the Framingham Study) Am J Cardiol. 1983 May 1;51(8):1375–1378. [PubMed] [Google Scholar]
- Singh JP, Evans JC, Levy D, et al. Prevalence and clinical determinants of mitral, tricuspid, and aortic regurgitation (the Framingham Heart Study) Am J Cardiol. 1999 Mar 15;83(6):897–902. [PubMed] [Google Scholar]
- Steinwachs DM, Collins-Nakai RL, Cohn LH, Garson A, Jr., Wolk MJ. The future of cardiology: utilization and costs of care. J Am Coll Cardiol. 2000 Apr;35(5 Suppl B):91B–98B. [PubMed] [Google Scholar]
- Stewart BF, Siscovick D, Lind BK, et al. Clinical factors associated with calcific aortic valve disease. Cardiovascular Health Study. J Am Coll Cardiol. 1997 Mar 1;29(3):630–634. [PubMed] [Google Scholar]

- Stewart BF, Siscovick D, Lind BK, et al. Clinical factors associated with calcific aortic valve disease. Cardiovascular Health Study. J Am Coll Cardiol. 1997 Mar 1;29(3):630–634. [PubMed] [Google Scholar]

- U.S. Census Bureau . U.S. Population Projections: 2010 to 2050. U.S. Department of Commerce; Washington, D.C.: [Accessed April 15, 2009]. 2008. Available at: www.census.gov/population/www/projections/summarytables.html. [Google Scholar]
- Yue NC, Arnold AM, Longstreth WT, Jr., et al. Sulcal, ventricular, and white matter changes at MR imaging in the aging brain: data from the cardiovascular health study. Radiology. 1997 Jan;202(1):33–39. [PubMed] [Google Scholar]

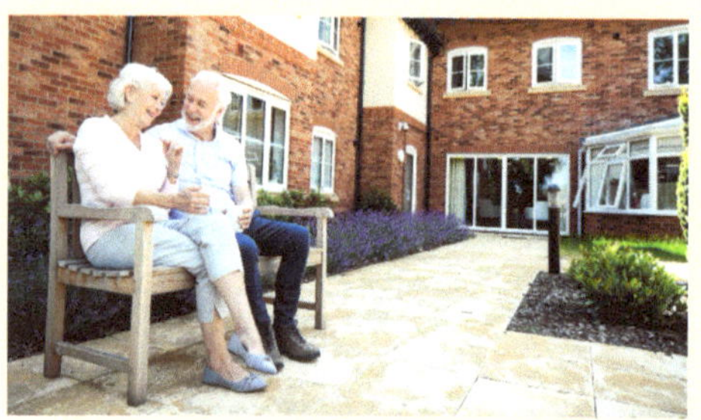

Regulation of Long-Term Care Homes for Older Adults in India

Demographic transition because of increased life expectancy has led to the rise of aging population resulting in huge demand for care. At the same time, there has been a decline in traditional familial, social support because of a reduction in fertility rates, small nuclear families, increased urbanization, a decline in traditional social networks, and migration of children to other cities and countries.This has contributed to the burgeoning of residential care homes for older adults, globally and in India.

In 1980, there was a national average of 54 beds per 1,000 elderly in the USA, while older people aged 65 and over were 25.5 million.Around 13% of people above the age of 85 years needed residential care in 2010. A Dutch economic survey between 2007 and 2009 found residential care to be expensive than home-based care. Resource limitations deter governments from operating elderly care facilities to meet the increasing demand, leaving the management of elderly care facilities to charities, nongovernmental organizations (NGOs), or the for-profit private sector.

The need to regulate the management of elderly care homes was recognized in Western countries. In 1984, the Department of Health and Social Security in England introduced the Registered Homes Act, Registered Care Home Regulations, Registered Homes Tribunal Rules, and a Code of Practice for residential care home life..With the majority of homes in the UK being run by the private sector, the government had to step in and develop legislations, monitor through regulations, and ascertain the care needs and outcome of long-term care in these homes. Unstructured, unaccounted growth of the number of residential care homes for older adults in India necessitates that similar regulations and regulatory framework would be required in India,5 and this article aims to study the relevant regulations and legislation of older adults' long-term residential care homes and explores the lacunae in the Indian system to make appropriate recommendations.

History of Residential Homes for Older Adults in India

The first documented residential care facility for older adults in modern India dates back to 1814. It was founded in erstwhile Madras (current Chennai) where a friend-in-need society comprising British merchants and bankers started to house Anglo-Indians and domiciled Europeans in difficulties. This was followed nearly 70 years later in 1882 when home for the aged was established in Kolkata by "Little Sisters of the Poor" as a focussed initiative from a Maltese man Asphar. These two homes for the aged and needy provided shelter, clothing, and medical care.

The initial focus was on providing basic needs such as shelter and clothing for those capable of taking care of their personal or nursing needs but could not live independently. Several religious organizations also opened ashrams for the elderly, which provided basic care in a spiritual environment. It is only later that nursing care, nutrition, physical and mental health care were incorporated into the care facilities for the elderly. Currently, residential care homes for the elderly are a non-formal sector in India, and the exact official numbers are not available. Nevertheless, in 2009, HelpAge India estimated 1,176 senior living facilities, with Kerala having the highest (182), followed by West Bengal (164), and Tamil Nadu (151). Tata Trusts and the United Nations Population Fund and NGO Samarth, surveyed on a sample size of 480 old age homes and 60+ senior living developments in 84 cities in 2018, concluded that these numbers were low when the actual demand is high.

Defining Residential Care Homes

Residential care homes involve caring for elderly persons who cannot manage themselves partially or wholly, supported by unregistered or unqualified support staff who have gained some experience. Care needs mainly involve personal, supportive care, as prompted or requested by the residents themselves. The term Nursing home is generally used when there is a nursing care need for the person with a medical ailment, usually provided by registered nurses. Some care homes are specialized in offering long-term rehabilitation care with the help of a multidisciplinary team involving specialists in medicine, psychiatry, neurology, speech therapists, dietician, physiotherapists, nurses, social workers, pharmacists, etc. for older adults with complex physical, cognitive, or behavioral problems. These are a step down from hospitals providing acute care. The need for such facilities is also increasing because of the high costs of hospitalization. Retirement homes are homes built by private builders in India as a community living where the neighborhood comprises older adults who buy or rent the property. Some of the risks of independent living are managed or aided by the retirement home society. These homes allow the elderly to live autonomously with privacy, exactly similar to living in their own house.

Home-Based Care Versus Residential Home Care for Elderly

A systematic review of studies from high-income settings concluded that there is insufficient quality published research to effectively compare institutional care with community-based care for functionally dependent older people. Institutional care may be associated with reduced risk of hospitalization, better activities of daily living, while community-based care may be associated with improved quality of life and physical function. The impact of both the care models on mortality, healthcare utilization, economic correlations, and caregiver burden needs further research.A meta-synthesis of ten studies from USA, Europe, and Asia found that culture impacts the decision making for a residential care facility, adjustment process, and eventual adaptation thereIn the South Asian cultural context, home is the preferred residential setting. The residential option is considered when there is no family member (or male offspring) or when the complex physical and mental health needs overwhelm the caregivers (respite care or long-term care) or when neglect or abuse by familial caregivers exists. Hence, the conditions of elderly and their outcomes in-home care versus residential care home are not comparable in India.A literature review from India reported that the experiences and perspectives of older adults living in residential facilities are heterogeneous. Several older adults residing in residential facilities view them favorably, citing security, medical attention, and a sense of independence. Still, most prefer their own homes and families despite having experienced neglect or abuse by them.The common stressors associated with living in residential facilities include difficulty in adjusting to the new environment and rigid time schedules, declining functional ability, separation from their family and community, social alienation, sense of powerlessness, and repeated witnessing of death and illness in such settings.

Health Concerns in Residential Care Homes for Older Adults and Their Implications

Older age is associated with multiple physical and psychiatric comorbidities. Assessment and management of comorbidities are major challenges for residential care providers. The needs of the residents are complex and multisectoral, and one has to look at addressing various issues than one particular specific health need.There is a lack of data on rates of comorbidities in Indian residential care facilities for older adults, but the trends are likely to be similar to residential care facilities in other countries.

To understand the care needs, the UK national census of care home residents survey (n = 16043 residents in 244 care homes) showed that medical morbidity with an associated disability was the cause for admission in over 90% of cases. Over 50% of residents had dementia, stroke, or another neurodegenerative disease. Around 76% of residents required assistance with their mobility, 71% were incontinent. Twenty seven percent had multiple issues of immobility, confusion, or incontinence. Only 40% of those in residential care were ambulant without assistance. It was concluded that care needs in long-term residential care homes were determined by progressive and chronic illnesses.Similarly, up to two-thirds of residents in care homes in USA have cognitive impairment, with many diagnosed with dementia.The care need issues imply residential care facilities for older adults need-specific adaptations for toilet facilities to ensure hygiene, nutrition planning taking into account specific nutritional needs of the elderly as well as individual comorbidities requiring customized diets, physiotherapy and exercise to maintain range of motion, balance, endurance, strength, and flexibility environmental adaptations for easy mobility and prevent falls, specific measures to prevent pressure ulcers in nonambulatory residents,periodic medical consultation as well as immunization. In addition, the elderly in old age homes have high rates of psychiatric morbidity. Indian studies have reported high rates of depression, anxiety, and psychotic disorder in residents of old age homes In addition to dementia.Apart from pharmacotherapy, addressing the mental health care needs of the elderly residents may range from providing cognitive stimulation, pro-social environments, ensuring sleep hygiene to managing agitation and frank aggression. Effective nonpharmacological management can reduce the need of dosage of pharmacotherapy. This requires specialized training. There are only a few centers like the National Institute of Social Defence under the Ministry of Social Justice and Empowerment, which runs courses in geriatric care. However, the number of human resources trained in this and similar settings is minuscule as compared to the requirements of residential care facilities. In addition, the requirement of trained manpower in multiple domains can escalate the cost of services. At the same time, there is no framework for periodic evaluation, inspections, certification, and recertification of such service providers.

Complaints and Litigations

Elderly care facilities in India do not have any formal mechanisms for feedback, appraisal, complaints, or grievance redressal. When the care becomes business, or there is no regulatory framework, there is always a scope for disagreements and complaints against the care-providers by the consumers, with scope for formal lawsuits. Some of the outcomes of such litigation may be beneficial for the residents. For example, malpractice litigation threats have led to an increase in registered nurse to staffing ratios. These may reduce issues like pressure sores among residents and improve quality.33 High-risk malpractice lawsuits have also led to the change of managers of nursing homes.

Since there is no regulatory body or licensing authority, it becomes difficult for the residents and their families, as they are unsure of where to complain if there are disagreements over the care and the responses from care home management. Even for the care providers, it becomes difficult to prove their quality of care when there are no benchmark standards. In the absence of defined regulatory frameworks, complaints against residential care facilities or individual care providers in such facilities have been made to elder's helpline or Human Rights Commission or the Local Health Authority.Choking, wandering and related risk, falls and related injuries, physical or chemical restraints, malnutrition, pressure sores, medication errors are a common source of litigation against the nursing homes.A study of claims against 1465 nursing homes in USA demonstrated that best-performing nursing homes providing quality care were sued less than low-performing ones.Repeated ongoing complaints or litigations may lead to the closure of poorly performing ones. Thus, there is an incentive to improve business by improving the quality of care and having good working relationships with the residents.

Need for Regulation

Aging-related issues coupled with living in an institutional environment may impact individuals' autonomy, especially if they have never experienced living in institutionalized spaces earlier. This issue was debated, and consensus that it can be a "relational autonomy" related to the care home policies. The boundaries of assertive care versus boundary violation to depriving someone of their rights can lead to conflict and stress amongst residents and the staff in the absence of policies.

There is also a concern about complex biopsychosocial needs of the elderly not being met in some of the residential care facilities through oversight, neglect, or deliberate measures. Various stakeholders to address the needs are the care providers, family members and friends of residents, advocacy groups, and State Health Authorities and Departments of Social Justice. Independent regulators have been proposed to regulate older adults' residential care facilities. Furthermore, regulation requires laws, rules, and minimum standards for such facilities. Unfortunately, such a framework does not exist in India as yet.

In contrast, the Department of Health in the UK established National Care Standards Commission in UK 2002, which has powers to regulate and inspect under the Care Home Regulations (2001) and National Minimum Standards (2001). Standard setting, self-regulation as well government regulation are important.40 Similar provisions are found in other high-income countries.

Case studies from high-income settings have also highlighted the challenges of over-regulation. The Ontario Nursing Homes Study concluded though the regulations and accountability scrutinizing objective was predominantly to improve quality of care, it, unfortunately, ended up increasing workload and paperwork. This meant reduced time to provide direct physical care and missing out on scrutinizing top management such as funding and staffing levels.41 This indicates that any form of licensing or regulations will come with minimum norms to provide care that can only be scrutinized by examining the documentation in the resident records. Audits are likely to pick up deficiencies and therefore will further increase the workload.

More human resources could be directed towards record keeping, and these issues of regulations not serving the real purpose need to be considered while preparing regulatory policies. Another study report from Quebec province, after regulation, found that some smaller care homes were closed; however, the quality of care provided by the private care homes saw improvement.

A survey on the status of old age homes in India was conducted by Tata Trusts and assessed 480+ old age homes and 60+ senior living developments in 84 cities, towns, and districts. The report concluded a wide gap between expectations and delivery of services at most elder care facilities, with no mechanism for evaluating the quality and appropriateness of the services leaving the elderly inmates vulnerable and providing no incentive for improvement of services to the facility owners and managers.

Quality of Care

Quality of care involves adequate and proper staffing, regular assessments, minimum standards, care planning and provision, appropriate management of behavior and psychological symptoms of dementia (BPSD), physical environment characteristics, innovations, and quality of care provided to residents. A review of adverse events in skilled nursing care facilities in the USA who were medicare beneficiaries by the Office of Inspector General found 22% of the residents had adverse incidents. Half of them were preventable. This was not different from previous studies showing poor safety culture and indicated a need for regular inspection.

In England, residential care for adults including for older adults is provided by public, not-for-profit, and for-profit organisations. A study of 15,000 homes showed that quality of care was significantly lower in the private for-profit organization that managed 74% of the total homes, with the highest quality in the not-for-profit charity organizations that managed 18%. Public sector managed only 8% of homes. The study concluded that regulation would help improve the quality of care.

There is attention being paid now for improving the residential care facilities for the elderly and those with dementia. The focus has been to ensure a safe environment, designs that will assist way-finding, orientation, navigation, and access to nature and the outdoors although there is an ongoing need to sensitize policy makers and construction firms on age-friendly design practices.

The only comparable initiative is by the Kerala Government Department of Social Justice, which has prepared a manual for old age homes. . It describes in detail the procedure for designing and maintenance of old age home, admission procedures, mechanisms for the protection of residents, provision of basic services (food, health care), safety and security, caregivers, rules, procedures, documentation, and rights framework of inmates and family members. No other Indian state has developed any such framework as yet.

Relevant Legislative Framework in India

The National Programme for the Health Care for the Elderly (NPHCE), National Policy on Older Persons (NPOP) in 1999, and Section 20 of the Maintenance and Welfare of Parents and Senior Citizens Act, 2007, all deal with provisions for health and social care of older adults. NPHCE aims to provide accessible, affordable, and high-quality long-term comprehensive care services to the aging population and build a framework to create an environment for older adults to function well. However, both NPHCE and NPOP have not discussed the need for residential care facilities for older people and their regulations. According to the provisions of the Maintenance and Welfare of Parents and Senior Citizens Act of 2007, the responsbility of health and social welfare lies with the legal heirs. The regional state government, where the responsibility of health lies as per the Indian Federal Structure, manages some of its citizens' health and social needs, including senior citizens. The states may provide staff salaries or funding for training caregivers. Also, there are provisions in some of the regional governments to offer financial assistance to NGOs to run old age homes to take care of the elderly persons providing all the basic amenities and care protection to life. A systematic review indicated 48% of long-term care residents had dementia, within which 78% had BPSD and 10% had major depression.49 Depression was found in one third and dementia in two thirds in care home survey in England.50 In a study of the prevalence of health conditions of elderly in residential homes, 93% had a mental or behavioral disorder, including dementia 58% and depression 54%.51 In a study of old age homes in Lucknow, it was found that depression was present in 37.7%, anxiety in 13.3%, and dementia in 11.1%.29 Dementia, with its complications that includes BPSD, depression, anxiety, is common in care homes that need access to mental health care. Therefore, such residential care facilities fall within the purview of the Mental Healthcare Act (MHCA) 2017.

According to Section 66 of MHCA 2017, any residential care home caring for person/s with mental illness comes under the definition of Mental Health Establishment (MHE). So, it must be registered with the State Mental Health Authority (SMHA). The SMHA needs to make regulations for the operation of MHE, including the minimum standards of facilities and services, the minimum qualifications for the staff personnel, and maintenance of a registry. There is no data in the public domain whether any residential facility for older adults with or without psychiatric morbidity has been registered under SMHA in any state. Admissions to care homes when they have locked facility when the older adult is not willing or not having competence to decide will have to be under the MHCA 2017 .National Accreditation Board for Hospitals and Healthcare Providers (NABH) Accreditation, a constituent of the Board of Quality Council of India, manages quality control and certifies hospitals in India. There is nothing specific for the long stay care homes, specific for the elderly in NABH. The Union Ministry of Housing and Urban Affairs in 2019 developed guidelines for developing regulations for retirement homes but there is no information in the public domain regarding the compliance of these guidelines by retirement homes.

The prevalence of elder abuse is high in India and was found to be around 50%, which during the covid lockdown period went up as high as 71%, and the general factors found were increase in age and lack of formal education. The elderly population is vulnerable, particularly when dependent and staying in institutional settings. WHO data on institutional elder abuse suggests that 64% of staff members perpetrated it in institutional settings. These acts include physically restraining inappropriately, depriving them of dignity, such as not changing soiled clothes or washing them, withholding or overmedicating them, and inadequate care to cause pressure sores.The vulnerability of dependent elderly residents can increase the risk of abuse and neglect because of their physical and cognitive functioning limitations in addition to their fear and anxiety. Examples include aggressiveness, yelling in anger, making threats, punching, slapping, kicking, hitting, speaking in a harsh tone or words, or humiliating. Neglect involves not providing food, water, assisting with toilet needs, or medicines. A report from Atlanta ombudsmen long-term residents program in 2000 found 44% of residents reported experiencing abuse.The challenges faced by the staff of the care homes must be addressed by regulation, by ensuring the training needs are met. The majority of the staff members and almost half of them reported violent incidents towards them from residents or their families. They expressed that poor working conditions compelled them to offer inadequate quality of care for the residents. Many thought such incidents of violence happened during their duty as careworkers. Staff training should include techniques and strategies to prevent and manage any form of violence from residents and their families.

When it was found out that the proportion of vulnerable patients or residents could not come under the purview of the Mental Capacity Act of 2005 of England and Wales, which could have impacted their human rights, another legislation called Deprivation of Liberty Safeguards was introduced. This was to ensure the vulnerable elderly persons were not deprived of their liberty to safeguard rights under Article 5 of Human Rights Act and that most of the elderly care homes are locked facilities. No such provision exists in India.

Regulations can be state-mandated by an independent public body, or there could be forces of market competition or self-regulation with accreditation by service providers associations.61 A Swedish study of the economics of care homes between 1990 and 2009 showed privatization with the associated increase in market competition significantly improved quality as measured by mortality rates.

The Karnataka Private Medical Establishment Act rules of the state of Karnataka from 2009 (amended 2018) includes details of the process of registration of private medical establishments, renewal, different types of hospitals, minimum standards for accommodation, equipment, facilities, staffing requirements and their qualification, and maintenance of records. The space requirement for the inpatients or examination room has also been mentioned.However, the act does not include old age homes/elderly care facilities.

The study by Tata Trusts published in 2018 explored the need for minimum compulsory standards for infrastructure and management to ensure attention given to physical needs, safety and security, dignity and respect for elderly persons. Lack of regulation was evident, and they recommended compulsory registration, annual filings, and periodic inspections. They highlighted few broader themes in terms of home healthcare, personal supportive care, social activities, complaints and safeguards, environment, staffing, and management. In addition, they also highlighted the need for a third-party regulator and ombudsmen for safeguards, certification for staff, and establishing model care homesSystem in Place for

Prevention of Elder Abuse

In December 2019, Indian Central Government proposed a bill to amend the Maintenance and Welfare of Parents and Senior Citizen Act, 2007, which proposes registration of senior citizens care homes/home care service agencies along with maintenance of minimum standards for senior citizen care homes. However, implementing the regulatory framework will be with nodal police officers for senior citizens in every police station and district-level special police unit. This framework is not satisfactory. The authors propose that regulations for residential care facilities for older adults must define minimum standards for living, nutritional care, medical care, palliative, and end-of-life care. There should be ongoing staff training in elderly care, ethics and human rights, and documentation of medical management, including any adverse drug events/complications with an evaluation of care to help improve services.

There should be a system to report incidents. All staff members must be trained in filling the incident reporting form, which is to be regularly reviewed by the named senior clinician Prevention strategies include public and professional awareness, training, screening before employing the staff of residential care home, and caregiver training on dementia. Mandatory reporting of abuse to a central independent agency is to be considered. Perpetrators need to be identified, and in the first instance, appropriate education, training program, and work should be supervized until confidence is built. If the abuse is severe, this may need to be informed to social services or senior citizen helpline for appropriate action by the judiciary. The homes may not record or report abuse may try to underplay the issue, for wary of receiving tag of a poor quality care home, despite the obligation to report. The managers of the care home must ensure there are enough safeguards. There could be regular monitoring of common areas with closed-circuit television recording, regular review of the residents, and feedback.Long-term social care is also the responsibility of the state. Since the government alone cannot meet the huge demand in this area, policies to expand health insurance schemes to include long-term care in a residential care home can be considered.

Conclusion

There is a need for health and social care reforms to manage the rapid aging process, which may help expand services through home care or

reforms to manage the rapid aging process, which may help expand services through home care or residential care.66 With demand rising, India is likely to see more residential care homes in the future. Although MHCA 2017 has provided some legislative framework when the care home has any one or more residents with a mental disorder, it is not enough to regulate and safeguard the residents. The government authorities could take the lead and bring in geriatric experts, NGOs, private care providers, and the main stakeholders, the elderly community, and their children on board to ensure consultations and discussions take place periodically. Appropriate quality control measures in terms of registry, licensing, periodic inspections, and developing minimum standards for all kinds of old age homes should be instituted. At the same time, under-or over-regulation should be avoided. Until the regulations are formulated, the residential care homes must follow general work ethics, safeguard the human rights of residents, provide compassionate care, self-regulate by regular review of their care and impact, and handle complaints and feedback and work on the shortcomings. There must be an appropriate care needs assessment endorsed by specialists and attempts to provide home-based care before admission to residential homes. The government should take the lead by setting up model residential care homes to train the staff in as many regions as possible and then serve as a mentor to the private or NGO bodies.

Abstract

The rising aging population in India has led to an increased caregiving burden, and accordingly, the number of residential care facilities is also burgeoning. There is no regulatory framework or registration authority specifically for residential care homes in India. The article's objective is to understand the need for a regulatory framework in India in the context of historic and global experiences in the UK, USA, and Europe. Although there is a lack of literature comparing the community home-based care and residential care, one study reported a preference for home-based care in the South Asian context. Elder abuse and deprivation of rights of seniors are common, and there is a need to bring in more safeguards to prevent these from the perspective of the older adults, their family members, the care providers, and the state. While the main priority of meeting care needs in long-term care is a challenge given the lack of trained care staff, the quality control mechanisms also need to evolve. A review of adverse incidents, complaints, and litigations also highlights the need for regulation to improve the standards and quality of care.

Bibliography and Acknowledgement

- Akbar S, Tiwari SC, Tripathi RK, et al. Reasons for living of elderly to in old age homes: An exploratory study. Int J Indian Psychol, 2014; 2(1). [Google Scholar]
- Atlanta Long-Term Care Ombudsman Program The silenced voice speaks out: A study of abuse and neglect of nursing home residents. Atlanta Legal Aid Society; National Citizens Coalition for Nursing Home Reform, 2000. [Google Scholar]
- Banerjee A and Armstrong P. Centring care: Explaining regulatory tensions in residential care for older persons. Stud Pol Economy, 2015; 95(1): 7–28. [Google Scholar]
- Chetty L, Ramklass S, and McKune A. The effects of a structured group exercise programme on functional fitness of older persons living in old-age homes. Ageing Soc, 2019; 39(9): 1857–1872. [Google Scholar]
- Dening T and Milne A. Depression and mental health in care homes for older people. Qual Ageing Older Adults, 2009; 10(1): 40–46. [Google Scholar]
- Fisher LH, Edwards DJ, Pärn EA, et al. Building design for people with dementia: A case study of a UK care home. Facilities, 2018; 36(7/8): 349–368. [Google Scholar]
- Gaugler JE, Yu F, Davila HW, et al. Alzheimer's disease and nursing homes. Health Aff, 2014; 33(4): 650–657. [PMC free article] [PubMed] [Google Scholar]
- Hearle D, Rees V, and Prince J. Balance of occupation in older adults: Experiences in a residential care home. Qual Ageing Older Adults, 2012; 13(2): 125–134. [Google Scholar]
- Henwood M. Through a glass darkly: Community care and elderly people. Research report 14. London: King's Fund Institute; 1992. [Google Scholar]
- Institute of Medicine (US) Toward a national strategy for long-term care of the elderly: A study plan for evaluation of new policy options for the future. National Academies Press (US), 1986. [PubMed] [Google Scholar]
- John R, Kerby DS, and Hennessy CH. Patterns and impact of comorbidity and multimorbidity among community-resident American Indian elders. Gerontol, 2003; 43(5): 649–660. [PubMed] [Google Scholar]
- Kerrison SH and Pollock AM. Regulating nursing homes: Caring for older people in the private sector in England. BMJ, 2001; 323(7312): 566–569. [PMC free article]
- Konetzka RT, Park J, Ellis R, et al. Malpractice litigation and nursing home quality of care. Health Serv Res, 2013. December; 48(6): 1920–1938. [PMC free article] [PubMed] [Google Scholar]
- Kumar R, Satapathy S, Adhish VS, Nripsuta S. Study of psychiatric morbidity among residents of government old age homes in Delhi. J Geriatr Ment Health [serial online], 2017;4:36–41. https://www.tatatrusts.org/upload/pdf/report-on-old-age-facilities-in-india.pdf (accessed March21, 2021)
- Kumar R, Satapathy S, Adhish VS, Nripsuta S. Study of psychiatric morbidity among residents of government old age homes in Delhi. J Geriatr Ment Health [serial online], 2017. [cited 2021. June 18]; 4:36–41. [Google Scholar]
- Kumar S. Economic security for the elderly in India. J Aging Soc Policy, 2003; 15 45–65. [PubMed] [Google Scholar]
- Kumar Y. Understanding the frontiers of human longevity in India: Imperative and palliative care. Indian J Palliat Care, 2019; 25(3): 455–461. [PMC free article] [PubMed] [Google Scholar]
- Loi SM, Westphal A, Ames D, et al. Minimising psychotropic use for behavioural disturbance in residential aged care. Aust Fam Physician, 2015. April; 44(4): 180–184. [PubMed] [Google Scholar]
- Mah JC, Stevens SJ, Keefe JM, et al. Social factors influencing utilization of home care in community-dwelling older adults: A scoping review. BMC Geriatr, 2021; 21: 145. [PMC free article] [PubMed] [Google Scholar]
- Menezes S and Thomas TM. Status of the elderly and emergence of old age homes in India. Int J Soc Sci Manag, 2018; 5(1): 1–4. [Google Scholar]
- Ministry of Health and Family Welfare National Program for Health Care of the Elderly (NPHCE): Operational Guidelines, 2011. Director General of Health Services, MOHFW, Government of India, 2011. [Google Scholar]

- Mah JC, Stevens SJ, Keefe JM, et al. Social factors influencing utilization of home care in community-dwelling older adults: A scoping review. BMC Geriatr, 2021; 21: 145. [PMC free article] [PubMed] [Google Scholar]
- Menezes S and Thomas TM. Status of the elderly and emergence of old age homes in India. Int J Soc Sci Manag, 2018; 5(1): 1–4. [Google Scholar]

- Nayar PKB. Manual on old age. Department of Social Justice, 2016. 12150.pdf (kerala.gov.in) (accessed April29, 2021)
  Paddock K, Wilson CB, Walshe C, et al. Care home life and identity: A qualitative case study. Gerontologist, 2019: 59(4); 655–664. [PMC free article] [PubMed] [Google Scholar]
- Reed J, Klein B, Cook G, et al. Quality improvement in German and UK care homes. Int J Health Care Qual Assur, 2003; 16(5): 248–256. [Google Scholar]
- Ramalingam A, Sarkar S, Premarajan KC, et al. Prevalence and correlates of elder abuse: A cross-sectional, community-based study from rural Puducherry. Natl Med J India, 2019; 32(2): 72–76. [PubMed] [Google Scholar]
- Ribbe MW, Ljunggren G, Steel K, et al. Nursing homes in 10 nations: A comparison between countries and settings. Age Ageing, 1997; 26(2): 3–12. [PubMed] [Google Scholar]
- Ross RB. Regulation of residential homes for the elderly in England and wales. J Soc Welf Law, 1985; 7(2): 85–95. [Google Scholar]
- Singh AP, Kumar KL, and Reddy CMPK. Psychiatric morbidity in geriatric population in old age homes and community: A comparative study. Indian J Psychol Med, 2012; 34(1): 39–43. [PMC free article] [PubMed] [Google Scholar]
- Sonawat R. Understanding families in India: A reflection of societal changes. Psicol: Teoria e Pesquisa, 2001; 17(2): 177–186.
- Tiwari SC, Pandey NM, and Singh I. Mental health problems among inhabitants of old age homes: A preliminary study. Indian J Psychiatry, 2012. April; 54(2): 144–148. [PMC free article] [PubMed] [Google Scholar]
- Unroe KT, Ouslander JG, and Saliba D. Nursing home regulations redefined: Implications for providers. J Am Geriatr Soc, 2018; 66(1): 191–194. [PubMed] [Google Scholar]
- World Health Assembly, 69 The global strategy and action plan on ageing and health 2016–2020: Towards a world in which everyone can live a long and healthy life. World Health Organization; 2016. https://apps.who.int/iris/handle/10665/252783 [Google Scholar]
- Young C, Hall AM, Gonçalves-Bradley DC, et al. Home or foster home care versus institutional long-term care for functionally dependent older people. Cochrane Database Syst Rev, 2017. April 3; 4(4): CD009844. [PMC free article] [PubMed] [Google Scholar]

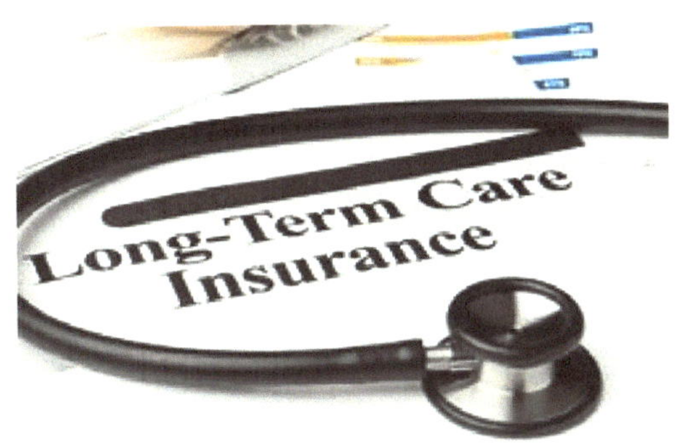

Long-Term Care Insurance for the Elderly

It feels good to imagine living all of your senior years without any worry. That's why the topic of long-term care insurance for the elderly is worth learning more about. After all, some people eventually need help with basic activities of daily living—things like eating, bathing, getting dressed, using the bathroom, taking care of personal hygiene, or moving from place to place. You may never need that sort of help, but wouldn't it be nice to know that you could access care if it ever became necessary?

For those who need it, long-term care (LTC) is a saving grace. Of course, the longer you live, the greater your chances of eventually needing LTC—as well as a reliable way to pay for it. (If you're wealthy, paying for care is probably not an issue. If you're financially disadvantaged, you can use Medicaid for certain types of care. But if your financial situation falls somewhere between those two extremes, your options may be a little less clear.)

That's where long-term care insurance (LTCI) comes in. Under the right circumstances, it can provide peace of mind and the ability to pay for extended help if you ever need it. But this care-funding option isn't right for everybody.

What Is LTC Insurance?

Long-term care (LTC) insurance is a type of financial product that can help you cover the costs of home care services or an extended stay in a nursing home, assisted living residence, memory care facility, or hospice. It provides a way to ensure that you and your family will be able to afford your care in the event that you eventually need assistance with two or more activities of daily living. When you purchase an LTC policy from an insurance company, you pay a certain amount of money (i.e., a premium) each month in exchange for a guarantee that your future care costs will be covered in accordance with the specific terms of your particular agreement.

Many families and individuals decide to buy LTC insurance because of the fact that Medicare only pays for long-term care under very limited circumstances and Medicaid is designed for people with low incomes and low-value assets. Plus, Medicaid programs vary from state to state in terms of what they do or do not cover. So, for example, your state may or may not cover assisted living. By purchasing an LTCI policy that covers the types of care you may need in the future, you can give yourself more options if a time ever comes when you or your family have to pursue long-term care.

However, it's important to know the potential limitations of LTC insurance. Most policies include a lot of exclusions. For example, services that are not covered by long-term care insurance usually include:

- Hospital care
- Care for self-inflicted injuries
- Paid care from an immediate family member
- Care for illnesses or disabilities caused by war or participation in illegal activity
- Treatment for alcohol abuse or self-induced drug addiction
- Care for certain pre-existing conditions such as diabetes, dementia, mobility problems, or HIV-related illnesses

Most LTCI policies are comprehensive, which means that, aside from exclusions, they cover a wide range of services, including home care and assisted living. But some policies only provide coverage for facility care. That's why you always need to read all the terms of any policy you're considering very carefully before buying it. Here are other terms that are crucial to understand:

- **Benefit amounts:** LTCI policies generally specify how much compensation you can receive for the cost of care on a daily or monthly basis. That amount can vary greatly from policy to policy. So you need to make sure It's high enough to cover your potential future costs if you want to avoid paying anything out of pocket.

Your policy will also have a maximum life benefit, which is the total amount of coverage it will provide over your lifetime. That dollar amount is sometimes represented as a period of time (based on the daily or monthly benefit). For example, if your monthly benefit is $9,000 and your maximum life benefit is $324,000, then your coverage would probably be good for three years. Alternatively, you can purchase an LTCI policy with unlimited or lifetime coverage, but your premiums will be much higher.

•**Elimination period:** This works kind of like a health insurance deductible. But instead of having to pay a certain amount of money before the policy provides benefits, you have to wait a certain amount of time. That means you'll be on the hook for your long-term care costs during the waiting period. Every policy is different, but elimination periods generally range from as little as 20 days to as much as a full year. Shorter elimination periods generally come with higher premiums.

•**Inflation protection:** Most of today's LTCI policies include a clause guaranteeing that the value of your benefits will increase by a certain percentage each year in order to account for the rising costs of senior care. Without this protection, your benefits (in today's dollars) may only cover a fraction of your future costs since inflation erodes your purchasing power. For example, the cost of long-term care in the U.S. rose by at least three percent a year between 2012 and 2017, according to Genworth.

Health Insurance for Senior Citizens Over 70 Years in India

At the age of 70 and above, individuals are more prone to health-related issues and medical emergencies. Having the right health insurance can significantly ease the financial burden of healthcare expenses. Let's take a closer look at the key aspects of health insurance for senior citizens in India.

As our loved ones age, their health becomes a priority, and ensuring they have access to adequate healthcare is essential. For senior citizens over 70 years in India, having comprehensive health insurance is crucial for their well-being and peace of mind.

In this chapter we will explore various health insurance options tailored for seniors in India, providing valuable insights into the best coverage and benefits. Let's delve into the world of health insurance for senior citizens over 70 years in India.

The importance of health insurance for seniors

As we age, the risk of developing chronic illnesses and age-related health conditions increases. Health insurance provides a safety net, covering medical expenses and hospitalisation costs, allowing seniors to receive timely and quality healthcare without worrying about the financial implications.

Understanding the specific needs of senior citizens

Seniors have unique healthcare requirements, including coverage for pre-existing conditions and a higher sum insured for comprehensive medical treatments. Tailored health insurance plans cater to these specific needs, ensuring seniors receive adequate care when they need it most.

Key features to look for in health insurance for seniors

When selecting health insurance for senior citizens over 70 years in India, certain features are vital to consider. These include:

Pre-Existing Conditions Coverage: Ensure the policy covers pre-existing medical conditions that are common among seniors.

Cashless Hospitalisation: Look for plans that offer cashless hospitalisation to eliminate financial stress during emergencies.

Sum Insured: Opt for a higher sum insured to cover expensive medical treatments and hospitalisation.

Renewal Age Limit: Check the renewal age limit to ensure continued coverage in the later years.

Waiting Period: Understand the waiting period for pre-existing conditions and other specific treatments.

Here are some useful tips to get the most suitable health plan for senior citizens.

Know Their Health Needs

Take a moment to understand your senior citizen's healthcare needs. Consider their medical history and existing conditions, so you can find a plan tailored to their requirements

Go for Comprehensive Coverage

Look out for plans that offer all-around coverage, including hospitalisation expenses,pre and post-hospitalization costs, ambulance charges, and critical illness benefits. Comprehensive plans mean peace of mind during tough times

Mind the Age-Related Limitations:

Some plans have age-related restrictions. Make sure to read the terms carefully to be aware of any limitations that may arise with age.

Compare Premiums and Deductibles: It's always a good idea to compare premiums and deductibles of different policies. Find a plan that strikes the right balance between affordability and benefits.

Accessible Network Hospitals and Cashless Facilities: Opt for a plan with a wide network of hospitals for easy access to medical facilities. Cashless claim facilities also make life easier during emergencies.

Watch Out for Waiting Periods: Waiting periods for specific illnesses or treatments are common. Be sure to know the details to avoid surprises later on.

Understand Sub-Limits and Co-Payment: Check if the plan imposes sub-limits on certain expenses or requires co-payment. Knowing these details will help you choose wisely.

Lifelong Renewability Matters: Look for plans with lifelong renewability. You want your loved one to have continuous coverage during their golden years.

Check the Claim Settlement Ratio: Higher claim settlement ratios mean a more reliable insurer. Do your research to make an informed decision.

Be Aware of Exclusions: Take the time to read and understand the policy's exclusions. Knowing what's not covered helps manage expectations.

Seek Expert Advice: If you're feeling overwhelmed, don't hesitate to seek advice from insurance experts or financial advisors. They can guide you towards the right plan.

Opt for Critical Illness Coverage: As age advances, it's smart to consider a plan with critical illness coverage to protect against unexpected health challenges.

Read Customer Reviews: Hear from others who have firsthand experience with the insurance company. Positive feedback is always a good sign!

Explore Additional Riders: Riders can offer extra benefits for specific conditions or treatments. Consider ones that align with your needs.

Go Digital for Convenience: Buying health insurance online is easy and often comes with discounts. Plus, you can compare multiple policies effortlessly.

Be Honest about Pre-Existing Conditions: When applying for insurance, provide accurate information about pre-existing conditions to avoid future claim issues.

Use the Free-Look Period: Take advantage of the free-look period to review the policy in detail. If it doesn't fit, you can get a refund within this time.

Consider Family Floater Plans: If you have multiple family members to insure, a family health plan can be cost-effective and efficient.

Prioritise Customer Service: Efficient customer service is crucial during emergencies. Make sure the insurance company has a good reputation for support.

Age-Specific Plans: Look for plans designed specifically for senior citizens, as they may offer more relevant benefits and premiums.

Avoid Unnecessary Add-Ons: While riders can be helpful, skip any add-ons that don't align with your needs to keep costs in check.

Understand Policy Renewal: Know the policy renewal process to ensure seamless coverage without any gaps.

Check for Copayment Waiver: Some insurers offer copayment waivers after a certain period of claim-free premiums, which can be beneficial.

Cover Pre and Post-Hospitalization: Make sure the plan covers both pre and post-hospitalization expenses, as they can be substantial.

Lifetime Renewability Matters: Confirm that the plan offers lifetime renewability for long-lasting coverage.

Health Insurance for senior citizens in India

From April 1, 2024, the insurance regulator removed the age cap on purchasing health insurance policies. Health Insurance for senior citizens: The recent amendments by the Insurance Regulatory and Development Authority of India (IRDAI) regarding health insurance rules are set to benefit senior citizens significantly. By removing the age ceiling of 65 years for purchasing health insurance, IRDAI has expanded access to health insurance products for individuals of various age There is also a notification from ministry of Health and family welfare that from April 25,2024 ,it will provide free health insurance for senior citizens over 50 yrs old

Securing health insurance for senior citizens over 70 years in India is a decision that promises peace of mind and comprehensive medical coverage. With specialised plans designed to meet the unique needs of seniors, such as coverage for pre-existing conditions and cashless hospitalisation, our elderly loved ones can age gracefully without worrying about medical expenses.

Laws for Protection And National Welfare Programmes For Elderly In India

Since time immemorial, aged persons in India have been accorded a place of honour and importance in the family and community. Ancient literature in India is replete with reverent references to the elderly. Long life was cherished, old age was viewed with deference and the elderly played an important role of advisors and counsellors. On the other hand, the family and community looked after them regardless of their productive capacity. To a society, and culture, that has long prided itself in its veneration of the elderly, the existential reality of the aged may come as a surprise. Our older citizens, on a daily basis, are reminded both of their expendability as also of the depending coarseness society displays against them. Be it the way they are treated within the family, the woeful inadequacy of the health care provisions or glaring problem of economic security and Þ nancial sustenance. It is evident that modern Indian society is ill-prepared to meet the challenges posed by the graying of its population.

The rapid advances in science and medicine and better quality of life are leading to increase in longevity of populations in several regions of the world.1 The ageing of the world population is a matter of concern for policy makers and administrators who are thinking in terms of the demographic, social, psychological, economic, and health aspects of ageing. According to Population Census 2011 there are nearly 104 million elderly persons (aged 60 years or above) in India; 53 million females and 51 million males.2 A report released by the United Nations Population Fund and HelpAge India suggests that the number of elderly persons is expected to grow to 173 million by 2026.3 Both the share and size of elderly population is increasing over time. From 5.6% in 1961 the proportion has increased to 8.6% in 2011. For males it was marginally lower at 8.2%, while for females it was 9.0%. As regards rural and urban areas, 71% of elderly population resides in rural areas while 29% is in urban areas. The life expectancy at birth during 2009 13 was 69.3 for females as against 65.8 years for males. At the age of 60 years average remaining length of life was found to be about 18 years (16.9 for males and 19.0 for females) and that at age 70 was less than 12 years (10.9 for males and 12.3 for females).4 Kerala has got the highest life expectancy at birth, followed by Maharashtra and Punjab. The life expectancy at birth in Kerala is 71.8 years and 77.8 years for males and females respectively.5 There are few studies in India that relate to the multidimensional problems of ageing. Research is needed to formulate, implement and evaluate policies and programmes for the elderly and their needs.Given the nature of socio-cultural changes under way and severe decline in the state s capacity to meet the welfare needs of the vulnerable sections of the society, betterment of the quality of life of this rapidly increasing segment of India s population emerging as a formidable task. The problem is further compounded because of greater longevity of the elderly. Hence, there arises a need to understand the socio-economic as well as demographic dynamics of the elderly population in general.

The Indian society is undergoing fast transformation under the impact of various forces. The forces of industrialization, urbanisation, modernisation and technological innovation have affected practically all aspects of life. Traditional safeguards of family care for the elderly are being threatened and becoming weak because of change in family structure from joint to nuclear, migration, dual careers, growing consumerism and so on. Contemporary culture poses serious challenges to us as great transformations have modiÞ ed the coping mechanisms and values that were prevalent for our making sense of the world and If our own selves. The consumer culture has modiÞ ed the symbolic insertion of individuals in the collective action in that the logic of consumption has overrun the centrality of production as a dominant structuration of social life. All these make the well-being of the elderly a growing challenge of the present era. Thus, it is of utmost importance to and probable solution to this emerging problem of old age.

This chapter will deal with an assessment of policies and programmes for welfare of the elderly in India on the basis of available information from government published sources and from the survey of review of related literature on various dimensions of social support of silver India.

Policies and Programmes for Elderly

Over the years, the government has launched various schemes and policies for elderly persons. These policies and schemes are meant to promote the health, well-being and independence of elderly people around the country. Some of these provisions have been discussed in this paper as follows:

1.Relevant Constitutional Provisions

2.Legislations

3.Various policies and programmes of Central Government for Elderly People

4.Some other important activities

5.Specific Measures Schemes implemented by other ministries

Relevant Constitutional Provisions

Article 41 of the Constitution:

Article 41 of Directive Principles of State Policy has particular relevance to Old Age Social Security. According to Article 41 of the constitution of India, the state shall, within the limits of its economic capacity and development, make effective provision forsecuring the right to work, to education and to public assistance in cases of unemployment, old age, sickness and disablement and in other cases of undeserved want.

Article 47 of the Constitution

Article 47 of the constitution of India provides that the state shall regard the raising of the level of nutrition and the standard of living of its people and improvement of public health as among its primary duties.

Some Other Constitutional Provisions

Entry 24 in list III of schedule VII of constitution of India deals with the welfare of labour, including conditions of work, provident funds, liability for workmen's compensation, invalidity and old age pension and maternity benefits.

Further, item 9 of the state list and item 20, 23 and 24 of concurrent list relates to old age pension, social security and social insurance, and economic and social planning. The right of parents, without any means, to be supported by their children having sufþ cient means has been recognized by section 125 (1) (d) of the Code of Criminal Procedure 1973, and section 20 (1 & 3) of the Hindu Adoption and Maintenance Act, 1956.

Among the administrative setup, the Ministry of Social Justice and Empowerment focuses on policies and programmes for the elderly in close collaboration with State Governments, Non-governmental Organisations and Civil Society. The programmes aim at their welfare and maintenance especially for indigent elderly, by supporting old age homes, day care centres, mobile medical units etc.

Legislations

Maintenance and Welfare of Parents and Senior Citizens Act, 2007

The Maintenance and Welfare of Parents and Senior Citizens Act, 2007 was enacted in December 2007, to ensure need based maintenance for parents and senior citizens and their welfare. Section 19 of the Maintenance and Welfare of Parents and Senior Citizens Act, 2007 envisages provision of at least one old age home for indigent senior citizens with a capacity of 150 persons in every district of the country. The objectives of the Act are:

- Revocation of transfer of property by senior citizens in case of negligence by relatives.
- Maintenance of Parents/senior citizens by children/ relatives made obligatory and justiciable through Tribunals.
- Pension provision for abandonment of senior citizens.
- Adequate medical facilities and security for senior citizens.
- Establishment of Old Age Homes for indigent Senior Citizens.

The Act was enacted on 31st December 2007. It accords prime responsibility for the maintenance of parents on their children, grandchildren or even relatives who may possibly inherit the property of a facilities for poor and destitute older persons.

The Act has to be brought into force by individual State Government. Himachal Pradesh is the first state and Punjab is the fifth state where old parents can legally stake claim to financial aid .

from their grown-up children for their survival and a denial would invite a prison term. As on 03.02.2010, the Act had been notified by 22 states and all UTs

Various Policies and Programmes of Central Government for Elderly People

Several initiative steps for various policies and programmes for the elderly have been taken by the government. Some of them have been discussed as below:

National Policy for Older Persons (NPOP) 1999

The National Policy on older Persons was announced by the Central Government of India in the year, 1999 to reafÞ rm the commitment to ensure the well-being of the older persons. It was a step to promote the health, safety, social security and well-being of elderly in India. The policy recognizes a person aged 60 years and above as elderly. This policy enables and supports voluntary and non-governmental organizations to supplement the care provided by the family and provide care and protection to vulnerable elderly people. It was a step in the right direction in pursuance of the UN General Assembly Resolution 47/5 to observe 1999 as International Year of Older Persons and in keeping with the assurances to elderly people contained in the Constitution. The policy envisages state support in a number of areas · financial and food security, healthcare and nutrition, shelter, education, welfare, protection of life and property etc. for the wellbeing of elderly people in the country. The primary objectives of this policy are to:

- Ensure the well-being of the elderly so that they do not become marginalised, unprotected or ignored on any count.
- Encourage families to take care of their older family members by adopting mechanisms for improving inter-generational ties so as to make the elderly a part and parcel of families
- Encourage individuals to make adequate provision for their own as well as their spouse;s old age.
- Provide protection on various grounds like financial security, health care, shelter and welfare, including protection against abuse and exploitation.
- Enable and support voluntary and non-governmental organizations to supplement the care provided by the family and recognising the need for expansion of social and community services with universal accessibility.
- Provide care and protection to the vulnerable elderly people by ensuring for the elderly an equitable share in the beneÞ ts of development.
- Provide adequate healthcare facility to the elderly. Promote research and training facilities to train care givers and organizers of services for the elderly.
- Create awareness regarding elderly persons to help them lead productive and independent life.

This policy has resulted in the opening of new schemes such as

- Promotion of the concept of healthy ageing
- Setting up of Directorates of Older Persons in the States.
- Training and orientation to medical and paramedical personnel in health care of the elderly.
- Assistance to societies for production and distribution of material on elderly care.
- Strengthening of primary health care system to enable it to meet the health care needs of older persons.
- Provision of separate queues and reservation of beds for elderly patients in hospitals.
- Extended coverage under the Antodaya Schemes especially emphasis for elderly people.

National Council for Older Persons (NCOP)

A National Council for Older Persons (NCOP) was constituted in 1999 under the chairpersonship of the Ministry of Social Justice and Empowerment to operationalize the National Policy on Older Persons. The NCOP is the highest body to advise the Government in the formulation and implementation of policy and programmes for the elderly. The basic objectives of this council are to:

- Advise the Government on policies and
- Suggest steps to make old age productive and interesting.
- Provide feedback to the government on the implementation of the NPOP as well as on speciifc programme initiatives for elderly.
- Suggest measures to enhance the quality of inter-generational relationships.
- Provide a nodal point at the national level for redressing the grievances of older persons which are of an individual nature provide lobby for concessions, rebates and discounts for older persons both with the Government as well as with the corporate sector.

- Work as a nodal point at the national level for redressing the grievances of elderly people.
- Undertake any other work or activity in thebest interest of elderly people.

The council was re-constituted in 2005 and met at least once every year. At present there are 50 members in it, comprising representatives of Central and State Governments, NGO· s, citizens· group, retired persons· associations, and experts in the Þ elds of law, social welfare and medicine.

Central Sector Scheme of Integrated Programme for Older Persons (IPOP)

An integrated Programme for Older Persons (IPOP) is being implemented since 1992 with the objective of improving the quality of life of senior citizens by providing basic amenities like food, shelter, medical care and entertainment opportunities and by encouraging productive and active ageing. Under this scheme Þ nancial assistance up to 90 percent of the project cost is provided to Non-Governmental Organizations for running and maintenance of old age homes, day care centres and mobile medicine units. The scheme has been made ß exible so as to meet the diverse needs of the older persons including reinforcement and strengthening of the family, awareness generation on issues pertaining to older persons, popularisation of the concept of lifelong preparation for old age etc. Several innovative projects have also been added which are as follows:

- Maintenance of respite care homes and continuous care homes.
- Sensitizing programmes for children particularly in schools and colleges.
- Regional resource and training centres for Helplines and counselling centres for older persons.
- Awareness Generation Programmes for elderly people and caregivers.
- Running of day care centres for patients of Alzheimer's Disease/Dementia, and physiotherapy clinics for elderly people.
- Providing disability and hearing aids for the elderly people.

The eligibility criteria for beneÞ ciaries of some important projects supported under IPOP Scheme are:

- Old age homes for destitute elderly persons.
- Respite care homes and continuous care homes for elderly persons who are seriously ill and require continuous nursing care and respite.
- Mobile Medicare units for older persons living in slums, rural and inaccessible areas where proper health facilities are not available.

The scheme has been revised in April, 2008. Besides an increase in amount of financial assistance for existing projects, Governments/ Panchayati Raj institutions/local bodies have been made eligible for getting Þ nancial assistance.

Inter-Ministerial Committee on Older Persons

An Inter-Ministerial Committee on Older Persons comprising twenty-two Ministries/Departments, and headed by the secretary, Ministry of Social Justice and Empowerment is another coordination mechanism in implementation of the NPOP. Action Plan on ageing issues for implementation by various Ministries/Departments concerned is considered from time to time by the committee.

National Old Age Pension (NOAP) Scheme

Under NOAP Scheme, in 1994 Central Assistance was available. The amount of old age pension varies in the different States as per their share to this scheme. It is implemented in the State and Union Territories through Panchayats and Municipalities. The assistance was available on fulfilment of the following criteria:-

65 years or more should be the age of the person

The Ministry is now implementing the Indira Gandhi National Old Age Pension Scheme (IGNOAPS). Under this scheme Central assistance in form of Pension is given to persons, above 65 years @ `200/-per month, belonging to a below poverty line family. This pension amount is meant to be supplemented by at least same contribution by the States so that each applicant gets at least `400/-per month as pension. The number of beneÞ ciaries receiving central assistance, in the form of pension, was 171 lakh as on 31st March, 2011. Further the Ministry has lowered the age limit from the existing 65 years to 60 years and the pension amount for elderly of 80 years and above has also been increased from `200/-to `500/-per month with effect from 01.04.2011. This decision of the Government of India has been issued to all States/UTs vide letter no. J-11015/1/2011-NSAP dated 30th June, 2011.

National Programme for Health Care of Elderly (NPHCE)

National Programme for Health Care of Elderly (NPHCE) is an articulation of the international and national commitments of the government as envisaged under (UNCRPD), National Policy on older Persons (NPOP) adopted by the Government of India in 1999 and Section 20 of The Maintenance and Welfare of Parents and Senior

Citizens Act, 2007 dealing with provisional for medical care of senior citizen. Ministry of Health and Family Welfare (MOHFW) has taken appropriate steps in this regard by launching the National Programme for Health Care of Elderly (NPHCE) as a centrally sponsored scheme under the new initiatives in the XI five years plan. Presently, it is being rolled out in 100 districts. The vision of the NPHCE is:

- To provide accessible, affordable and high quality long-terms comprehensive and dedicated care services to an Ageing population.
- Creating a new architecture for Ageing
- To build a frame-work to create an enabling environment for · a society for all ages·
- To promote the concept of Active and Healthy Ageing.
- Convergence with National Rural Health or through fiancial support from family members or others.
- To identify the health problems in the elderly and provide appropriate health interventions in the community with a strong referral backup support.

Our seniors are our responsibility. Intergenerational equity is a principle of natural justice. A generation which neglects its elders and aged commits crime and shall be mate with same fate in their elder years. Ageing is a natural process, which inevitably occurs in human life cycle. It brings with a host of challenges in the life of the elderly, which are mostly caused by the changes in their body, mind, thought process. Ageing refers to a decline in the functional capacity of the organs of the human body, which occurs mostly due to physiological transformation. The senior citizens constitute a precious reservoir of such human resource as is gifted with knowledge of various sorts, varied experiences and deep insights. May be they have formally retired, yet an overwhelming majority of them are physically and mentally capable of contributing to the well being of the society. Hence, given an appropriate opportunity, they are in a position to make significant contribution to the socioeconomic development of their nation. Our seniors are our responsibility. Intergenerational equity is a principle of natural justice. A generation which neglects its elders and aged commits crime and shall be mate with same fate in their elder years. Ageing is a natural process, which inevitably occurs in human life cycle. It brings with a host of challenges in the life of the elderly, which are mostly caused by the changes in their body, mind, thought process. Ageing refers to a decline in the functional capacity of the organs of the human body, which occurs mostly due to physiological transformation. The senior citizens constitute a precious reservoir of such human resource as is gifted with knowledge of various sorts, varied experiences and deep insights. May be they have formally retired, yet an overwhelming majority of them are physically and mentally capable of contributing to the well being of the society. Hence, given an appropriate opportunity, they are in a position to make significant contribution to the socioeconomic development of their nation

Laws for Senior citizens in India

Our seniors are our responsibility. Intergenerational equity is a principle of natural justice. A generation which neglects its elders and aged commits crime and shall be mate with same fate in their elder years. Ageing is a natural process, which inevitably occurs in human life cycle. It brings with a host of challenges in the life of the elderly, which are mostly caused by the changes in their body, mind, thought process. Ageing refers to a decline in the functional capacity of the organs of the human body, which occurs mostly due to physiological transformation. The senior citizens constitute a precious reservoir of such human resource as is gifted with knowledge of various sorts, varied experiences and deep insights. May be they have formally retired, yet an overwhelming majority of them are physically and mentally capable of contributing to the well being of the society. Hence, given an appropriate opportunity, they are in a position to make significant contribution to the socioeconomic development of their nation.

Growing Population:

By 2025, the world will have more elderly than young people and cross two billion mark by 2050. In India also, the population of elder persons has increased form nearly 2 crores in 1951 to 7.2 crores in 2001. In other words about 8% of the total population is above 60 years. The figure will cross 18 % mark by 2025.

Problems of The aged as follows:

(i) Economic problems, include such problems as loss of employment, income deficiency and economic insecurity.

(ii) Physical and physiological problems, include health and medical problems, nutritional deficiency, and the problem of adequate housing etc.

(iii) Psychosocial problem which cover problems related with their psychological and social maladjustment as well as the problem of elder abuse etc.

International Efforts:

The question of ageing was first debated at the United Nations in 1948 at the initiative of Argentina.

The issue was again raised by Malta in 1969.

International Efforts:

The question of ageing was first debated at the United Nations in 1948 at the initiative of Argentina. The issue was again raised by Malta in 1969.

In 1971 the General Assembly asked the Secretary General to prepare a comprehensive report on the elderly and to suggest guideline for the national and international action. In 1978, Assembly decided to hold a World Conference on the Ageing. Accordingly, the World Assembly on Ageing was held in Vienna from July 26 to August 6, 1982 wherein an International Plan of Action on Ageing was adopted. The overall goal of the Plan was to strengthen the ability of individual countries to deal effectively with the ageing in their population, keeping in mind the special concerns and needs of the elderly. The Plan attempted to promote understanding of the social, economic and cultural implications of ageing and of related humanitarian and developed issues. The International Plan of Action on Ageing was adopted by the General Assembly in 1982 and the Assembly in subsequent years called on governments to continue to implement its principles and recommendations. The Assembly urged the Secretary General to continue his efforts to ensure that followup action to the Plan is carried out effectively.

(i) In 1992, the U.N.General Assembly adopted the proclamation to observe the year 1999 as he International Year of the Older Persons.

(ii) The U.N.General Assembly has declared "Ist October" as the International Day for the Elderly, later rechristened as the International Day of the Older Persons.

(iii) The U.N.General Assembly on December 16, 1991 adopted 18 principles which are organizedinto5clusters, namely independence, participation, care, selffulfillment, and dignity of the older persons.

These principles provide a broad framework for action on ageing. Some of the Principles are as follows

(i) Older Persons should have the opportunity to work and determine when to leave the work force.

(ii) Older Persons should remain integrated in society and participate actively in the formulation of policies which effect their wellbeing.

(iii) Older Persons should have access to health care to help them maintain the optimum level of physical, mental and emotional wellbeing.

(iv) Older Persons should be able to pursue opportunities for the full development of their potential and have access to educational, cultural, spiritual and recreational resources of society.

(v) Older Persons should be able to live in dignity and security and should be free from exploitation and mental and physical abuse

National Efforts:

(I) Constitutional Protection:

Art. 41 : Right to work, to education and to public assistance in certain cases : The State shall, within the limits of economic capacity and development, make effective provision for securing the right to work, to education and to public assistance in cases of unemployment, old age, sickness and disablement, and in other cases of undeserved want.

Art. 46: Promotion of educational and economic interests of .... and other weaker sections : The State shall promote with special care the educational and economic interests of the weaker sections of the people.....and shall protect them from social injustice and all forms of exploitation.

However, these provision are included in the Chapter IV i.e., Directive Principles of the Indian Constitution. The Directive Principles, as stated in Article 37, are not enforceable by any court of law. But Directive Principles impose positive obligations on the state, i.e., what it should do. The Directive Principles have been declared to be fundamental in the governance of the country and the state has been placed under an obligation to apply them in making laws. The courts however cannot enforce a Directive Principle as it does not create any justiciable right in favour of any individual. It is most unfortunate that state has not made even a single Act which are directly related to the elderly persons.

(II) Legal Protections:

Under Personal Laws: The moral duty to maintain parents is recognized by all people. However, so far as law is concerned, the position and extent of such liability varies from community to community.

(I) Hindus Laws: Amongst the Hindus, the obligation of sons to maintain their aged parents, who were not able to maintain themselves out of their own earning and property, was recognized even in early texts. And this obligation was not dependent upon, or in any way qualified, by a reference to the possession of family property. It was a personal legal obligation enforceable by the sovereign or the state. The statutory provision for maintenance of parents under Hindu personal law is contained in Sec 20 of the

Hindu Adoption and Maintenance Act, 1956. This Act is the first personal law statute in India, which imposes an obligation on the children to maintain their parents. As is evident from the wording of the section, the obligation to maintain parents is not confined to sons only, and daughters also have an equal duty towards parents. It is important to note that only those parents who are financially unable to maintain themselves from any source, are entitled to seek maintenance under this Act.

(II) Muslim Law:

Children have a duty to maintain their aged parents even under the Muslim law. According to Mulla :

(a) Children in easy circumstances are bound to maintain their poor parents, although the latter may be able to earn something for themselves.

(b) A son though in strained circumstances is bound to maintain his mother, if the mother is poor, though she may not be infirm.

(c) A son, who though poor, is earning something, is bound to support his father who earns nothing.

According to Tyabji, parents and grandparents in indigent circumstances are entitled, under Hanafi law, to maintenance from their children and grandchildren who have the means, even if they are able to earn their livelihood. Both sons and daughters have a duty to maintain their parents under the Muslim law. The obligation, however, is dependent on their having the means to do so.

(III) Christian And Parsi Law:

The Christians and Parsis have no personal laws providing for maintenance for the parents. Parents who wish to seek maintenance have to apply under provisions of the Criminal Procedure Code.

(III) Under The Code of Criminal Procedure:

Prior to 1973, there was no provision for maintenance of parents under the code. The Law Commission, however, was not in favour of making such provision.

According to its report:The Cr.P.C is not the proper place for such a provision. There will be considerably difficulty in the amount of maintenance awarded to parents apportioning amongst the children in a summary proceeding of this type. It is desirable to leave this matter for adjudication by civil courts.

The provision, however, was introduced for the first time in Sec. 125 of the Code of Criminal Procedure in 1973. It is also essential that the parent establishes that the other party has sufficient means and has neglected or refused to maintain his, i.e., the parent, who is unable to maintain himself. It is important to note that Cr.P.C 1973, is asecular law and governs persons belonging to all religions and communities. Daughters, including married daughters, also have a duty to maintain their parents.

(IV) Governmental Protections:

1. The Government of India approved the National Policy for Older Persons on January 13, 1999 in order to accelerate welfare measures and empowering the elderly in ways beneficial for them. This policy included the following major steps :

(i) Setting up of a pension fund for ensuring security for those persons who have been serving in the unorganized sector,

(ii) Construction of old age homes and day care centers for every 34 districts,

(iii) Establishment of resource centers and reemployment bureaus for people above 60 years,

(iv) Concessional rail/air fares for travel within and between cities, i.e.,30% discount in train and 50% in Indian Airlines.

(v) Enacting legislation for ensuring compulsory geriatric care in all the public hospitals.

2. The Ministry of Justice and Empowerment has announced regarding the setting up of a National Council for Older Person, called agewell Foundation. It will seek opinion of aged on measures to make life easier for them.

3. Attempts to sensitise school children to live and work with the elderly. Setting up of a round the clock help line and discouraging social ostracism of the older persons are being taken up.

4. The government policy encourages a prompt settlement of pension, provident fund (PF), gratuity, etc. in order to save the superannuated persons from any hardships. It also encourages to make the taxation policies elder sensitive.

5. The policy also accords high priority to their health care needs.

6. According to Sec.88B, 88D and 88DDB of Income Tax Act there are discount In tax for the elderly persons.

7. Life Insurance Corporation of India (LIC) has also been providing several scheme for the benefit of aged persons, i.e., Jeevan Dhara Yojana, Jeevan Akshay Yojana, Senior Citizen Unit Yojana, Medical Insurance Yojana.

8. Former Prime Minister A.B.Bajpai was also launch 'Annapurana Yojana' for the benefit of aged persons. Under this yojana unattended aged persons are-being given 10 kg food for every month.

9. It is proposed to allot 10 percent of the houses constructed under government schemes for the urban and rural lower income segments to the older

persons on easy loan.The policy mentions:
The layout of the housing colonies will respond to the needs and life styles of the elderly so that there is no physical barriers to their mobility; they are allotted ground floor; and their social interaction with older society members exists.
Despite all these attempts, there is need to impress upon the elderly about the need to adjust to the changing circumstances in life and try to live harmoniously with the younger generation as for as possible.
It may be pointed out that recently the Madurai Bench of the Madras High Court has ruled that the benefits conferred on a Government employee, who is disabled during his/her service period, under Section 47 of Persons with Disabilities (equal opportunities, protection of rights and full participation) Act, 1995 cannot be confined only seven types of medical conditions defined as 'disability' in the Act. The seven medical conditions are blindness, low vision, leprosycured, hearing impaired, locomotor disability, mental retardation and mental illness. A Division Bench comprising Justice F.M.Ibrahim and Justice K.Venkataraman said : "We feel that the court cannot shut its eyes if a person knocks at its doors claiming relief under the Act. In a welfare State like India, the benefits of benevolent legislation cannot be denied on the ground of mere hyper technicalities. It may be noted that this Act is not directly related to aged person but seven medical conditions which prescribed in this Act are the common symptom of the aged person.

Need For A Change In Approach:

In the older times, after the completion of 50 years of life, one had to detach oneself from the responsibilities of a 'Grihastha' and switch over to the third stage of human life which was known as 'Vanpristha' which referred to the devotion of the next 25 years of life by the 'Vanpristhi' by mana, vachana and karma to the selfless service of the suffering humanity and the larger society in return to the services received form society during the first 50 years of life.
Certain strategies and approaches at different levels of policy making, planning and programming etc. will have to be adopted in order to harness this vast human resource for promoting the involvement and participation of senior citizens in socioeconomic development process on a much larger scale.This participation must result in an end to their social isolation and an increase in their general satisfaction with their life. Any attempt to secure the help of the elderly in offering their service to the nation must simultaneously ensure some sort of package of services aimed at arranging for them a better quality of life and a well designed social security network for the senior citizen. The society and the state in India need to accept the challenge of their effectively focusing their attention on the following twin issues of:
(i) How to provide a fair deal to the senior citizens so that they are able to peacefully, constructively and satisfactorily pass their lives; and
(ii) How to utilize the vast treasure of knowledge and rich life experience of the older people so that they are able to utilize their remaining energies and contribute to the all round development of their nation.
Palliative Care: Need of the hour : According to a pilot survey, 70% of city's elderly population is undergoing some kind of medication. The average spending per day ranges between Rs. 3 to 200. However, nearly half of the money goes waste. The reason is absence of proper palliative care in the country. World Health Organization has marked October 7 as a day to create awareness about the importance and need for hospice and palliative care. "Access to the best quality care, while facing terminal illness is a human right. Ironically, many people in the world are denied this right. The bitter side is that government in many countries does not even realize the important of this right" said geriatric physician Dr. Abhishek Shukla.

Conclusions

It may be conclude by saying that the problem of the elderly must be addressed to urgently and with utmost care. There is urgent need to amend the Constitution for the special provision to protection of aged person and bring it in the periphery of fundamental right. With the degeneration of joint family system, dislocation of familiar bonds and loss of respect for the aged person, the family in modern times should not be thought to be a secure place for them. Thus, it should be the Constitutional duty of the State to make an Act for the welfare and extra protection of the senior citizen including palliative care.

References

1.Survey of the old reveals human rights violations., The Hindu. Accessed 20 October 2015.UNAgeinghttp://www.un.org/en/globalissuesageing/
2.Agewell Study on Human Rights of Older Persons in India." United Nations: Department of Economic and Social Affairs (DESA) - Economic and Social Council (ECOSOC)
3.Singh, Rakesh K. "Rights Of Senior Citizen: Need Of The Hour. Allahabad Law House, 2011

10 Government Schemes Launched for the Benefit of Senior Citizens

Senior citizens in India are undeniably a vital part of the nation, with their wisdom and experience being invaluable to the younger generations and the economy in general. As such, understanding the senior citizen benefits that are available to the venerable elderly population of the country is an important topic that needs to be discussed.

From pension schemes and retirement benefits to healthcare and travel concessions, senior citizens can access a range of services and resources to help them lead a more comfortable and secure life in the arms of their motherland. That said, with ever-changing policies and regulations, it is critical to stay up-to-date on the latest senior citizen benefits available in India.

As life expectancy increases, the geriatric population in India is set to experience a dramatic increase. According to statistics given by trusted sources, by 2050, it is estimated that the elderly population will account for around a quarter of the total population. In this situation, savings play a critical role in making their lives merry and content.

As one's income diminishes during retirement, it becomes difficult to manage medical expenses. Elderly people are more prone to various ailments, and this increases the need for a steady flow of income to cover the costs of both treatment and prevention. In order to protect the rights of senior citizens and ensure their wellbeing, the Indian government has launched several schemes. The following are some of the best and top government schemes for senior citizens in India 2022 and 2023:

1. Pradhan Mantri Vaya Vandana Scheme

The Pradhan Mantri Vaya Vandana Scheme is a pioneering senior citizen welfare fund for Indian citizens over the age of 60. This pradhan mantri yojana for senior citizens is designed to provide financial security and assurance to the senior citizens of India.

It offers an attractive interest rate of 8% per annum, and pensioners can choose their own payment frequency: monthly, quarterly, half-yearly, or annually. The monthly minimum and maximum pension caps are Rs. 3,000 and Rs. 10,000, respectively. With this scheme, the government ensures that senior citizens' futures are secure and that they have the opportunity to live a dignified life.

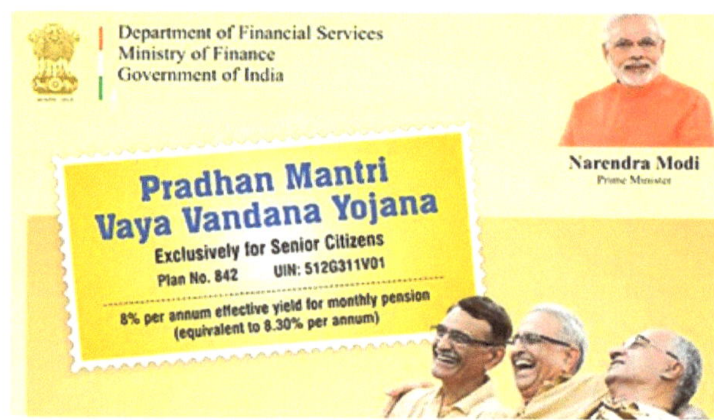

Fig. 29.1 Govt announced Pradhan mantri vaya vandana yojna to senior citizen

In other words, the PM Vaya Vandana Yojana upsc is a government scheme designed to ensure the financial security of senior Indian citizens. This pension plan, administered by the Life Insurance Corporation (LIC) of India, offers a safe and secure post-retirement financial planning option.

Senior citizens can benefit from this welfare fund by receiving assured returns, tax benefits, and life insurance.

The scheme also offers the option of withdrawing a lump sum at the time of maturity or opting for a pension to meet regular expenses.

With PMVVY, senior citizens can enjoy a secure retirement with the added peace of mind that comes from being covered by government schemes for senior citizens. This senior citizen welfare fund provides a much-needed safety net for those who want to enjoy a comfortable life after retirement.

2. Indira Gandhi National Old Age Pension Scheme (IGNOAPS)

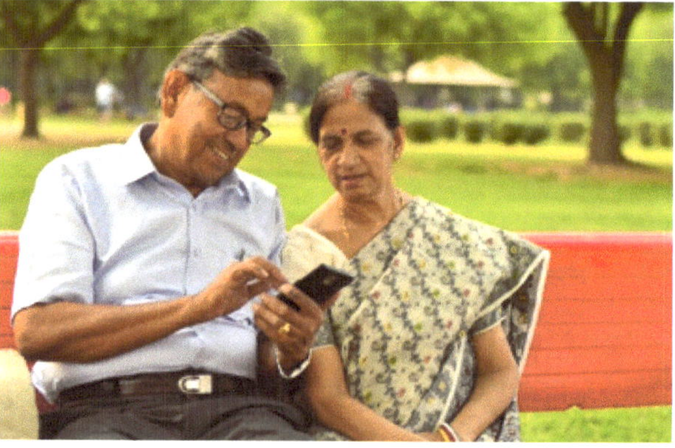

Fig. 29.2 Elders are studying Indira Gandhi National Old Age Pension Scheme (IGNOAPS)

The Indira Gandhi National Old Age Pension Scheme (IGNOAPS) is a government-backed program in India that provides financial support to senior citizens. It is one of the most popular programs for elderly in the country. It is specifically designed for those aged 60 and older who fall below the poverty line as per government guidelines. Through this scheme, senior citizens can receive a pension of up to Rs. 200 per month if they are between the ages of 60 and 79 and up to Rs. 500 per month if they are over the age of 80. This important senior citizen benefit in India provides much-needed financial support to the elderly and helps them to lead a better quality of life. All in all, IGNOAPS is one of the many programs for the elderly available in India, and it is an essential part of the government's efforts to ensure the welfare and safety of senior citizens.

3. National Programme for the Health Care of Elderly (NPHCE)

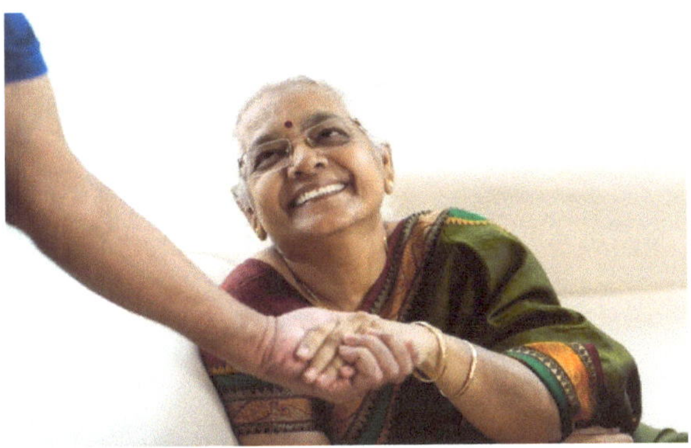

Fig. 29.3 Old er women is feeling happy on annousment of National Programme for the Health Care of Elderly (NPHCE)

The National Programme for Health Care of Elderly (NPHCE) was established in 2010 to offer senior citizens the advantages of preventive and promotive health care services. This initiative provides elderly citizens with access to health and wellness services so they can maintain their physical and mental wellbeing. In other words, the programme was launched to ensure that senior citizens are provided with the necessary medical care they require and to enable them to live healthier and more independent lives.

The NPHCE is committed to providing quality health care services to those living in district hospitals, community health centres (CHC), primary health centres (PHC), and sub-centres (SC) across the nation. The programme strives to facilitate access to necessary health care facilities and resources at all levels through the State Health Society. These senior citizen benefits from government or health facilities could be free or heavily subsidised, allowing the elderly population in the country to access quality health care services at reasonable prices.Moreover, this programme is part of the government's senior citizen pension yojana and is a comprehensive program designed to ensure that senior citizens are provided with the necessary medical care they need. On the whole, our venerable senior citizens now have the opportunity to access quality health care services at a more affordable cost due to the implementation of the National Primary Health Care Expansion (NPHCE).

4. Varishta Mediclaim Policy

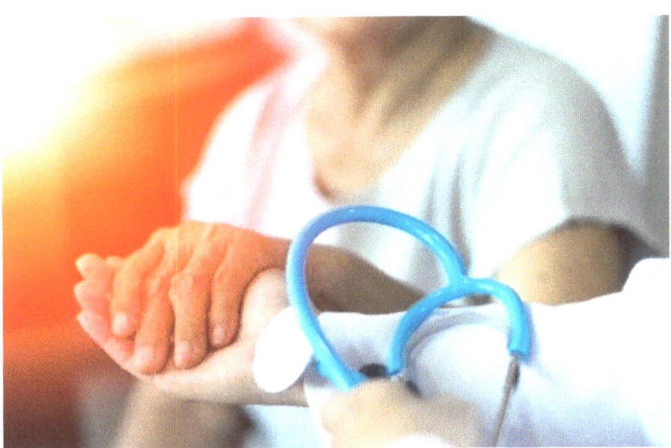

Fig. 29.4 Doctor is informing elderly women about the Varishta Mediclaim Policy

For elderly citizens in India, the Varistha Mediclaim Policy offers comprehensive health coverage and is one of the best national health programmes in India. This policy is customised to provide specialised medical care to senior citizens aged between 60 and 80 years. It covers the costs of medicine, blood transfusions, ambulance services, and other diagnosis-related charges. It is basically designed in a way that it can meet the unique needs of the elderly population in the nation and ensure their wellbeing.

Even though the policy is valid for a year, it can be renewed up to the age of 90 and comes with additional benefits, such as an income tax rebate under Section 80D. This policy is designed to promote the health and well-being of senior citizens. With the Varistha Mediclaim Policy, elderly citizens can avail quality healthcare services without having to worry about astronomical medical bills.Long story short, this policy is a great way to secure the health of elderly citizens in India and provides them with much-needed financial support at a time when the cost of medical care is skyrocketing. It ensures that elderly citizens can enjoy their retirement without worrying about medical expenses or bills, as the government will provide coverage for them. This provides a sense of security and peace of mind, allowing them to relax and make the most of their leisure time.

5. Rashtriya Vayoshri Yojana

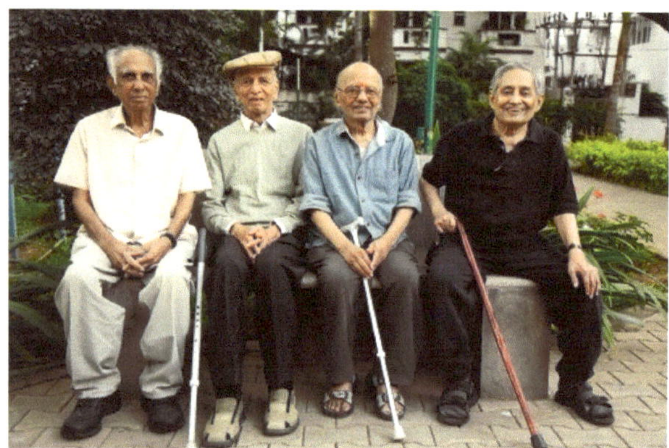

Fig. 29. 5 A group of senior citizen are feeling happy after knowing about Rashtriya Vayoshri Yojana

The Government of India has recently launched the Rashtriya Vayoshri Yojana, a government scheme for senior citizens over the age of 60. This initiative is designed to help those senior citizens living in poverty lead a more comfortable and independent life by providing physical aids and assisted-living devices. This scheme specifically targets those who belong to the Below Poverty Line (BPL) category, granting them much needed access to the resources and products that can help them in their everyday lives.In addition, the central government is funding this scheme entirely, making it a "central sector scheme." In order to avail themselves of the benefits of this scheme, a senior citizen must have a BPL card. This scheme helps support and sustain the livelihood of senior citizens who are living below the poverty line. Moreover, it furnishes them with the essential and appropriate assistance and tools to enhance their quality of life and empowers them to live with respect and autonomy. Overall, the Rashtriya Vayoshri Yojana is an excellent government scheme for senior citizens above the sr citizen age of 60 who are living below the poverty line. It is an excellent initiative taken by the government of India to ensure the well-being of its citizens and to empower them to live a comfortable and independent life.

6. Varishta Pension Bima Yojana

This pension scheme, launched by the Ministry of Finance, is for senior citizens above 60 years. The LIC of India has the authority to operate this scheme. You don't need to get any medical check-ups done to avail this policy. It offers assured pension with a guaranteed interest rate of 8% per annum for up to

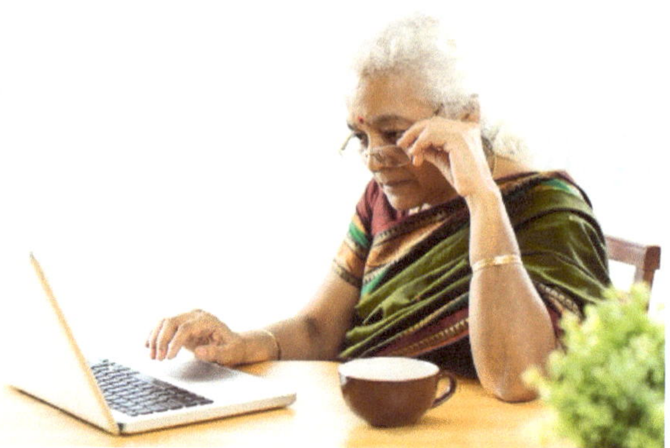

Fig.29. 6 Elderly women wanted to know every aspect of Varishta Pension BimaYojana through social media Govt.channel..

10 years – you can opt for monthly, quarterly, half-yearly, and yearly pension – depends on how you'd like to receive it.

7. Senior Citizens' Welfare Fund

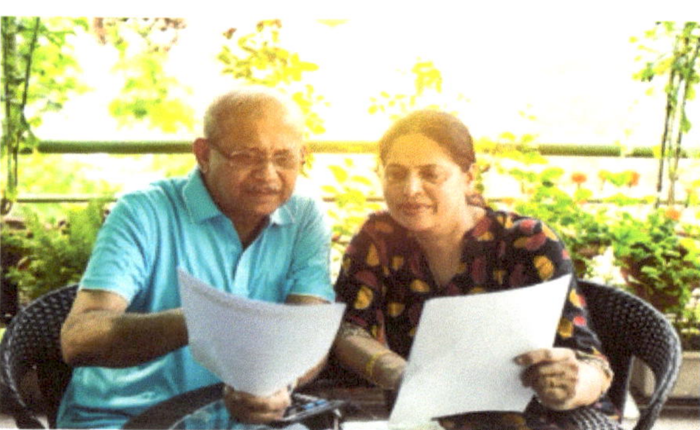

Fig.29.7 A Senior couple is analyzing Senior Citizens' Welfare Fund scheme.

The government of India has recently established the Senior Citizens' Welfare Fund under the Ministry of Social Justice and Empowerment to ensure the welfare of its elderly citizens. This fund is intended to provide financial assistance to elderly citizens by tapping into the unclaimed sums from small savings and savings accounts in the government's schemes. The aim is to guarantee that seniors have the means to sustain their physical and mental health and wellbeing.

The scheme provides various government benefits to senior citizens, such as subsidised healthcare, financial assistance for medical treatments, and pensions for needy seniors. This government scheme for senior citizens is a welcome step for the welfare and protection of our elderly population and will ensure that no one is deprived of the basic necessities of life.

8. Vayoshreshtha Samman

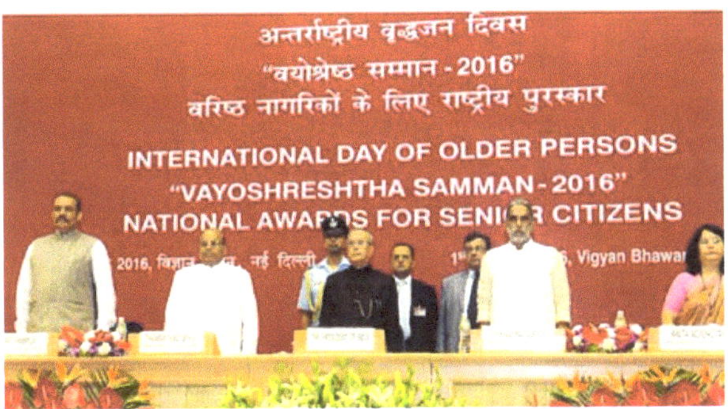

Fig. 29.8 Govt is announcing national Vayoshreshtha Samman to senior citizens on international Day of Older Persons .

The Vayoshreshtha Samman is a prestigious government senior citizen award program in India that was established in 2012 to recognize and reward senior citizens for their significant contributions to their respective fields. This annual initiative of the Government of India was elevated to a national award in 2013, and since then, recognition has been given in thirteen distinct categories.

The district panchayats providing exemplary services and facilities to senior citizens will be rewarded with a citation, a memento, and a cash award of Rs. 10 lakh. Similarly, the best institution undertaking research in the field of ageing will receive a citation, a memento, and a cash award of Rs. 5 lakh. These awards aim to recognize and encourage the selfless service of individuals and institutions towards the welfare of the elderly.

The most esteemed institution for providing services to senior citizens and increasing awareness will be given a citation, a memento, and a cash award of Rs. 5 lakhs. This award will be presented to celebrated individuals aged 90 and above who are still active and independent, and making a valuable contribution to society. The awardee will also receive a citation, a memento, and a cash award of Rs. 2 lakh 50 thousand.

On the other hand, the Iconic Mother Award will be conferred on senior women citizens who, despite all hardships, raised their children and supported them in achieving great success in any field of their choice. The recipient of this award will be presented with a citation, a memento, and a cash award of Rs. 2 lakh fifty thousand. The Vayoshreshtha Samman is an incredible government senior award program that recognizes and rewards the hard work and dedication of seniors by recognizing their exemplary service. By awarding these individuals and institutions, the Government of India is showing its appreciation for those seniors who have made significant contributions to their respective fields.

9. Reverse Mortgage Scheme

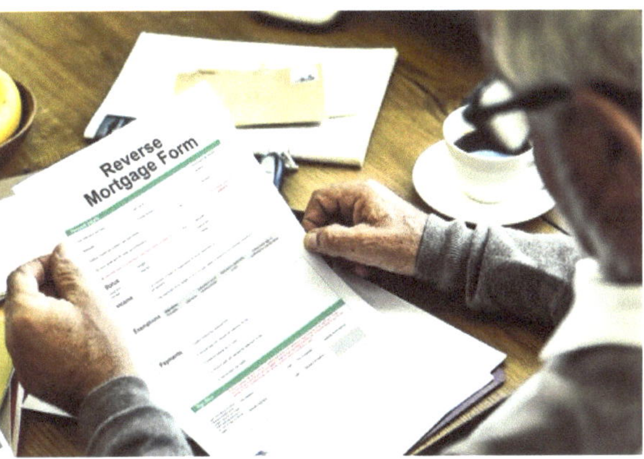

Fig.29.9. Senior citizen is studying Reverse Mortgage Scheme

The Reverse Mortgage Scheme is an innovative program designed to support senior citizens in India that was introduced in 2007 by the Indian Ministry of Finance. It is a loan scheme that enables senior citizens to mortgage their residential property in order to avail themselves of a loan of up to 60% of the value of the house. The loan must be maintained for a minimum period of 10 years. This scheme provides great financial assistance to senior citizens, enabling them to access funds from their homes without having to sell their property. This senior citizen loan program is a great way for retired individuals to access the funds they need for their daily or special needs.

This scheme provides seniors with a financial security blanket, allowing them to remain at home and maintain their independence despite facing economic challenges in their golden years. It also encourages seniors to remain within their local communities by providing them with access to funds that can be used to cover medical bills, utility bills, and other expenses. All in all, this scheme provides senior citizens with the financial security they need to live comfortably and with dignity.

10. Pradhan Mantri Jan Arogya Yojana

Pradhan Mantri Jan Arogya Yojana (PMJAY), launched by the Ministry of Health and Family Welfare in 2018, is an ambitious scheme that has revolutionised the healthcare system in India. It has provided coverage of up to Rs. 5 lakhs per family for secondary and tertiary hospitalisation to 10 crore people belonging to poor and vulnerable families.With this scheme, the government has taken a major step towards making healthcare more accessible and affordable.

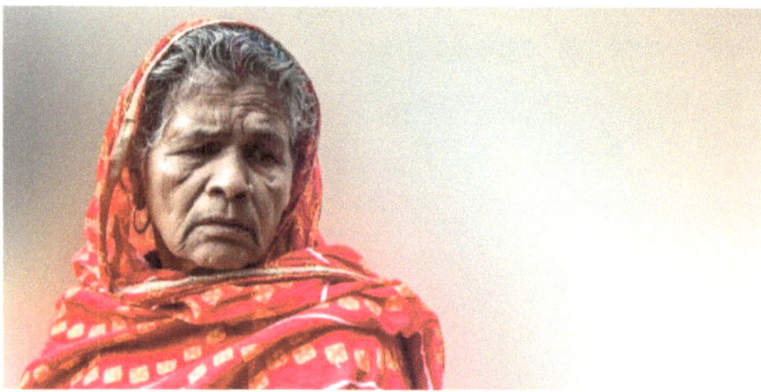

Fig. 29.10 Elderly women is listening about Pradhan Mantri Jan Arogya Yojana

In addition to PMJAY, the government of India has launched several other schemes that have been of great help to the elderly population in particular. These include schemes that aid in the planning of medical and other expenses. Such measures have given a much-needed boost to the healthcare system in India and have made it easier for people to access quality healthcare

Credit Cards for Senior Citizens in India – Eligibility, Challenges & Popular Options

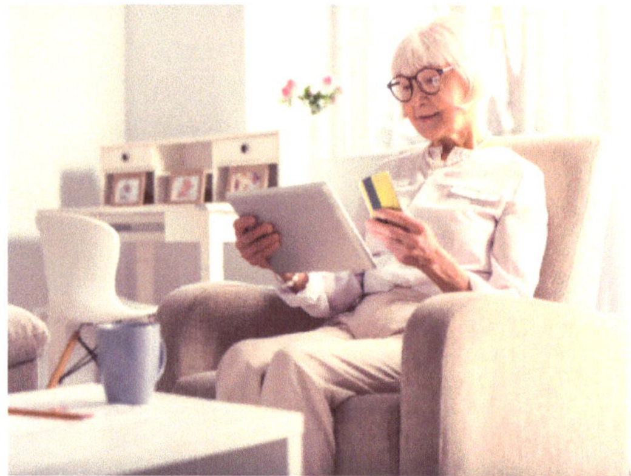

Fig.29.11 Many banks are thankfully offering new products that make it easier for seniors to avail of credit card and personal loan services.

Credit cards offer credit for a short duration and are often are used for transactions, especially when you do not want to part with cash-in-hand. When used cautiously, credit cards can be of great benefit, especially when you wish to protect your liquidity. Some senior citizens also choose to keep the loom running after retirement by being self-employed or offering consultancy services. For such industrious folks, credit cards can prove to be a blessing that helps meet capital expenses or sudden business needs.

Why Is It Hard for Senior Citizens to Get Credit Cards?

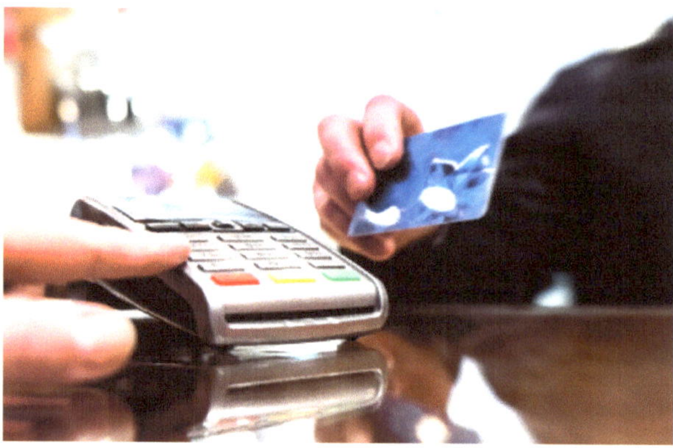

Fig. 29.12 Credit Cards for Senior Citizens in India

Credit Scores - It is a no brainer that your credit scoring affects your eligibility for credit cards. As a majority of senior citizens do not necessarily have a steady source of income, availing the facility of plastic money becomes difficult due to the risk of default.

The Age Factor – Most credit cards are offered to the customer segment in the age group of 18 years to 60 years. Card issuers perceive older applicants as financial dependents and often take business decisions accordingly. This makes it difficult for those above 60 years to enjoy the benefits of credit. Yet, thanks to the booming financial services industry in India, even customers with low-income as well as seniors with non-consistent income are being covered and are offered credit cards with attractive features and benefits.

Conclusion

The Indian government has launched many schemes to benefit senior citizens living in the country. These (above-mentioned) schemes are designed to provide a range of benefits such as financial security, healthcare, access to pension schemes, and other social welfare benefits. Most of these schemes, or senior citizen benefits in India, have provided a much-needed lifeline to elderly citizens, helping them to live with dignity and financial security. The government has shown a great deal of commitment to providing a secure future for senior citizens and has taken several steps to ensure the welfare of this important segment of the population. The government's efforts in this regard are commendable and should be appreciated by all citizens of India. Do you have an opinion on this? Let us know in the comment section below! We'd love to hear from you!

Summary Of Performing Everyday Routines To Remain Physically & Mentally Fit .

Expert-approved ways to help seniors keep up with everyday routines

Senior care experts share their best tips for supporting seniors in keeping up with everyday tasks and staying active and healthy.Daily routines can be beneficial for people of any age, but they are especially vital to the mental and physical health of seniors. For seniors, daily routines offer a way to stay motivated, a regular schedule of activities and things to look forward to and a roadmap for accomplishing tasks that keep them feeling healthy and productive.

"Keeping a routine decreases stress and keeps seniors from becoming overwhelmed," says Nicole Brackett, a care delivery and education manager at Homewatch CareGivers in Greenwood Village, Colorado. "Consistency with the activities of daily living can also bring a sense of calm and safety, and staying active can help ward off the effects of immobility."

But as important as daily routines may be, sticking to them isn't always easy for seniors. Changes in health status and other difficulties that come with aging can create physical and emotional challenges to staying active. Caregivers have a unique opportunity to work closely with seniors to establish routines that meet their unique needs and to support them in following through with those routines.

Here's what experts say you can do to help older adults develop and maintain the right kind of daily routine for them.

What are the benefits of a daily routine for seniors?

A daily routine is the usual series of things people do to take care of themselves each day. This includes basic hygiene and self-care tasks, but it may also include daily exercise, chores, hobbies and time for socializing. Each senior's routine will depend on their interests, lifestyle and abilities, says Gabrielle Juliano-Villani, a therapist and licensed clinical social worker who specializes in senior and disability care at Colorado In Home Counseling in Denver, but maintaining some kind of daily routine, even if it's just a few brief tasks, is profoundly important for seniors' mental wellness and independence."We know our older adults and seniors are at high risk for depression," says Juliano-Villani. "Many of them aren't working anymore, and some have chronic health conditions that can be exacerbated by depression and isolation. If they aren't taking care of themselves, their mental health can decline and those health conditions can get worse."

In addition to staving off depression and illness,
Brackett says seniors who keep a daily routine and stay active also benefit from:

- Increased mobility.
- Higher energy levels.
- Improved mood.
- Reduced stress.
- Improved cognitive function.

How caregivers can support a senior's daily routine

1. Start small

Yes, routines and activity have benefits, but it's important to move at the senior's pace. "There are so many different levels of ability," Juliano-Villani says. "If someone is able to get themselves out of bed and ready for the day, they should do that. Or maybe they are bedridden, but can they make calls independently or read a book?"

Juliano-Villani recommends picking simple tasks together that seniors can manage, such as:

- Getting dressed and combing their hair.
- Making themselves coffee or breakfast.
- Making a weekly call to a friend or relative to check in.
- Making a grocery list and shopping.
- Doing some deep breathing, chair yoga or mindfulness exercises.

"Find things that work for them and allow them to still have control over that piece of their lives," she adds.

2. Focus on the cans versus the can'ts

Many seniors are dealing with changes to their health and mobility, and it's normal for them to feel overwhelmed and even frustrated by that, says Juliano-Villani. "Many times I'll hear from patients saying, 'I , 'I can't drive. I can't do this or that. Why should I even bother?'"

When this happens, there are two steps to take:

- Reframe the conversation to focus on what they can do.
- Modify the activity.

"I might reframe by saying, 'That's true. You can't drive, and that's really hard,'" Juliano-Villani says, "'But you still walk well. You can take a walk around the block, and you have a caregiver who is there to make sure you're safe and don't fall. That's really great.'"

Iris Waichler, a licensed clinical social worker, patient advocate and the author of Role Reversal: How To Take Care of Yourself And Your Aging Parents, says to modify by finding new ways for seniors to do the things they enjoy. "If they can't dance, maybe you can play their favorite music and sing together to create new memories," she says. "Music is a wonderful form of reminiscence therapy for people with memory issues. If they can't walk, maybe you can sit together in a beautiful garden

3. Dive into their routine with them

Sometimes helping a senior stay motivated is as simple as diving into their routine along with them. "If a senior does an activity with a caregiver, then they know, like, 'OK, Jessica gets here at this time. When Jessica gets here, we make breakfast together,'" Juliano-Villani says. "It gives them something to look forward to and a way to take ownership of that activity."

Amy Graber, a physical therapist and the co-owner of Fit Family Physical Therapy in Phoenix, says having caregiver support is also important to keeping seniors safe and helping them feel more confident during activities. "It's a huge determinant of participation in exercise, and it may take away some of the anxiety associated with being active," she says.

Most importantly, Waichler adds, doing things together is an opportunity for joyful bonding with caregivers. Seniors are more willing to do things that are fun, says Waichler who adds, "And incorporating daily activities, like walking to enjoy a beautiful day or dancing, can create beautiful shared moments for all involved."

4. Use schedules and reminders

Giving seniors tools to manage parts of their routine can help them take ownership of their daily tasks and feel more in control, says Juliano-Villani. Some tools the experts recommend to help seniors keep track of their daily activities include:

•Writing reminders on a white board where seniors can see them.

•Setting hourly timers to remind them to get up and move.

•Creating a schedule for simple household chores.

•Making to-do lists for tasks like grooming and errands.

5. Make movement a priority

"Strength and mobility loss don't have to be commonplace for seniors," Graber says. "While muscle loss is a natural occurrence as we age, we can do activity to combat these losses."

To begin a movement practice with a senior, Graber says to start by:

•Checking with a medical provider about what can be done safely.

•Finding movements seniors feel comfortable doing.

•Supervising or joining in with seniors for safety.

•Remembering that even a few minutes of movement has benefits.

"Staying active, even for 20-30 min a day can lead to so many positive health changes," Graber says. "One 30-minute brisk walk a day can ensure seniors are continuing to challenge their cardiac, respiratory, muscular and skeletal system."

6. Find a social group

If a senior has a hobby they enjoy and they like socializing, Graber says finding a group dedicated to that activity can give them an opportunity to mingle and feel supported in doing something they love. "There are so many wonderful senior groups out there that can support an active lifestyle," she says. "There are senior hiking groups, walking groups, fitness classes, yoga classes. Finding a social circle of like-minded, active individuals can go a long way."

Of course, not every senior is an extrovert. If a group isn't the right fit for seniors, Juliano-Villani says to find more personal social opportunities that feel comfortable for them, whether that's visiting with a close friend, family member or people from their place of worship. "Just some social contact, even if it's really small, can be beneficial," she adds.

7. Focus on what they love

"Staying active works best when we're engaging in things we enjoy," Brackett says. "Keeping a routine has its benefits, but too much structure can begin to feel sterile or institutional, and that doesn't sound appealing to anyone."

Rather than treating a routine like a daily checklist, Brackett says to connect with seniors, really get to know them and find ways to add personalization, fun and comfort to their daily activities. "For example, a normal bath can become more like a spa day if you add some scented bath soaps, dimmer lighting, soft music and maybe a heated robe to put on afterwards," Brackett says. "Honor all the things that bring them meaning and joy, and infuse those things into the activities of daily living as much as possible."

8. Don't force it

Waichler believes it is important to acknowledge that maintaining a daily routine may be challenging for some seniors. If a senior is dealing with a medical condition or struggles with mental health, the idea of maintaining routine can cause additional stress. Rather than turning the routine into a battleground, she suggests making space for seniors' feelings and working together to find a solution.

"Caregiving is always more successful if the dynamic is one of collaboration rather than confrontation," Waichler says. "People tend to push back more if they are forced to do something they don't want to do. I would use a trusted physician to recommend activities and explain why they are beneficial for health and quality of life."

9. Honor their independence

Brackett says routines should center the senior's needs and take their unique interests, abilities and desires into account. Some seniors may have fears about losing their independence or bodily function. Honor those fears, Brackett says, and reassure them that their independence and well-being is your priority.

"It is key to convey that we want to honor their personhood and all the things that are important to them and actually encourage independence," says Brackett. "Doing everything for a person strips them of all they still have to contribute. The focus needs to be on how much life the person has lived and what they still have to contribute."

The Benefits of Setting a Daily Routine for Seniors

The truth of the matter is the older we get, the less in command we feel, especially in certain parts of our lives. For seniors, this is something way too common. For older adults, they can lose their ability to function correctly, whether it be cognitively, emotionally, or physically. They need help in focusing on a task or concentrating on doing routine chores. However, there is a simple solution. Whether you are a caregiver of an elderly patient or a concerned loved one caring for older parents, establishing a daily routine can be very helpful. Add tasks that are easy to do and simple to structure around other important tasks that need to be done. For example, playing a short game of checkers before settling down for an afternoon nap. If possible, ask for the senior's input on what to add to the routine, including types of activities. Just remember that a daily routine for seniors should not feel like a rigid regimen.Below is a sample of what a daily routine could look like:

- •Wake up at 7:30 a.m.
- •Take care of personal hygiene needs and get dressed
- •Enjoy a balanced breakfast in the sunroom while listening to favorite music
- •Take a walk around the neighborhood
- •Tackle a puzzle or create artwork to share with family
- •Pack a picnic lunch to take to the neighborhood park
- •Run an errand
- •Spend some quiet time reading or take a short nap
- •Make dinner together and clean up afterwards
- •Prepare and take a bath
- •Watch a relaxing movie
- •Go to bed at 10:30 p.m.

4 TOP BENEFITS OF A DAILY ROUTINE FOR SENIORS

Many seniors can benefit from creating and sticking to a daily routine. It provides several benefits to the senior and helps the caregiver maintain stability throughout the day. Although there may be several benefits, here are the three main benefits for seniors who stick to a daily routine.

1. Reduced stress and anxiety

When seniors keep to a routine, they are more likely to lower stress levels and kick anxiety to the curb. Routines can also keep seniors calm and comfortable while eliminating chances of wandering about what to do next. Caregivers should be there to assist throughout the day and make sure everything goes as planned. Even when there is no plans but to relax and enjoy the day.

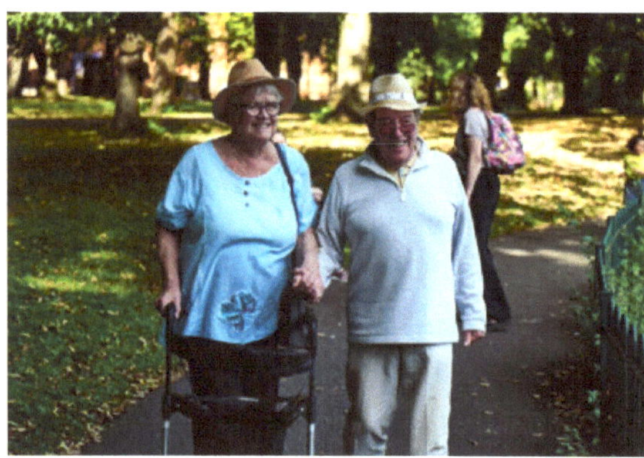

Fig 30.1 Elderly couple are on routine morning walk

2. Safety and security Increased

It is important to create a safe and secure environment for seniors, especially for those who are mentally struggling, due to memory and cognitive issues that have developed. It is also easier for seniors to cope with everyday challenges when they are aware schedules. For those who are beyond understanding of schedules or daily plans because of dementia or other cognitive declines, keeping to a routine can still help with unpredictable events and provide security.

3. Improved sleep

The next benefit to discuss is improved sleep, which is a big one. Everyone needs sleep, yet for seniors, this is essential. According to national studies, sticking to a daily routine will improve the quality of a senior's sleep patterns. In fact, a WebMD article called "Daily Routines Help Seniors Sleep Better", stated, "doing the same basic activities, like eating, dressing, and bathing at the same time every day, improves sleep quality." It can also help seniors to fall asleep and remain asleep better.

4. Benefits Caregivers

Routines do not only benefit the senior, but it can help caregivers to do their job. Taking care of a loved one or a patient that needs constant care can be overwhelming at times. The amount of tasks or duties needed to care for the senior may seem a lot, and is also a big responsibility to take on. However, when there is a daily routine in place, then things can go much more smoothly throughout the day. It may often reduce the burden in the planning process for each day. Plus, it takes a lot of pressure off the caregiver

A summary of the benefits that a daily routine for seniors can do:

- Increased mobility.
- Higher energy levels.
- Improved mood.
- Reduced stress.
- Improved cognitive function.

The Importance of Maintaining a Daily Routine for Seniors

Below are six successful tips to help seniors maintain a daily routine:

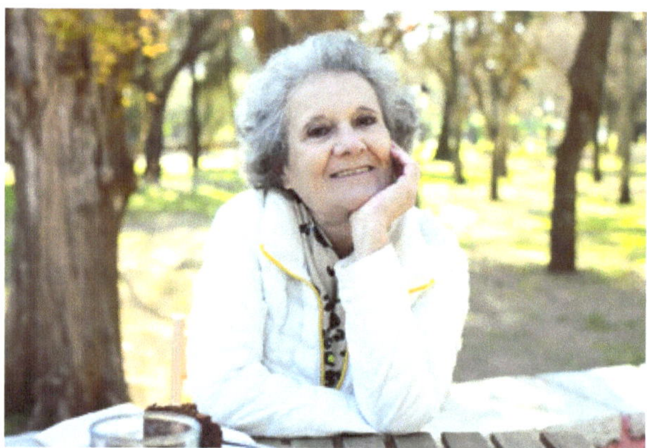

Fig 30. 2 Older women is enjoying pollution free out door weather

Plan a day outdoors: Getting some Vitamin D and sunshine is good for everyone. But for seniors, it could help their bodies become align with nature. We all benefit from the fresh air and sunlight. But enjoying a day outdoors can also help seniors to get a better night's sleep and wake up refresh.

Make meaningful moments: Every day should be full of meaning. Stay consistent throughout the day. Make sure you have time to spend with close family, a loved one that you haven't seen in a bit, or talk to a neighbor that you've been meaning to share a new recipe. Take time to write in a journal, read a book, or just do things that will brighten your day.

Move your body: The moment seniors get up, they should move their bodies. This will help them keep their activity levels high. It can also improve their heart rate up, blood flowing, oxygen moving, and their muscles, organs, and brain functioning well. Exercising also helps us detox our body and keeps the heart pumping strong.

Be consistent: Do the same task daily and do it at the same time. For example, keep your wake time, meal time, and sleep time consistently at the same time, each day. Things do happen throughout the day that are unexpected and there will be peaks and dips in a daily routine; but for the most part, try to keep to the schedule. By doing so, you will align your body with nature and won't feel bogged down when mishaps in the schedule do happen. Being consistent can help seniors plan ahead and feel more relaxed when unexpected situations happen.

Restore your mental health: It's true, that when we sleep, your bodies get recharged for another day, but there are other ways as well to recharge your body and mind. Whenever we do physical activities as part of a daily routine, we not only benefit our bodies, but we keep our mind active too. Engaging in activities helps give us a sense of purpose, rejuvenates the spirit, and calms our soul. Just by taking a short 10-minute walk in the cool of the afternoon or doing yoga off the porch can recharge your body and renew your energy.

Scheduling Routine in an Assisted living facility

A daily routine for those who are residents of an assisted living home or facility may be more structured than a senior living in their own home. For one, seniors who live there usually have a morning wake-up call or a caregiver that assists them in morning routines. This includes, personal hygiene, dressing, and providing a balanced breakfast. Some assisted living facilities have all meals prepared for all residents in the cafeteria or dining areas.

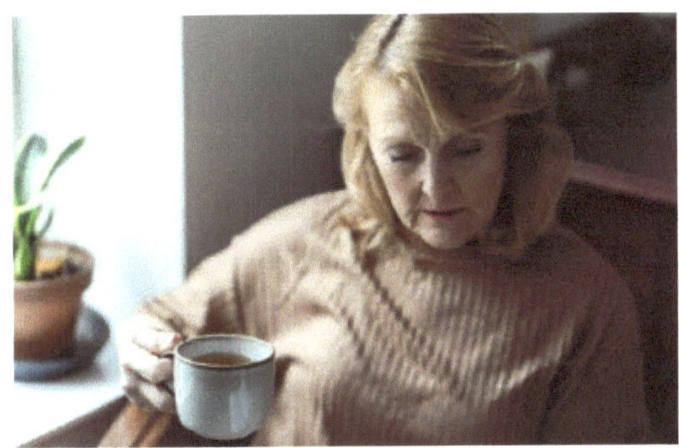

Fig.30.3 Elderly women is enjoying morning tea in an assisted living home

After breakfast is done, there may be arts and craft time, Bingo, or morning worship, depending on the day. Seniors may receive help with light housekeeping and laundry as well. Some assisted living homes offer transportation help, such as going to the grocery store, shopping centers, doctor visits, and other errands. Sometimes, transportation is available for specific outings on certain days of the week, like visiting family and friends that live nearby.

At assisted living places or even nursing homes, the staff is usually in charge of medication. However, seniors who can handle there own pills, may just be reminded to take them. There is often specific times for medication reminders or distribution of pills during the day and evening. So, as you can see, daily routines in assisted living facilities are definitely more structured and on a specific time schedule for senior living.

Keeping to a Schedule for Seniors with Dementia

Not knowing what to expect throughout the day is often common for those with dementia. When working with people that have been diagnosed with dementia, keeping to a schedule is one of the best ways to provide order and stability to their lives. Routines can help them stay on track with average every day tasks and give them a sense of comfort, especially when they can't always anticipate what is next. Similar to seniors living in assisted living facilities, dementia patients need a familiar routine every day. Keeping to the same daily habits, like taking a bath before bed or eating dinner at 5 pm each night helps seniors or older adults with dementia feel safe and secure. Seniors with dementia would also be less likely to become disoriented or confused when an established daily routine is in place.

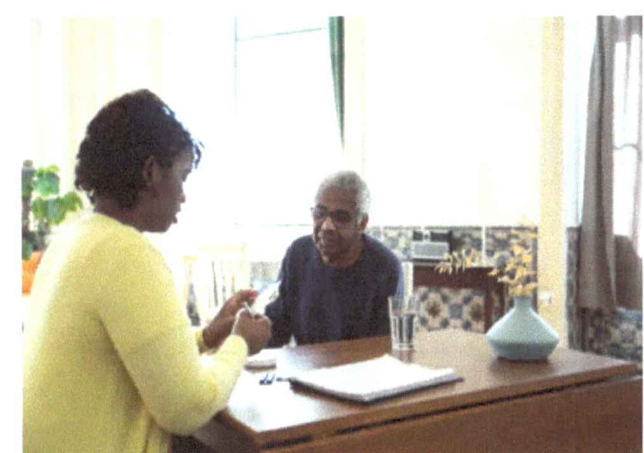

Fig.30 .4 Elderly person with dementia is taking daily instructions from health worker to assist him to perform better

According to the Alzheimer's Project, "Persons with dementia thrive on familiarity." Being familiar to their surrounding and what they do daily will help, since most people with dementia gradually decline both physically and cognitively. It become a challenge to do simple tasks. So, keeping to a schedule or a routine will help them retain a sense of control and independence, to a degree. It may even help build up their long-term memory in their brain. Just like remembering to brush their teeth or use the bathroom.

Coaching your Loved Ones to Good Health with Positive Outcomes

Sometimes seniors are stubborn or refuse to do simple tasks that you know they should. This is common among those who have been diagnosed with dementia or Alzheimer's disease. The worst thing to do is pester or command them to do a task. By doing so, it an cause the senior to become even more upset or annoyed at the caregiver. What a caregiver should do is simply suggest or mention if they have done what you ask them to do, like taking an afternoon walk or brush their teeth before heading to bed. If their responds is no, them simply suggest it, without coming across harsh or demanding. Maybe if you walk with them, the "task" will be easier to complete for the senior. Caregivers can also coach their loved ones by encouraging them and explaining how good they will feel afterwards.

Coaching is sometimes difficult, especially if the senior has experienced cognitive declines, due to their condition. Sometimes they just may not want to do part of their routine for that day. This often happens with some senior adults that have been living alone for some time before needing a caregiver. Be patient and never give up. Continue to show compassion and be flexible with the daily routine. Offer to do something you know they will enjoy instead. Things do not always go as planned, and that's okay. Every day will be an adventure and a new journey for the older adult. Having open "slots" throughout the day makes room for unexpected changes, because of a senior's behavior. Below is a sample daily schedule for older adults and caregivers. Feel free to copy and paste. A Medication promping sheet is included.

Date: ________________

A.M.

12:00 (midnight)________________________________

1:00________________________________

2:00________________________________

3:00________________________________

4:00________________________________

5:00________________________________

6:00________________________________

7:00________________________________

8:00________________________________

9:00________________________________

10:00________________________________

11:00________________________________

P.M.

12:00 (noon)________________________________

1:00________________________________

2:00________________________________

3:00________________________________

4:00________________________________

5:00________________________________

6:00________________________________

7:00________________________________

8:00________________________________

9:00________________________________

10:00________________________________

11:00________________________________

Medication Prompting

Medication:

____

Dose:

____

Scheduled times to take:

____

Prescribing doctor:

____

Additional notes about medication (take with food, etc.):

____

For those who are contemplating on becoming a caregiver, know that this is a very honored and worthy job, even when you may not always feel that way. It can be hard to cope with seniors who need extra help. Many caregivers do burnout. Here are some simple tips and resources for caregivers that need a helping hand.

Coping Strategies for Caregivers:

Walk 20-30 minutes a day- when you have time, get away and take a walk. get your mind away from work and just breathe in the fresh air. Doing this, it will lower your blood pressure, regulates your blood sugar, can improve your brain function. Making you energized to do your job well.

Take a short break- even for 5 minutes, look out the window, water a plant, or just go in a vacant room to breathe, slowly. If you are tech saavy, there is an app called Headspace that can provide short meditation breaks and help you focus.

Emergency Preparedness for Seniors

When an emergency happens, seniors are among the most vulnerable. Seniors are not vulnerable to emergencies just because of their age but also because of the challenges of aging, such as frailty, memory loss, and mobility problems. Even independent seniors are at significant risk if they are cut off from their support systems. Seniors and those who look over them must therefore be prepared for emergencies.

For those looking for answers on how to take care of their older loved ones in emergencies and how to prepare them for emergencies, some of the answers lie below.

These answers benefit:

- Senior adults
- Their families
- Caregivers who care for seniors

It's important to know helpful information, tips, and recommendations that assist families with senior emergency preparedness and emergency elderly care

How Do Seniors Modify Their Homes for Emergencies?

According to the U.S. Centers for Disease Control and Prevention:

•About 3 million older adults are hospitalized in emergency departments for fall injuries.

•Falls are the most prominent cause of traumatic brain injuries (TBI).

With the right knowledge, caregivers can help themselves and an elderly loved one to be safer and equipment, etc. keep them from joining this alarming statistic.

Safety is the foremost concern for any senior, as well as for their family. To make the home suitable for senior family members, caregivers must prioritize safety above all else while designing and adjusting the following rooms for them which are:

- Anti-slip rugs
- Wide doorways for wheelchair mobility
- Safety bars in the bathtub or shower
- Rearrangement of kitchen cabinets and the refrigerator for easy accessibility
- Space for their favorite chair, medical

How Do Seniors and Loved Ones Create an Emergency Plan?

Every part of the world is vulnerable to some dangerous events. Hurricanes, tornadoes, wildfires, earthquakes, landslides, floods, and winter storms pose genuine threats to millions of people annually. Safety and survival depend on careful planning and preparation for the likelihood of these emergencies.

Following these steps can help families and seniors get ready:

•**Have an emergency communications plan:** Create a chain of mobile phone calls or group texts amongst family members caring for the elderly. Making the first call to someone, who then calls the next person, and so on, is known as a phone call chain. This makes sure that everyone in the family and circle of acquaintances is informed of the situation in an emergency.

•**Keep contact details complete and up to date:** Have the most recent contact details for everybody they'd need to call in an emergency. Make sure seniors have family members' and neighbors' phone numbers. Put a copy of this in their travel wallet, bag, or suitcase.

•**Get local emergency plan in advance:** Obtain the local community's disaster/emergency plan. Find out where evacuees go to receive medical care or emergency packages. Get a map of evacuation routes to put in the person's car.

•**Decide on a meeting place for evacuation:** When an emergency happens, friends and family might not be together. Select two feasible meeting locations—one near their home, the other outside of the neighborhood, where they can wait and family members can find them. Make sure they know the location name, address, and contact information. Caregivers should check where seniors will be taken during an evacuation if they are taking care of elderly people who live in apartments.

Depending on the situation, keep in mind that the road network may not be safe and that internet and telecommunications lines may be down for a while. Create a list of local shelters' phone numbers and aid groups and save them in an emergency folder.

•**Exercise mock-disaster situations:** Review and practice their emergency plan with their family and friends to make sure it can be executed if necessary.

•**Obtain a medical ID bracelet:** Request a medical ID bracelet for elderly people with chronic health challenges. It is possible to engrave the surface with details about their medical conditions, sensitivities, and emergency contacts. Put identification information, diagnoses, and treatments in a wallet that travelers can carry with them at all times.

How Do You Keep Seniors Calm Ahead of An Emergency?

When they have time to prepare for how they'll handle a natural disaster, seniors won't worry as much. Making a plan in advance to help everyone feel prepared to withstand the emergency can reduce the possibility that seniors will feel alone if and when it does strike.

If a natural disaster is imminent, there are a few things that can help keep seniors calm:

- Maintain contact. In the days before the disaster, call them twice or three times every day, or more frequently depending on the event's severity.
- Maintain regular routines, eating patterns, and sleeping schedules as much as possible.
- Stay off any news programs about the imminent natural disaster.
- Explore exciting activities to have fun, such as games or other things they like.
- If they are capable and willing, seniors can volunteer and provide support to others. Finding means to contribute to society helps reduce feelings of hopelessness.

If an individual has Alzheimer's disease or another kind of dementia, they can still detect an emergency if they are elderly and have cognitive impairment. They won't be able to remember all the details, so convey what is happening in clear terms. Validate their concerns but make an effort to remain as composed as possible. Give clear directions without condescending or rushing the process.

It is essential to put together a thorough emergency plan and supplies pack to make sure that seniors and their families are well-prepared for any unforeseen risks. These actions not only assist seniors practically and logistically but can also boost their self-assurance, which reduces anxiety

What Makes Up a Senior Medical Kit?

A senior emergency kit should include:

•**Medications:** A 3–6-day supply of their medications, as well as a current list of all the medications they are taking, including the dosage and generic and brand names.

•**Medical equipment**: Seniors must bring their own durable medical equipment (DME) because the majority of local shelters lack it. These include any portable DME their loved one requires to maintain their health, such as blood sugar monitors, specific pillows to prevent skin damage, and therapeutic oxygen equipment.

•**Mobility Aids:** Plan how a senior will move around and leave the house if they are bedridden, wheelchair-bound, or have mobility issues. If someone uses a motorized wheelchair, for example, make sure a manual wheelchair is available as a backup.

•**Visual Aids**: Keep an extra walking stick with a whistle attached for an elderly relative who is blind or visually impaired. Tell them to be cautious when moving during or right away after an emergency because things in the house might have been moved around or blocked paths. Make sure to include extra eyeglasses or any other necessary visual aids in their medical kit.

•**Hearing Aids:** Hearing-impaired people should keep extra hearing aid batteries on hand and keep their hearing aids in a designated location, such as their nightstand, so they can be found quickly in an emergency.

•**Legal and Health Documents:** Keep copies of important medical documents in a designated folder that is accessible to both seniors and their caregivers. Ask their healthcare provider for a list of all their current medical issues, a description of any ongoing therapies, as well as their medical history. Other essential documents include a comprehensive medication list. In cases of evacuation, copies of the deed or lease to one's home, as well as insurance plans, may be helpful.

Senior Emergency Kits are also known as Senior Survival Kits or Senior Citizen Survival Kits. A senior emergency kit should include senior medical kit equipment, as listed above, and:

•**Drinking Water:** Seniors or people who take care of them should plan for at least 1 gallon per person daily, or at most for three days.

•**Food:** It should contain at least a three-day supply of non-perishable canned and dried goods. Soups, smoothies high in protein, and juices can be particularly beneficial.

•**Prescription Medications:** Request the healthcare professional caring for an elderly loved one to provide an extra supply of their prescriptions. This enables their loved one to stick to their regimen despite bad weather and closed or inaccessible pharmacies. Recall that both prescription and over-the-counter medications have expiration dates, so dispose of any that have already passed their expiry dates.

•**Essential Supplies:** Lighting devices, batteries, knife, basic cooking utensils, whistle, power bank should be added to the kit.

•**Clothing:** A complete set of clothing for each individual, including a long-sleeved shirt, long trousers, footwear and weather-appropriate outerwear can be of great help.

•**Basic Personal Hygiene Products:** Seniors constantly require specialized goods for their convenience and personal hygiene. Adult briefs, pads, bath soaps, toothbrushes, toothpaste, latex gloves, and toilet paper are all emergency supplies for older adults that enable them to maintain as much of their normal daily routine and level of care as possible during and after an emergency. Don't forget to include items like face masks, paper towels, disposable trash bags, disinfectants, hand sanitizers, etc.

•**Contact Information and Important Documents:** Have the phone numbers and addresses of relations and neighbors they might need to contact, their healthcare provider, and any medical practitioner they see. Include copies of their identification and credit cards.

•**Cash:** Keep emergency cash on hand and ensure seniors have at least $100 available in case the power goes out and access to electronic cash isn't available.

•First Aid Kit

What Makes Up Senior First Aid Kits?

One of the main priorities during an emergency is to stay safe and take care of any sustained injuries as medical assistance may not be accessible. Seniors first aid kits should have the essential supplies to treat minor and major wounds.

Their first aid kit should include the following items.

Sanitation and Cleaning

- Hydrogen Peroxide
- Liquid Antiseptics
- Methylated Spirit
- Eye drops
- Saline solution
- Oral analgesic gel

•Essential oils
•Eye wash solution
•Hydrocortisone cream or calamine lotion for the treatment of bug bites, itchiness, and inflammation
•Aloe Vera
•Antibiotic ointment to avoid infections, such as Neosporin
•Burn Cream

Wounds Treatment

•Tourniquet
•Medical tape
•Compression bandage
•Flexible splint
•Medical-grade super glue
•Butterfly bandage
•Non-adhesive pads to protect wounds or arrest bleeding
•Iodine
•Flexible bandage with clips
•Latex-free adhesive bandages

Medicinal

•Their personal prescription and over-the-counter medications
•Digestive disorders' medication and laxatives
•Pain-relievers such as Ibuprofen, Aspirin, Benadryl, and Tylenol
•Cough syrups
•Antacids. Consult their physician if they have any health challenges that could interfere with the administration of antacids
•Activated charcoal pills
•Immune system boosters

Protection

•Sunglasses
•Lip gloss
•Insect Repellants
•Instant cold ice packs
•Salt packets for water and electrolyte retention

Tools

•Tweezers
•Thermometer
•Scissors or Trauma Shears
•CPR Masks
•Surgical gloves
•Safety pins
•Cotton balls and swabs
•Fingernail cutter
•Needles and Threads
•Magnifying lens
•First-aid booklet or manual

How Much Should Senior Survival Kits and First Aid Kits Weigh?

First aid kits weigh less when only the basic things are included. For senior survival kits, minimize the contents, since seniors don't have the strength to carry many items. They may need a helping hand to transport emergency supplies. To make things easier, for example, seniors can store all their emergency supplies in a backpack they can connect to the back of their wheelchairs.

What Is The Best Evacuation Option For Seniors?

Staying with relatives or friends outside the emergency zone is the best evacuation option for elderly relatives. Staying in a hotel can be an excellent substitute.

Attempting to weather the storm at a public emergency shelter is the absolute last thing a senior should do. Most shelters don't have facilities to house evacuees with special needs. People with special needs are frequently not accommodated in these shelters. Make a plan for transportation if a senior cannot drive alone, and make sure they have a nearby caregiver who can accompany them during the evacuation.

Families must make arrangements for pre-admittance prior to departure if their loved one has unique medical needs and their doctor advises evacuating to a hospital or other medical facility. They will need a pre-admission letter from their doctor stating that their loved one is to be sent to a certain hospital or nursing home in order to accomplish this. As they evacuate, make sure seniors bring this letter with them.

How Do They Take Care of Their Pets In Time of Emergency?

Make sure the pet is microchipped if their loved one has one so that, in the event that they become separated during the evacuation, they may be found more quickly. The ideal situation for elderly pet owners is to stay with family and friends, but if there are no close family or friends, booking a room at a pet-friendly hotel might be a wonderful alternative. Public emergency shelters do not allow pets, with the exception of service animals.Seniors could also think about boarding their pets if that is an option. Study the out-of-town lodging possibilities along the intended evacuation route, and make sure to phone ahead to confirm there is space before dropping off the pet. Include pet care materials like a leash and enough pet food in the senior's emergency kit, along with vaccination records and other necessary papers

Is It Better To Buy A Kit Or Make Their Own?

For people unable to gather all the various items ontheir own, purchasing a kit can be the preferred choice. Although purchasing a kit saves a ton of time and work, some people decide to make their own kit with their chosen brands. It's worth the time and trouble to acquire a kit.

What Can Seniors Do During A Building Fire Emergency?

DON'T IGNORE THE FIRE ALARM: The first thing they should do is grab their room keys, tell everyone around, and leave.

•Act quickly but try to stay calm.

•Stay low in case of smoke or fumes. If in bed, roll off the bed and crawl towards the door.

•Save time by not getting dressed or searching for valuables.

•If they aren't adequately trained, don't attempt to put out a fire. Leave firefighting to the experts.

•To alert anyone who may be asleep, shout. "Fire! Everyone out!"

•Place newspapers, clothing, or towels in the door cracks to keep smoke out.

•Open the door gently even if it's cool. In case smoke or fumes leak around the entrance, take a low stance to one side.

•If heat and smoke enter, slam the door firmly, fill any spaces with clothing, towels, or newspaper to keep the smoke out, and use a different exit.

•To escape by a window, ensure the room's other windows and doors are shut tightly. If not, the draft from the open window may bring fire and smoke into the space.

These fire safety outreach materials can provide even more examples of senior fire safety.

If there is no smoke in the corridor, calmly head toward the closest fire exit and leave the building.

•Take the stairs rather than the elevator. Elevators are typically connected to a fire detection system, and if the alarm goes off, residents cannot use them.

•Keep low to avoid any possible smoke, fumes, or highly heated gases.

•As they leave, shut doors to help contain fire as much as possible.

•Pull the fire alarm while exiting the building if it isn't already going off.

Senior survival kits and emergency evacuation plans can give seniors and their caregivers peace of mind. That could make all the difference to seniors in poor health and with limited resources.

Indoor Gardening for Seniors

Seniors looking for enjoyable, low-impact activities can consider gardening a top choice. Gardening is a leisurely past-time that has monumental impacts on older adults' physical and mental health, emotional well-being, and life goals and meaning. Unfortunately, many older adults believe they cannot take up gardening due to a lack of outdoor space or mobility issues. Yet, indoor gardening activities for seniors can be an excellent way to develop gardening skills and nurture living plants. Likewise, it can be beneficial for individuals to relax and enjoy the fruits of their labor in the comfort of their own homes.

Older adults looking forward to a thriving green space, beautiful year-round blooms, or a flourishing vegetable garden may wonder how to begin their new hobby. This informative FAQ will answer all the important questions about indoor gardening for seniors.

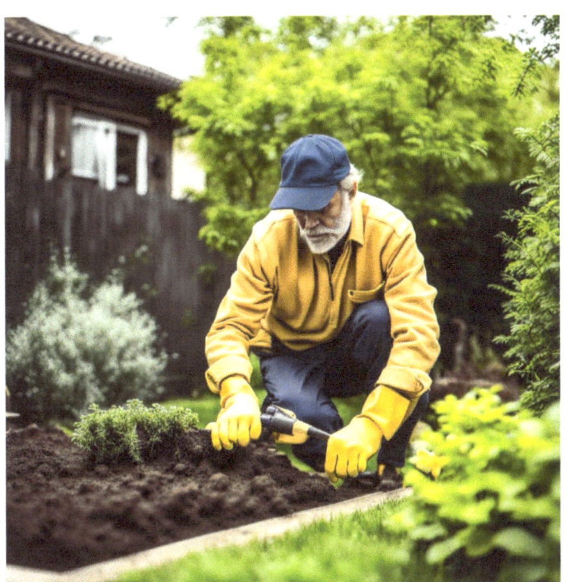

Fig 30.5 Elderly person is doing indoor gardening to have some physical activity

What Is Indoor Gardening?

Indoor gardening is a popular way to grow plants, flowers, and produce inside a residence or greenhouse. It requires similar tasks as outdoor gardening only hobbyists must create and maintain suitable conditions for their preferred plants. The most important elements include soil, water, temperature, humidity, and sunlight. While many gardening enthusiasts have extensive systems to house many plants and produce, indoor gardening for seniors can be easy and uncomplicated. They simply need to ensure their preferred plants are perfect for the given environment and tend to their plants regularly. There is an ideal plant for everyone, from fruit trees to herb gardens to pretty potted plants to cacti.

What Are the Types of Indoor Gardens?

Anyone can achieve the garden of their dreams, even in an indoor environment. There are plenty of gardens for seniors that start or flourish as:

•**Herb Gardens:** Herb gardens are one of the easiest ways to start indoor gardening. Once they have grown, individuals can regularly pick a few leaves to spice up delicious dishes.

•**Potted Plants:** Potted green plants, flowers, cacti, and trees are an excellent way to set up a living garden around the house. They double as decorative pieces, providing pleasant balance to any room.

•**Terrariums:** Terrariums are perfect for plants that thrive in humid conditions. They are also ideal for elderly gardening as all plants are in one enclosed space.

•**Air Plants:** Air plants are a stylish, unique way to garden and decorate indoor spaces. Tillandsias grow without soil, taking in their nutrients from the air and moisture.

•**Fruit and Vegetable Gardens:** Fruit and vegetables can be a little harder to grow indoors, but nothing that the proper conditions and an experienced hand cannot accomplish well. Root vegetables and fruit trees may be the best beginner options as they require less care.

•**Plant Walls:** If individuals genuinely are interested in elderly gardening but lack space in their homes, they may wish to try vertical gardening. The set-up may require assistance if mobility issues are a concern. However, maintenance can be effortless when all chosen plants need similar conditions.

•**Community Gardens:** Adults without space for indoor gardens may consider a lot in a community garden or greenhouse. Social interaction and shared purpose may be motivating for some older adults.

What Are Gardening Benefits for Seniors?

Gardening for the elderly is an incredibly beneficial activity. Whether hands-deep in a vegetable garden or carefully tending to indoor flowers, older adults can realize the advantages of long-term engagement with the hobby. A few of the top gardening benefits for seniors include:

Better Mental Health

Indoor gardening activities for seniors can be therapeutic, especially for those afflicted by mental health issues. The exercise can reduce stress, anxiety, and depression. In fact, daily gardeners have 6.6% higher well-being and 4.2% lower stress than non-gardeners. Additionally, gardening links to a lower prevalence of dementia, reducing the risk of developing the condition by 36%. Since indoor gardens allow older adults to access their plants readily, they are well-poised to reap these benefits.

Improved Physical Health

Gardening for seniors is a low-impact exercise, making it ideal for those with mobility issues. Indoor gardening may be even more beneficial to those who suffer from physical conditions making it challenging to move around, as they do not have to kneel or dig into the earth. That said, indoor gardening can still be beneficial for physical health. Gardening can elevate the heart rate, improving cardiovascular fitness. It can also improve hand functioning and strength, as seniors need to tend to the plants regularly.

Indoor gardens can also improve living environments, indirectly affecting health. Depending on the preferred plants and size of the garden overall, individuals may benefit from better indoor air quality. Further, simple exposure to green plants can positively affect health, particularly heart rate and mood.

Greater Emotional Well-Being

Along with improved mental health, elderly gardening can help regulate emotions. Studies find reduced anger, fatigue, and depression levels and increased overall mood. Likely, this is due to the relaxing activity providing a boost in serotonin and reduction in cortisol, a stress response hormone. Ultimately, when older adults experience better moods, they have greater overall health and life satisfaction.

Sense of Purpose

Seniors working towards goals or engaging in their interests maintain an excellent sense of meaning in their lives. Planting a garden, tending to the plants, and watching the garden thrive can help individuals develop a sense of responsibility and reward. Additionally, the creativity in planning and creating an indoor garden is mentally stimulating. If older adults need to learn about plants, ideal growing environments, and gardening techniques, they will also have plenty of mental stimulation.

What Do Seniors Need To Start Indoor Gardening?

After reading through all the gardening benefits for seniors, the activity may look very appealing. Fortunately, it is relatively easy to start indoor gardening. Simply follow these steps to start the new hobby on the right foot:

Find Ideal Plant Spots

Seniors or their loved ones should evaluate the residence for optimal gardening areas. There are plants for every type of condition, but natural sunlight marks an ideal spot for most plant life. Temperatures and humidity levels should be relatively stable for a flourishing plant. It is also important to look for secure and easily accessible spaces for safe elderly gardening.

Select the Perfect Plant

Plant buying can be one of the most enjoyable activities, but seniors need to consider a few factors. They should check the ideal growing location and ensure their indoor conditions are a good fit for the plant. They should also research the specific plant care, blooming season, maximum growth, and toxicity for pets or young children. Additionally, they have the choice of growing plants from seeds and bulbs, sprouts, or mature stages.

Purchase Supplies

If individuals are novice gardeners, they only need a few basic supplies to begin the activity. Plant pots and trays, potting soil, a handheld shovel, a small watering can, pruning shears, and gardening gloves are all important pieces of equipment to have on hand. As gardeners build expertise and experience, they may opt for more elaborate supplies and set-ups.

Consider a Subscription

Gardening for the elderly can be a simple hobby or an enjoyable learning experience for seniors. They may like to sign up for a gardening magazine, newsletter, or website to learn more about the activity. They could also benefit from an annual gardening seed or bulb magazine, allowing them to browse potential additions to their gardens. Social individuals may like to participate in a gardening class or club.

What Are Easy Indoor Gardening Activities for Seniors?

When older adults start a new activity, it is crucial to start small. There is a higher chance that they will keep up with the hobby if it is accessible, and they can build on their knowledge as their interest grows. Accordingly, it may be advantageous to know some easy gardening projects:

Succulents

Succulents are hardy plants, surviving in many types of

environments. They are ideal for beginners, as they do not take a significant amount of care. Additionally, they do not take up much room and can easily sit in small pots on a windowsill or coffee table.

Herbs

Herbs are another excellent choice in indoor gardens for seniors. Small pots or long trays can accommodate basil, mint, chives, parsley, rosemary, thyme, and other cooking favorites. If gardeners are feeling adventurous, they can add some vegetables like garlic, tomatoes, or peppers in deeper pots.

Cacti

Cacti require sunny environments with warm temperatures. If seniors live in warmer climates, they may enjoy the aesthetic and easy care. Some even have beautiful, colorful blooms. Choosing cacti with soft or small glochids may be necessary, as sharp spines may be dangerous for certain individuals.

Smart Gardens

Smart gardens are small gardening systems with everything needed to maintain the plant. They come with plant pods with plant seeds, nutrients, and soil. A connection to WiFi takes care of temperature, humidity, light, and water. While seniors may not receive all the gardening benefits for seniors from these all-inclusive packages, they will have a flourishing garden in no time.

Terrariums

Terrariums are the perfect way for older adults to create ideal plant environments. They can make and maintain tropical or desert biomes. They can even add decorative stones or fountains to their set-ups to enhance their aesthetic appeal. However, individuals may need to invest in equipment such as heaters, LED lights, and misters.

What Are Low-Maintenance Indoor Plants?

Gardening for seniors can be made easy with low-maintenance indoor plants. While beginners can benefit from plants that are easy to care for, it can also be good for seniors with memory problems to have adaptable plants. A few excellent indoor plants include:

•**Snake Plant:** These long green stem plants are incredibly hardy. They can thrive in low lighting and withstand long dry periods.

•**Spider Plant:** The spider plant will grow fast if placed in bright sunlight or low lighting. While it enjoys regular watering, it can retain water well.

•**Pothos:** Pothos grows well in all lighting and only requires water when the top of the soil becomes dry.

•**Air Plants:** Air plants take all their nutrients from the air, so gardeners need to ensure they have ample moisture or humidity.

•**Aloe:** Apart from an ideally warm environment, these tiny plants do not require much care. They also thrive in dry conditions, so regular waterings are not necessary.

Seniors – Keep Your Mind Active By Writing and Journaling!

The first person you probably think about when you hear the word journal is a young adult or even a teenager. Yet the truth of the matter is many seniors or older adults could also benefit from writing in a journal or diary. Journaling provides advantages at all ages, but for seniors, it can help improve both their mental and physical health. The purpose of journaling will depend on each person's specific reasons. This article will introduce the many benefits to journaling, journal prompts that can help inspire creativity, and what seniors gain out of journaling. We will also provide the differences from writing in a journal by using pen and paper, compared to using a computer to type, whether it be online or offline. To get started, all you need is a notebook, writing utensil, and some dedication to do this fun activity every day. Now let's talk about the five main benefits to writing in a journal for seniors.

1. Writing down experiences can preserve Memories.

Seniors have had many more experiences to share or talk about when they travel down memory lane. But as seniors get older, sometimes their memory is not as sharp it used to be. However, by writing in a journal they can preserve these memories and reminisce about them as they jot them down in a journal. It is also a great way to refresh their memory of activities that had occurred the night before. Although journals are often kept private, when seniors share their memories to their kids or grandkids, it can open a meaningful conversation. It can also help loved ones learn about their ancestry or heritage.

2. The act of writing in pen will keep your brain sharp and may also improve coordination skills.

When you write using a pen, you use more of your senses. You can hear the strokes of the pen or pencil, feel your hand brush against the paper, smell the paper, and even think about what you want to write as you write. You are using your fine motor skills, which benefits seniors as they age. We will discuss more of this later in Typing vs. Handwriting.

3.Using a computer to keep a journal allows seniors to become more tech savvy. In today's world, there are more opportunities to keep a journal online by using computer software.

Seniors can also write about their inspirations on the internet. Seniors can link almost anything, from inspirational quotes, favorite recipes, or even ideas you may want to share to the world. Journaling on a computer can also benefit seniors that may have limited mobility by using special features such as talk to text and touch keyboards. Seniors can also use journaling apps on the phones. For more information, read on to Typing vs. Handwriting: Which is better?

4. Journaling is a stress reliever.

Journaling is also a therapeutic method to lowering stress levels. When writing down your thoughts, whether from the day or the week, it can help relax and calm your mind. In fact, many therapist encourage their mental health patients to journal, helping them organize their thoughts in their mind on paper. By doing this, it can allow seniors see more clearly and focus on what's more important. Journaling can also help senors that may be facing anxiety or depression, due to a loss of a loved one. The mental benefits is very proactive and can also give seniors a separate outlet and help them write how they feel, instead of just verbalizing it with a therapist. As a result the power of grief can be lifted.

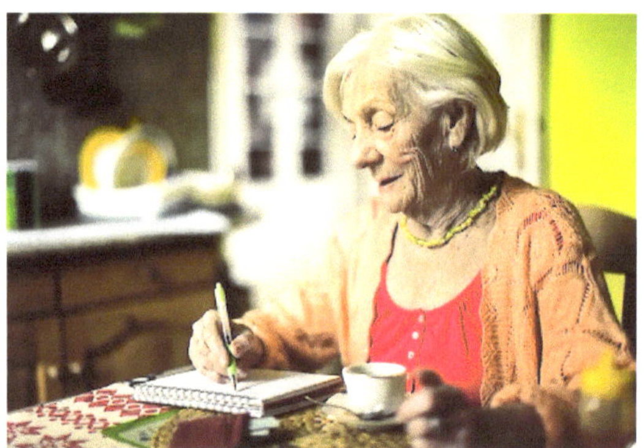

Fig. 30.6 Women is buisy in journalism to keep her anxiety free

5. Writing can boost creativity.

There are many ways to use a journal. Many seniors use one for art therapy by doodling or drawing in one. It could be just as fun as writing in it. Some seniors that keep a journal may also write poetry or keep secret family recipes in one. According to the National Institute of Aging, creative writing can improve the quality of life and well-being in older adults. Other times a senior that uses a journal might just use one to compile family photos or even record your favorite sports team wins and loses. Be creative; the benefits are endless.

Journal Prompts That Inspire Seniors

When starting to journal, sometimes you need a little help in how to get started. This is common for seniors that haven't picked up journaling before. As mentioned earlier, sometimes you need to be creative. Seniors should consider journaling prompts that can help them get in the swing of writing. Whether writing using a pen and paper, on the computer, or by using a typewriter, journaling prompts can give seniors a fresh start to a great hobby. It can also help those that suffer from writer's block. Below are some of the most common journaling prompts that will inspire seniors get moving with writing in a journal.

1. Movies and music

Here's a quick way to journal about your favorite movies or music bands. Write down which movies or music bands are your favorites. Then explain what makes them your favorite. Or, you can provide a brief summary of each movie you have watched the most and share in your journal how you felt about the movies or music you listen to. You can also jot down the lyrics to your favorite songs of the bands. Seniors that do this "exercise" can help improve their cognitive thinking and boost their memory!

2. Day-to-day reflections or fun activities

Another great way to journal is to write about current events in your community. Write down about what your opinions are about the latest trends in fashion, new businesses that are popping up in the town, or events specifically to your own town. For example, in the City of Commerce, TX; every September they have a Bois Arc Bash, which brings out the whole town for fun activities, music, and food! Seniors can also reflect on meaningful events of when they felt the happiest or even strange things that happen around you.

3. Anything random or fun

Seniors can write about anything in their journal, from what scares them the most, to places they have been to or visited, to what are their biggest pet peeves. Seniors may also write about their favorite time of the year to what are their favorite candle scents and why. The point is to make it random and fun. Sometimes just writing about your body or writing 20 things that makes you smile can also be fun.

4. Enhancing Your Memories

As we see, there are many types of journal prompts that seniors can use to get started in journaling. Choosing ways that can enhance your memory and your life is one the best types of journaling. For example, Seniors could write about their first love or important people that have impacted their lives. They can also write on recurring dreams that they may recently been having or even nightmares. Seniors can also write on how they felt when they were lied to by a loved one or when someone showed an act of kindness to you. Doing these types of writing exercises can help seniors who may be struggling with memory issues or have been diagnosed with dementia.

Typing vs. Handwriting: Which is Better?

With the boom of the technology advancements, it's hard to think of a time when we didn't communicate without using a computer, iPhone, laptop, or tablet. For centuries, people only had one option to take notes or write in a journal with; and that was by simply using a pencil or pen and a pad or notebook. However, now we can choose which one we feel more comfortable with. Whichever one you choose, it can help sharpen your memory, relieve stress, and possibly ward off any symptoms you may have of depression or isolation. Here are a few examples of each type of writing styles, and which one could be right for you.

Typing: Most young people use this form of writing; however, as technology is becoming more readily available, some seniors are pulling out the laptop and enjoying writing using an online format to journal in. In fact, there are benefits to using electronic devices compared to just picking up a pen and paper. When using a computer, seniors can check their spelling or grammar much easier by installing a grammar checker, such as Grammarly. The software will notify he senior if a word is misspelled right away before they move on to the next word or paragraph. Plus, typing on a computer can help seniors become more comfortable with technology.

Handwriting: For those that enjoy writing with a pen and paper, there are just as much benefits to it than typing on a computer. For one, writing by hand pushes the senior to boost the brain power. Seniors will be able to visualize and imagine what they see better when the handwrite. It can also help seniors increase their fine motor skills. Including, improving their hand-eye coordination, which many seniors do sometimes suffer from as they get older and may experiencing some cognitive declines. *Food for thought- Whichever learning style you prefer, be aware that taking breaks is highly recommended. Taking a 10-15 minute break away from the computer or desk can help seniors relax their hand muscles and also get a better perspective on what their wring about.

Some believe that handwriting is a better option for several reasons. Here are some of these reasons. Those who use an electrical device like a computer or laptop for long periods of time can develop carpal tunnel syndrome, poor posture, or eye strain. For seniors that may already have symptoms like this, it may be suggested to try handwriting first.

Going above and beyond in writing: Brain Training

When using a journal, your brain is constantly working, no matter if you're typing or handwriting. Some may consider this as training your brain. There are some studies that prove when drawing out letters or taking notes can actually increases the effects of brain movement. In fact, it is believed that doing longhand is more effective in than if one was to type words on a computer. Basically, your brain is learning more effectively when handwriting.

Risks to writing for seniors

Although uncommon to some, there are a few risks for journaling for seniors. Here are just some of possible risks, whether handwriting or typing for seniors.

Seniors may Reinforce their Own Storytelling

When you journal, you create a point of view in your mind, and it can help you understand situations around you. However, sometimes seniors get stuck in their own opinions or ideas of had write down other solutions that contradict what really occurred when they journal. They may also look to blame someone for situations that they had no control of. The best thing to do is focus on your own point of view and not on others.

Writing can be introspective

Overall, this is not exactly a bad thing. Some people that are introspective or contemplate their life decisions can help see things in a new perspective. However, there is a downside to this. Spending too much time writing about everything you do, or overthinking every decision they make, it can cause a person to not get things done. To solve this issue, seniors should have a specific time of day to journal. It is a good idea to add it into the routine of the day. For instance, setting aside 30 minutes a day to journal.

What Can Seniors Gain from Keeping a Personal Journal?

In closing, we want to express and relterate what can seniors really gain from journaling. For one, it will build or enhance memory, especially if it has already started to decline. Two, it can improve technological abilities for seniors, especially for those who are not digital savvy. And last, it can reduce stress and balance out any emotional strains of the senior. Bottom line, if you have something to say or share, even to yourself, just pick up that pen and write about it. When you do this, it will bring it to life.

Biking for Seniors

Exercising provides many benefits to the human body. These benefits include physical, psychological, social, and mental health wellbeing. For seniors, this a big win, since their abilities, both physical and mental start to decline as they age. When older adults incorporate exercise in their routine, they can improve cognitive function and may even prolong life expectancy. Exercising can also reduce the risk of cardiovascular disease, stroke, diabetes, and other health conditions that often occur in seniors.

One of the best ways for seniors to incorporate exercise into their daily routine is by biking. Biking is a low impact workout that most seniors can easily pick up. Most bikes come with a comfortable seat, durable material, and can sometimes provide special features for those with limited mobility. Plus, biking is an affordable choice as well. Below are the best bikes for seniors. Take a look to see which bike may be the best choice for you!

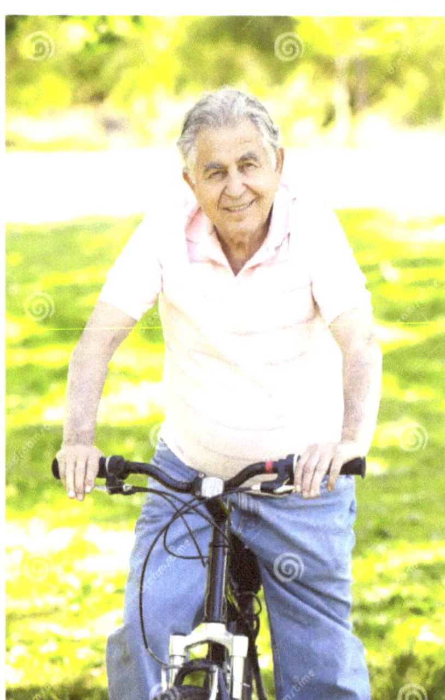

Fig 30.7 older man is cycling to have physical exercise.

How to Choose the Bike for you

Some believe that the best options for bikes for seniors is a hybrid model. The reason for this is that it can help seniors get the exercise they need while also providing the opportunity to run some errands around town with ease. A hybrid bike can offer seniors more features too. From better comfortable seating, to having a higher weight capacity, to a better overall ride on almost any terrain. Whichever model that seniors choose, making sure it offers the best height, weight, or physical needs for each senior. Below are some other features that seniors should consider.

•**Adjustable handlebars** — Handlebars should be high enough to be comfortable for cruising, yet easy for gripping firmly, no matter the speed.
•**Contoured seats** — Saddles, as some call them, should be padded and shaped for both male or female riders. Giving them a more comfortable feel.
•**Seat adjustment** — Upright seat positions give the rider a better ride and less pressure on the back.
•**Shock absorbers** — Choose the "road feel" that is preferred but still buffers bumps on the road.
•**Tires** — Seniors should choose tires with anti-slip grooves for wet weather and wider tires for more comfort.
•**Terrain** — If you live in a hilly area, get a bike that's lighter but with good handling ability on inclines.

What kind of bike is the easiest to ride?

For seniors or older adults, most people will agree that the easiest bikes to ride are lightweight and provides dual brakes, making it simple and easy to stop fast. A bike with a good suspension system is also a plus. Most bikes that are made for seniors have about 3 to 7 speeds, making it convenient to ride on smooth rides, hilly terrain, or rough pathways. Having all weather tires are also a must! They can help seniors to improve their traction while cruising around town. Both hybrid and cruisers are a great option for seniors.

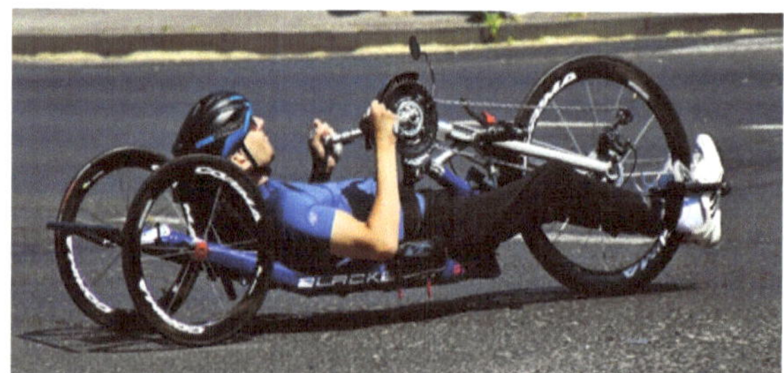

Fig.30.8 A particular type of cycling as shown here is done by a person with spine problem

Safety Tips on how to Stay Safe while cycling

•Always put a helmet on, even if you are going around the neighborhood.
•Wear closed-toe shoes, this is to protect your feet and grip the pedals.
•Attach bike lights to the front and back of your bike for greater visibility.
•Be sure to have a working bell so you can warn pedestrians ahead.
•You should wear reflective or light-colored clothing, so motorists can see you easily at night.
•Signal well ahead of when you intend to turn, and check for traffic.
•Add a patch kit and a pump to your bike frame, and know how to use them.
•Avoid cycling at night if your night vision is poor.
•Carry a mobile phone and battery charger in case of emergency.
•Always have some form of ID on your person.

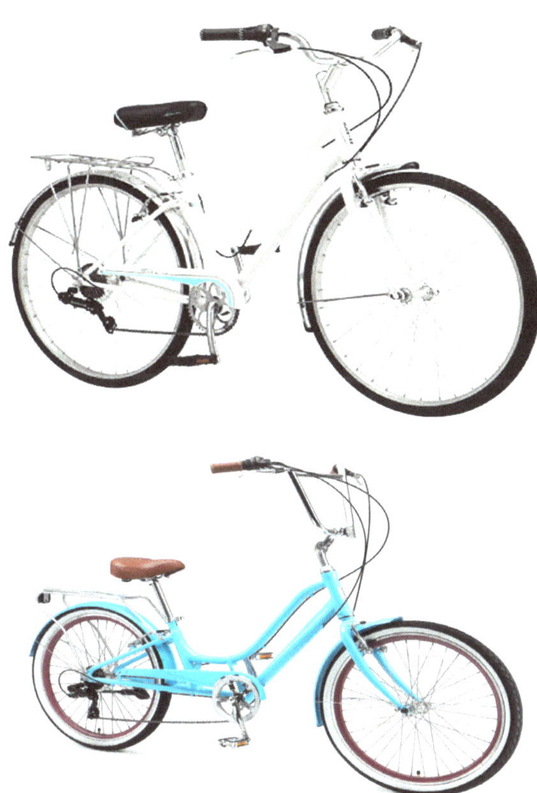

Fig.30.9 (Top) Best Inexpensive Step-Through Bikes for Seniors: Schwinn Wayfarer Step-Through Bike(Bottom)Best Women's Step-Through Cruiser Bikes for Seniors:SixThreeZero Relaxed Body Hybrid Bike

Bikes designed for seniors with mobility issues

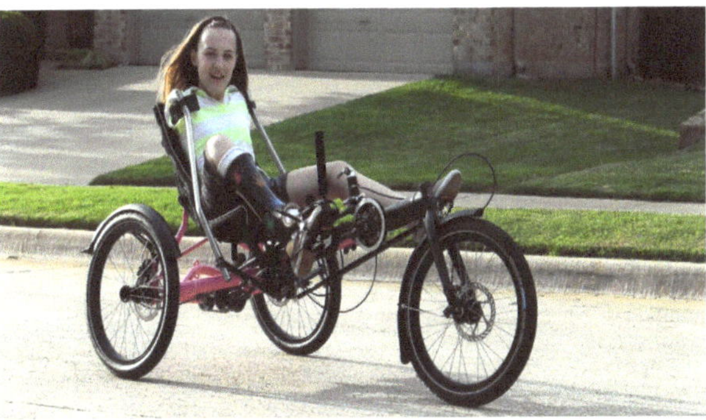

Fig.30.10 Disability affects each and every one of us. Chances are good that you already know - or will soon meet - someone with a disability who could benefit from adaptive cycling equipment.

Although the previous bike options are some of the best for seniors overall, the bikes in this section are better designed for those that have mobility issues or concerns. Here is a small list of the best choices for disabled or physically-challenged seniors.

Recumbent Bikes

Recumbent bicycles are a great alternative for seniors who still need to exercise, yet may have some mobility issues. The average recumbent bike will help seniors to burn up to 300 calories per hour, depending on the person's weight. It also gives the senior a more comfortable seat, while getting them in shape, all at the same time. Since the senior is sitting while riding, and lower to the ground, the bikes provide a less of a chance for seniors to tumble off the bike, making it a safer ride. Seniors with balance issues should also choose this type of bike, since there is no need for them to balance while riding. Cycling in a recumbent bicycle is also good for the heart and lungs, lowering the senior's chances of heart disease and stroke. The bikes are for all people that have problems with the tissue or cartilage in their knees or ankles, not just seniors. Recumbent bikes come with both 2 and 3 wheels, and in all shapes and sizes, so seniors can choose which one is right for them.

Trikes

The trike is second on this list, although some believe it is easier to balance on than the recumbent bikes. These three-wheeled cruisers give seniors and disabled individuals an great alternative than your average two-wheel traditional bicycle.

The trike offers wide tires and handlebars, comfortable saddle to keep senior sitting upright, and both front and rear fenders for a classy look while riding down the street or through the neighborhood. Most model trikes provide rear wire basket, easy to control pedals, and a bell on the handlebars for walking pedestrians to notice them riding by. The trike is ideal for short trips, such as taking a stroll down to the beach, making a quick trip to the grocery store, or just walking the family dog. The trike also helps seniors raise their heart rate and gets the blood flowing for a good workout. Even though the trikes do provide good balance, seniors should avoid going to fast around corners, to prevent the risk of rolling out. The price are trikes are more affordable than the recumbent bikes. They range from a few hundred dollars to couple thousand dollars, depending on where you buy it.

The Alinker

Our last bike that works well for seniors with mobility issues is the Alinker. It is designed with two large wheels in front and a smaller one in the back. It is often called a “walking bike” built specifically for those with balance and mobility limitations, or have been sedentary for some time. The bike works by requiring the senior to propel it with their feet, instead of using pedals. The Alinker offers an adjustable saddle, strong aluminum frame, and a hand brake on the right handle bar, making it very easy to stop if need be. It is also a great choice for seniors with arthritis, sore joints, or other physical impairments related to balance. If you are looking for physical assistance, then the Alinker is the right bike for you. It can help with rebuilding muscles and boost your cardiovascular health, and stimulate circulation for those who have been wheelchair-bound for some time. It holds up to 265 pounds and is available in 3 sizes.

Final Notes

The older we get, the harder it is to ride a traditional bicycle. Many traditional bikes can put unnecessary strain on the back, hips, and knees, making it uncomfortable to do long trips. For seniors, comfort is probably the main feature that they look for in a bike. Seniors also want to find a bike that will support their back and reduce knee pain while pedaling. The width of the tires are also important, since they want to be able control where they ride and get a smoother ride. Riding a bike improves your physical and mental wellbeing, so seniors should consider this activity. Plus, riding offers a low impact workout for seniors, which is exactly what they need. For those who choose the recumbent bikes, it will provide the perfect combination of comfort with a good cardio workout without straining the muscles. Stability is also important to seniors. So choosing the Alinker may be the best choice for you.

For those who still have their balance yet want an easy ride, then choosing a hybrid bike would probably be a good option. Look through all the features that each bike offers when choosing the right one for you. Pricing is always a factor as well. There are some sites that do offer bikes for those on a budget. Lastly, always choose a bike that comes with a warranty, even if it a small one, just in case you might need to repair it or if something breaks on it. It may be helpful to choose a bike with some extra features to help you enhance your workouts. This could be like having a Bluetooth app that can track your workouts or adding resistance levels to boost your physical fitness. Whichever you choose, make sure you are comfortable with the changes on the bike.

Sensory System and the Senior Adult

It is no surprise that as we age, our senses are not as sharp as they once were. In fact, the Aging process can affect sensory changes in a variety of ways. But first, let’s get a better picture of what the sensory system does. People percieve the world around them by sight, sound, touch, taste, and smell through the sensory nervous system. The system converts sensory information into nerve signals that are then carried to the brain. Once there, the signals are turned into sensations, useful for the specific sense it is targeting. The two most common senses that are affected in seniors is their sight and hearing; however, other senses can also be a factor to some. Our sensory system can affect how we live and what we do. Seniors may not notice simple details or not hear what was said correctly in a conversation. Having sensory issues can also lead to isolation; the senior may feel embarrassed, so they stop socializing with family and friends. And begin to isolate themselves.According to the National Institutes of Health, almost 67 percent of seniors suffer from two or more sensory deficiencies nationwide. Like sight and hearing, some seniors may also suffer from a loss of taste or spatial awareness. Although sensory impairments can affect anyone, it is more prevalent within older adults, men, African Americans, and

Hispanics, according to the NIH. Below are the five senses that can be affected due to age and what seniors can do to help manage their loss

Sense Organs

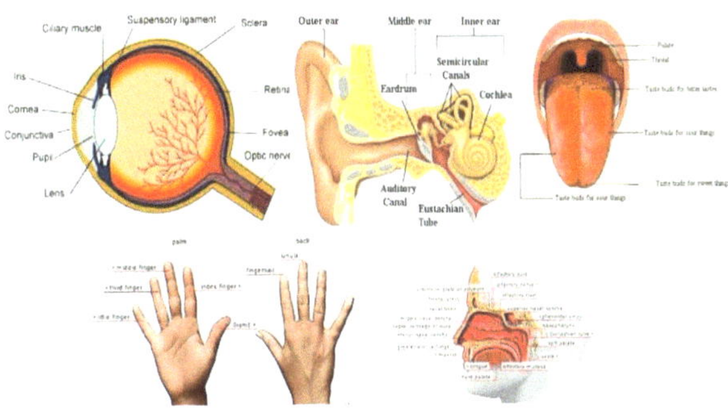

Fig 30.11 Photograph shows five sensory organs that can help seniors to perform coordinated bodly functions.

Hearing

There are two primary purposes of the ears; one, is to hear, and two, is to help maintain balance. We hear through small sound vibrations as they enter the eardrum and into the inner ear. The vibrations then convert into nerve signals, which fluid and small hairs within the inner ear stimulate the auditory nerve, and are finally carried to the brain to help maintain balance. Unfortunately, as we age the structures of what our ears are made of and their function will start to decline. It becomes much harder to hear certain sounds or even maintain proper balance when simply walking, sitting, or just standing still. Some people, including seniors, may develop hearing loss called presbycusis, which can affect both ears.

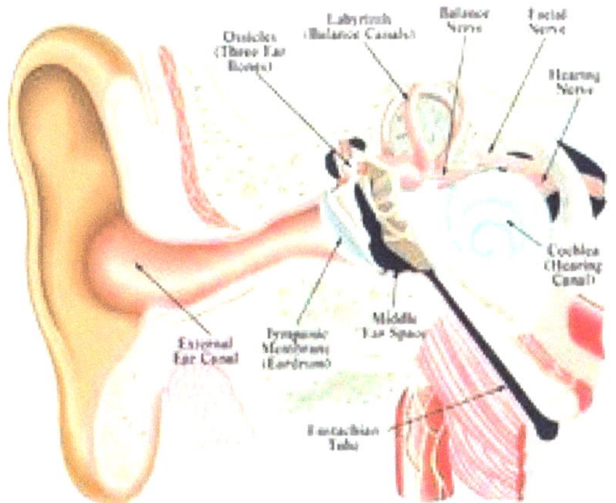

Fig 30.12 Photograph shows inner structure of organ of hearing

Presbycusis is the inability to hear high-frequency sounds, such as speech. Someone with this also may have trouble differentiating between certain sounds. There are a few things that seniors can do to help fix this condition. One is by removing any excess ear wax buildup. This is common for older adults, so stay on top of it. Seniors can manage it by getting a hearing aid as well. If you have this condition, it is recommended to speak with your health care provider soon.

Vision

When you age, sometimes it can affect your vision. How you see things around you can change. Your cornea can become less sensitive to light, preventing a person to not be aware of eye injuries. Over time your pupils may decrease. For Example, an individual in their 60's may have smaller pupils compared to when they were in your 20's. Most seniors react slower to light changes, such as if a room is too bright or too dark.

Sometimes older adults have difficulty in seeing the difference between colors. Seniors may find it hard to know blue from green. Or having trouble walking in your own home. If this happens, switching out regular lights to red, dim lights may help.

Blurry vision is also common in the elderly. There's not many older adults walking around town without glasses on. In fact, many seniors may experience a condition called presbyopia, which is when seniors or individuals have difficulty focusing their eyes on close-up objects. Your eye doctor may suggest reading glasses, bifocal glasses, or contact lenses to help with this condition. In some older adults other conditions can arise. Many seniors as they age will develop eye disorders.

These include: Cataracts (clouding of the lens of the eye), Glaucoma (rise in fluid pressure in the eye), Macular degeneration (disease in the macula (responsible for central vision) that causes vision loss), and Retinopathy (disease in the retina often caused by diabetes or high blood pressure). Anyone that may be experiencing any of these symptom should seek their primary care physician.

Taste and Smell

The sense of taste and smell actually work together. When tasting food, you will smell what is presented in front of you before taking the first bite. In fact, most people use all 5 senses when they eat. When you smell, it begins at the nerve endings located in the lining of the nose.

you sit down with family or friends for a nice meal and there's a pleasant aroma coming out from the kitchen. Your total mood just changed. You automatically feel happy, relaxed, and enjoying life. On the other hand, your taste and smell can also detect negative outcomes, such as spoiled food, harmful gasses or smoke

Tasting

Babies are born with about 30,000 taste buds. By the the time we become adults we lose about two-thirds of them, leaving the average adult with only 10,000. Your taste buds do get replaced every two weeks. So, some people may have more or less at a given time. Your taste buds can sense sweet, salty, sour, bitter, and umami flavors. Most of your sense of taste is linked with odors. As adults become older, their taste buds stop growing or may shrink in size. By the time adults become senior citizens, they are left with only 5,000 taste buds, making it difficult to distinguish between certain smells. By the time seniors are over 60, their five senses start to decline and become more sensitive. You produce less saliva in your mouth as you age as well.

Smelling

A senior's sense of smell also diminishes as they age, especially after turning 70. This can happen due to the loss of nerve endings and less mucus in the nose. For adults that lose their sense of taste or smell, it can be due to diseases or exposure to smoking or other particles in the air. As a result, an individual over 70 may not be able to sense dangers, such as smoke or natural gas leaks. Sometimes your loss of taste or smell is due to medicine you are taking. Talk to your doctor if you detect this may be a reason. There are a few things you can do to help with this problem. Switching medication might help. Start using different spices in the home that are stronger while preparing food. Seniors can also replace or buy a gas detector with an alarm so you can hear it go off in an emergency.

Touch

The older we get, our skin can become sensitive to touches or vibrations. This is because the skin is much more thinner than when we were younger. Our sense of touch also allows us to be aware of pain, pressure, and even the temperature of an object or person close to you. It is the skin, muscles, joints, tendons, and organs that detect these sensations through the nerve endings inside of them. Our brain will then interpret the type or amount of touch sensation is either pleasant (warm), unpleasant (too hot), or just neutral (like giving you a simple signal that you are touching something). For seniors, these sensations may change with age and become less noticeable. This is because the blood flow to the nerve endings are decreasing and it may not reach the brain as fast. The signal receptors to the brain are slower. Those with touch sensitivity should not be left alone in places where they may be in harm's way. Caregivers may need to check the water heater temperature in the home, lowering it down to no higher than 120°F (49°C) to avoid burns. Many senior may find it hard to know the difference between hot and warm or cool and cold. If this happens, it can increase the risk of frostbite,burns, or hypothermia, which is very low body temperature.

In some seniors with sensitivity issues, health problems may develop. Having a lack of the right nutrients can cause sensation changes to increase. Other issues can affect sensation changes, such as problems in the brain, confusion, or nerve damage from a previous injury or long-term disease, which can make sensation changes worst.

Products that help people with sensitivity issues

There are some people that find it difficult to address sensitivity problems or issues. Sometimes, anxiety or stress may develop in seniors with specific sensation impairments or issues. However, there are now products that have proven to assist seniors with these conditions by relieving stress and provide both comfort and calmness. One place to buy these products are at Stacy's Sensory Solution. They are an online store that offers a variety of products designed to calm and comfort those with sensitivity issues. Each product helps seniors keep their hands and minds active and engaged, no matter what stage of the aging process they find themselves in. The site offers cognitive engagement products, such as puzzles, arts and crafts, and other games to keep seniors alert and focused. Those struggling with touch or pressure may consider buying a weighted blanket, neck wrap, or a lap pad. They also provide items for those struggling with anxiety, restlessness, auditory impairments, and much more. Stacy's Sensory Solution also has a traditional store located in Dallas, TX, where they originated.

Tips for Helping Seniors with Sensory Impairment

As a caregiver, you may notice that certain daily tasks become difficult to accomplish as seniors age. This is especially true to those struggling with sensory impairments. However, there are ways to help seniors regain or remain independent throughout their daily lives. Here are five tips for helping seniors with sensory impairments

1. Approach seniors slowly

Many seniors who have sensory issues may get spooked or feel uneasy if you approach them to fast.

When coming behind them, walk slow and lightly touch their shoulder to let them be aware of your presence. It may be wise to keep children out of the room for those with sensory impairments.

2. Provide all electrical devices with screen readers

Seniors can sometimes have visual impairments as they age. Adding a screen reader software to computers, tablets, and smartphones may help them read better. They are especially useful for those who are completely blind. There are some screen readers where braille can be displayed. Some companies are more expensive than others. However, there are a few inexpensive types, such as ChromeVox and Apple VoiceOver, which assists seniors to navigate through their system swiftly and easily.

3. Talk with your mouth visible to the senior

Some seniors or older adults with sensory impairments find it hard to hear someone talking if they are facing a different way or direction. If they can see you move your mouth while talking to them, this can help them understand what you are saying and be able to focus on the conversation better. With Covid 19 still looming, many caregivers or home health aides still wear face masks. However, there are some clear faceguards available to those in the healthcare field.

4. Be patient with seniors

For those with hard of hearing, you may need to repeat or rephrase a saying a few times. Always be patient, giving the senior time to respond to the question or task. Some caregivers may need to speak up or raise their voice for a senior with hearing issues to understand or comprehend the conversation. Sometimes just writing down what you want them to do is a better option.

5. Present foods that look like they would taste

Sometimes seniors loose their sense of taste as they age. However, they may be able to still enjoy and smell the flavors of certain foods. Choosing foods that offer simple and natural flavors in the foods you serve to seniors with taste sensitivity.

How to help Seniors stay connected

Losing any of the senses can be difficult for seniors. The best thing to do is letting seniors know you are always there when they need you most. Caregivers may want to keep them connected with a senior center that provides hands-on approaches for those with sensory impairments. You can also search for local sensory impairment support groups

Self Defense For Seniors

Self-defense for seniors does not necessarily require intense training like martial arts or Taekwondo, though, learning them to defend yourself could help. After all, everyone deserves to feel safe and secure whenever they leave their home or just walking down the street. For seniors that live alone, being aware of their surroundings and knowing how to protect themselves is essential in today's society. This is especially helpful as seniors age. As older adults get older, their response time may not be as sharp. Unfortunately, some seniors do fall prey to acts of crimes. Many seniors tend to walk slower and can be vulnerable to attacks by criminals. In fact, a report from the CDC states that the rate of nonfatal assaults to both men and women over 60 continues to rise each year, with burglary and theft as the highest crimes against seniors. Seniors are not as susceptible to actual violent crimes, however, elder abuse from either a family member or even a caregiver does happen. It is also estimated that 1 in 10 older adults have experienced some form of elder abuse. And the biggest targets are those who have degenerative diseases or cognitive disabilities.

Basic Techniques to Protect Yourself

1. Avoid Escalation

If someone is really determined to take your possessions, just let them. It is better to not escalate a situation, causing you to possibly get hurt, than to just throw down your purse or wallet and run. Especially if they are holding a knife. It would be better to lose some cash and freeze your accounts than end up in an ambulance. Resisting can cause an unnecessary fight, and more danger to you

2. Be aware of your Surroundings

Some older adults are not as alert to people or objects in their way or around them when they leave their home

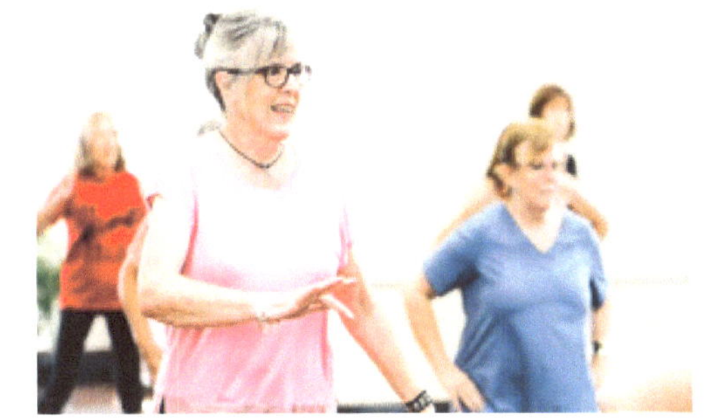

Fig30.13 Elderly women is learning techniques of self defence to protect herself from sudden attack by street bulger

Some older adults are not as alert to people or objects in their way or around them when they leave their home. As seniors age, their reaction time may be slower; they may also experience changes in the vision or hearing. Seniors who do run errands or shop by themselves should always watch who is near or behind them as they are coming out of stores or approaching their car after shopping. The best thing to do is scan your surroundings. This can help avoid getting in trouble while also keeping you safe.

3. Leave and Get Help

The goal here is to get away, fast. Teaching an attacker who's boss doesn't solve anything and may make things worse. Self-preservation is the key. Find an opportunity to get away as quick as possible; such as distracting him by pointing in one direction, then running (if you can) the other way. Once safe and out of harm's way, track down or call the police.

4. Use a Weapon

Never forget, almost anything can be used as a weapon. For seniors this is important to know. You can conflict pain to an attacker, leaving you enough time to get away. Even if it is just a small jab in the stomach, seniors will leave the person on the ground and in pain. Or throwing ars keys into their eyes, causing them to become unfocused on you and more on themselves. Seniors could also carry around some mace or pepper spray in their purse to be used in case of an unexpected attack.

Here is a small list of possible items to use as weapons:

- Cane/walking stick (see above for more information)
- Car keys
- Groceries
- Handbag
- Newspaper
- Pen
- Pepper spray
- Scarf
- Umbrella

5. Aim for the most vulnerable areas

There is always a possibility that the attacker is going to be bigger, taller, and stronger than you. However, there are still ways to defend yourself. Hitting them in very sensitive or vulnerable areas are a good choice. These include the eyes, nose, neck, groin, and knees. Depending on the position of where they are from you, and how agile you may be, depends on where will be the best place to do damage. . For example, if the person is about a few feet from you, it may be good to kick them in the side or on the knee, giving you time to escape.

6. Make noise

If you still got a voice, this is the time to use it! However you can; shout, yell, use a whistle, send off an alarm using your phone. Whatever it takes. Some alarms can be on a keychain and fit in your pocket or purse. And many can be heard from over 300 feet away. When seniors do use an alarm, it can let bystanders near by hear it. This is an effective way in having a criminal run from you.

7. Practice the Art of Deception

For women, leaving the house without a purse is nearly unheard of. However, there are ways to get things done around town without looking like you are even carrying anything with you. For one, having a small travel wallet instead of a bulky purse can prevent any criminals from bothering you in the first place. Seniors can find some these other tips very helpful through the art of deceiving attackers from grabbing your personal possessions.

1.Carry a small purse around your neck and tucked under a jacket. This way a criminal may not even perceive you are carrying anything on your person. Or, if you have deep pockets on the jacket, slip the wallet inside, instead of having them visible to those around you.

2.For men, sometimes carrying a dummy wallet in their pockets while having their actual money placed elsewhere can deter criminal also.

3.Seniors should also keep their keys in their hand or in a pocket of your clothing, instead of in your purse. This way, when you do escape, you can still get in your car and drive away.

4.Seniors should always avoid getting pushed into a corner of a room. You never want an assailant to have the upper hand. Stay in an open area as much as possible and always look for the exits when in unfamiliar places.

5.Try to avoid places that are not well lit or dim, such as back alleys or parking lots with no lighting. Though some seniors do live alone, they should make a priority to shop with close friends, family members, or a caregiver whenever possible.

6.If for any reason you do find yourself grabbed from behind, try not to struggle. Instead push yourself against the person while throwing your head back, this will make the attacker lose his or her balance and possibly fall, and giving you time to run.

Benefits of Self-Defense Training

Although some physical limitations can hinder seniors from doing certain activities, this does not mean it will prevent them from learning how to protect themselves. Studying basic self-defense techniques will give seniors the capabilities to defend themselves against attackers or criminals. It can also boost their confidence and self-esteem. It can also help with stamina, coordination, range of motion, and mental acuity. Many seniors also pursue simple martial arts training to help them become stronger and able to properly defend themselves. Studying these moves can also empower seniors to help others in need as well Martial arts training is available to all ages and ability levels. Below are just some of the most common martial arts techniques for seniors to learn.

Types of Self-defense Martial Arts for Seniors

Krav Maga

Our first on the list is Krav Maga. Developed by the Israeli Military, it focuses on the willingness to survive an attack by using street fighting techniques, rather than martial arts itself. However, it is one of the best types of martial arts for self-defense purposes. In this form of martial arts, seniors will learn to quickly neutralize an assailant by the use of simple and natural movements. Example of Krav Maga is kicking an attacker in the groin or poking them in the eye in order to get away quickly. This type of technique is highly useful for all ages, even seniors since you do not need much strength or speed.

For this reason, it is never too late to learn some self-dense techniques. All it takes is really learning some simple moves to protect yourself from a dangerous situation. Below are some basic self-defense moves or techniques that any senior can learn in order to protect themselves.

Judo

Our next technique is called Judu. Judo will help seniors to take action against an opponent by throwing them down or lodging after them their strength. In order to do this correctly, seniors will need to build up enough dexterity to be able to hold or pin down an adversary or assailant. Those that teach this method of martial arts can offer classes geared to specifically seniors, making sure each person feels comfortable in each lesson learned.

Wing Chun

Wing Chun is a type of Kung fu, which uses open-handed strikes and low kicks to the opponent. For this reason, it is a great form of defense that seniors should use. The form teaches seniors how to defend themselves by focusing on precision and posture. It is also a low-impact activity that can be easy for seniors to do, since it requires not much movements or jumping around.

Aikido

The next one to share is the art of Aikido, which is a great option for people who have disabilities. Since some seniors do have physical impairments, learning Aikido can help them redirect damage back onto the assailant instead of the senior citizen; similar to Judo. However, Aikido doesn't involve kicks or big punches, compared to the other martial art trainings mentioned. This type of self-defense training can also teach seniors how to avoid injuries, especially to their knees.

Jiu Jitsu

The last one is the Jiu Jitsu technique. This form of martial arts derives from the Japanese word "Jū", which means "gentle", and "Jutsu", meaning "art". So therefore, a "gentle art". This type of martial arts uses the principles of pressure, angles, leverage, and timing, in order to subdue an opponent. Sometimes knowledge of the human anatomy is also taught, so the person can take down the assailant quickly and with more force. However, this is not done by use of kicks or strikes, but rather it focuses on close contact holds, and techniques. This is a great form of martial arts that would definitely be great for seniors. Giving them an adequate time to do damage while getting away quickly.

Being Confident in Your Abilities

As we see, self-defense can provide many benefits to seniors through many forms of martial arts training that is available. Seniors who participate in self-defense training will be better equipped to handle almost any type of situation. Whether it be an intense class of Judo or a learning street combat course like Krav Maga, seniors will be able to protect themselves from an assailant and get away safely as quick as they can.There are other types of martial arts available. Seniors should find the best one that will work them and their personal capabilities. They should train hard in becoming well acquainted with it. Talk to the instructor that knows what you are comfortable with and understands your physical abilities, as well as your limitations. Tip to all seniors: Always take it slow whenever you are learning a new technique. The worst thing to do is hurt yourself before truly learning something completely.

Locate Senior Self-defense Classes in your Area

The purpose of self-defense classes is not to exercise or receive some high-intense physical workout or training. It is to educate people on how to better protect themselves, both physically and mentally. Many towns and cities who have a high population of elderly will have several places to learn self-defense training. For those who come from smaller towns, or rural areas may still have one or two places to choose from. For those who are more tech savvy, you will find some courses available on the internet, such as YouTube.

- Here are some common places to find martial arts training or self-defense courses:
- Local martial arts studios
- Free online instructional videos (like on YouTube)
- Community senior centers
- Police stations
- R.A.D. for Seniors program
- YMCA
- Public Library

Best Fitness Trackers for Seniors

Seniors are aging better than they ever have, and part of that reason is due to a willingness to commit to regular exercise routines. Engaging in low-impact and gentle exercise maintains strength and keeps the body functioning at its best. Using a fitness tracker helps seniors get the most out of their efforts by tracking their fitness data.

Fitness trackers for seniors are great for tech-savvy seniors, those who want to get a baseline on their vitals, and many provide safety features including a fall sensor. These features can be tracked by seniors and their children or caregivers who want to keep an eye on their seniors without being obtrusive. Another benefit of getting a fitness tracker for seniors is the fact that many can act as an emergency communication device without the need for a subscription.

Last, but not least, fitness trackers run for at least a week before needing a recharge. That means a senior can wear a watch for long periods of time and regularly keep in touch with their fitness data and alerts without worry. It's also a benefit for adult children of seniors in that they don't have to be concerned with their parents going without the watch for long periods of time.

The Benefits of Getting a Fitness Tracker for Seniors

A fitness tracker is a multi-purpose device that helps monitor physical health and strength for a better quality of life. Buying a fitness tracker for seniors and having them wear it helps them determine their personal health baselines. It also gives them access to information about their own body that's more comprehensive than going to the doctor's office. Here are some of the benefits of getting a fitness tracker for seniors.

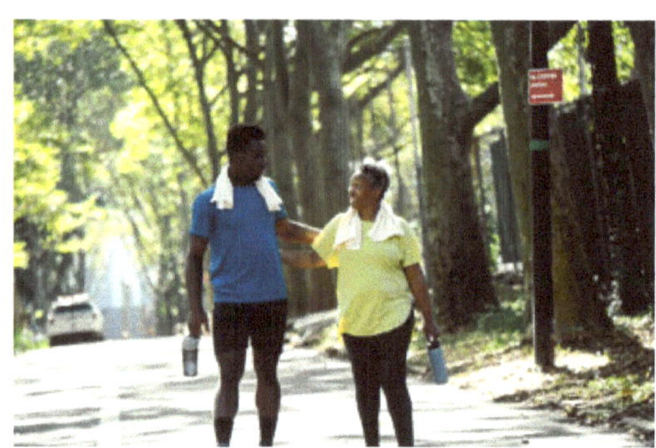

Fig.30.14 Eldery couple is going for hiking to have moderate physical exercise.

Encourages exercise

Part of aging gracefully is staying in shape and maintaining strength. That doesn't mean a senior needs to head to the gym and do a full weightlifting routine, but they should get regular walks and engage in activities that get them moving. Simple exercise routines go a long way towards maintaining fitness, preventing falls, and maintaining normal body functionality.

A tracker such as a Fitbit for seniors gives them a "reward" in the form of a record that shows they did something that day. It's a simple premise, but it's a way of encouraging a senior to step outside on a nice day and enjoy a walk. The tracker also helps them figure out a regular distance goal that's right for them and have a visual that shows them what their body is experiencing.

Senses falls and can act as a medical emergency device

One of the unfortunate facts of aging is that the risk of a fall increases due to various health conditions. It's not unusual for a senior to fall in their home and no one be the wiser for an extended period of time. Medical alert devices that call emergency services are available, but they typically have subscription fees, something seniors on a fixed income tend to resist. Getting a tracker is a one-time cost and you don't need a subscription unless there's a desire to access more features. Many of them have a fall-sensing feature, GPS location tracking, and the ability to to handle playing music and phone calls.

These features typically require the use of a smartphone, but are otherwise free.

Easy to use

One of the challenges seniors face is understanding technology. They didn't grow up with technology as part of their daily lives, and they tend to be more resistant to learning new things. Fitness trackers get around these issues by being simple and intuitive in their use. A senior doesn't have to put a lot of effort into figuring out how the tracker works. All they have to do is swipe the screens or press buttons to get to the tracker they're looking for. They get real-time data for the function they're looking to track and don't have to worry about how to collect it going forward.

Seniors can take their data collection a step further by uploading the information to an app on their computer or phone. The app makes it easy for them to read their historical health data, something that can be used to show their physician.

Improves eating and sleeping habits

Fitness trackers also work as sleep monitors and can be used to remind the wearer that it's time to eat. Fitbits have excellent sleep tracking software, which makes getting a Fitbit for seniors a good idea. Simply program the Fitbit, or any other fitness tracker, to alert the wearer that it's time to eat or go to bed. This stimulates the wearer to get up and take care of their needs at regular times throughout the day.

Seniors frequently fall off their habits due to a lack of stimulation or desire to take care of themselves. A fitness tracker helps overcome this by getting the wearer to think about their needs and the fact they need to be taken care of.

You can help your senior parents with their healthcare

Adult children with senior parents face the challenge of taking care of their senior parents' needs, even though their parents still maintain a large degree of independence. In turn, their senior parents may resist their children's efforts to actively monitor their activities or get them to use emergency alerts. Getting a fitness tracker for seniors serves to take care of the need to monitor a senior parent while helping them retain their independence. their independence.

The data collected by a fitness tracker is easily understood and can help you be your parents' advocate for their healthcare. You can also see how active they're being, make sure they're taking care of themselves, and if you need to be more proactive in helping them with aspects of their lives. The GPS and fall detection helps you respond more quickly to an emergency situation no matter where they happen to be. A fitness tracker offers peace of mind for children of elderly parents.

Best Fitness Trackers for Seniors

The following list covers the best fitness trackers for seniors, their features, and what you can expect from different brands and price points.

Galaxy Watch4 ($199.99)

The Galaxy Watch4 delivers great value in comparison to the number of innovative features it contains. It has GPS fall detection, tracks sleep cycles, and counts steps and does a lot more. It also has an ECG monitor, body composition analysis that includes readings for body fat, skeletal muscle, water retention, and more. It also acts as a smartwatch and can be used for phone calls, notifications, streaming music, and texts. The Galaxy Watch4 also comes in two different watch face sizes. It's one of the best fitness trackers for seniors due to its comprehensive suite of features.

Apple Watch 7 ($619.99)

The Apple Watch 7 is the most expensive of the group, but it makes sense for seniors whose devices are from the Apple ecosystem. The Apple Watch 7 can take an ECG, measure blood oxygen levels, and has irregular heart rhythm notifications. It also features fall detection and will call emergency services if needed. The phone features a cell phone connection along with GPS location, features that eliminate the need to carry a phone. The watch also contains the expected fitness tracking features, including movement and exertion. It's also built to resist dust, cracking, and is waterproofed for swimming. Refurbished watches cost about $300 less than new, and work as well as a brand-new device that's just out of the box.

Amazfit Bip U Pro ($69.99)

The Amazfit Bip U Pro is a budget-priced fitness tracker that's loaded with features that are great for a senior's needs. It has GPS tracking, 60 sport modes, tracks blood oxygen levels, has a sleep monitor, and is waterproof up to 50 meters. It also handles phone calls, alerts, and messages, and can also be used for music. The watch is on the smaller side at 1.43" square and is lightweight, making it comfortable to wear. In terms of its use, it's one of the easy fitness trackers for seniors with its bright display and responsiveness. The watch also features Amazon's Alexa technology, further helping a senior take care of their life.

Fitbit Inspire 2 ($99.95)

The Fitbit Inspire 2 is priced at the lower end of the range, but it's one of the best Fitbits for seniors because it's very user-friendly, has a long battery life, and an easy-to-ready display. The battery lasts for 10 days before needing a recharge, tracks activity, and also tracks sleep. The Inspire 2 features a slim design and simple display that's touch responsive. A wearer can easily tap through the screens to find the data they're looking for.

The only major drawback to finding the best Fitbit for the elderly is the fact the brand does not include emergency communication on any of its devices. That may change in the future, but it's still one of the best fitness trackers for seniors due to its low-key profile and comprehensive data collection.

Wyze Smart Watch ($39.98) and Band Fitness Tracker ($32.99)

The Wyze Smart Watch is another affordable fitness tracker that's great for seniors. Wyze offers both a smart watch and a fitness tracker that are similar to each other, but have different features in key areas. The watch connects to iPhones and Androids to receive smartphone features and functions, but also has the ability to collect blood oxygen levels, heart rate, monitor sleep, and even track sleep position. Wyze's Smart Watch also connects to the manufacturer's smart home products, enabling the wearer to see what's going on at home while they're out.

The Wyze Band Fitness Tracker is capable of doing many of the same functions as the Smart Watch, but features a slender design and also has Amazon Alexa connectivity. It can control a smart TV, keep the wearer on track for a nighttime routine, and play music. The Band Fitness Tracker connects with iPhones and Androids, and is capable of delivering alerts and notifications to the wearer.

Eye Care for Seniors

Getting older comes with different effects on the body. One of the most prevalent changes occur with the eyes. Some seniors may start having a loss of vision, resulting in the need for an eye exam. There are many different senior eye care programs available that can assist in handling these expenses because some insurance plans require a special senior eye care insurance policy, and Medicare Part B does not pay for routine eye exams, glasses, or contact lenses.

The good news is, there are multiple places that cater to eye care for seniors. In fact, there are places that provide free eye exams for seniors to ensure they are getting the resources and care they need. Eye care insurance for seniors is needed because most of them are already on a fixed income. With the cost of senior eyeglasses being out of reach for some, subsidiary costs are welcome.

How important is eye care for seniors?

As seniors get older, regular eye care should be a high priority. While there are several factors that can affect vision, paying attention to maintaining a healthy diet and some form of exercise can assist in preventing progressive vision loss. As the eyes worsen, driving could become an issue. People rely on their vision to function. As the aging process continues, the mind and body start experiencing changes that can be scary. When vision becomes impaired, it creates a snowball effect that may result in depression, anxiety, slip and falls, withdrawal from activities, and other conditions.

Getting regular vision checkups is vital because underlying issues can also be detected during the exam. Depending on the condition of the eye and the age of the senior, annual or bi-annual eye exams may be required.

What could happen if the eyes are not checked?

There are a few things that can occur. Some eye care issues involve age-related conditions like glaucoma. There may be no warning for those who get glaucoma. This is why it is very important to get eye exams as recommended. Another condition is age-related macular degeneration, which occurs by blurring the central vision. People who smoke should refrain, exercise regularly, eat healthy diets with leafy green vegetables and fish, and watch their blood pressure and cholesterol.

Cataracts are also a common occurrence. Some symptoms include trouble seeing at night, seeing double, sensitivity to light, blurred vision, halos around lights, and colors that aren't as clear anymore. Surgery is available that can assist.

Dry eye is another common occurrence that can impact vision. Burning eyes or irritation of the eyes, red eyes, blurred vision, light sensitivity, and watery eyes are symptoms of dry eye. This is very common in older adults.

Ways to maintain eye health

There are ways to help maintain good eye health. First, get routine medical and vision care and senior eye exams. Additionally, if the senior is experiencing additional changes in their body or starts experiencing problems with their eyes, they can wear eye protection, increase lightingin the room, exercise in some way, wear sunglasses, get sleep and rest, and eat healthily.

What is a senior eye care program?

A senior eye care program is one where qualified individuals can get a comprehensive senior eye exam at no cost. In fact, EyeCare America is one of the providers that offer a free eye exam for seniors who are 65 or older and eligible for the program. These individuals are also vulnerable to getting glaucoma.

The program is designed to increase awareness about age-related eye disease while providing senior eye care and free eye exams to prevent diseases of the eyes. Qualifications include being a US citizen or legal resident aged 65 or older, not have seen an ophthalmologist in at least three years, and they do not belong to the VA or an HMO.

Additional senior eye care programs include:

- Lions' Club
- New Eyes for the Needy
- While Medicare Part B does not pay for routine vision exams or glasses, there is certain eye-related vision care that is covered:
- Annual exam testing for diabetic retinopathy
- Annual glaucoma test for at-risk individuals (diabetes, African-Americans 50+, Hispanics 65+, and those with a family history of glaucoma)
- Macular degeneration diagnostic tests and screenings
- Cataract surgery, including a pair of post-surgery eyeglasses or contact lenses

There are Medicare Advantage plans (Plan C) that do cover some vision benefits. This is another way to get coverage for Medicare through a private vision insurance policy. These plans offer benefits that aren't covered by Medicare. An additional solution that may work is a MediGap plan, which is a Medicare supplement plan. This covers basic eye exams, eyeglass lenses, frames, and contact lenses.

What is Vision Insurance?

Vision insurance is a plan to help policyholders have lower costs for routine eye care. These policies may cover corrective surgery and procedures. It does not work the same way as standard medical insurance, but they do cover most, if not all, eye exams, frames, lenses contact lenses, LASIK, and other procedures. These policies have different criteria and the costs are different based on the type of policy acquired by the senior. Seniors who have vision insurance have the advantage of being able to get eye exams whenever they are recommended to get them without worry that they won't be able to cover their needs.

Senior Eye Care Insurance Options

There are a few eye care insurance for seniors policies available to help maintain healthy eyes and prevent or detect the occurrence of eye disease. This helps in lessening costs for seniors to make it more affordable to take care of their eyes. These senior eye care plans can make a difference:

•VSP

A VSP plan is used in conjunction with Medicare to help seniors get the vision care they need. These are available through a larger network provider. VSP is well known and has the largest independent provider network in the country. There is full coverage for routine eye needs after meeting the required deductible.

•UnitedHealthcare

UnitedHealthcare is known for its seniors' eye care program that has several benefits for reasonable rates. This helps seniors in getting eye care exams and eyeglasses from retailers like Target and Costco along with thousands of other eye care providers. One of the advantages of this insurance plan is that there are no enrollment fees and there are out-of-network benefits that are highly lauded. They are generous with their eyeglass frame allowance, and they are known throughout the industry to be solid when it comes to filing claims.

•Direct Vision Insurance

This insurance has a network of opticians and ophthalmologists accessible through discounts and other savings on aids to help correct vision, and other standard services. Pricing varies, but they have flexible, affordable plans that don't have waiting periods and no claim forms to fill out. They also have discounts if the senior needs LASIK surgery.

•Spirit Vision

While a smaller company, Spirit Vision has generous policy limits and other types of insurance policies that may benefit seniors. There are very small co-payments for routine services, there are customized plans based on the senior and what's needed. Major procedures do not have to wait, and they have bundled plans.

Getting to the information is just as important as having the information. There are hubs that help seniors find eye care insurance. eHealth is one of those hubs. A marketplace where seniors can find eye insurance, they have one of the largest networks of providers to assist. They have a user-friendly website where side-by-side comparisons can be made. Seniors who need assistance from a loved one to determine the right policy can easily acquire the information. Another advantage of using this hub is that it carefully explains each section and gives the coverage types to make informed decisions.

Additional resources that can assist with senior eye care include the AMD resource through the American Academy of Ophthalmology; the National Federation of the Blind; Glaucoma Foundation; VisionAware, and the National Eye Institute.

Understanding the pros and cons of senior eye care insurance

Having access to free insurance and programs is helpful, but private vision insurance is also a good solution for saving money on eyeglass frames and lenses. There are some insurance programs that have great networks and are accessible to seniors. There are also networks that have limitations that limit the senior from getting an in-network doctor. This could put the seniors at a disadvantage because they have to switch doctors they are comfortable with. In most cases, seniors have been with their doctors for many, many years, creating anxiety if they must go see someone new.

Getting the right senior eye care discounts

Many seniors do not know there are discounts available to them. Pricing can get very steep when attempting to pay for these eye care services. A senior eye care discount can have huge discounts when it comes to prescription eyewear. Eye doctors are very concerned with senior eye care and promote healthy vision and doing the work to make sure their eyes are in the best condition they can be. Giving seniors the option to get those eye exams and other resources at a reduced cost.

Beyond the eHealth hub, there are ways seniors or their guardians can find discounts on eye care. The first step is to ask eye care providers if they have senior discounts. If they don't have senior eye care discounts, they can probably help point the senior in the right direction. Senior-based organizations like AARP also have resources and information on senior eye care discounts and affordable options that help in getting the vision services they need. Vision Source is a website resource that lists eyecare providers and their senior discounts.With any senior vision insurance plan, thoroughly reviewing all the benefits and what it offers is key. Every plan must be carefully scrutinized to ensure the senior is getting everything they need at the best possible cost. Senior vision discounts and insurance plans can help save hundreds, if not thousands of dollars on all the services they need. The qualifications to get into these plans or get discounts vary based on the provider. In most cases, these discounts start at age 55, but there are some that have a requirement of being 65 or older.

It's important for everyone to care about their eyes as they age, but seniors experience much more if their eyesight starts failing. Keeping up with regular eye appointments can help get their eyes functioning correctly if the symptoms are caught early enough to be rectified. Once a senior starts picking up reading glasses at the drugstore, it's time to seek additional eye care from a licensed doctor specializing in eye treatment. While some people go once a year, there may be a need to visit more than once if the eyes are starting to always feel tired or vision is getting poor.

It can be surprising knowing that an eye prescription can change in the middle of a year, but it really depends on eye strain, diet, and exercise. Seniors should make getting their eye checked a priority, especially when things just don't seem right, or they start having problems seeing during the day and at night.

Here are a few things seniors can do to help in practicing good eye care:

- Know the eye history within the family
- Be mindful of how contact lenses are worn – clean them as recommended and discard them based on instructions
- Wear sunglasses when going outdoors or get transitions lenses to protect the eyes
- Do not smoke
- Get adequate exercise, which should be about 150 minutes a week according to the AHA
- Wear protective gear when necessary
- Eat leafy greens
- Take Vitamin A

Even if it seems like the senior has good vision, it never hurts to visit an eye doctor to check things out. Again, other underlying conditions can be identified through an eye exam. Putting eye health first is the key to getting the benefits of a healthy lifestyle where vision is unimpaired.

Shingles and the Senior Adult–Am I At Risk?

Have you ever had the childhood disease called chickenpox? If you are over 50, chances are you had it.The good news is most people only get it once, due to your body becoming immune to the virus afterwards, which the actual name is called the varicella-zoster virus. The bad news is that the virus is still with you, it's just dormant or inactive within your nerve cells since when you were young. And unfortunately, this virus can turn into shingles later in life. According to the CDC, about one third of the nation's population will get shingles, especially those over 60. That's almost one million seniors! However, there are ways to take care of your health and prevent you or your elderly parents from getting this painful disease. First, let's talk about what really is shingles.

What is Shingles?

Shingles is actually a viral infection, which will affect your nerves and can cause a rash that is both unpleasant and very painful to the person dealing with it. For those who had chickenpox, the risk of shingles is even higher. In fact, your chances of getting it increases the older you become. Many scientists and medical professionals still do not understand what causes the shingles virus to become active, especially being dormant for so many years. Some believe it may be connected to a person's immune system and how it responds to infections.

Nearly all cases of the viral disease are of adults older than 60 years of age. According to the National Institute on Aging, the chances are even greater for those who are over 70. Approximately, one in three adults will get shingles as they age. Fortunately, for some, the virus never becomes active throughout the body, and thus, does not develop into shingles. Now, let's talk about the symptoms or signs that are common to have if you get shingles.

Common symptoms and signs of Shingles

There are several signs and symptoms to look out for if you suspect you have the shingles. Below are just a few common symptoms that people with Shingles may have:

- Fluid-filled blisters
- Burning, shooting pain
- Sensitive to touch, tingling, mild itching, or numbness of the skin
- Chills, fever, headache, or upset stomach
- Fatigue
- Sensitivity to light

Some elderly people may experience mild symptoms of shingles, while others are more intense. If you get blisters, they can show up on the face, such as near the eyes or ears. If this happens, it may cause eye damage, blindness, paralysis, or hearing loss during the time you have the shingles. Some symptoms do last even after the shingles are gone. In some cases, the symptoms may be mistaken as heart, lung, or kidney problems, depending on where the pain is located. If this occurs, call your doctor. It is also advised to talk to your doctor the moment signs or symptoms occur. Next, we will explain some of the primary causes of shingles.

The Causes of shingles

As mentioned above, Shingles comes from a virus called the varicella-zoster virus (VZV), which is the same virus that caused chickenpox in children. If you were one to have chickenpox as a child, the virus is already in you. This is why anyone who had chickenpox when they were little has a greater chance of contracting shingles as an older adult. Most people who have the VZV virus may not get shingles themselves. Here is one common reason for the elderly to get shingles: a weakened immune system. And when you don't have a strong immune system, fighting off infections is even harder. Another reason is our age. For instance, the older we are, the higher are the chances of getting shingles. This is why about half the population of people over 80 will get shingles. Stress and other conditions can also play apart in getting the shingles disease as well. Many people who have higher chances of cancer, have underwent organ transplants, or experienced excessive exposure to the sun also can get the shingles.

How is shingles diagnosed and treated?

If you suspect that you have shingles, talk to your doctor as soon as possible; or, preferably no later than three days after a rash starts. Sometimes the quickest way to know you have the shingles is by just getting a visual examination or a shingles test itself . To determine the result, a small pice of skin tissue will be sent to a lab where they can test it and confirm that the patient has been diagnosed with shingles or if it something else entirely. Unfortunately, there is no cure for shingles. However, antiviral medications can help treat the condition. The virus medication can also help clear up blisters faster and can limit any pain you may be having. The best way to prevent the shingles virus is by getting the shingles vaccine. Other vaccines may also help prevent older adults from certain diseases like shingles, such as COVID-19, flu, pneumonia, tetanus, and whooping cough.

How long does shingles last?

Shingles often lasts between three to five weeks. Most people feel slight numbness, burning, or tingling as the first signs. After about a week, redness may occur on or in the area of where the tingling first occurred. In most cases, the rash or redness may turn to blisters with fluid inside. About a week to 10 days later, the blisters will dry up and a scab will appear. Within two weeks, the scab tends to fall off. The good news is that most people only get the shingles once; however, there have been some cases of seniors who have gotten the shingles again.

Is shingles contagious?

One thing that's good news is you can't pass on the symptoms of Shingles to others. Plus, the risk of spreading shingles is low if the rash is covered. So, you probably won't get it just because a close friend or family member already has it. However, for those who may not had chickenpox are more likely to get Chickenpox itself if they are in direct contact with the person with a fluid-filled rash. This is also true for those who did not get the chickenpox vaccine. They too may be more susceptible of getting the chickenpox virus once again.

Who should get the shingles vaccine?

For those who have already had chickenpox, the chickenpox vaccine, or shingles itself, should go ahead and get the shingles vaccine. In fact, if you don't remember having chickenpox, then getting the shingles vaccine is highly recommended. This also includes seniors who have had the shingles vaccine called Zostavax, which is the older, and original shingles vaccine. Doctors now recommend the Shingrix shingles vaccine, which is a safer, newer, and more effective vaccine to the shingles. The Shingrix vaccine is FDA-approved, and aimed to prevent shingles infection in adults 50 years and older. It is believed to also help adults 18 and up that are prone to have immunity problems, due to prior disease or therapy concerns. The vaccine will protect seniors that get it at least 85 percent of the time, and during the first four years after having the vaccination. According to the U.S. Department of Health and Human Services (DHHS), it is recommended that those living with HIV or AIDs, and are 50 years and older, should get the Shingrix vaccine, regardless of their CD4 count. The shingles vaccination may cause some side effects, such as headaches and injection-site reactions. However, most of them are mild.

Who should not get the Vaccine

Here are some reasons to not get the shingles vaccine: Seniors who are already suffering with shingles, are sick, have a fever, or had some type of allergic reaction to a prior shot of the shingles vaccine, should not get the vaccine again. Those who are breastfeeding or pregnant should also not have the shingles vaccine. For anyone who have not had the chance to get vaccinated yet are experiencing some symptoms of the virus, there are a few medications available to ease the pain and reduce symptoms. The shingles medications available to seniors are acyclovir (Zovirax), valacyclovir (Valtrex), and famciclovir (Famvir). Each one must be prescribed by a doctor.

Common side effects of the Shingles vaccine

Some have reported that after vaccination they may feel the following:

- Pain and redness at the injection site
- Swelling at the injection site
- General malaise, muscle pain, and tiredness
- Systemic symptoms such as headache, shivering, fever, and upset stomach

Tips for coping with shingles

Having Shingles can make a person feel agitated and uncomfortable for the duration of the time they have it. However, there are some ways to get through the pain. Here are a few handy tips to make you feel better:

- Wear loose-fitting, natural-fiber clothing.
- Take an oatmeal bath or use calamine lotion to soothe your skin.
- Apply a cool washcloth to your blisters to ease the pain and help dry the blisters.
- Keep the area clean and don't scratch the blisters; it can become infected or leave a scar.
- Try simple exercises like stretching or walking.
- Get plenty of rest and eat well-balanced meals.
- Distract yourself by doing other activities, such as watch TV, read, talk with friends, listen to relaxing music, or work on a hobby such as crafts or gardening.
- Avoid stress, doing so, can worsen the pain.
- Let your family know how you are feeling and ask for support while going through the shingles

Chances of Long-term Pain

In some cases, the pain of shingles can linger on. This can become a permanent condition to certain seniors. This ongoing pain is referred as PHN, postherpetic neuralgia. PHN leaves seniors with pain in the areas where the rash occurred. Sometimes, the older you are when you get shingles, the greater the chance of PHN and the more severe the pain can be. For some, PHN can cause other conditions, such as anxiety and depression, weight loss, and sleeplessness. Seniors can also find it difficult to do ADLs, such as cooking, dressing, and even eating. If you or have a senior parent suffering from PHN, contact your family physician immediately. Fortunately, PHN usually lessens over time

.Another possible long-term effect of the shingles is bacterial skin infections, especially the older the individual is when they are diagnosed. These skin infections can cause scarring of the skin and may affect a person's vision and hearing as well. Sometimes, the Bacterial infection may bring on more serious conditions, such as Bell's palsy, which may paralyzes the nerves in the face.

Does Insurance companies pay for the Shingles Vaccine?

For most healthcare plans, as long as you are over 60, then the shingles vaccine should be covered. However, it is recommended to check with your provider to see if you meet their criteria. Some factors may apply, such as your age, the type of plan you have, and your health history. For those with no insurance, the average cost of the shingles vaccine is between $200 to $250, per injection. If you choose the two-shot vaccine option, the average cost is about $350. Most people that choose the two doses of Shingrix, need to wait about two to six months between doses, to prevent shingles and complication from the disease.

Anyone over 50 should contact their healthcare provider and insurance to know their options and how to prevent the shingles virus. Those with Medicare Part D may have their shingles vaccine partially or fully covered. On the other hand, those with Medicare Part B may not have their shingles vaccine shot covered. Seniors who have Medicaid, may or may not have the shot covered, it just depends on the provider.

Other Resources Available

Getting older can bring on some unpleasant conditions. However, there are many online resources for seniors to find everything they can on diseases or conditions that affect the elderly. For more information on the shingles virus or the shingles vaccination, contact the Centers for Disease Control and Prevention, National Shingles Foundation, and the National Institute on Aging.

Fall Prevention and Safety for Seniors

Let's face it, the older we get, the more prone we are to accidents. Whether it be just from losing our footing or something much worse, like falling down a staircase. Seniors can easily break a bone, which could take a long time to heal. When seniors do experience broken bones, it can be the start of more serious health conditions or lead to joint problems. It may possibly lead to a long-term disability. For those that have fallen or had problems with their balance, know that you are not alone in this. It is estimated that about one in four seniors over 65 fall each year. In fact, the risk of falling increases the older you get. The good news though, is that there are ways to prevent seniors from falling. For example, having your vision checked regularly and making your home safer is a good start. In this article you will find a list of some of the best ways to prevent falling and keep seniors safe in their homes. But first, let's talk about what causes a senior to fall.

What causes falls in older adults?

There are several factors of what can cause an older adult to lose their balance and fall. In many cases, a senior may experience more than one of these factors to why they fell. In fact, the older they are, the more chances of falling. Below are the most common risk factors that can contribute to falling.

1. Declines in Physical Fitness

It's true that as we age, we become less active and lose the energy to do simple activities or a workout to stay in shape and keep us moving. Sometimes seniors may feel tired and less motivated. Even mild exercises can become hard to achieve or cause other problems to occur, such as low flexibility, loss of muscle mass and the lack of strength. Sometimes these declines can affect our coordination, balance, and increase the likeliness of a severe injury, which may cause a senior to recover much slower.

2. Impaired Vision

Another factor to falling is impaired vision. Many older adults are affected by loss of sight or vision issues that are common as we age. In fact, according to the American Optometric Association, by the time seniors reach 60 years of age, there is a greater chance of eye disorders or conditions, such as cataracts, diabetic retinopathy, glaucoma, or other age-related macular degenerations. These eye diseases can cause a senior to have impaired sight, and making it hard to detect fall hazards. If these occur, contact your doctor for the right treatment as soon as possible.

3. Environmental Hazards

Many falls that happen to seniors is due to their own environment at home. Some environmental factors include poor lighting, loose carpets, and slick floors. Other factors may be the lack of safety equipment,

, such as no grab bars in the shower, no outdoor ramps and stair lifts, or just too much clutter around the home. All these can jeopardize the safety of a seniors's safety and cause them to fall and lead to accidents.

4. Chronic Diseases

There are several types of chronic diseases that can cause a person to fall and lose their balance. Examples of these are Parkinson's disease, Alzheimer's disease, arthritis, and other problems that affect a person's mobility to get around. Many can also increase a senior's risk of falling, slipping, or tripping. Sometimes conditions like neuropathy or having nerve damage can also contribute to falls. Seniors who have problems with their balance may also find it difficult to respond to accidents quickly.

5. Medication Side Effects

There are many over-the-counter medications and dietary supplements that tend to have strong side effects and can cause imbalance issues with seniors. These may include drowsiness, dizziness, and low blood pressure, which can cause a senior to fall or loose their footing. Other types of medications, such as sedatives, opioids, antipsychotics,antidepressants, and cardiovascular drugs can also cause side effects and increase the risk of accidents or falls. Sometimes polypharmacy drugs can increase adverse reactions in seniors taking them, causing drug-related falls.

6. Surgical Procedures

For anyone that has had surgery knows it can be an unpleasant procedure. For seniors, it can sometimes leave them immobile for quite some time. Especially that the healing process can take longer than for a young person. For example, having a hip replacement can leave a senior with lots of discomfort and pain; as well as difficulties in getting around, compared to before the surgery. Seniors might also find it hard to recover as fast. Surgeries may also affect seniors not only physically, but also cognitively. For some, surgical procedures are just a temporary discomfort; however, it is crucial to get seniors up and moving around quickly as possible. This is when physical therapy or rehabilitation is often suggested.

7. Behavioral Hazards

The risk of falls can also happen due to behavioral hazards. Types of these hazards include participating in normal daily routines that could put a strain on a senior's level of physical demand to do certain activities. Some seniors may feel exhausted just putting up laundry or can find it hard to walk a basket of clothes up and down stairs. Caregivers should work with seniors when adapting new safety protocols, especially after a fall. Seniors should also invest in non-skid shoes, to help prevent falls and so they don't lose their balance.

Nine Tips To Help Prevent Falls

There are a variety of reasons why falls happen among seniors. For instance, your senses are not as sharp as they once were. You may have poor eyesight, hearing loss, or your reflexes may be declining. Whichever it is, know that there is help in preventing falls that you can do; whether it be in your home r when you are out on the town. Below are a handful of simple tips to help seniors from falling.

1. Remove Clutter

By the time we get into our 60s or older, we tend to accumulate lots of things. Some seniors have many items within their home that they have collected over the years. And there's nothing bad about that. But it can become a problem, if you have mobility issues and find it hard to move from one room to the next. Seniors with mobility concerns should put up things in its right place and off the floor. Having a clear path will help prevent falls, and also make the home less cluttered.

2. Stay physically active

Seniors who participate in an exercise routine or workout on a regular basis can lower their chances of falling and lesson the risk of a serious injury. Staying active and healthy builds good bone structure and increases your mobility as you age. An exercise workout, such as walking, can also slow the chance osteoporosis, which is a disease that can make bones weak and break easily.

3. Get into balance and strength training exercises.

Along with a good exercise routine, seniors should also consider strength training. Examples of these include Yoga, Pilates, and tai chi. All of which is known to improve balance and muscle strength. Some seniors who have good strength may also want to try lifting weights. Seniors can also use resistance bands to help build strength.

4. Improve your sleep habits

The average person needs about seven to eight hours of sleep each night to feel well rested for the next day. However, each person's sleep patterns may vary. A young adult may feel fine after only six hours of sleep. For seniors, getting enough sleep can help them focus better throughout the day. On the other hand, seniors who lack the right amount of sleep, can feel tired and uncoordinated while moving in and around the house, which increases your chances of a stumbling or falling. When seniors, or anyone for that matter, does get a good night's sleep, you are more cognitively aware of your surroundings, which can help prevent you from a fall.

5. Have regular medical exams

Getting routine health checkups can help seniors avoid unnecessary problems as they get older. Most doctors encourage their senior patients to receive annual hearing and vision exams. For seniors who makes vision care a priority will see better and with more clarity. The same goes with your hearing. Scheduling routine ear exams are important because it is your inner ear that maintains balance. When you have an ear infection or some form of deterioration in the ear canals, you are more prone to falls.

6. Be aware of medications

Every type of medication has some side affects. However, staying on top of what kinds of problems they can have on your health is important. Some types of meds may have short term affects, while others may linger much longer. Examples of side affects are blurred vision, drowsiness, dizziness, and incoherent speech. Each one may affect how a person walks, speaks, or sleeps. Sometimes all three can be present, making it more likely for seniors to fall or lose their balance, and possibly hurt themselves as well.

7. Use mobility aids

Many seniors try to avoid using mobility aids, such as canes and walkers because they strive to look independent and may feel they that they have no use for them. However, it is better to use these assistance devices, even temporarily, because it can prevent you from falling. Those that use either canes, walkers and wheelchairs can provide you with something to lean on, improve your balance, and can lower the risk of a fall. There are many types of assisted devices; choosing the right fit and size is important for seniors to maintain good balance. If you are using a walker, make sure the wheels roll smoothly. Speak with your doctor on which devices are best for you and how to correctly use the equipment.

8. Invest in nonslip walking shoes

It may be nice to wear some soft slippers while hanging around the house, but investing in some good slip-resistant shoes can keep you from falling, especially on slippery floors, such as tile, concrete, and wood surfaces. Seniors should look for good walking shoes with low or no heels and rubbery soles to reduce the risk of falling. In fact, using unsafe footwear can increase the risk of falling, especially for shoes with no backs. Seniors should stay indoors during bad weather. However, if you must go outdoors, seniors should invest in a good pair of boots, especially where snow and ice are present.

9. Slow down and stop rushing

Most people fall simply because they are moving too fast. For seniors, moving fast can lead to falls. You can lose your balance when you are too much in a rush, and that can lead to even more serious problems like a broken bones or fractures. Taking one step at a time is the key. Also, when you are sitting, do not get up too fast. If you stand too quickly, there is a higher chance of falling. Plus, getting up fast can affect your blood pressure and you may feel dizzy afterwards. If you do feel dizzy, sit down and rest immediately.

How to keep your bones strong

Taking a fall can leave a person in lots of pain and possibly immobile, especially if the fall turns into a serious injury. Those who do have an injury from falling, it can put them in the hospital or send them to a nursing home. However, if you have strong bones, the fall may not be as bad. Studies suggest seniors to get enough calcium and vitamin D in their diet to keep their bones strong. Another way seniors could keep your bones strong is by staying physically active. To maintain good bone heath, seniors should also consider quitting smoking and avoid drinking alcohol. Both tobacco and alcohol use may decrease your bone mass, increase the chances of fractures, and can also lead to balance problems or falls.

The Importance of Sleep for the Older Adult

Reasons why older adults may not get enough sleep

The older we get, there is a less chance of a good night's sleep. It's true. Many people over 50 do not get enough sleep compared to when they were younger. There are a variety of reasons for this. Older adults that have been diagnosed with a sleeping disorder, such as insomnia, may find it hard to relax and close their eyes to sleep. Sometimes seniors that are sick or ill, may experience sleep deprivation, which can leave a person up for hours. In fact, if you suspect you have sleep deprivation, talk to your doctor as soon as possible; since it can lead to more serious problems like depression, schizophrenia, and chronic pain syndrome.

Other reasons may be because of the medications an elderly person is taking. There are some that is known to cause restlessness and keep a person irritable, which then will keep you from getting a good night's sleep. Whatever your reason, rest assure that there are ways to get your body calm and relaxed, so you can sleep well.

What could happen if I don't get enough sleep?

Here are a few symptoms that seniors may feel if they do not get enough sleep:

- Become irritable in the morning
- May experience memory problems or forgetfulness
- Feel depressed
- More chances of falls or accidents
- May experience sleeping disorders

How to get better sleep

Getting enough sleep is important for everyone, especially seniors. There are several things that seniors can do to make sure they receive the best sleep they can, and need. Here are just a few ideas to help older adults to do for a good night's sleep:

1.Use low lighting- It is said that when you lower the lights around the house and in the bedroom may help prepare your mind for bedtime.

2.Develop a bedtime routine- Taking time to relax before getting into bed can help seniors get a good night's sleep. This includes reading a book, listening some soft music or taking a bath before bed. You should also go to sleep at the same time, no matter what day it is. Keep this bedtime schedule even on the weekends or when traveling.

3.Avoid electronics, such as TVs and Computers- There have been many studies that state watching TV, playing on the computer, or using your phone can easily distract you from getting a good night's sleep. The best thing to do is put them away or shut them off at least 30 minutes before you are ready to sleep.

4.Reduce consumption of Alcohol and Caffeine- A little red wine is nice with dinner, but not before bed. Those that drink alcohol find it hard to fall asleep. This is the same as caffeine. Avoid eating chocolate, coffee, soda, and tea before heading to bed. Unless, of course it is decaf.

5.Keep your house temperature comfortable- Have your home comfortable to sleep well. Not too hot, but also not too cold. This can keep you from moving around at night or waking you up.

6.Avoid large meals before bed-Studies show that a person's last meal (dinner/supper) should be the smallest one of the day. Plus, it should be consumed at least one to two hours before going to bed. If you eat right before laying down for the night, you won't be able to sleep, or at least sleep well.

More on Sleeping disorders

Sleeping disorders are quite common among the elderly. One reason is that most seniors have trouble relaxing their minds as the day goes on, so they may find it difficult to stay rested and calm by the time it's bedtime. There are several types of sleeping disorders that seniors may develop. Here is a list of the most common types of sleeping disorders that can affect older adults.

Sleep Apnea

Those who have been diagnosed with sleep apnea tend to experience short pauses in between their breathing as they sleep. The pauses can go on throughout the night, and can cause a person to stop breathing at times. If not treated correctly, the sleeping disorder may cause other problems to occur, such as a stroke, memory loss, or even high blood pressure. Some seniors who do have sleep apnea may also have a tendency to snore loudly. Most individuals may not be aware that they even have this sleeping disorder. Common symptoms of sleep apnea are:

- Loud snoring
- Disturbed sleep
- Morning headaches
- Sleepiness or lack of energy during day time
- Waking up with dry mouth or sore throat
- Irritability
- Mood changes
- Loss of libido (loss of interest in sex)
- Insomnia

Talk to your doctor as soon as you notice symptoms of sleep apnea. There are treatments available for sleep apnea. One type is using a continuous positive airway pressure (CPAP) device. Most seniors who use this device find it very useful. Sometimes, surgery can also help seniors cope with sleep apnea.

Insomnia

Insomnia is common among older adults, especially those over 60 years of age. Many with this condition have trouble sleeping, staying asleep, or falling asleep; it can last for a number of days, months, or even years. Treatment is available by talking to your family doctor. Sometimes, family history of insomnia may increase the likelihood that you will have it yourself. There are many causes of insomnia. A few common causes are overactive mind; mental health or illnesses, such as depression, bipolar disorder, anxiety, and psychotic disorders; being jet lag from traveling; or environmental noise.

Narcolepsy

Narcolepsy is a neurological condition known to disturb the wake cycles of those affected. Many people with this condition find themselves sleepy throughout the day and can easily fall asleep while doing every day activities. Narcolepsy is a rare condition, with less than 20,000 cases throughout the nation. Most people are between the ages of 18 to 35; however, seniors can also be affected by this condition. Diagnosis is available by getting a lab test by your doctor. Treatments include the following: Polysomnography-measuring signals and electrical activity of the brain during sleep using electrodes; Multiple sleep latency test- measuring a person's tendency to fall asleep and activity of isolated elements of REM sleep; and the Epworth sleepiness scale- questions given to the patient to determine the degree of sleepiness. There is currently no cure for narcolepsy.

The Connection between Sleep and Movement Disorders

There are several types of sleep movement disorders that can affect the way people sleep or lack there of. These sleep movements are known to disturb your sleep schedule or sleep pattern, making it difficult for people to stay asleep at night or cause daylight sleepiness when awake. Common movement disorders include Parkinson disease, dystonia, myoclonus, Huntington disease, rapid eye movement syndrome, and ataxias. Treatment for each one will vary.

Below are some examples of what these movement disorders can do to your sleep. Each one is common among seniors or older adults with sleeping problems.

Restless legs syndrome: also known as RLS, can cause tingling, crawling, or pins and needles in one or both legs. The feeling is often worse during the night than the day.

Periodic limb movement disorder: PLMD, can cause jerking or kicking with their legs, some do this every 20 to 40 seconds while sleeping. There is medication for it. You can also take warm baths, exercise, and relaxation exercises to help.

Rapid eye movement: aka, REM. This is a sleep behavioral disorder. Normally, when a person is in REM sleep, their body and muscles don't move; so they can stay fast asleep. However, if you have a disturbance in your REM sleep, your muscles may move involuntary and can keep you up at night, disturbing your sleep pattern.

The Link between Alzheimer's Disease and Sleep

People who have been diagnosed with Alzheimer's disease can also have trouble with sleep. They can often sleep too much, or, in some cases, do not get enough sleep. Many Alzheimer's patients can be found wondering around the house at night or yelling for someone or something. In many cases, the person with Alzheimers is not the only one not getting enough sleep. Caregivers that live with the person can also lose sleep, due to many sleepless nights and worrying about the Alzheimer's person. For those who are Alzheimer's caregivers, here are a few tips to help keep them safe while giving you a better good night's sleep:

- Attach grab bars in the bathroom.
- Make sure the floor is clear of objects.
- Place a gate across the stairs.
- Lock up any medicines.

Quick Tips to Help You Fall Asleep

There are many ways to get your body and mind rested enough for you to fall asleep. The old adage of counting sheep doesn't necessity work for all people, so here are a few tips that seems to work better, especially for seniors who find it hard to relax and fall fast asleep.

1.Counting down slowly: Instead of sheep, just think of numbers itself. Some believe counting slowly can help calm your mind and make you sleepy at the same time. Whether you are counting up or down, it doesn't matter. It can still work the same.

2.Use your bedroom only for sleep: when you feel sleepy, go to the bedroom, close he door, shut off the lights, and get in bed. You should give yourself about 20 minutes to fall asleep. If you are still awake, go to another room til you feel sleepy again.

3.Meditate before bedtime: sometimes, seniors find that if they relax their body and mind through meditation, they can fall to sleep much easier. Try it about 30 minutes before going to bed.

4.Play a mind game: Some people that play an activity where they need to concentrate, may feel tired or sleepy after a while. For example, playing a game of chess or trying to complete a jigsaw puzzle can make a person so relaxed, they can get tired and fall asleep.

5.Trying relaxation techniques: Some seniors that have a hard time sleeping may need to try some relaxation techniques to calm their bodies. The best way to do this is by starting from your toes, then slowly moving up the body, til your whole body is completely relaxed. Concentrate on relaxing your toes, then the feet, ankles, knees, and so on. Most people will fall fast asleep before they even get to their head.

For those who still feel tired, yet unable to get a good night's sleep for more than two to three weeks, you may have a sleeping disorder. Talk to your doctor as soon as possible if this persists.

Safety tips for older adults when preparing to sleep

Here is a short check list of to do's when you are getting ready to lay down for the night. These can not only help you sleep better, but can also keep you safe while you sleep.

- Make sure all windows and doors that lead outdoors are locked before going to bed.
- Find a safe place to sleep and get rested for the night.
- Make sure smoke alarms are working correctly and are on each floor of the house.
- Keep your phone with emergency numbers by the side of your bed.
- Have a lamp that is easy to turn on within your reach.
- Put a glass of water next to the bed, just in case you wake up thirsty.
- Remove area rugs so you won't trip if you get out of bed during the night.
- Do not smoke, especially in bed.

Still having trouble Sleeping?

Some older adults who struggle with falling asleep try over-the-counter sleeping aids, others use prescribed medication from a doctor, while others may use natural remedies to help with sleeping. Whichever method you choose, know that medicines are meant for temporary use and are not necessary a cure. If being unable to sleep continues, talk to your doctor about the best treatment or method for your own health and wellness when it comes to sleep

The Holidays and The Senior Adult

As the holidays are fast approaching, many seniors can feel overwhelmed with lots of emotions. Some are joyful, pleasant, and filled with gratitude. However, with more seniors living alone or with no family nearby, it can also be a challenge to stay positive and happy when the holidays are here. Loneliness can lead to feelings of despair, due to social interaction or isolation. This is more prevalent in older adults over 65 with no connection to others Sometimes this happens because of the social demographics around them, such as loved ones passing away, no neighborhood community involvement, or they may not have the mobility to get out to be apart of the holiday season around them. Having holiday activities set in place for seniors is especially important. This can help seniors feel wanted or needed. Being apart of holiday activities, whether with family or within a community can also help them feel like they are part of something bigger than themselves.

Why Some Seniors Experience Holiday Loneliness

There could be a variety of reasons why seniors become lonely during the holidays. One may because of depression. According to the National Institute of Mental Health (NIMH), those that are higher risk for depression are socially isolated seniors. Below are three reasons why loneliness sets in during the holidays for seniors.

1.Missing loved ones: This could be a close friend that has moved away and you no longer talk to, a family member who has passed on, or a combination of both. Whatever it is, the holidays have made you miss them and this has made you feeling sad.

2.Memories of past holidays: This could be pleasant memories of special events, traditions, or the people in your life. Or it may be past memories that was not so pleasant and you want to forget. Whichever it is, these can trigger many emotions that can make a person feeling sad and alone.

3.Feeling social pressure: What you see on social media is usually portrayed as social gatherings of happy and loving individuals with no arguments, no yelling, and no disagreements- this picture of goodness is not always the best image of reality. Things go wrong, food can burn, and friends or family members that don't show up can cause the holidays to become very stressful for the elderly.

Tips for Reducing Loneliness During the Holidays

Although the holiday season is often filled with joyful events and good memories, it can also cause stress to those living alone. Many seniors may live a great distance from the ones they care about. Some may mourn a loss of a spouse. This season could even be the first time without them. To help cope with this loneliness, here are some tips to help reduce loneliness during the holidays.

1. Start your holiday planning early

Plan out a holiday schedule of what needs to be done for next few weeks before the big day arrives. Make sure the majority of the week keeps you busy. Discuss your plans for the holidays with loved ones and close friends. It may also be nice to Invite them over to help plan your holiday as well. If you are alone, then seek out new ways to make meaning memories for yourself.

2. Volunteer whereever and whenever possible

Although it is often seniors that need help as they age, many older adults who can still get around and are mobile have a strong desire to help others in need as well. This will not only lesson the feelings of loneliness, it is also nice to help those who are less fortunate than yourself. Many seniors can volunteer in soup kitchens, homeless shelters, and retirement homes. Some seniors may also enjoy making animal balloons for children in a pediatric wing of a hospital during the holidays.

3. Join social and community gatherings

One of the best ways to combat loneliness as a senior is to join social gatherings, especially during the holiday season. You are more than likely will enjoy being around others than home all by yourself. Meet up at coffee shops or libraries, such as a book club. Surround yourself at local events where people you know will be present.

4. Stay connected to loved ones

During the pandemic, the only way to stay connected to loved ones safely was virtuality through online. It was sometimes hard to be away from those we care about. Now that most things have got back to normal, staying connected to the ones we love is easier. Especially during the holiday season approaching, seniors should reach out to close family and friends to help with being alone. For those who have family not near, don't worry. With advanced technology, seniors can now video chat by using skype or Facetime the ones you care about. Even after the holidays, continue to communicate with loved ones and share your experiences.

5. Invite family and friends over for a fun cooking or baking day

Bake some traditional and seasonal goodies and treats for the family and close friends to enjoy. Have them come over to participate in the cooking/baking, as long it is safe for them to be together in the kitchen. Use seasonal spices in the food, such as gingerbread, apple cinnamon, and pumpkin spice. Decorate the home with holiday decor. For those seniors who live in assisted living facilities or nursing homes, ask thestaff if it would be ok to take your loved one home for the holiday. If not, you can always bring the treats to them so they can still enjoy in the festivities.

Celebrating holidays with Seniors in Assisted living facilities

The holidays should be fun for all ages, even if your loved ones are living in an assisted living facility. Many people that live in these places feel isolated and alone. Especially if their loved ones do not always are around to visit them. The mental wellbeing of seniors who are alone in these homes can make them feel depressed and isolated. But there are ways for caregivers to reduce their loneliness and make the holidays positive and fun for all in the assisted living home. Here are some good tips to help ease their pain and lift their spirits.

•**Decorate their room-** Caregivers or loved ones who come to visit can participate in making their room filled with holiday cheer by adding garland to the walls, getting a mini tree with little ornaments, and hanging a wreath on the door.

•**Arrange family visits-** When family or friends come to visit, make sure there are presents for everyone to open. This allows the senior to feel included in the holiday event.

•**Plan a holiday-themed movie to watch-** If the assisted living facility has a great room or living room for all the residents, then plan a holiday movie night (or afternoon) that is joyful, funny, and filled with love.

•**Plan video chatting-** For those with family away, arrange video chats or Facetime, so residents can see their family members virtually.

•**Keep it low-key for those mentally-challenged-** If you have a loved one with dementia, make the holiday celebration simple and stress-free. Too much overstimulation can cause confusion and may agitate the older adult. It is also wise to make the holiday gathering small. The least amount of people, the less stress for the dementia patient. For more information on those with dementia or Alzheimer's disease, please check out our other articles.

•**Plan a gift exchange party-** Many families share in holiday traditions by doing a big gift exchange. In fact, everyone loves to open presents or watch as their love ones receive packages on this joyous occasion. This is fun not only for your older parents, but also when the grandkids come over and enjoy in this great pastime of exchanging gifts. If your older parents need help in knowing what to get for the grandkids, you can always send them a small suggestion list of what the grandkids favorite hobbies are or what is trending online.

Other Ideas for Seniors during the holidays

Participate in social activities through local organizations

Whether at churches, temples, or mosques, participating in social events through nonprofit and local organizations are a great place to meet new people and enjoy the holidays. Even if you are not religious, there are plenty of social activities that seniors can do through charity events. For example, some churches open their doors to the homeless when the weather is cold. They may also feed the homeless during the holidays. These acts of kindness can help seniors feel good about helping others and keep their minds off of feeling alone.

Tap into your inner creative side while hanging with friends or family

Figure out what you like to do to, whether it's exploring a new hobby or working on a craft you haven't done in a while, and do it with the family during the holiday season. You can participate in a knitting or sewing class, a candle making course, or an authentic cooking class. Chances are, other people in the family will want to join in on the fun as well. It can turn into a night that no one will ever forget.

Be aware of your spending

It is so easy to go a little overboard with your finances, especially during the holiday season. Between buying gifts for the grandkids or close friends, some people may lose control of how much they spend in just a few weeks before Christmas day even arrives. Seniors should plan ahead of how much they should spend for each member of the family, including close friends that come over for the holiday. Seniors can also get organized with their finances making a list of only close friends and family, and only buying presents for those on the list. By staying organized with a holiday budget, seniors can not only reduce stress, but also refrain from over spending.

How Seniors with Alzheimer's disease can still enjoy the Holiday season

Some adult children that have older parents living in a nursing home or an assisted living facility may wonder of it is safe to bring home their elderly parent, especially if they are mentally challenged. If they have been diagnosed with dementia or Alzheimer's disease, it may be better to celebrate the holiday in their room at the nursing home. To help decide, it may be a good idea to ask her first, that is if she is responsive. Here are some things to consider before you make the final decision.• Depending how long the stay will be, your loved one may feel too tired to stay for long periods of time and may need a helping hand with personal care.

•Adult children should make the elderly parent welcomed and reassure her that all will be okay while she is there.

•If the older parent feels afraid or her emotions seem to be off a bit, remind her that she is not a burden and that everyone is excited to see her this holiday.

•If your loved one does have Alzheimer's, dementia, or any other type of cognitive impairment, it may be best to not take her out of a familiar environment, such as a nursing home. They could easily become disoriented and confused, which you don't want to happen.

•Keep in mind, certain elderly people with dementia may enjoy the holiday events, and look forward to them throughout the year. However, there are others who can become easily rattled when it comes to routine or schedule changes. SOme also do not not load music or busy, crowded rooms of people.

Creating an atmosphere that is uplifting and positive is what seniors need and truly want during the holiday season. This will prevent them from having feelings of doubt, loneliness, or hopelessness. Focus on what really matters: being together during the holidays. When we keep the true meaning of the season as an exciting pastime, it will bring good cheer to seniors for yeears to come.

Exercises for seniors at home for all ability levels

There's no doubt about it: Regular exercise is key for older adults and beneficial for many aspects of aging. In addition to reducing the risk of chronic diseases and improving cardiovascular health, "physical activity builds strength, enhances flexibility and range of motion and improves balance and coordination," explains Linda Borgmeyer, founder of the Wisdom Warrior Challenge and owner of Novoleo Therapy and Fitness in Palm Beach Gardens, Florida.

And as a byproduct of the strength and balance seniors gain from exercise, their fall risk reduces while their overall well-being increases, notes Dr. Bob Mirsky, chief medical officer at Nymbl and former vice president of medical operations at Aetna Medicare. "When older adults have strong balance, they're more apt to leave their homes and get out into the community and engage in activities they truly enjoy," he says. "This helps combat loneliness and depression and contributes to their sense of purpose.

Whether you're an older adult or a family or professional caregiver, check out our list of expert-vetted exercises for seniors at home.

Exercises for seniors at home:-

Here, Borgmeyer, Mirsky and other experts share exercises older adults of all abilities can do at home.

NOTE: Before starting any new exercises, make sure to consult with your healthcare provider or that of your loved one or client. You should also practice safety precautions for exercising at home, by wearing proper footwear, staying hydrated and exercising in an open space to reduce fall risk.

Warm-up exercises

Before engaging in more vigorous exercises, Borgmeyer recommends warming up. Here are two of her favorite warm-up exercises for older adults.

Neck stretches

- Sit or stand tall with your shoulders relaxed.
- Gently tilt your head to one side, bringing your ear closer to your shoulder. Hold for a few seconds and then repeat on the other side.
- Next, slowly turn your head to the left, looking over your shoulder. Hold for a few seconds and then repeat on the right side.
- Finally, lower your chin towards your chest, feeling a stretch in the back of your neck. Hold for a few seconds before returning to the starting position.

Hip circles

Did you know how amazing hip circles are? Such an easy movement to add to your daily movement.

- Stand with your feet hip-width apart and place your hands on your hips.
- Begin rotating your hips in a circular motion, moving them forward, to the side, back and then to the other side.
- Perform hip circles 5-10 times in one direction and then switch to the opposite direction.

Balancing exercises

Both Borgmeyer and Mirsky agree that maintaining balance is key for reducing the risk of falls. Here, two of Borgmeyer's favorite balancing exercises.

Heel and toe raises

1.Stand upright with your feet hip-width apart and arms by your sides.

2.Slowly raise your heels off the ground, lifting your body weight onto your toes.

3.Lower your heels back to the ground. Repeat 10-15 times.

4.Next, shift your weight to your heels and raise your toes off the ground. Lower them back down.

5.Repeat as many times as you can in 30 seconds.

Heel-to-toe walk

1.Find a clear space where you can walk in a straight line.

2.Position your heel against the toes of the opposite foot, creating a heel-to-toe stance.

3.Take small, deliberate steps, maintaining balance with each step.

4.Walk along the counter for safety if needed

5.Repeat for a distance of 10-15 feet.

Strengthening exercises

In addition to balancing exercises, strength-enhancing activities are "vital for maintaining independence and reducing the risk of falls," Borgmeyer explains.

"Weight-bearing activities are key," Mirsky agrees. "They increase muscle mass, which can help with balance.

Here are a few exercises recommended by both Borgmeyer and Josh York, a certified personal trainer and founder and CEO of GymGuyz in-home personal training.

Chair squats

1.Begin by standing in front of a sturdy chair with your feet shoulder-width apart.

2.Extend your arms forward for balance.

3.Slowly lower yourself toward the chair as if you were going to sit down.

4.Pause briefly, stand back up. Repeat as many times in 30 seconds.

Side leg raises

1.Stand behind a chair, using it for balance if needed.

2.Lift one leg out to the side, keeping it straight.

3.Return the leg to the starting position and repeat on the other side.

4.Repeat as many times as you can in 30 seconds.

Wall pushups

If you're struggling with regular push-ups, try these wall push-ups instead

How to do wall push-ups:

- Stand an arm's length away from a wall with your feet shoulder-width apart.
- Place your hands shoulder-width apart on the wall at chest height.
- Lean forward until your chest is almost touching the wall.

- Push back to the starting position using your chest, shoulders, and triceps.
- Stand facing a wall at arm's length, feet hip-width apart.
- Stand facing a wall at arm's length, feet hip-width apart.
- Place palms flat against the wall at shoulder height.
- Bend elbows to lower your chest toward the wall, then push back to starting position.
- Repeat for 10-15 repetitions, 2-3 sets.

Leg raises

- Sit tall in a chair with feet flat on the floor and hands resting on the sides for support.
- Lift one leg straight out in front of you, keeping it parallel to the floor.
- Hold for a few seconds, then lower it back down.
- Alternate legs and repeat for 10-15 repetitions on each side, 2-3 sets.

Tension-releasing exercises

MirandaEsmonde-White, author of "Aging Backwards" and founder of Essentrics, a fitness program that focuses on strength, posture, mobility and flexibility in older adults, recommends the following exercises in order to relieve tension and even pain in targeted areas.

Slow shoulder rotations

- Stand with your feet wider than your hips, and let your arms relax at your sides.
- Keep your arms relaxed and hanging at your sides throughout the shoulder rotations. Do these shoulder rotations smoothly; don't jerk through the movements.
- Pull both shoulders in front of you as far as possible.
- Slowly lift your shoulders as high as possible.
- lowly drop your shoulders backward, imagining you are putting your shoulder blades into your back pockets.
- Take your time to slowly rotate through your entire range of motion. If your shoulders are tense or blocked, take deep breaths to help you release the tension.
- Allow your muscles to release tension with every move. Give them time to release before continuing in the rotation.
- Repeat 4 to 6 times in each direction (forward and back).

Embrace yourself sequence

1. Stand with your feet apart and your arms relaxed.
1. Wrap your arms around your body, embracing yourself.
2. Gently rock your body side to side as though you were comforting yourself, shifting your weight from one leg to the other.
3. Rock yourself slowly about 8 times.

How often should older adults exercise?

Older adults should aim for at least five days a week, dedicating at least 15 minutes to each session, notes Borgmeyer.

"It's fine to mix and match exercises to keep the routine varied and enjoyable," she continues. "Just remember to stay hydrated by drinking water before, during and after exercise sessions; and monitor your progress and celebrate your achievements, no matter how small!"

Arthritis in the Older Adult

Why does Arthritis cause people so much pain

According to the National Institutes of Health, "Arthritis" basically means joint inflammation. Anyone can be diagnosed with arthritis; however the elderly are most often the victim of this debilitating disease. The joints, which are placed between two bones, such as your elbow or knee, over time can develop pain, swelling, or stiffness, making hard for a person to easily move them. This pain develops into inflammation and can last for a long time if not treated properly.

For example, a common type of arthritis is Rheumatoid arthritis. It is a disease known to attack the immune system and the joints, by first attacking the lining of joints. When a person has too much uric acid in their blood, uric acid crystals will develop, causing gout to show up. A person with Infections or underlying disease, such as psoriasis or lupus, can also lead to other types of arthritis. Now let's talk about the signs and symptoms commonly associated with arthritis.

Signs and Symptoms of Arthritis

There are many signs and symptoms that relate to arthritis. Sometimes the symptoms may also share similarity to other diseases. In fact, because of this, it is sometimes hard to know if a person has arthritis or something else is wrong. Arthritis can look like other conditions, so speaking to your primary care physician is recommended when these signs and symptoms occur. Symptoms will vary from person to person. However, here is a list of the most common symptoms to look for if you expect to have arthritis:

- Joint pain- either or both the knee or hip pain
- Swelling, especially around the joints
- Redness in the joints
- Tenderness in joints
- Loss of appetite
- Fever

What are the common types of Arthritis?

Just like there are different signs and symptoms of arthritis, there is also many types of the disease as well. In some cases, it is possible to experience two types of arthritis at the same time. As a reminder, most elderly will experience arthritis, however, it can affect younger people as well; even children. Below is a list of the most common types of arthritis that people are diagnosed with.

Osteoarthritis

Osteoarthritis is one of the most common types of arthritis, affecting millions of Americans nationwide. This type of arthritis occurs when the cartilage around the bones starts to wear down, which can happen over time. The cartilage stops protecting the bones and can begin to cause mild to severe joint pain for older adults. It can affect any part of the body; however, it affects often the joints in your hands, knees, hips and spine. People with Osteoarthritis may experience pain or aching in the area affected, stiffness, decreased range of motion (or flexibility), bone spurs, and swelling.

How does a person treat this form of arthritis?

At the moment, there is no cure for OA. However, some doctors have experienced with different forms of therapies that have helped patients suffering with OA. Some have increased physical activity to help manage the symptoms of OA, while others have used physical therapy with strength-training exercises. The CDC encourages seniors facing OA to stay physically active as long as they can. It may also help reduce the chances of chronic diseases, such as heart disease, strokes, and diabetes. Sometimes medications and weight loss are also useful.Medical devices, such as canes, walkers, and crutches are used. Lastly, surgery is also an option, if the pain persists.

Rheumatoid Arthritis

RA, as it is often called, is another common chronic inflammatory disease. There are on average about 200,000 cases of RA per year in the United States. The signs and symptoms of Rheumatoid arthritis is similar to OA, however, it may affect more than one area at a time. Common symptoms of this type of arthritis is pain or aching in more than one joint, stiffness in several joint areas, and tenderness and swelling in more than one joint. Many times it can affect both hands or knees at the same times. Other signs may be weight loss, fever, fatigue or tiredness, and occasionally weakness throughout the body.

What can individuals do to lessen their symptoms of RA?

The good news is that through specific medications and self-management strategies, RA can be very treatable and give a person their life back. Medications for RA can slow down the disease process and reduce inflammation and pain. These strategies include:

- Quit smoking: that is, if you are a smoker.
- Lose weight: extra pounds can cause the pain to be worse.
- Increase or get better sleep: bad sleep habits can make RA uncomfortable.
- Exercise regularly: this can help with all types of arthritis.
- Improve dental hygiene: those with gum disease are at a higher risk of RA.
- Manage stress levels: Stay calm and relax, worrying about things is not healthy, physically and mentally.

Fibromyalgia

The condition called Fibromyalgia is also a type of arthritis that affects senior citizens. Seniors can get pain and stiffness throughout their whole body with this form of arthritis. Other symptoms may include fatigue, headaches or migraines, and can also develop sleeping disorders, depression and anxiety. Some people can develop problems with thinking, memory, and concentration. Usually, a rheumatologist (doctor specialized in treatment of arthritis) can diagnose the affected person if they feel the senior has the condition. However, the treatment of fibromyalgia is often done in conjunction of other treatments. For example, those with osteoarthritis, rheumatoid arthritis, systemic lupus erythematosus, and ankylosing spondylitis may also be dealing with fibromyalgia.

Dealing with Fibromyalgia

It's important for those with fibromyalgia to stay physically fit. Seniors should try to get up to 150 minutes of exercise per week. Walking, swimming, or even biking are good ways to exercise when dealing with this form of arthritis. Doing regular exercises can also reduce any risk of chronic diseases, such as heart disease and diabetes.

Complications of Fibromyalgia

Fibromyalgia can also cause pain, disability, and lower the quality of life in those diagnosed with it. Complications can sometimes arise as well. Older adults living with fibromyalgia may experience complications such as:

- Extended hospital stays
- Higher levels of depression
- Higher risk of suicide
- Higher risk of rheumatic conditions

Gout

According to the Mayo Clinic, Gout is another form of arthritis that tends to be very complex and common among male seniors. However, some women can also experience this as well. The symptoms and signs of gout can happen very suddenly. Examples of gout are intense pain, swelling, redness (especially around the big toe), and heat sensitivity. Many times the pain can be so intense that nonsteroidal anti-inflammatory drugs (NSAIDs) or colchicine will be administered to deal with the flare ups.

How can seniors treat Gout?

As mentioned above, anti-inflammatory drugs are suggested for treatment; however, there are other options. Some elderly choose to use self-management strategies to help with the pain of Gout.These strategies can be similar to self-managed strategies mentioned from the other types of arthritis conditions in this article. Diet and lifestyle changes is a good start. Limiting alcohol and red meat in your diet can also help. Sometimes living with Gout can affect your kidneys by causing kidney stones to appear. Especially that some types of medications can cause high levels of uric acid to develop in the body while dealing with Gout and other forms of arthritis. Talk to your primary care doctor if you suspect you may have gout.

Lupus

Our last type of arthritis being mentioned in this article is Lupus. Unlike Gout, it is more common among women than men. But that does not mean men can't be diagnosed with it. Lupus is an immune disease that can damage any place within the body. Common signs and symptoms for a person with Lupus are muscle and joint pain, fever, rashes, chest pain, and sensitivity to light. Some people may also experience hair loss, kidney problems, memory issues, and extreme fatigue. Mouth sores and blood clotting issues also may develop if you have Lupus. Sometimes Anemia may develop due to the extreme fatigue, and for the lack of red blood cells to bring oxygen throughout your body.

How can people lessen their symptoms of Lupus?

One of the best ways to manage Lupus is by staying on a good treatment plan and taking care of yourself the best you can. Here are some tips to help manage Lupus:

- Learn how to tell if and when a flare is coming.
- Limit the time you spend in the sun and in fluorescent and halogen light.
- Make regular checkups with your doctor.
- Get enough sleep and rest.
- Build a strong support group of trusted and caring people.

How adult children or caregivers can help their loved ones deal with their variation of Arthritis illness

Taking care of a loved one with arthritis can be challenging at times. Especially since their many types of arthritis and a variety of signs and symptoms to look out for. It is sometimes hard to manage the healing process as well. Being there for your elderly parent or loved one suffering from arthritis is important. Each person will have a different experience with it. Their pain may be mild on some days and intense on other days. Their mobility may be limited, such as having difficulty walking, and moving their hands, arms, and legs; or trouble with fine motor skills. It is common to notice stiffness in the joints as well. Always show compassion and let the patient know you care. If you are the one with arthritis, do not be afraid to open up and share to your loved ones what you are going through. There are always plenty of support groups or systems that can provide you with many resources. Below are a few of these resources for people with arthritis.Learn about their condition to understand what they are truly going through. Encourage loved ones to continue walking each day, even when it's hard to. Physical therapy is often considered for those suffering from any form of arthritis. Caregivers can also help manage their medications, especially if the patient is also going through memory conditions, such as dementia. Some patients with arthritis feel very anxious and depressed, so caregivers should know when to step back and give the person some space.

Important Vaccinations for Seniors

The older we get, the more susceptible we become to illnesses and diseases. The reason is that seniors have a more weakened immune system compared to when they were younger. Seniors may also have a harder time fighting off the common cold as quick as someone in their teens. This is why it is so important to get the right vaccines or vaccinations to stay healthy, while protecting yourself from sickness or death. There many types of vaccines, but first let's talk about why do people, especially seniors, need to get a vaccine.

Why do I need to get vaccines?

As just mentioned, vaccinations can help people stay healthy and offer some protection from certain diseases or illnesses. Not getting these vaccinations may cause serious implications to your help. Seniors may also develop certain complications related to their health if they don't get vaccinated. However, not all vaccinations are right for every person. Speak with your primary care provider on which vaccines are right for you. Keep in mind, many diseases are common among the elderly, so having vaccines or vaccinations could help prevent or at least reduce the chances of being diagnosed with a serious condition. Seniors should also be aware the protection that certain vaccines provide wear off over time. Sometimes a booster is necessary to stay protected from diseases or illnesses. Always stay up to date with the vaccines that your doctor recommends for you.

Which vaccines should older adults get?

Flu vaccine

The Flu, which is short for influenza, is a virus that may cause another of symptoms to occur throughout your body. Examples of these symptoms are fever, chills, headaches, sore throat, stuffy nose, and muscle aches. Most of the time the flu will affect the respiratory system, specifically the lungs. Anyone can get the flu; however, seniors or older adults over 65

Most of the time the flu will affect the respiratory system, specifically the lungs. Anyone can get the flu; however, seniors or older adults over 65 are more inclined to develop and experience serious complications, such as pneumonia if diagnosed. There are some vaccines which may only be necessary once in a life, like the polio vaccine.Unfortunately, the flu strand changes every year. So, it may be a good idea to get the vaccine each season. Especially that it is often easy to pass the virus from person to person.

Shingles vaccine

It is estimated that one in 3 people will get shingles, especially after the age 50. Shingles comes from the childhood disease or condition known as Chickenpox. Many children who ever had chickenpox as a child, are more susceptible to getting the Shingles virus as an older adult. It could be a very unpleasant disease, affecting millions each year nationwide and globally. The good news is that not everyone who had Chickenpox gets shingles. However, to keep you safe and healthy, it is highly recommended for people over 50 to get the Shingles vaccine, so they are protected from the virus. If you believe that you may shingles, contact your primary care doctor as soon as possible. Treatment is available to those going through this disease. Common symptoms of the Shingles are Fluid-filled blisters; Burning, shooting pain; Sensitive to touch, tingling, mild itching, or numbness of the skin; Chills, fever, headache, or upset stomach; Fatigue; Sensitivity to light. There are a few potentially dangerous complications to the shingles virus to be aware of; these include Pneumonia, Depression, Hearing problems, Vision problems, Toxic shock syndrome, and Brain inflammation. To learn more about the Shingles disease and how it affects the body, click the link!

MMR vaccine

The acronym MMR stands for measles, mumps, and rubella. The MMR vaccination will help a person be protected against these diseases. The vaccine is often given to a child within their first year of life, and a second dose from 4 through 6 years of age; however, seniors can also benefit from this vaccine, since they are at a higher risk for these diseases and can develop serious complications if found diagnosed with any combination of MMR. Some serious complications to measles mumps and rubella are Pneumonia, brain damage, deafness, and inflammation of the brain.

Swelling around the genital areas are also possible. Most of the time one dose is enough; however, some seniors will need 2 doses of the vaccine, if they have a weakened immune system. Certain adults and mid-life individuals should also consider getting the MMR vaccine, such as those working as healthcare personnel or international travelers.

Pneumonia vaccine

Pneumococcal disease is an airborne disease that is easily spread from one person to another. Although anyone can catch this, older adults are highly susceptible to this condition. The disease can cause pneumonia to build up in the lungs, and also spread through the rest of the body. Many seniors can get seriously sick or die from this condition. Those with a pneumonia disease may experience several infectious disorders. These include Sinusitis (sinus infection), Otitis media (ear infection), Meningitis(affecting the brain or spinal cord) , and Bacteremia (blood infection). According to the CDC, seniors over 65 are recommended to get this vaccine, since there are multiple forms of the disease that are fatal to the elderly. The pneumococcal conjugate vaccine, as some call it, is sometimes given to children. Children receive the PCV13 or PCV15, whereas adults more likely will receive the PCV20. Seniors who had the PCV15 when they were younger should then follow-up by taking a dose of PPSV23.

Tdap: Tetanus, dipheria, and pertussis

Another vaccine that is common for seniors to consider is the Tdap. Also called Td, the Tdap can provide protection against some diseases that can be fatal to the older adult, especially if they do not seek proper care or treatment right away. This is a 3-part vaccination. Tetanus, is the first part of the vaccine. It is sometimes referred to lockjaw. Symptoms of Tetanus is tightening of the muscles, making it hard to swallow, move, or even breathe. The second part is diphtheria, causing a thick coating of mucus to form in the back of the throat. Commonly affecting the tonsils, throat, nose, or skin. This too can cause people with it find it impossible to breathe. The last and third part of the vaccine is pertussis. Many healthcare professionals commonly refer this to whooping cough. Severe and violent coughing is common and can lead to many complications, such as rib fractures, difficulty breathing, vomiting, and pneumonia. All these illnesses can be passed from person to person and can enter the body through a deep cut or burn. The Tdap or Td vaccine should be offered at least once every 10 years to help prevent sickness or death. Talk to your health provider if you may need a booster shot for it.

COVID-19 vaccines

COVID-19 is a respiratory disease that plagued the world over the last couple years.There is no known cure for this disease, however, there are different vaccines to help protect you from the disease. Symptoms of the disease can reflect the common cold, in some cases. Especially if you have mild signs of the virus.Getting the vaccine can help ease the pain it has on a person's health. If you are diagnosed with COVID, the disease can cause symptoms such as fever, coughing, hot sweats, and shortness of breath. Although anyone can get this disease, it does affect the elderly or those with compromised health conditions more. The CDC states that the COVID-19 vaccines may reduce the risk of getting it.

There are four types of COVID-19 vaccines that are available to the public. One comes from Novavax, one from Pfizer-BioNTech, one from Johnson & Johnson, and one from Moderna. However, most Americans have received the Moderna or Pfizer ones. Johnson & Johnson is used in certain situations. Booster shots are required on some of the vaccines, such as the Novavax, Moderna and Pfizer options. However, the vaccine of COVID-19 is still new, and scientists are still learning about the effectiveness of the vaccine. This includes learning about the affects of the disease and its variants of the virus as well. Seniors may also need to have booster shots of the vaccine to stay protected from the disease.

Other reasons why You may need vaccines:

- Have a long-term health condition like diabetes or heart, lung, or liver disease
- Didn't get all your vaccines when you were a child
- Have a health condition that makes it harder for your body to fight off infections — like HIV or problems with your spleen
- Are a man who has sex with men
- Smoke
- Drink heavily or have alcohol use disorder
- Spend time with infants or young children
- Travel outside the United States

Important information about Vaccines for Travelers

We all know that when seniors hit retirement age, many of them love to travel, whether by visiting family or just taking a vacation. However, seniors should still be aware of who they may come in contact while traveling. Always check with your primary doctor before you travel, even if it is just domestically. Ask questions, like which types of vaccines you may need, especially when going to visit certain countries. If you do travel globally, take with you a list of medications you are presently on, any allergy reactions you may have to certain foods or medications, and a record of all the vaccinations you need or had in the past. If you do need a vaccine to travel, it is best to have them done at least four to six weeks before leaving on your trip. This is important, because while you wait, your body will have time to build up immunity to the vaccine and stay protected longer. Depending where you are heading, multiple doses may be required.

Working professionals may need a vaccine if they work at:

- Hospital or clinic
- Nursing home
- Prison
- School or daycare center

Other vaccines for Seniors

•**Hepatitis A vaccine:** This disease is known to affect the liver. Those 50 and older are more at risk of the disease, especially if they have been around infected individuals. The vaccine is offered in two doses, about six months apart. The disease is common among travelers who visit other countries, where the hepatitis A virus is easily transmittable.

•**Hepatitis B vaccine:** It is transmitted through bodily fluids, such as blood, semen, and saliva, from a person who is already infected with the hepatitis B virus. There are three doses of the Hepatitis B vaccine. The second dose is offered four weeks after the first, then the third one is given five months after the second.

•**Polio vaccine:** many people in the early 20th century got polio, and there was no vaccine for it until the 1950s. So, if you feel you may be susceptible to this disease, you should get the Polio vaccine.

•**Lyme disease vaccine:** according to the CDC, there is currently no cure or vaccine for this terrifying disease. However, there are some new studies being done and both Valneva and Pfizer are working on a vaccine to help protect people from it.

•**Measles and Chickenpox vaccine:** most senior will not necessary need these, since most people their have had measles or chickenpox as a child, and they probably have become immune to the disease.

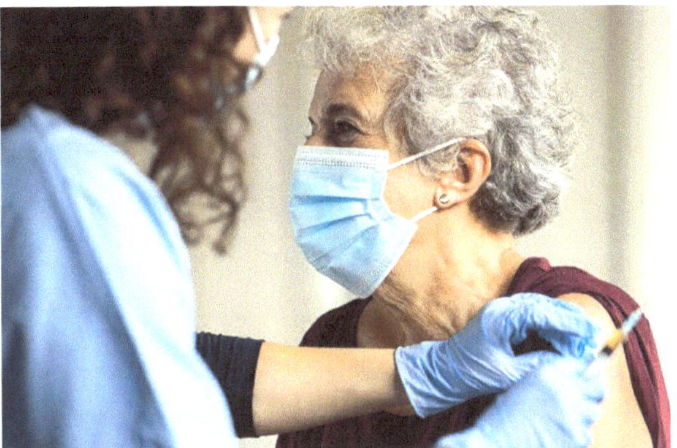

Fig.30.15 Nurse is injecting one of the travellers"vaccine in a passenger

Vaccine safety and side effects

In most cases, vaccines are very safe. People who get vaccinated will have a less chance of getting serious or life-threatening diseases.The most common side effects to vaccines are usually mild. A person may experience pain and notice swelling or redness where the vaccine was given. Those who have an allergic reaction to yeast must talk to their doctor before getting a vaccination; since components of yeast may be in the vaccine. Everyone should consult their doctor if a vaccine is necessary for them to have. Make sure your doctor knows your health history, including any past illnesses or treatments, as well as allergic reactions to foods or medications. Seniors could also keep a log of their own vaccinations they may had previously, including dates of the shots and if their was any side affects that may occurred.

Are vaccines free?

Many insurance plans will cover the recommended vaccines for senior adults, according to the Affordable Care Act. Depending on your plan, it may be little to no cost. Check your insurance company for more details.

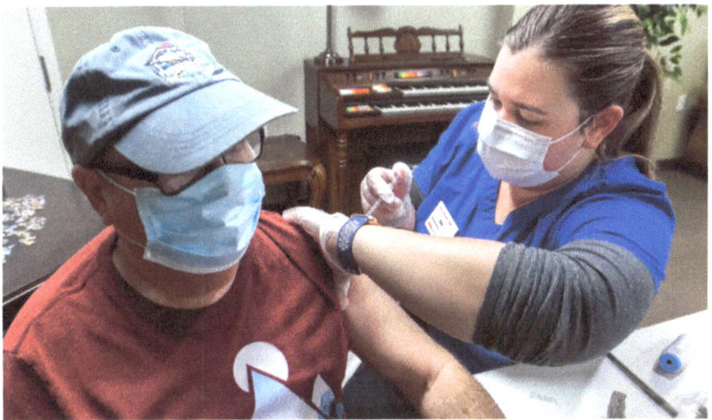

Fig.30.16 Nurse is injecting COVID-19 vaccine in a passenger

INDEX

A

B

C

D

E

F

G

H

I

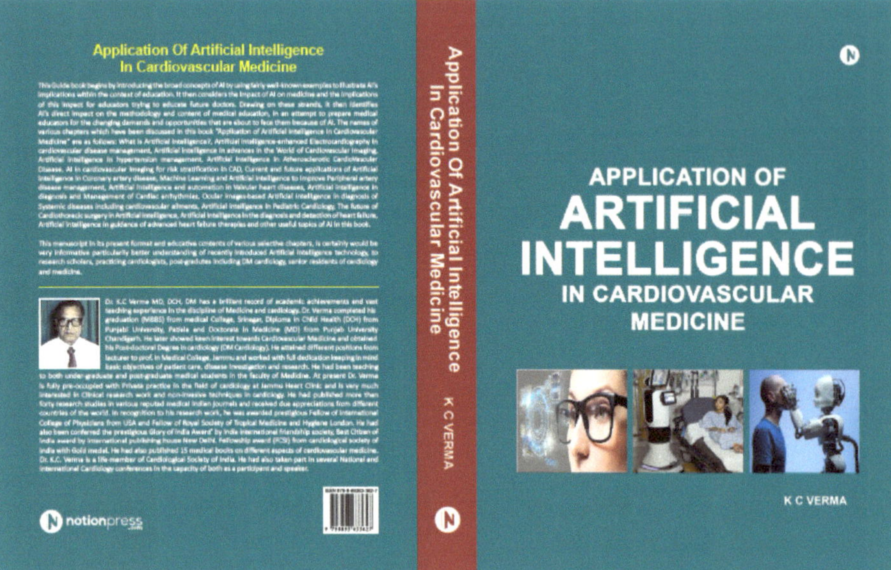
Application Of Artificial Intelligence
In Cardiovascular Medicine
notionpress
Application Of Artificial Intelligence In Cardiovascular Medicine
K C VERMA
APPLICATION OF
ARTIFICIAL
INTELLIGENCE
IN CARDIOVASCULAR
MEDICINE
K C VERMA

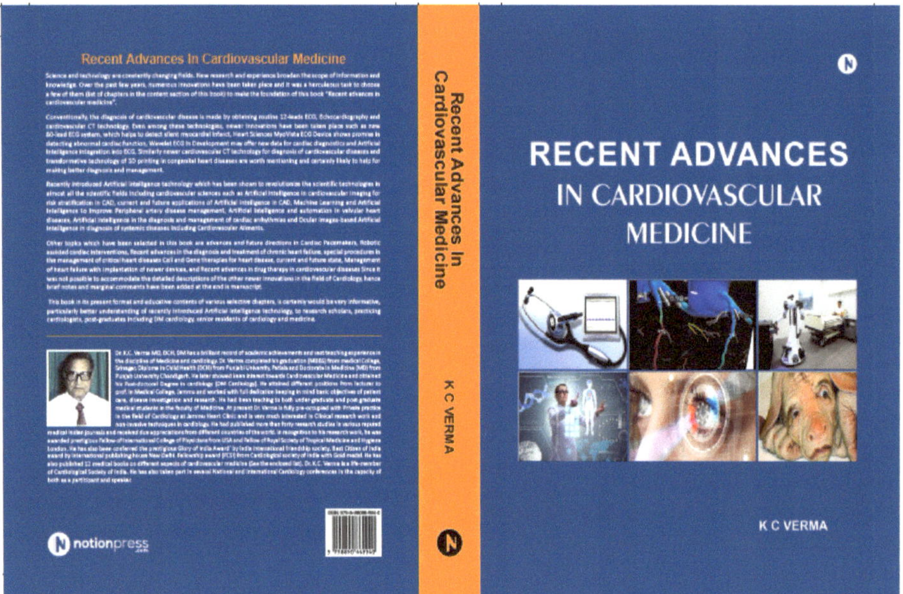
Recent Advances In Cardiovascular Medicine
notionpress
Recent Advances In Cardiovascular Medicine
K C VERMA
RECENT ADVANCES
IN CARDIOVASCULAR
MEDICINE
K C VERMA

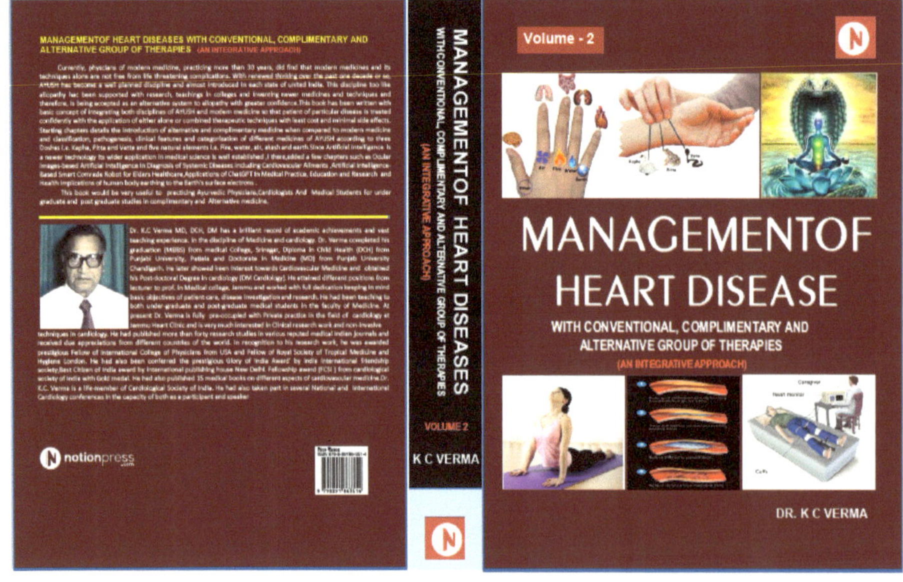
MANAGEMENTOF HEART DISEASES WITH CONVENTIONAL, COMPLIMENTARY AND ALTERNATIVE GROUP OF THERAPIES (AN INTEGRATIVE APPROACH)
notionpress
MANAGEMENTOF HEART DISEASES
WITHCONVENTIONAL, COMPLIMENTARY AND ALTERNATIVE GROUP OF THERAPIES
(AN INTEGRATIVE APPROACH)
VOLUME 2
K C VERMA
Volume - 2
MANAGEMENTOF
HEART DISEASE
WITH CONVENTIONAL, COMPLIMENTARY AND
ALTERNATIVE GROUP OF THERAPIES
(AN INTEGRATIVE APPROACH)
DR. K C VERMA

Recognition And Management Of Congenital Heart Diseases

This book discusses the anatomy and physiology of congenital heart diseases and the transition from fetal to adult circulation. Physical examination, clinical history, signs and symptoms in pre-operative and post operative children and adults. It also discusses the management of intra-uterine and critically ill newly born infants., the pre and post-operative complications in children and adults and rehabilitation of operated adults with congenital heart diseases. A brief account of ECG features of Acyanotic and cyanotic congenital heart diseases including athletes has been discussed. This book in its contents would help:

- Post-graduates of Internal medicine
- Diploma /Postgraduates of pediatric medicine
- Resident doctors in pediatric cardiology and pediatric cardiac surgery.
- It would also be a handy book for physicians practicing cardiology
- Resident doctors preparing for their DNB/DM/M.Ch examinations.

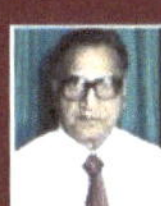

Dr. K.C Verma MD, DCH, DM has a brilliant record of academic achievements and vast teaching experience. In the discipline of Medicine and cardiology. Dr. Verma completed his graduation (MBBS) from Medical College, Srinagar, Diploma in Child Health (DCH) from Punjabi University, Patiala and Doctorate in Medicine (MD) from Punjab University Chandigarh. He later showed keen interest towards Cardiovascular Medicine and obtained his Post-doctoral Degree in Cardiology (DM Cardiology). He attained different positions from lecturer to prof. in Medical College, Jammu, and worked with full dedication keeping in mind the basic objectives of patient care, diseaseinvestigation, and research.He had been teaching both undergraduate and post-graduate medical students in the Faculty of Medicine.

At present Dr. Verma is fully pre-occupied with Private practice in the field of Cardiology at Jammu Heart Clinic is very much interested in Clinical research work and non-invasive techniques in cardiology. He had published more than forty research studies in various reputed medical Indian journals and received due appreciation from different countries of the world. In recognition of his research work, he was awarded the prestigious Fellow of the International College of Physicians from the USA and Fellow of the Royal Society of Tropical Medicine and Hygiene London. He has also been conferred the prestigious Glory of India Award' by India International friendship society. Best Citizen of India award by International publishing house New Delhi. Fellowship Award (FCSI) from the cardiological society of India with a Gold medal. He has also published 15 medical books on different aspects of cardiovascular medicine. Dr. K.C. Verma is a life member of the Cardiological Society of India. He has also taken part in several National and International Cardiology conferences in the capacity of both a participant and speaker.

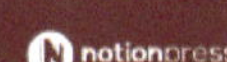

Recognition & Management Of Congenital heart Diseases

K C VERMA

RECOGNITION AND MANAGEMENT OF CONGENITAL HEART DISEASES

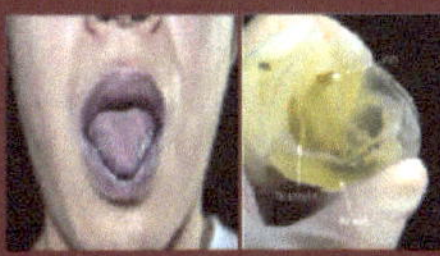

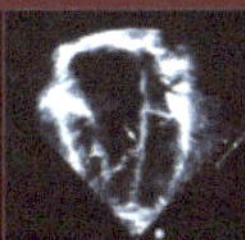

K C VERMA

ESSENTIALS OF LEARNING IN MODERN EDUCATIONAL SYSTEM

This book starts with the historical basis of origin of our earth and first couple to land on it. Futhermore, it also explains as how sperm and egg meet to initiate the process of fertilization and finally to produce their offerings to maintain their future generations. One would also like to know that When Your Baby Can hear in the Womb? Does Music around the fetus has Positive Effect on IQ. One may also acquire the knowledge about formation of the black holes in space and gravity holes in the Indian ocean and their geographic effects on this earth. There may not be many peoples who know about the history of past civilizations like. Maya, Chola and Indus civilizations and their language, living standards, administration, their rise and fall. Through this book, one would get almost entire and much needed information. Since many common people including students may not know about our Solar system, planets and type and nature of life, therefore, a separate chapter on ISRO, Chandrayaan-3, lunar-1 and future missions of ISRO and about Aliens. Proof Of Existence of Aliens have been written with utmost care, Just to add further knowledge of students and general public,two chapters regarding prominent personalities, firstly from cinema, art and culture and secondly about the worldly famous scientists of India alongwith their brief biographies have been appended. This manuscript, to my understanding would certainly prove a treasure house of knowledge to common people, undergraduate and postgraduate students of history, geography, mathematics, Science, architectural designing, yoga and Vedic Cosmology students.

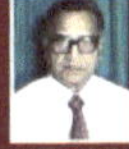

Dr. K.C. Verma MD, DCH, DM has a brilliant record of academic achievements and vast teaching experience. In the discipline of Medicine and cardiology. Dr. Verma completed his graduation (MBBS) from medical College, Srinagar, Diploma in Child Health (DCH) from Punjabi University, Patiala and Doctorate in Medicine (MD) from Punjab University Chandigarh. He later showed keen interest towards Cardiovascular Medicine and obtained his Post-doctoral Degree in cardiology (DM Cardiology). He attained different positions from lecturer to prof. in Medical college, Jammu and worked with full dedication keeping in mind basic objectives of patient care, disease investigation and research. He had been teaching to both under-graduate and post-graduate medical students in the faculty of Medicine. At present Dr. Verma is fully pre-occupied with Private practice in the field of Cardiology at Jammu Heart Clinic and is very much interested in Clinical research work and non-invasive techniques in cardiology. He had published more than forty research studies in various reputed medical Indian journals and received due appreciations from different countries of the world. In recognition to his research work, he was awarded prestigious Fellow of International College of Physicians from USA and Fellow of Royal Society of Tropical Medicine and Hygiene London. He had also been conferred the prestigious Glory of India Award' by India international friendship society,Best Citizen of India award by International publishing house New Delhi. Fellowship award (FCSI) from cardiological society of India with Gold medal. He had also published 12 medical books on different aspects of cardiovascular medicine. Dr. K.C. Verma is a life-member of Cardiological Society of India. He had also taken part in several National and International Cardiology conferences in the capacity of both as a participant and speaker.

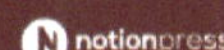

Essentials Of Learning In Modern Educational System

K C VERMA

ESSENTIALS OF LEARNING IN MODERN EDUCATIONAL SYSTEM

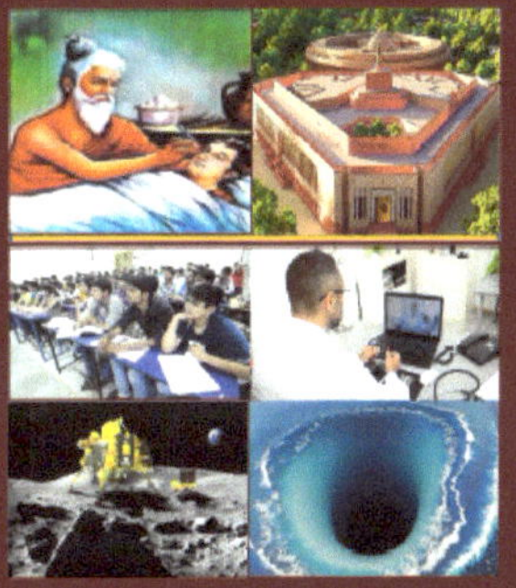

K C VERMA

Management of Heart Diseases with Non-Invasive & Endovascular Techniques

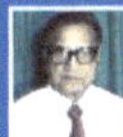

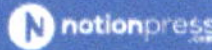

Management of Heart Diseases with Non-Invasive And Endovascular Techniques

K C VERMA

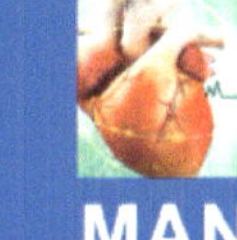

MANAGEMENT OF HEART DISEASES WITH NON-INVASIVE & ENDOVASCULAR TECHNIQUES

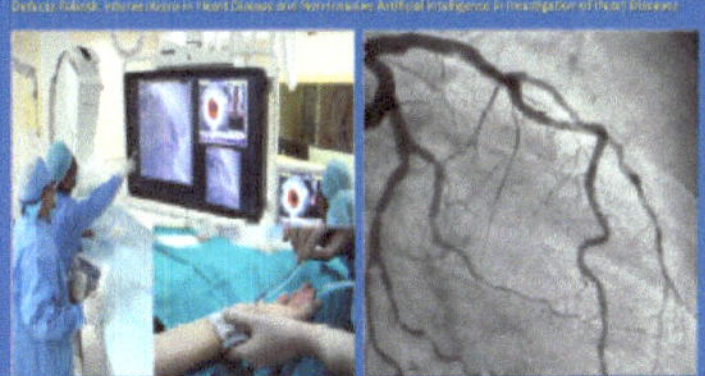

K C VERMA

www.ingramcontent.com/pod-product-compliance
Ingram Content Group UK Ltd.
Pitfield, Milton Keynes, MK11 3LW, UK
UKHW060118300726
14090UKWH00002B/258

* 9 7 9 8 8 9 4 7 5 3 9 8 0 *